CLINICAL CASES
IN ANESTHESIA

CLINICAL CASES IN ANESTHESIA

THIRD EDITION

Edited By

Allan P. Reed, MD

Associate Professor
Department of Anesthesiology
Mount Sinai School of Medicine
New York, New York

Francine S. Yudkowitz, MD, FAAP

Associate Professor
Departments of Anesthesiology and Pediatrics
Mount Sinai School of Medicine
New York, New York

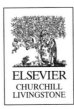

ELSEVIER
CHURCHILL
LIVINGSTONE

ELSEVIER
CHURCHILL
LIVINGSTONE

The Curtis Center
170 S Independence Mall W 300E
Philadelphia, Pennsylvania 19106

Clinical Cases in Anesthesia
Third Edition

Notice

Anesthesiology is an ever-changing field. Standard safety precautions must be followed, but as new research
and clinical experience broaden our knowledge, changes in treatment and drug therapy may become
necessary or appropriate. Readers are advised to check the most current product information provided by
the manufacturer of each drug to be administered to verify the recommended dose, the method and
duration of administration, and contraindications. It is the responsibility of the licensed prescriber, relying
on experience and knowledge of the patient, to determine dosages and the best treatment for each
individual patient. Neither the publisher nor the author assumes any liability for any injury and/or damage
to persons or property arising from this publication.

The Publisher

Previous editions copyrighted 1989, 1995.

ISBN-13: 978-0-443-06624-5
ISBN-10: 0-443-06624-8

Publisher: Natasha Andjelkovic
Editorial Assistant: Rachel Poyatt
Publishing Services Manager: Joan Sinclair
Project Manager: Cecelia Bayruns
Marketing Manager: Emily McGrath-Christie

Printed in the United States of America.

Last digit is the print number: 9 8 7 6 5 4 3 2

To Michael and Becky, of whom I have always been proud.

—Allan P. Reed

In loving memory of my mother, Lea, and to my father, Herman, who were my strongest supporters and inspired me to be the best I could be.

—Francine S. Yudkowitz

CONTRIBUTORS

Mark Abel, MD

Assistant Professor
Department of Anesthesiology
Mount Sinai School of Medicine
New York, New York

Sharon Abramovitz, MD

Instructor in Anesthesiology
Weill Medical College of
    Cornell University
New York, New York

Barbara Alper, MD

Assistant Professor
Department of Anesthesiology
Mount Sinai School of Medicine
New York, New York

Arthur Atchabahian, MD

Assistant Professor
Department of Anesthesiology
Columbia University College of Physicians and Surgeons
New York, New York

Adel Bassily-Marcus, MD

Clinical Instructor
Critical Care
Mount Sinai School of Medicine
New York, New York

Yaakov Beilin, MD

Associate Professor
Departments of Anesthesiology and Obstetrics,
    Gynecology, and Reproductive Science
Mount Sinai School of Medicine
New York, New York

Howard H. Bernstein, MD

Associate Professor
Departments of Anesthesiology and Obstetrics,
    Gynecology, and Reproductive Science
Mount Sinai School of Medicine
New York, New York

JoAnne Betta, MD

Department of Anesthesiology
Englewood Hospital and
    Medical Center
Englewood, New Jersey

Michael E. Bilenker, DO

Department of Anesthesiology
Mount Sinai School of Medicine
New York, New York

Levon M. Capan, MD

Professor
Department of Anesthesiology
New York University School
    of Medicine
New York, New York

Michael Chietero, MD

Associate Professor
Departments of Anesthesiology and Pediatrics
Mount Sinai School of Medicine
New York, New York

Isabelle deLeon, MD

Assistant Professor
Department of Anesthesiology
Mount Sinai School of Medicine
New York, New York

James B. Eisenkraft, MD

Professor
Department of Anesthesiology
Mount Sinai School of Medicine
New York, New York

Dennis E. Feierman, PhD, MD

Associate Professor
Department of Anesthesiology
Mount Sinai School of Medicine
New York, New York

Gordon Freedman, MD

Associate Professor
Department of Anesthesiology
Mount Sinai School of Medicine
New York, New York

George V. Gabrielson, MD

Associate Professor
Department of Anesthesiology
Mount Sinai School of Medicine
New York, New York

Mark Gettes, MD

Assistant Professor
Department of Anesthesiology
Mount Sinai School of Medicine
New York, New York

Cheryl K. Gooden, MD

Assistant Professor
Departments of Anesthesiology and Pediatrics
Mount Sinai School of Medicine
New York, New York

Laurence M. Hausman, MD

Assistant Professor
Department of Anesthesiology
Mount Sinai School of Medicine
New York, New York

Andrew Herlich, MD

Professor
Department of Anesthesiology
Temple University School of Medicine
Philadelphia, Pennsylvania

Ingrid Hollinger, MD

Professor
Department of Anesthesiology
Mount Sinai School of Medicine
New York, New York

Ronald A. Kahn, MD

Associate Professor
Department of Anesthesiology
Mount Sinai School of Medicine
New York, New York

Dan A. Kaufman, MD

Assistant Professor
Department of Anesthesiology
Mount Sinai School of Medicine
New York, New York

James N. Koppel, MD

Assistant Professor
Department of Anesthesiology
Rockville Center
New York, New York

David C. Kramer, MD

Assistant Professor
Department of Anesthesiology
Mount Sinai School of Medicine
New York, New York

Joel M. Kreitzer, MD

Associate Professor
Department of Anesthesiology
Mount Sinai School of Medicine
New York, New York

Merceditas M. Lagmay, MD

Assistant Professor
Department of Anesthesiology
Mount Sinai School of Medicine
New York, New York

Andrew B. Leibowitz, MD

Associate Professor
Department of Anesthesiology
Mount Sinai School of Medicine
New York, New York

Gregg Lobel, MD

Department of Anesthesiology
Englewood Hospital and Medical Center
Englewood, New Jersey

Ilene K. Michaels, MD

Assistant Professor
Department of Anesthesiology
Mount Sinai School
   of Medicine
New York, New York

Sanford Miller, MD

Associate Professor
Department of Anesthesiology
New York University School of Medicine
New York, New York

Alexander Mittnacht, MD

Assistant Professor
Department of Anesthesiology
Mount Sinai School of Medicine
New York, New York

Neeta Moonka, MD

Department of Anesthesiology
Englewood Hospital and Medical Center
Englewood, New Jersey

Steven M. Neustein, MD

Associate Professor
Department of Anesthesiology
Mount Sinai School of Medicine
New York, New York

Irene P. Osborn, MD

Associate Professor
Department of Anesthesiology
Mount Sinai School of Medicine
New York, New York

Michael Ostrovsky, MD

Attending Anesthesiologist–Cardiac Anesthesiologist
Seton Medical Center
Daly City, California

Allan P. Reed, MD

Associate Professor
Department of Anesthesiology
Mount Sinai School of Medicine
New York, New York

David L. Reich, MD

Horace W. Goldsmith
Professor and Chairman
Department of Anesthesiology
Mount Sinai School of Medicine
New York, New York

Jodi L.W. Reiss, MD

Assistant Professor
Department of Anesthesiology
Mount Sinai School of Medicine
New York, New York

Navparkash S. Sandhu, MD

Assistant Professor
Department of Anesthesiology
New York University Medical Center
New York, New York

Arthur E. Schwartz, MD

Associate Professor
Department of Anesthesiology
Mount Sinai School of Medicine
New York, New York

Aryeh Shander, MD

Professor
Department of Anesthesiology
Mount Sinai School of Medicine
New York, New York
Chairman
Department of Anesthesiology
Englewood Hospital and Medical Center
Englewood, New Jersey

Linda J. Shore-Lesserson, MD

Associate Professor
Department of Anesthesiology
Mount Sinai School of Medicine
New York, New York

Leon K. Specthrie, MD

Assistant Professor
Department of Anesthesiology
Mount Sinai School of Medicine
New York, New York

Marc E. Stone, MD

Assistant Professor
Department of Anesthesiology
Mount Sinai School of Medicine
New York, New York

Celeste Telfeyan, DO

Assistant Professor
Department of Anesthesiology
Mount Sinai School of Medicine
New York, New York

Carolyn F. Whitsett, MD

Associate Professor
Departments of Medicine, Hematology and
    Medical Oncology, and Pathology
Mount Sinai Hospital
New York, New York

Francine S. Yudkowitz, MD, FAAP

Associate Professor
Departments of Anesthesiology and
    Pediatrics
Mount Sinai School of Medicine
New York, New York

PREFACE

Preface to the Third Edition

Why a third edition?

Following the success of the second edition, this new edition expands and updates the previous text, and also includes more solutions to frequently occurring practical problems. The new text adds numerous important topics. The cardiovascular section offers new cases relating to cardiac tamponade, cardiomyopathy, noncardiac surgery after heart transplantation, coronary artery bypass grafting, and do-not-resuscitate. Also, cardiovascular pharmacology and new practice guidelines will be incorporated into the appropriate cases. The respiratory section features new cases on post-thoracotomy complications and thoracoscopy. The central nervous system part is enriched with cases on monitoring in spinal injury, transsphenoidal hypophysectomy, and magnetic resonance imaging. In the abdominal section readers will find valuable new cases on endovascular surgery, morbid obesity, laparoscopy, carcinoid, and kidney transplantation. Various other important topics such as hemophilia, infant anesthesia, lower extremity anesthesia, and celiac plexus blocks also appear in this new edition. Postanesthesia care is expanded to include pulmonary function testing, respiratory failure, delayed emergence, coma and brain death, and anaphylaxis.

Besides numerous new cases, the existing cases are thoroughly revised to include the new treatments, treatment guidelines, and the relevant pharmacology. Basic science research that seems poised for clinical applications is also included. In all, it is hoped that the new edition will follow in the footsteps of its predecessors as an important and useful clinical reference on all aspects of anesthesia practice.

Allan P. Reed, MD
Francine S. Yudkowitz, MD, FAAP

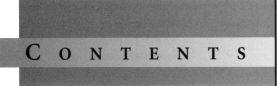

Contents

PART I   THE CARDIOVASCULAR SYSTEM

CASE 1   Cardiopulmonary Resuscitation   1
Alexander Mittnacht, MD
David L. Reich, MD

CASE 2   Coronary Artery Disease   11
Alexander Mittnacht, MD
David L. Reich, MD

CASE 3   Recent Myocardial Infarction   15
Alexander Mittnacht, MD
David L. Reich, MD

CASE 4   Congestive Heart Failure   21
Alexander Mittnacht, MD
David L. Reich, MD

CASE 5   Aortic Stenosis   27
Alexander Mittnacht, MD
David L. Reich, MD

CASE 6   Mitral Stenosis   31
Alexander Mittnacht, MD
David L. Reich, MD

CASE 7   Eisenmenger Syndrome
(Subacute Bacterial Endocarditis
Prophylaxis)   35
Alexander Mittnacht, MD
David L. Reich, MD

CASE 8   Hypertrophic
Obstructive Cardiomyopathy   39
Alexander Mittnacht, MD
David L. Reich, MD

CASE 9   Cardiac Pacemakers and
Defibrillators   43
Alexander Mittnacht, MD
David L. Reich, MD

CASE 10   Cardiac Tamponade   47
Michael Ostrovsky, MD
Linda J. Shore-Lesserson, MD

CASE 11   Cardiomyopathy Managed
with a Left Ventricular Assist
Device   51
Marc E. Stone, MD

CASE 12   Noncardiac Surgery after Heart
Transplantation   59
Marc E. Stone, MD

CASE 13   Coronary Artery Bypass
Grafting   65
Linda J. Shore-Lesserson, MD

CASE 14   Do-Not-Resuscitate Order   69
Linda J. Shore-Lesserson, MD

PART II   THE RESPIRATORY SYSTEM

CASE 15   One-Lung Anesthesia   73
Steven M. Neustein, MD
James B. Eisenkraft, MD

CASE 16   Thoracoscopy   85
Steven M. Neustein, MD
James B. Eisenkraft, MD

PART III   THE CENTRAL NERVOUS SYSTEM

CASE 17   Intracranial Mass,
Intracranial Pressure, Venous
Air Embolism, and
Autoregulation   89
Irene P. Osborn, MD

CASE 18   Intracranial Aneurysms   97
Arthur E. Schwartz, MD

CASE 19   Carotid Endarterectomy   101
Arthur E. Schwartz, MD

CASE 20   Electroconvulsive Therapy   105
David C. Kramer, MD
Michael E. Bilenker, DO

CASE 21   Spine Surgery   109
Irene P. Osborn, MD

CASE 22   Transsphenoidal
Hypophysectomy   113
Irene P. Osborn, MD

PART IV   THE NEUROMUSCULAR SYSTEM

CASE 23   Depolarizing Neuromuscular
Blockade   117
Mark Abel, MD

CASE 24   Nondepolarizing Neuromuscular
Blockade   125
Mark Abel, MD

CASE 25   Antagonism of
Nondepolarizing Neuromuscular
Blockade   129
Mark Abel, MD

CASE 26   Monitoring the Neuromuscular
Junction   133
Mark Abel, MD

CASE 27   Myasthenia Gravis   137
Mark Abel, MD

CASE 28   Malignant Hyperthermia   143
Mark Abel, MD

PART V   THE ENDOCRINE SYSTEM

CASE 29   Diabetes Mellitus   149
Leon K. Specthrie, MD
Allan P. Reed, MD

CASE 30   Thyroid Disease   155
Leon K. Specthrie, MD

CASE 31   Calcium Metabolism   161
Leon K. Specthrie, MD

CASE 32   Perioperative Corticosteroid
Administration   165
Andrew B. Leibowitz, MD
Adel Bassily-Marcus, MD

CASE 33   Pheochromocytoma   169
George V. Gabrielson, MD
Leon K. Specthrie, MD

PART VI   THE ABDOMEN

CASE 34   Full Stomach   175
Laurence M. Hausman, MD

CASE 35   Liver Disease   181
Dennis E. Feierman, PhD, MD
George V. Gabrielson, MD

CASE 36   Abdominal Aortic
Aneurysm   195
Ronald A. Kahn, MD

CASE 37   Endovascular Aortic Stent
Placement   201
Ronald A. Kahn, MD

CASE 38   Transurethral Resection of the
Prostate   205
Laurence M. Hausman, MD

CASE 39   Morbid Obesity   211
Allan P. Reed, MD

CASE 40   Laparoscopy   217
Ilene K. Michaels, MD

CASE 41   Carcinoid Syndrome   225
Barbara Alper, MD

CASE 42   Kidney Transplantation   231
Barbara Alper, MD

PART VII   EYE, EAR, AND THROAT

CASE 43   Open-Eye Injury and Intraocular
Pressure   235
Andrew Herlich, MD

CASE 44   Retinal Detachment   239
Andrew Herlich, MD

CASE 45   Tympanomastoidectomy   243
Andrew Herlich, MD

CASE 46   The Difficult Airway   247
Allan P. Reed, MD

CASE 47   Adenotonsillectomy   261
Andrew Herlich, MD

CASE 48   Laser Laryngoscopy   265
Andrew Herlich, MD

PART VIII   BLOOD

CASE 49   Transfusion Reaction   269
Carolyn F. Whitsett, MD

CASE 50   Intraoperative Coagulopathies   279
Carolyn F. Whitsett, MD

CASE 51   Blood Replacement   287
Mark Gettes, MD

CASE 52   The Jehovah's Witness Patient   297
Cheryl K. Gooden, MD

CASE 53   Hemophilia A   303
JoAnne Betta, MD
Neeta Moonka, MD
Aryeh Shander, MD

PART IX   ORTHOPEDICS

CASE 54   Total Hip Replacement   307
Dan A. Kaufman, MD

CASE 55   Local Anesthetics   313
Isabelle deLeon, MD
Allan P. Reed, MD

CASE 56   Spinal Anesthesia   323
Isabelle deLeon, MD
Allan P. Reed, MD

CASE 57   Brachial Plexus
Anesthesia   335
Jodi L.W. Reiss, MD

CASE 58   Lower Extremity Anesthesia   341
Dan A. Kaufman, MD

PART X   OBSTETRICS

CASE 59   Labor and Delivery   347
Yaakov Beilin, MD

CASE 60   Preeclampsia   355
Yaakov Beilin, MD
Celeste Telfeyan, DO

CASE 61   Abruptio Placenta and Placenta
Previa   363
Howard H. Bernstein, MD
Yaakov Beilin, MD

CASE 62   Anesthesia for Nonobstetric Surgery
During Pregnancy   371
Yaakov Beilin, MD

CASE 63   Thrombocytopenia in
Pregnancy   379
Yaakov Beilin, MD
Sharon Abramovitz, MD

PART XI   PEDIATRICS

CASE 64   Neonatal Resuscitation   387
Francine S. Yudkowitz, MD, FAAP

CASE 65   Gastroschisis and Omphalocele   393
Gregg Lobel, MD

CASE 66   Congenital Diaphragmatic
Hernia   399
Francine S. Yudkowitz, MD, FAAP

CASE 67   Pyloric Stenosis   403
Francine S. Yudkowitz, MD, FAAP

CASE 68   Tracheoesophageal Fistula   405
Michael Chietero, MD

CASE 69   Congenital Heart Disease   409
Ingrid Hollinger, MD

CASE 70   Preterm Infant   419
Gregg Lobel, MD

CASE 71   MRI and the Down Syndrome Child   425
Cheryl K. Gooden, MD

PART XII   **PAIN**

CASE 72   Acute Postoperative Pain   429
Joel M. Kreitzer, MD
Gordon Freedman, MD

CASE 73   Low Back Pain   439
Gordon Freedman, MD
Joel M. Kreitzer, MD

CASE 74   Postherpetic Neuralgia   443
Joel M. Kreitzer, MD
Gordon Freedman, MD

CASE 75   Complex Regional Pain Syndrome   447
Gordon Freedman, MD
Joel M. Kreitzer, MD

CASE 76   Cancer Pain Management   451
Gordon Freedman, MD
Joel M. Kreitzer, MD

PART XIII   **AMBULATORY ANESTHESIA**

CASE 77   Ambulatory Surgery   455
Laurence M. Hausman, MD
James N. Koppel, MD

CASE 78   Office-Based Anesthesia   475
Merceditas M. Lagmay, MD
Laurence M. Hausman, MD

PART XIV   **TRAUMA**

CASE 79   Thoracic Trauma   481
Levon M. Capan, MD
Navparkash S. Sandhu, MD
Sanford Miller, MD

PART XV   **POSTANESTHESIA CARE UNIT**

CASE 80   Asthma   495
Andrew B. Leibowitz, MD
Arthur Atchabahian, MD

CASE 81   Shock   503
Andrew B. Leibowitz, MD
Arthur Atchabahian, MD

CASE 82   Bradycardia and Hypertension   509
Andrew B. Leibowitz, MD
Arthur Atchabahian, MD

CASE 83   Hypothermia   513
Andrew B. Leibowitz, MD
Arthur Atchabahian, MD

CASE 84   Postanesthesia Care Unit Discharge Criteria   517
Andrew B. Leibowitz, MD
Arthur Atchabahian, MD

CASE 85   Respiratory Failure   521
Arthur Atchabahian, MD
Andrew B. Leibowitz, MD

CASE 86   Delayed Emergence, Coma, and Brain Death   527
Arthur Atchabahian, MD
Andrew B. Leibowitz, MD

CASE 87   Anaphylaxis   531
Arthur Atchabahian, MD
Andrew B. Leibowitz, MD

Index   535

1

CARDIOPULMONARY RESUSCITATION

Alexander Mittnacht, MD

David L. Reich, MD

An 86-year-old woman with congestive heart failure, coronary artery disease, and syncopal episodes presents for elective permanent pacemaker insertion. A recent 24 hour ambulatory electrocardiogram recording demonstrated multiple episodes of severe sinus bradycardia associated with pre-syncopal symptoms. Monitored anesthesia care is requested in light of the patient's advanced age and associated medical conditions. The infiltration of local anesthesia and isolation of the cephalic vein in the left deltopectoral groove proceeds uneventfully. During placement of the ventricular pacing lead, ventricular ectopy occurs as the lead encounters the right ventricular endocardium. Subsequently, as the lead is repositioned, ventricular tachycardia is induced and rapidly deteriorates into ventricular fibrillation.

QUESTIONS

1. What is the initial response to a witnessed cardiac arrest?
2. How do chest compressions produce a cardiac output?
3. What are the recommended rates of compression and ventilation?
4. What are the complications of CPR?
5. What is the optimal dose of epinephrine?
6. What is the indication for vasopressin in CPR?
7. What are the indications for sodium bicarbonate (NaHCO₃) administration?
8. What are the indications for calcium salt administration?
9. What is the antidysrhythmic therapy of choice in VF/pulseless VT?
10. What are the management strategies in bradycardias?
11. What is the treatment of supraventricular tachydysrhythmias?
12. What are the indications for magnesium therapy?
13. What are the indications for a pacemaker?
14. Why is it important to monitor serum glucose?
15. What are the indications for open cardiac massage?
16. What is the management strategy for pulseless electrical activity (PEA)?

1. What is the initial response to a cardiac arrest?

The initial response to a witnessed cardiac arrest is to confirm the diagnosis. Patients in arrest are unresponsive, apneic, and pulseless. Assistance should be called for immediately prior to any intervention. In the past, it was recommended to call for assistance after the initiation of cardiopulmonary resuscitation (CPR), but since 80–90% of patients with sudden cardiac arrest have ventricular fibrillation (VF), which is the most treatable dysrhythmia but which requires urgent defibrillation, the rescuer is advised to call first so that a defibrillator can be brought to the scene. The only exception is in the case of children less than 8 years of age, who usually arrest because of airway problems. In that case, an attempt at securing the airway should first be made.

Monitored patients should be treated according to the Advanced Cardiac Life Support (ACLS) protocol devised for their dysrhythmia. This includes basic life support (BLS), usually in the form of CPR, as well as adjunctive equipment for airway control, dysrhythmia detection and treatment, and post-resuscitation care. Unmonitored, unresponsive patients should have their airway assessed first followed by two breaths and a pulse check. In a witnessed cardiac arrest, a precordial thump may be indicated but CPR must be started immediately if the patient remains pulseless. As soon as possible, paddles or electrocardiogram (ECG) leads should be placed on the patient to determine the rhythm. If pulseless ventricular tachycardia (VT) or VF is the initial rhythm, the patient should receive up to three uniphasic countershocks of increasing power: 200 joules (J), 200-300 J, and 360 J, respectively. Biphasic equivalents are approximately half that of uniphasic doses. If VF or pulseless VT is not the initial rhythm, or if the countershocks are unsuccessful, then chest compressions and ventilation should be continued and the patient treated accordingly (Figure 1.1).

The essential element in treating cardiac arrest is rapid identification and treatment. The goal of CPR is to provide oxygenated blood to the heart and brain until ACLS procedures are initiated. The best results (survival of approximately 40%) are achieved in patients receiving CPR within 4 minutes and ACLS within 8 minutes of arrest, whereas survival is less than 6% when CPR and ACLS are started after 9 minutes.

The groups of patients most likely to be resuscitated include patients outside the hospital with witnessed arrests due to VF, hospitalized patients with VF secondary to ischemic heart disease, arrests not associated with coexisting life-threatening conditions, and patients who are hypothermic or intoxicated. Patients with severe multisystem disease, metastatic cancer, or oliguria do not often survive CPR.

2. How do chest compressions produce a cardiac output?

It used to be assumed that chest compressions produced a cardiac output by directly compressing the ventricles against the vertebral column. This was thought to produce systole, with forward flow out of the aorta and pulmonary artery, and backward flow prevented by closure of the atrioventricular (AV) valves.

This explanation is probably not completely valid. Echocardiographic images during arrest show that the AV valves are not closed during chest compressions. There are reports of patients who, during episodes of monitored VF, have developed systolic pressures capable of maintaining consciousness by coughing. This demonstrates that chest compressions per se are not necessary to maintain a cardiac output. Furthermore, CPR is frequently ineffective in patients with a flail chest until chest stabilization is achieved. If direct compression were the etiology of blood circulation in CPR, then a flail chest would be an advantage by increasing the efficiency of the "direct" compression. These observations have led to the proposal of the "thoracic pump" theory of CPR.

The "thoracic pump" theory proposes that forward blood flow is achieved because of phasic changes in intrathoracic pressure produced by chest compressions. During the downward phase of the compression, positive intrathoracic pressure propels blood out of the chest into the extrathoracic vessels that have a lower pressure. Competent valves in the venous system prevent blood from flowing backwards. During the upward phase of the compression, blood flows from the periphery into the thorax because of the negative intrathoracic pressure created by release of the compression. With properly performed CPR, systolic arterial blood pressures of 60–80 mmHg can be achieved, but with much lower diastolic pressures. Mean pressures are usually less than 40 mmHg. This only provides cerebral blood flows of approximately 30% and myocardial blood flows of about 10% compared with pre-arrest values.

3. What are the recommended rates of compression and ventilation?

Animal models of CPR have shown that the optimal blood flows are achieved when chest compressions are performed at 80–100 times per minute and the chest is compressed 1.5 to 2 inches (3–5 cm). The new Guidelines for Cardiopulmonary Resuscitation published by the American Heart Association in 2000 recommend a chest compression rate of 100 times per minute. The proportion of time spent during the compression phase should be 50% of the relaxation phase.

Artificial ventilation is preferentially given by endotracheal tube (ETT) at a rate of 10–12 breaths per minute. Nevertheless, the new ACLS guidelines de-emphasize endotracheal intubation during CPR due to a high incidence of incorrectly placed ETTs. Mask ventilation or alternative airways, such as the laryngeal mask or the esophageal-tracheal Combitube, may be preferable in situations where the rescuer is not properly trained or skilled in ETT placement. It is now mandatory to confirm correct ETT placement by both physical examination and a secondary device, such as capnography, a colorimetric carbon dioxide (CO_2) detector, or an esophageal detector device. During two-person CPR, ventilation in the intubated patient should be performed with every fifth compression. With an unprotected airway or during one-rescuer CPR the compression to ventilation

Primary ABCD Survey

Focus: basic CPR and defibrillation

- **Check** responsiveness
- **Activate** emergency response system
- **Call** for defibrillator

A **Airway:** open the airway
B **Breathing:** provide positive-pressure ventilations
C **Circulation:** give chest compressions
D **Defibrillation:** assess for and shock VF/pulseless VT, up to 3 times (200 J, 200–300 J, 360 J, or equivalent biphasic) if necessary

↓

Rhythm after first 3 shocks?

↓

Persistent or recurrent VF/VT

↓

Secondary ABCD Survey

Focus: more advanced assessment and treatments

A **Airway:** place airway device as soon as possible
B **Breathing:** confirm airway device placement by exam plus confirmation device
B **Breathing:** secure airway device; purpose-made tube holders preferred
B **Breathing:** confirm effective oxygenation and ventilation
C **Circulation:** establish IV access
C **Circulation:** identify rhythm ⟶ monitor
C **Circulation:** administer drugs appropriate for rhythm and condition
D **Differential Diagnosis:** search for and treat identified reversible causes

↓

- **Epinephrine** 1 mg IV push, repeat every 3 to 5 minutes

or

- **Vasopressin** 40 U IV, single dose, 1 time only

↓

Resume attempts to defibrillate

1 × 360 J (or equivalent biphasic) within 30–60 seconds

↓

Consider antiarrhythmics:

- **Amiodarone** (IIb for persistent or recurrent VF/pulseless VT)
- **Lidocaine** (Indeterminate for persistent VF/pulseless VT)
- **Magnesium** (IIb if known hypomagnesemic state)
- **Procainamide** (Indeterminate for persistent VF/pulseless VT; IIb for recurrent VF/pulseless VT)

↓

Resume attempts to defibrillate

FIGURE 1.1 Algorithm for ventricular fibrillation and pulseless ventricular tachycardia. From ACLS Provider Manual, American Heart Association, 2001.

ratio is 15:2. Each breath should take about 2 seconds and should make the chest rise clearly. Animal studies demonstrate higher cerebral perfusion pressures when ventilation occurs simultaneously with compressions. However, improved survival has not been demonstrated in humans, and this technique is not recommended.

4. What are the complications of CPR?

Complications of CPR include skeletal injuries, especially rib fractures, visceral injuries, airway injuries, and skin and integument damage (skin, teeth, lips). Less than 0.5% of the complications are considered life-threatening. These include injuries to the heart and the great vessels. However, a significant number of complications could be expected to require therapy and prolong the hospitalization. These include rib and sternal fractures, myocardial and pulmonary contusions, pneumothorax, blood in the pericardial sac, tracheal and laryngeal injuries, liver and spleen ruptures, and gastric perforation and dilatation.

5. What is the optimal dose of epinephrine?

Pharmacologic therapy has been changed significantly from the previous ACLS protocols. Epinephrine is still the therapy of choice, but vasopressin has emerged as an alternative in the treatment of VF/VT. The vasoconstriction caused by the α-adrenergic effects of large doses of epinephrine that are administered during CPR increases arterial pressure and improves myocardial and cerebral blood flow. Studies have suggested that this is a dose-dependent phenomenon. Animal studies have shown better outcomes from cardiac arrest using 0.1–0.2 mg/kg of epinephrine rather than the present recommended dose of 0.01 mg/kg. Two recent large multicenter investigations, however, did not demonstrate survival differences in patients treated with larger doses of epinephrine. This lack of clinical efficacy may arise from the fact that the time elapsed prior to the initial dose of epinephrine was significantly longer than was the case in the animal studies.

The presence of coronary artery disease in many patients hinders coronary artery blood flow even in the presence of higher aortic diastolic pressures. The β-adrenergic effects of epinephrine may actually worsen the outcome by increasing myocardial oxygen requirements. Until further studies clarify this issue, the 2000 ACLS protocol recommends a standard dose of 1 mg epinephrine (0.01 mg/kg intravenous (i.v.) push) every 3–5 minutes. Higher doses up to 0.2 mg/kg may be considered, but these doses are not recommended and may be harmful.

6. What is the indication for vasopressin in CPR?

Vasopressin, also known as antidiuretic hormone, is a potent vasoconstrictor when used at higher doses. Vasopressin's vasoconstrictive effect increases blood flow to the brain and heart during CPR. The vasoconstrictive effect is mediated via V_1 receptors and thus independent of the adrenergic-receptor-mediated effect of epinephrine. Therefore, vasopressin seems to lack some of the β-adrenergic- mediated adverse effects of epinephrine, such as increased myocardial oxygen demand and tachycardia. Vasopressin currently holds a Class IIb recommendation in the treatment for pulseless VT/VF. It is not yet recommended for asystole and pulseless electrical activity, mainly because large studies showing improved outcome are still missing. Thus, vasopressin is currently recommended as a first-line alternative to epinephrine in patients with pulseless VT/VF, given as a single dose of 40 U i.v. push. Because of the longer half-life of vasopressin (10–20 minutes) compared with epinephrine (3–5 minutes), and lack of supportive evidence in human trials, a second dose is not recommended at this point. Following vasopressin administration and 10–20 minutes of continued CPR without the return of a perfusing rhythm, it is acceptable to return to 1 mg epinephrine every 3–5 minutes.

7. What are the indications for sodium bicarbonate (NaHCO₃) administration?

Before 1986, $NaHCO_3$ was routinely used during CPR, even without knowledge of the patient's acid–base status. Acidosis inhibits myocardial contractility and also inhibits the effects of catecholamines. However, this inhibitory effect on catecholamines does not appear clinically significant at the range of pH commonly encountered and the catecholamine doses administered during resuscitation. The myocardial depressant effect of metabolic acidosis is delayed compared with that produced by the intracellular acidosis that follows the administration of $NaHCO_3$. As is apparent from the equilibrium equation,

$$[HCO_3^-] + [H^+] \Leftrightarrow [H_2CO_3] \Leftrightarrow [CO_2] + [H_2O]$$

every 50 mEq of bicarbonate administered produces large amounts of CO_2 gas. CO_2 gas freely diffuses across cellular membranes, and causes a paradoxical worsening of the intracellular acidosis. Intracellular CO_2 tensions of greater than 300 mmHg and pH values less than 6.1 have been recorded.

Carbicarb, a buffering agent that does not produce as much CO_2, has also been tried without significant improvements in outcome following CPR. Another probable explanation for the ineffectiveness of these buffering agents is that they also cause hypernatremia and hyperosmolality. Hyperosmolar solutions may decrease aortic pressures, and compromise survival. Initially, the leftward shift in the oxyhemoglobin saturation curve following the administration of $NaHCO_3$ may theoretically decrease oxygen availability.

Thus, $NaHCO_3$ should only be given when the results of arterial blood gas analysis indicate a significant metabolic acidosis in the presence of severe acidemia (e.g., with an arterial pH <7.20). It currently holds a Class III indication in hypercarbic acidosis and thus may be harmful during CPR. $NaHCO_3$ is indicated in known hyperkalemia (Class I), bicarbonate-responsive acidosis (Class IIa), tricyclic antidepressant overdose (Class IIa), to alkalinize urine in aspirin or other drug overdose (Class IIa), and for intubated and ventilated patients with a long arrest time or return of circulation after prolonged CPR (Class IIb). When $NaHCO_3$ administration is planned, the correct full dose is calculated as follows:

$$\text{Patient's weight (kg)} \times \text{base deficit} \times 0.3$$

Many clinicians use half of the calculated dose initially. If blood gas results are unobtainable, an empiric dose of 1 mEq/kg can be administered in prolonged arrest situations.

8. What are the indications for calcium salt administration?

Routine calcium chloride or calcium gluconate administration has also been scrutinized. Studies indicate that intracellular calcium accumulation may be a final common mediator of cellular injury and death. Specific indications for calcium therapy during CPR include hyperkalemia, documented hypocalcemia, and calcium-channel blocker overdose. Calcium salts are not recommended in the routine treatment of electromechanical dissociation or asystole.

9. What is the antidysrhythmic therapy of choice in VF/pulseless VT?

After CPR has been initiated and the underlying rhythm recognized, immediate defibrillation is the mainstay therapy in the treatment of VF/pulseless VT. The choice of antidysrhythmic therapy has not been shown to influence outcome if repeated countershocks, epinephrine/vasopressin, and appropriately administered CPR are ineffective in a patient with refractory VF or VT. No drug has clearly proven superiority in most cases of intractable VT or VF. Despite this, the 2000 ACLS protocol contains many changes in drug administration in VF/pulseless VT compared with older recommendations. Lidocaine is no longer recommended as the antidysrhythmic drug of choice for the treatment of malignant ventricular ectopy, VT, or VF. Lidocaine and procainamide hydrochloride are now classified as drugs with intermediate evidence for this indication. Bretylium is no longer recommended and has been removed from the ACLS algorithm. Instead, amiodarone is now a Class IIb indication for cardiac arrest from VF/pulseless VT that persists after multiple shocks. Amiodarone has been shown to increase the intermediate outcome of admission-to-hospital following out-of-hospital refractory VF arrest in one prospective double-blinded randomized controlled study.

Nonetheless, amiodarone administration is not associated with improvement of long-term outcome. After attempts to defibrillate and epinephrine and/or vasopressin administration fail to establish a perfusing rhythm, the new ACLS guidelines indicate consideration of antidysrhythmics as follows (Table 1.1):

- amiodarone 300 mg i.v. push for persistent or recurrent VF/pulseless VT
- magnesium sulfate 1–2 mg i.v. when an underlying hypomagnesemic state is suspected or in torsades de pointes
- procainamide 50 mg/min in refractory VF (maximum 17 mg/kg)

10. What are the management strategies in bradycardias?

Most symptomatic bradycardias (e.g., sinus bradycardia and asystole) should be treated with atropine, transcutaneous pacing (TCP), and dopamine or epinephrine infusions. Patients with third-degree heart block and Mobitz type II second-degree heart block should not receive atropine because it may cause a paradoxical slowing of ventricular escape rates. Isoproterenol should not be used for the treatment of bradycardias because it increases myocardial oxygen consumption and may cause hypotension.

In the setting of an acute myocardial infarction, the ACLS protocol recommends that third-degree heart block and Mobitz type II heart block require transvenous pacing. TCP or epinephrine should be used in symptomatic patients until a transvenous pacemaker is inserted.

11. What is the treatment of supraventricular tachydysrhythmias?

The most important initial step is to evaluate whether the patient with an underlying tachycardia is stable or unstable. Tachycardias in unstable patients require immediate electrical cardioversion, whereas stable tachycardias are usually treated with drugs and/or electric cardioversion until further evaluation and diagnostic measures can be performed. It is extremely important to treat all wide complex tachydysrhythmias as VT. Clinical or ECG criteria used to differentiate wide complex supraventricular tachycardias from VT are problematic. Administration of verapamil to a patient with VT may cause irreversible hemodynamic collapse. However, since adenosine has almost no effect on blood pressure, it can be tried in stable patients who are suspected of having a wide complex supraventricular tachycardia. Adenosine is an endogenous purine nucleoside that depresses sinus and AV nodal activity that is extremely short-acting (the serum half-life is less than 5 seconds) and produces few significant side-effects.

In narrow complex supraventricular tachycardias, vagal maneuvers should be performed or adenosine (0.1 mg/kg

TABLE 1.1   Treatments Used in Cardiopulmonary Resuscitation

Modality	Description	Dose
Electrical	*Indications:*	
	VF/pulseless VT	200, 200–300, 360 joules
	Atrial fibrillation	100, 200, 300, 360 joules
	Atrial flutter/paroxysmal supraventricular tachycardia	50, 100, 200, 300, 360 joules
Amiodarone	*Indications:*	
	Cardiac arrest from persistent VF/pulseless VT	300 mg i.v. push
	Recurrent VF/pulseless VT	150 mg i.v. over 10 minutes
	Wide complex tachycardia (stable)	followed by 1 mg/min over 6 hours
	Supraventricular and ventricular tachycardias	and then 0.5 mg/min over 18 hours
		Maximum dose: 2.2 g per 24 hours
Procainamide	*Indications:*	
	Recurrent VF/pulseless VT	Up to 50 mg/min (maximum
	Wide complex tachycardia which cannot be	dose of 17 mg/kg)
	differentiated from VT	Once stabilized begin infusion
	Side-effects:	of 1–4 mg/min
	Hypotension, widened QRS complex, seizures	
Epinephrine	*Indications:*	
	Persistent or recurrent VT, VF, asystole,	1 mg bolus every 3–5 minutes (if unsuc-
	PEA, bradycardia	cessful higher doses of up to 0.2 mg/kg,
		but not generally recommended and
		may be harmful)
	Side-effects:	
	Hypertension, dysrhythmias, myocardial ischemia	If used for symptomatic bradycardia
		2–10 µg/kg titrated to effect
Vasopressin	*Indication:*	
	Persistent VF/pulseless VT arrest	Single, one-time dose of 40 U i.v.
		(half-life 10–20 minutes)
Atropine	*Indications:*	
	Bradycardia, asystole, slow PEA	*In asystole and slow PEA:*
	Side-effects:	1 mg repeat in 3–5 minutes up
	VT, VF	to 0.04 mg/kg
	NOTE: doses <0.5 mg may be	*In bradycardias:*
	parasympathomimetic	0.5–1 mg repeat in 3–5 minutes
	Contraindications:	up to 0.03 mg/kg
	Mobitz type II AV block and third-degree	
	AV block with a new wide QRS	
Magnesium sulfate (MgSO$_4$)	*Indications:*	
	Cardiac arrest from hypomagnesemia,	MgSO$_4$ 1–2 g diluted in 10 cc
	torsades de pointes	D5W i.v. push
	Torsades de pointes (not in cardiac arrest),	Load with 1–2 g in 50–100 cc D5W over
	dysrhythmia suspected to be caused by	5–60 minutes, then 0.5–1 g/hr up to
	hypomagnesemic state	24 hours
Adenosine	*Indications:*	
	Narrow complex supraventricular tachycardia	Initial bolus 6 mg over 1–3 seconds
	(diagnostic, may unveil underlying rhythm:	followed by 20 cc flush. If no response
	paroxysmal supraventricular tachycardia, junctional	within 1–2 minutes repeat with 12 mg
	tachycardia, ectopic, or multifocal atrial tachycardia)	
	Side-effects:	
	Transient sinus bradycardia or arrest, ventricular	
	ectopy, flushing, dyspnea, chest pain	

Continued

TABLE 1.1   **Treatments Used in Cardiopulmonary Resuscitation—cont'd**

Modality	Description	Dose
Diltiazem	*Indications:* Paroxysmal supraventricular tachycardia, control of ventricular response in atrial fibrillation, atrial flutter, and multifocal atrial tachycardia *Side-effects:* Myocardial depression, bradycardia, hypotension (less than veraramil)	0.25 mg/kg then 0.35 mg/kg Maintenance: 5–15 mg/hr
Dopamine	*Indications:* Symptomatic bradycardia, hypotension	Start at 2–5 µg/kg/min
Norepinephrine	*Indications:* Hypotension due to low SVR *Side-effects:* Hypertension, dysrhythmias, increased or decreased cardiac output (depending on contractile state and SVR), renal, mesenteric and myocardial ischemia	0.04–0.4 µg/kg/min
Dobutamine	*Indications:* Congestive heart failure *Side-effects:* Hypertension, dysrhythmias, myocardial ischemia	2.5–15 µg/kg/min
Calcium	*Indications:* Hypocalcemia, hyperkalemia, hypermagnesemia *Side-effects:* Bradycardia	250 mg of 10% calcium chloride solution, repeat as needed or 500 mg of calcium gluceptate
Sodium bicarbonate (NaHCO$_3$)	*Indications:* Pre-existing hyperkalemia, pre-existing bicarbonate-responsive acidosis, tricyclic antidepressant overdose, aspirin or drug overdose to alkalinize urine, long arrest interval, return of circulation after long arrest interval *Side-effects:* Hypercarbia, metabolic alkalosis, hyperosmolality, impairs oxyhemoglobin dissociation	# mEq NaHCO$_3$ = base deficit × weight kg × 0.3 (many give half the calculated dose initially) Empiric dose: 1 mEq/kg Subsequent empiric doses are administered at a rate of 0.5 mEq/kg
Nitroglycerin	*Indications:* Myocardial ischemia, pulmonary hypertension, systemic hypertension *Side-effects:* Hypotension, reflex tachycardia	0.5–1.0 µg/kg/min initially, then adjust according to response Usual dose range is 1–8 µg/kg/min
Nitroprusside	*Indications:* Systemic hypertension, induced hypotension, congestive heart failure *Side-effects:* Hypotension, reflex tachycardia, cyanide toxicity	Initially 0.2 µg/kg/min, then adjust accordingly Maximal dose: 10 µg/kg/min or 1–1.5 mg/kg over 2–3 hours
Milrinone	*Indications:* Congestive heart failure (especially right heart failure) *Side-effects:* Marked systemic vasodilation especially in hypovolemic patients	Loading dose (i.v.): 50 µg/kg over 10 minutes, infusion rate 0.375–0.75 µg/kg/min

VF, ventricular fibrillation; VT, ventricular tachycardia; PEA, pulseless electrical activity.

i.v. push) administered to help identify the exact underlying rhythm. Treatment also depends on the underlying cardiac function (preserved or impaired, ejection fraction (EF) <40%, congestive heart failure). Paroxysmal supraventricular tachycardias can be treated with calcium-channel blockers, β-blockers, digoxin, or amiodarone (the latter especially in the patient with impaired cardiac function). In junctional tachycardia or ectopic or multifocal atrial tachycardia, electrical cardioversion is not recommended.

If atrial fibrillation/flutter is suspected as the underlying rhythm, it is imperative to evaluate the patient before further management is initiated. If possible, the patient's cardiac function should be assessed, a Wolff-Parkinson-White (WPW) syndrome ruled out, and the time of onset of atrial fibrillation determined (<48 hours or >48 hours). The goals are to treat unstable patients urgently to control the rate, convert the rhythm, and to provide anticoagulation. Patients with an onset of symptoms > 48 hours should be evaluated for thrombi in the atria using transesophageal echocardiography (TEE) before electric cardioversion is attempted. WPW patients are preferably treated with electric cardioversion or amiodarone. In these patients, adenosine, β-blockers, calcium-channel blockers, and digoxin are contraindicated. These drugs can lead to an increased ventricular response or may precipitate VF by selectively blocking the AV node in patients with coexisting accessory conduction pathways. Once the diagnosis of atrial fibrillation/flutter is confirmed, treatment usually consists of electric cardioversion, β-blockers, calcium-channel blockers (e.g., diltiazem), or digoxin. Amiodarone is preferred in the unstable patient or the patient with impaired ventricular function (Table 1.1).

12. What are the indications for magnesium therapy?

Magnesium deficiency is associated with ventricular ectopy, sudden cardiac death, and CHF. It can also precipitate refractory VF and impede correction of hypokalemia. Hypomagnesemia should be corrected in cases of refractory VT or VF. Magnesium sulfate is the treatment of choice for torsades de pointes. Magnesium supplementation may also reduce the incidence of post-myocardial infarction ventricular dysrhythmias. Thus, some authorities suggest administering it prophylactically to patients after myocardial infarction.

13. What are the indications for a pacemaker?

The use of transcutaneous or transvenous pacemakers in ACLS is indicated in patients with symptomatic bradydysrhythmias (i.e., myocardial ischemia, hypotension, mental status changes, pulmonary edema), and for overdrive pacing in patients with refractory tachydysrhythmias. They are rarely indicated in asystolic patients who have had prolonged attempts at resuscitation.

14. Why is it important to monitor serum glucose?

Serum glucose levels may affect post-cardiac arrest neurologic function. Animal studies have shown less functional brain recovery after normothermic cerebral ischemia in hyperglycemic animals. The mechanism probably relates to increased lactic acid production secondary to availability of larger amounts of the precursor, glucose. Unfortunately, it is not clear what levels of glucose should be treated. Severe hypoglycemia as a result of overtreatment of hyperglycemia will cause neuronal injury.

15. What are the indications for open cardiac massage?

Open cardiac massage is probably indicated only in postoperative cardiac surgical patients (in case of pericardial tamponade), in the operating room if the heart is accessible, in patients with severely deformed thoracic cages, and in some cases of penetrating chest trauma. It should be considered in cases of cardiac arrest caused by hypothermia, pulmonary embolism, pericardial tamponade, abdominal hemorrhage, and blunt trauma with cardiac arrest. It has not been found to be of value in patients who have had prolonged closed CPR.

16. What is the management strategy for pulseless electrical activity (PEA)?

PEA refers to the clinical picture of cardiac electrical activity without a detectable pulse. VF, VT, and asystole are specifically excluded from the wide range of electrical activity that may present. The ACLS guidelines emphasize the search for reversible causes of PEA. This must not exclude basic resuscitation measures, which should be started as soon as possible. After VF/pulseless VT have been ruled out, securing an airway, oxygen administration, and chest compressions must be the primary task. The etiology of PEA must now be sought. Table 1.2 lists the most frequent causes of PEA.

First-line drugs in the continuing resuscitation algorithm include epinephrine 1 mg i.v. push every 3–5 minutes and

TABLE 1.2	The 5 "Hs" and 5 "Ts" as the most frequent causes of pulseless electrical activity (PEA)
Hypovolemia	Tablets (drug overdose, accidents)
Hypoxia	Tamponade (cardiac)
Hydrogen ion—acidosis	Tension pneumothorax
Hyper-/hypokalemia	Thrombosis (coronary)
Hypothermia	Thrombosis (pulmonary)

atropine 1 mg i.v. every 3–5 minutes as needed when the underlying PEA rate is slow. Nevertheless, treatment of PEA is not limited to these drugs and pharmacologic treatment of a patient with PEA must be customized to the suspected underlying cause. PEA is not an indication for defibrillation. "Shockable" rhythms have to be ruled out. Once a patient converts to VF/pulseless VT, however, the appropriate algorithm should be initiated immediately.

SUGGESTED READINGS

American Heart Association: Guidelines 2000 for cardiopulmonary resuscitation and emergency cardiovascular care. Circulation 102:Suppl I, 2000

Spearpoint KG, McLean CP, Zideman DA: Early defibrillation and the chain of survival in "in-hospital" adult cardiac arrest; minutes count. Resuscitation 44:165, 2000

Wenzel V, Krismer AC, Arntz HR, et al.: European Resuscitation Council Vasopressor during Cardiopulmonary Resuscitation Study Group: A comparison of vasopressin and epinephrine for out-of-hospital cardiopulmonary resuscitation. N Engl J Med 350:105, 2004

Xavier LC, Kern KB: Cardiopulmonary Resuscitation Guidelines 2000 update: what's happened since? Curr Opin Crit Care 9:218, 2003

Alexander Mittnacht, MD
David L. Reich, MD

A 65-year-old man with hypertension, familial hyper-cholesterolemia, type II diabetes mellitus, and angina pectoris presents for resection of a tumor of the sigmoid colon. A dipyridamole-thallium scan demonstrates an anteroseptal perfusion defect, which shows filling on the delayed image. Coronary angiography demonstrates a critical lesion of the left anterior descending coronary artery and a 50% stenosis of the proximal circumflex coronary artery. Percutaneous transluminal coronary angioplasty (PTCA) was performed successfully on the left anterior descending lesion 6 weeks prior to surgery.

General anesthesia is induced with etomidate, midazolam, and fentanyl, and maintained with oxygen, isoflurane, and fentanyl. Muscle relaxation is provided with vecuronium. During mobilization of the tumor, the heart rate increases from 70 to 120 beats per minute. The blood pressure remains stable at 130/70 mmHg. Two millimeters of horizontal ST-segment depression are noted on the V_5 electro-cardiogram (ECG) lead, but no abnormality is seen in lead II. An additional dose of fentanyl is associated with a decrease in the heart rate to 95 beats per minute, but no change in the ST-segment depression in V_5.

QUESTIONS

1. What are the determinants of myocardial oxygen supply?

2. What are the determinants of myocardial oxygen consumption (demand)?
3. What are the pharmacologic alternatives for treating myocardial ischemia in this patient?
4. What is coronary steal and what agents might induce it?
5. Should this patient receive perioperative β-adrenergic blockade?
6. How should this patient be monitored intraoperatively?

1. What are the determinants of myocardial oxygen supply?

The major concern in the anesthetic management of patients with coronary artery disease (CAD) is maintaining a favorable balance between myocardial oxygen supply and demand (Figure 2.1). The myocardial oxygen supply is tenuous in patients with CAD. It is preserved by maintaining both the coronary perfusion pressure and the length of the diastolic interval.

Coronary perfusion pressure is maintained by ensuring a normal to high diastolic arterial pressure along with a normal to low left ventricular end-diastolic pressure, which is usually estimated by measuring the pulmonary capillary wedge pressure.

2. What are the determinants of myocardial oxygen consumption (demand)?

Heart rate, contractility, and myocardial wall tension are the three major determinants of myocardial oxygen

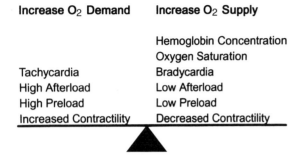

Increase O₂ Demand	Increase O₂ Supply
	Hemoglobin Concentration
	Oxygen Saturation
Tachycardia	Bradycardia
High Afterload	Low Afterload
High Preload	Low Preload
Increased Contractility	Decreased Contractility

FIGURE 2.1   The balance between myocardial oxygen supply and demand.

consumption. Heart rate is probably the most important parameter regulating the myocardial oxygen supply-demand balance. Decreasing heart rate both increases oxygen supply by prolonging diastole and decreases oxygen demand. The association between tachycardia and myocardial ischemia is well documented. Severe bradycardia should be avoided, however, as this will cause decreased diastolic arterial pressure and increased left ventricular end-diastolic pressure. β-Adrenergic blocking drugs are commonly used to maintain a mild bradycardia in patients with CAD.

Myocardial contractility is loosely defined as the intrinsic ability of the myocardium to shorten. This is a very difficult parameter to measure and is poorly described by the cardiac output or even the left ventricular ejection fraction. Decreased myocardial contractility is associated with decreased myocardial oxygen demand. Thus, "myocardial depression" may be beneficial in patients with CAD. Specifically, agents that depress myocardial contractility but are not potent vasodilators may be beneficial as long as coronary perfusion pressure is maintained. Thus, potent volatile anesthetic agents (halothane, enflurane, and isoflurane) are examples of "myocardial depressants" that could be useful for patients with CAD as long as coronary perfusion pressure is maintained.

Myocardial oxygen supply and demand are kept in balance by properly managing left ventricular preload, afterload, heart rate, and contractility. Major increases in preload (left ventricular end-diastolic volume) add to the volume work of the heart (increased demand) and decrease coronary perfusion pressure because of the associated increase in left ventricular end-diastolic pressure (decreased supply). Nitrates assist in maintaining a normal to low preload (see below). Excessive increases in afterload result in increased pressure work of the heart (wall tension) during systole (increased demand) despite the increase in coronary perfusion pressure. At the other end of the spectrum, extreme vasodilatation (decreased afterload) will lower the diastolic arterial pressure and decrease myocardial oxygen supply (see Table 2.1).

3. What are the pharmacologic alternatives for treating myocardial ischemia in this patient?

Nitroglycerin and other nitrates exert their anti-anginal effects by dilating epicardial coronary arteries and decreasing left ventricular end-diastolic pressure due to systemic venodilation. Nitrates also cause mild arterial vasodilatation and may decrease the pressure work of the myocardium on that basis. The limiting factor of nitrate therapy is that large doses cause hypotension, which would lower myocardial oxygen supply, and reflex tachycardia may occur.

β-Adrenergic blocking drugs slow the heart rate, which has two beneficial effects on myocardial ischemia. First, the

| TABLE 2.1 | Hemodynamic Goals in Myocardial Ischemia to Optimize Coronary Perfusion Pressure |

Parameter	Goal	Indicated	Contraindicated
Heart rate	Slow	β-Adrenergic blockers	Isoproterenol Dobutamine Ketamine Pancuronium
Preload	Normal to low	Nitroglycerin Diuretics	Volume overload
Afterload	Normal to high	Phenylephrine	Nitroprusside *High-dose* isoflurane
Contractility	Normal to decreased	β-Adrenergic blockers Volatile anesthetics	Epinephrine Dopamine

duration of diastole increases and improves coronary perfusion. Second, myocardial oxygen consumption is decreased. β-Adrenergic blockers also decrease myocardial contractility, and this also decreases myocardial oxygen consumption. Propranolol and metoprolol have been used for many years for intraoperative β-adrenergic blockade. Esmolol, a short-acting intravenous β-adrenergic blocker, has become increasingly popular among anesthesiologists because of its relative cardiac (β₁ receptor) selectivity and favorable pharmacokinetics.

Calcium-channel entry blockers are an important component of the medical therapy for patients with CAD. Their role as intraoperative agents for the management of myocardial ischemia is less clear. There is even some evidence that preoperative calcium-channel entry blocker therapy may increase the incidence of intraoperative myocardial ischemia.

Phenylephrine, a "pure" α-adrenergic agonist, is the agent of choice for the treatment of hypotension in myocardial ischemia because it increases diastolic pressure with no change (or a slight decrease) in heart rate. Drugs with β-adrenergic effects, such as ephedrine, dobutamine, and dopamine, would increase the heart rate, increase myocardial contractility, and decrease diastolic arterial pressure. All these β-adrenergic actions are undesirable during myocardial ischemia.

Clonidine is an α₂-adrenergic agonist, which is available only for the enteral route of application in the United States. Dexmedetomidine is a more selective α₂-adrenergic agonist than clonidine that can be intravenously administered. This class of drugs decreases sympathetic outflow from the central nervous system and plasma norepinephrine concentrations. α₂-Adrenergic agonists ameliorate episodes of "breakthrough hypertension" that occur with surgical stimulation and postoperative stresses, attenuate increases in heart rate, and reduce myocardial oxygen demand. α₂-Adrenergic agonists potentiate anesthetic agents, can be used as sedatives, and decrease postoperative pain medication requirements. Thus, their role in the perioperative treatment for patients with CAD seems to be very favorable. A review of recently published studies on the efficacy of α₂-adrenergic agonists in the perioperative treatment of cardiac risk patients indicates reduced risk of perioperative myocardial ischemia, but the incidence of myocardial infarction or death did not change. The exact role of this class of drugs in the cardiac risk patient has yet to be defined.

4. What is coronary steal and what agents might induce it?

Coronary steal may occur when a segment of the myocardium distal to a stenotic coronary artery receives its major blood supply from collateral vessels that originate from a "normal" segment of myocardium supplied by a normal coronary artery. Arteriolar vasodilators (e.g., isoflurane, sodium nitroprusside, and dipyridamole) may decrease the flow across the collateral vessels by dilating the arterioles in the normal segment of myocardium. However, there is no convincing evidence that isoflurane should be avoided in patients with CAD provided that excessive tachycardia and hypotension do not occur. It would be prudent, though, to avoid arteriolar vasodilators in patients with "steal-prone" anatomy.

5. Should this patient receive perioperative β-adrenergic blockade?

The following describes a randomized, double-masked, placebo-controlled trial to compare the effect of atenolol with that of a placebo on overall survival and cardiovascular morbidity in patients at cardiac risk who were undergoing noncardiac surgery. Atenolol was given intravenously before and immediately after surgery and orally thereafter for the duration of hospitalization. Patients were followed over the subsequent 2 years. Of 200 patients, 99 were assigned to the atenolol group, and 101 to the placebo group. One hundred ninety-four patients survived to be discharged from the hospital, and 192 of these were followed for 2 years. Overall mortality after discharge from the hospital was significantly lower among the atenolol-treated patients than among those who were given placebo, over the 6 months following hospital discharge (0 vs. 8%, $P < 0.001$), over the first year (3% vs. 14%, $P = 0.005$), and over 2 years (10% vs. 21%, $P = 0.019$). The principal effect was a reduction in deaths from cardiac causes during the first 6 to 8 months. Combined cardiovascular outcomes were similarly reduced among the atenolol-treated patients; event-free survival throughout the 2-year study period was 68% in the placebo group and 83% in the atenolol-treated group ($P = 0.008$). The incidence of diabetes mellitus may have had a confounding influence on this study, but the results suggest that perioperative β-adrenergic blockade is potentially quite beneficial in high-risk patients.

6. How should this patient be monitored intraoperatively?

The most important modality for monitoring this patient intraoperatively is a multiple-lead electrocardiogram (ECG) system. Up to 89% of the ECG changes of myocardial ischemia that are present on a standard 12-lead ECG will be detected by a V_5 precordial ECG lead alone. Since the late 1970s, it has been recommended that limb lead II and precordial lead V_5 be monitored simultaneously for the detection of intraoperative myocardial ischemia. This combination should enable >90% of ischemic episodes to be detected. In addition, this combination also monitors the distribution of both the right and left coronary arteries.

Operating room ECG systems nowadays are usually capable of continuous ST-segment monitoring. Generally, these determine the relationship of the ST-segment 60–80 msec after the J-point (junction between the QRS complex and the ST-segment) to the baseline (during the P-Q interval). Ischemia may be defined as >0.1 mV of horizontal or downsloping ST-segment depression or >0.2 mV of ST-segment elevation. These systems are rendered less effective by left ventricular hypertrophy and frequent electrocautery, and are not useful in left bundle branch block or ventricular pacing.

If only a three-lead ECG system is available it is still possible to intermittently monitor both the inferior (lead II) and the lateral (V_5) walls of the heart. The left arm lead is placed over the precordial V_5 position and the other leads are placed in their usual positions: the right shoulder and left leg. The modified V_5 lead is monitored by setting the ECG device to lead I. The monitor will display a modified V_5 lead known as the CS_5 (chest-shoulder 5). If the monitor is intermittently switched to lead II, the true lead II will be seen on the monitor. Thus, it is possible to intermittently use a multiple-lead ECG system even with a three-lead ECG system.

Transesophageal echocardiography (TEE), if available, is an extremely sensitive method of detecting myocardial ischemia. This is done by continuously imaging the transgastric short-axis view of the left ventricle. This images the distributions of the three major coronary vessels. The disadvantages are that it is difficult to pay continuous attention to the echo image and that changes in regional wall motion may not be specific for myocardial ischemia even if they are highly sensitive. Additionally, the cost of the equipment and need for specialized training are limiting factors in the use of TEE.

SUGGESTED READINGS

Chung F, Houston PL, Cheng DCH, Lavelle PA, McDonald N, Burns RJ, David TE: Calcium channel blockade does not offer adequate protection from perioperative myocardial ischemia. Anesthesiology 69:343, 1988

Gold MI, Sacks DJ, Grosnoff DB, Harrington C, Skillman CA: Use of esmolol during anesthesia to treat tachycardia and hypertension. Anesth Analg 68:101, 1989

Jorden VSB, Tung A: Dexmedetomidine: Clinical update. Semin Anesthes Periop Med Pain 21:265, 2002

Kaplan JA, King SB: The precordial electrocardiographic lead (V_5) in patients who have coronary artery disease. Anesthesiology 45:570, 1976

Kotrly KJ, Kotter GS, Mortara D, et al.: Intraoperative detection of myocardial ischemia with an ST segment trend monitoring system. Anesth Analg 63:343, 1984

Landsberg G, Mosseri M, et al.: Perioperative myocardial ischemia and infarction. Anesthesiology 96:264, 2002

Mangano DT, Layug EL, Wallace A, Tateo I: Effect of atenolol on mortality and cardiovascular morbidity after noncardiac surgery. Multicenter Study of Perioperative Ischemia Research Group. N Engl J Med 335:1713, 1996

Nishina K, Mikawa K, Uesugi T, et al.: Efficacy of clonidine for prevention of perioperative myocardial ischemia: A critical approach and meta-analysis of the literature. Anesthesiology 96:323, 2002

Park KW: Preoperative cardiology consultation. Anesthesiology 98:754, 2003

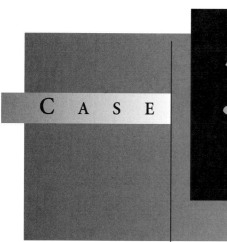

C A S E 3

RECENT MYOCARDIAL INFARCTION

Alexander Mittnacht, MD
David L. Reich, MD

A 68-year-old woman with multiple cardiac risk factors had sudden onset of crushing substernal chest pain. Despite aggressive thrombolytic therapy, the patient had electrocardiogram (ECG) evidence of a transmural antero-lateral myocardial infarction (MI). Three weeks following the MI, the patient develops acute cholecystitis, and presents for a cholecystectomy.

QUESTIONS

1. How do you evaluate the cardiac risk in a patient scheduled for noncardiac surgery?
2. What is the cardiac risk in this patient? What additional investigations should be performed?
3. What are the implications for anesthetic management when coronary revascularization is performed before noncardiac surgery?
4. What intraoperative monitors would you use?
5. What additional drugs would you have prepared?
6. What anesthetic technique would you use?
7. How would you manage this patient postoperatively?

1. How do you evaluate the cardiac risk in a patient scheduled for noncardiac surgery?

The preoperative cardiac evaluation and assessment of any patient includes a review of the history, physical examination, and laboratory results, and knowledge of the planned surgical procedure. The history should assess the presence, severity, and reversibility of coronary artery disease (CAD) (risks factors, anginal patterns, history of myocardial infarction), the clinical assessment of left and right ventricular function (exercise capacity, pulmonary edema, pulmonary hypertension), and the presence of symptomatic dysrhythmias (palpitations, syncopal or pre-syncopal episodes). Patients with valvular heart disease should also be asked about the presence of embolic events.

On physical examination, particular attention should be paid to the vital signs, specifically the heart rate, blood pressure, and pulse pressure (determinants of myocardial oxygen consumption and delivery), the presence of left- or right-sided failure (jugular venous distention, peripheral edema, pulmonary edema, or an S_3), and the presence of murmurs. Baseline laboratory tests include a chest radiograph to assess heart size, and an ECG. Further evaluation depends on the results of the above preliminary investigations, as well as the planned surgical procedure.

The significance of historical and laboratory data is the subject of much controversy. It is not really known how predictive these variables are of patient outcome. For example, a review of the literature suggests a variable contribution from patient age. In general, it is believed that age has no effect on resting parameters of cardiac function, such as ejection fraction, left ventricular dimensions, and wall motion. It is believed that older patients have decreased reserve and decreased response to stress. However, not all studies show a relationship between age and perioperative cardiac events (PCE). A PCE is generally defined as postoperative unstable angina, myocardial infarction (MI), congestive heart failure (CHF), or death from cardiac causes.

The current standard of care is defined by the most recent updated American College of Cardiology/American Heart Association (ACC/AHA) Guidelines for Perioperative Cardiovascular Evaluation for Noncardiac Surgery. The general paradigm is that patients are risk-stratified based upon patient-related clinical predictors of PCE, the risk imparted by the surgical procedure, and the appropriate use of noninvasive testing. In elective procedures, this algorithmic approach should be used by internists, surgeons, and anesthesiologists for the appropriate management of the cardiovascular evaluation strategy.

Unstable angina is a major clinical predictor of PCE in the ACC/AHA Guidelines, and chronic stable angina is an intermediate clinical predictor of PCE. Fleisher and Barash (1992) suggested that patients should be classified in a more functional way. They contended that not all patients with stable angina have the same disease process (i.e., coronary anatomy, frequency of ischemia, and left ventricular (LV) function). The number of ischemic episodes is especially difficult to quantitate without some sort of continuous monitoring (ambulatory ECG). This information is probably important since more than 75% of ischemic episodes are silent and more than 50% of patients with CAD (not just diabetics) have silent ischemia. It is not clear what the role of silent ischemia is in myocardial injury, although it seems to portend a worse prognosis if present in patients with unstable angina or post-MI patients.

Noninvasive studies are designed to determine the risk of ongoing ischemia (and the quality of LV function in some instances), and include ambulatory ECG (Holter monitoring), exercise stress tests, nuclear perfusion scans and function studies, and echocardiography. Exercise, steal-inducing drugs (dipyridamole or adenosine), or dobutamine are commonly used to induce reversible ischemia for noninvasive studies. Angiography may be performed if the noninvasive studies are highly suggestive of CAD and coronary intervention is logical for the patient from a global cardiovascular disease standpoint. A patient suspected of having mild disease may benefit from an aggressive investigation if the surgical procedure is associated with a high incidence of PCE. The same patient scheduled for a procedure with minimal cardiac risk probably does not warrant further testing.

The relationship between history of infarction and PCE varies significantly based upon the age of the infarction. Recent infarctions are defined by cardiologists as those within the last 7–30 days, and are acknowledged as a major clinical predictor of PCE. Prior MI by history or pathologic Q waves on the ECG is an intermediate clinical predictor. This is somewhat complicated to interpret in anesthesia practice because anesthesiologists traditionally refer to recent infarctions as those occurring within the preceding 6 weeks to 6 months. The classic "re-infarction" studies from data collected 20–40 years ago, found that patients with an infarct within 3 months had a 5.7–30% incidence of re-infarction. Between 3 and 6 months the risks vary from 2.3% to 15%, and an infarct more than 6 months prior to surgery is associated with a 1.9–6% incidence. The mortality of myocardial re-infarction was about 50%, and this figure varies very little among the various studies. The lower numbers in each group are from the study of Rao et al. (1983), in which aggressive hemodynamic monitoring was used and patients recovered in the intensive care unit postoperatively. The problem with applying these data to modern care is that they precede the widespread use of β-blockers, coronary interventions, and enzyme-based diagnosis of infarctions. Nevertheless, there is no doubt the more recent MIs represent a significant risk factor for PCE. The severity of the infarction must also be considered.

Medical literature distinguishes mortality in Q wave versus non-Q wave MIs, involving the right versus the left coronary artery distribution, uncomplicated versus complicated infarcts (recurrent pain, CHF, or dysrhythmias) and negative versus positive post-MI exercise stress test results. It seems reasonable to assume that mortality rates from (recent) MIs should not all be classified together based solely on the time since the infarction.

CHF in the general population has a poor prognosis. There is only an approximately 50% 5-year survival, although this may be improving with modern afterload-reduction and antidysrhythmic therapies. Patients with LV ejection fractions less than 30% have approximately 30% 1-year mortality. The ACC/AHA Guidelines include uncompensated CHF as a major clinical predictor and compensated or prior CHF as an intermediate clinical predictor.

Dysrhythmias are not an uncommon problem. They are usually benign, except in patients with underlying heart disease, in whom they serve as markers for increased morbidity and mortality. For example, many patients with LV dysfunction and dysrhythmias die from LV failure and not from a dysrhythmia. Acknowledged major clinical predictors include high-degree atrioventricular block, symptomatic ventricular dysrhythmias in the presence of underlying heart disease, and supraventricular dysrhythmias with uncontrolled ventricular rate. Minor predictors include abnormal

ECG (i.e., LV hypertrophy, left bundle branch block, and ST-T wave abnormalities). Rhythm other than sinus (e.g., atrial fibrillation) is also a minor clinical predictor.

Patients with valvular heart disease are difficult to evaluate because the lesions cause changes which are independently associated with increased risk (i.e., CHF, rhythm changes). Severe valvular disease, however, is considered a major clinical predictor.

Routine laboratory tests, such as ECG, chest radiography, electrolytes, BUN and creatinine, and complete blood counts may also have some predictive value. However, normal ECGs may be present in up to 50% of patients with CAD. The most common ECG findings in patients with CAD are ST-T wave abnormalities (65–90%), LV hypertrophy (10–20%), and pathologic Q waves (0.5–8%).

It is generally agreed that patients with a "combined" risk of PCE (based upon patient and surgical factors) of greater than 10% warrant further study. The noncardiac surgical procedures associated with the highest PCE rate are mostly vascular surgical procedures. Peripheral vascular and aortic surgeries have high PCE rates, while carotid artery surgery has PCE rates of about 5%. While the data are still emerging, it appears that endovascular repairs have low associated risk. The high PCE rate is usually attributed to the high incidence of CAD in vascular patients (estimated to be as high as 90%), and to the stress imposed on the myocardium by hemodynamic changes.

The metabolic changes induced by surgery, such as increased levels of stress hormones, and increases in platelet adhesiveness, are also implicated as factors that increase PCE. Nonvascular surgical procedures associated with higher morbidity and mortality include intrathoracic and intra-abdominal surgery. Presumably, the increased risks are because of the greater hemodynamic changes associated with large fluid shifts, and compression of the great veins, as well as aberrations in cardiopulmonary function during thoracic surgery. Emergency surgery is also associated with increased risk. Procedures associated with a lower risk of PCE include extremity surgery, transurethral prostate resections, and cataract surgery. Therefore, the risk of surgery must always be included in the estimation of patient risk, and this is constantly changing due to the emergence of less invasive techniques that cause less physiologic disturbance.

Thus, the assignment of "cardiac risk" to a particular patient for a particular surgical procedure is difficult, but there are guidelines that should be followed. Further evaluation should depend on whether the information gained would change the planned surgical or anesthetic management. These changes in management might include altering the surgical procedure to one associated with lower risk, medical or surgical treatment of CAD, perioperative anticoagulation, or perhaps more aggressive intraoperative and postoperative monitoring. Although many of these strategies sound logical, there is relatively weak evidence of outcome improvements with interventions. Interventions that are probably effective in reducing PCE include β-adrenergic blockade and prevention of hypothermia.

The use of myocardial revascularization by percutaneous coronary angioplasty/stent placement or coronary artery bypass grafting prior to elective noncardiac surgery for PCE risk reduction is a very controversial subject. If myocardial revascularization is considered appropriate from a cardiovascular disease management perspective then it may be beneficial, but the risks associated with the "preoperative" myocardial revascularization must be added to those associated with the planned noncardiac surgery. In many cases, the combined risk may be prohibitive. There is also emerging evidence that surgery in the early period following coronary artery stent placement is extremely risky (see below).

Predictors of Perioperative Cardiac Events (PCE)

Major
> Unstable angina
> Myocardial infarction within 7–30 days
> Uncompensated congestive heart failure
> Dysrhythmias
>> Symptomatic ventricular dysrhythmias in the presence of underlying heart disease
>> Supraventricular dysrhythmias with uncontrolled ventricular rate
>> High degree of atrioventricular block
> Severe valvular disease

Intermediate
> Chronic stable angina
> Prior myocardial infarction by history
> Q waves on electrocardiogram
> Compensated or prior congestive heart failure
> Diabetes mellitus
> Renal insufficiency

Minor
> Abnormal electrocardiogram
>> Left ventricular hypertrophy
>> Left bundle branch block
>> ST-T wave abnormalities
> Rhythm other than sinus (e.g., atrial fibrillation)
> Advanced age
> History of stroke
> Arterial hypertension (uncontrolled)
> Low functional capacity

Surgical Risk for PCE

High
   Intrathoracic
   Intra-abdominal
   Emergency
   Peripheral vascular
   Aortic

Low
   Extremity
   Transurethral prostate resections
   Cataract
   Carotid
   Endovascular

2. What is the cardiac risk in this patient? What additional investigations should be performed?

This patient is an elderly woman with known CAD, and a recent MI who is going for emergency surgery. There are several important factors that require consideration. The first of these is the post-MI course. If she has recurrent pain, CHF, or late ventricular dysrhythmias (>48 hours post-MI) she has a 15–30% risk of death or re-infarction in her first post-infarct year even without surgery.

Another issue is whether there was evidence of reperfusion following thrombolytic therapy. This would include pain relief, reperfusion dysrhythmias, large increases in creatine phosphokinase (CPK) enzyme levels, and an improvement in the ECG without evidence of MI. Anticoagulant therapy is of importance. Heparin therapy used for patients with recurrent chest pain would have to be stopped prior to surgery. Recent studies suggest that the timing may be very important. Patients whose heparin was stopped for more than 9.5 hours were more likely to develop recurrent ischemia requiring urgent intervention.

The majority of patients who have received thrombolytic therapy have significant residual stenosis in vessels that have been reperfused, and they are often investigated with early cardiac catheterization, especially if they had a complicated infarction. Some centers treat patients who are doing well as they do any patient with a recent uncomplicated infarct, that is they perform a modified symptom-limited stress test prior to discharge (on post-MI day 5–7), and a symptom-limited stress test 6 weeks later.

The presence of sepsis is an important issue. The hemodynamic changes associated with sepsis may significantly stress the myocardium. These include an increased cardiac output because of endotoxin-induced vasodilation, and myocardial depression from myocardial depressant factor.

If the patient must have an urgent surgical procedure and no additional cardiac studies have been performed (e.g., stress test or angiogram), one should assume the patient has significant CAD. If time permits, a transthoracic echocardiogram (TEE), specifically assessing wall motion, LV ejection fraction, and mitral valve function would provide useful information.

3. What are the implications for anesthetic management when coronary revascularization is performed before noncardiac surgery?

The ACC/AHA Guidelines for Perioperative Cardiovascular Evaluation for Noncardiac Surgery provide a stepwise algorithm for the preoperative assessment of the patient with an increased risk for PCE. According to these recommendations, patients with coronary revascularization within the last 5 years without significant change in symptoms or a favorable cardiac evaluation within the last 2 years may proceed for surgery without further testing. An increasing number of patients are presenting for noncardiac surgery with prior percutaneous coronary artery stenting (new drug-eluting stents have recently been introduced), and more patients are taking a combination of anticoagulant and antiplatelet medications, all of which may influence anesthetic management.

Recent data on coronary artery interventional therapy shows an increased incidence of PCE in patients with prior percutaneous coronary myocardial revascularization. A retrospective study by Posner et al. (1999) looked for adverse cardiac outcomes after noncardiac surgery among 686 patients with prior percutaneous transluminal coronary angioplasty (PTCA). Patients with prior PTCA had twice the rate of adverse cardiac outcomes compared with normal subjects, 7 times the rate of angina, almost 4 times the rate of MI, and twice the rate of CHF. Patients who underwent PTCA within 90 days of noncardiac surgery had twice the rate of perioperative MI compared with patients with uncorrected CAD. Kaluza et al. (2000) found a high number of MIs, major bleeding episodes, and fatal events in patients who underwent coronary stent placement less than 2 weeks before noncardiac surgery. Wilson et al. (2003) reviewed a larger cohort at the Mayo Clinic and found that the period of increased risk extended to 6 weeks following stent placement. It is unclear at present, but drug-eluting stents may extend the period of risk even longer by virtue of their inhibition of neointimal formation.

Antiplatelet drugs that prevent thrombosis of the newly stented coronary arteries, such as GPIIb/IIIa receptor antagonists and ADP inhibitors, have profound anticoagulative properties, and recommendations about when these drugs should be discontinued prior to neuraxial anesthesia have been created and periodically updated by the American Society of Regional Anesthesia and Pain Medicine (http://www.asra.com). In emergency procedures, these patients demonstrate increased risk of perioperative bleeding and platelet transfusions may be necessary to achieve hemostasis. When these antiplatelet regimens are discontinued for elective surgery shortly after coronary interventions, the risk of stent thrombosis is probably increased, especially in the setting of the hypercoagulable state that frequently is present in the postoperative period.

In summary, recently published data suggest an increased risk for patients presenting for noncardiac surgery who have undergone percutaneous coronary interventions with stent placement within the 2 months prior to surgery. While the data are preliminary, elective surgery should be undertaken with caution and attention should be paid to the management of anticoagulation in the perioperative period.

4. What intraoperative monitors would you use?

A general goal in these patients is to maintain intraoperative hemodynamics within 20% of preoperative values. Therefore, in addition to the standard intraoperative monitors, other monitors that should be considered include an intra-arterial line, a pulmonary artery catheter (PAC), and a TEE. An intra-arterial line would be the optimum way of monitoring blood pressure (BP) beat-to-beat. Although 40% of intraoperative ischemic episodes are not related to aberrations in hemodynamics, there are studies demonstrating that inadequate management of hemodynamic abnormalities may increase risk. Hypotension (BP <30% baseline for greater than 10 minutes) has been shown to be a strong predictor of PCE in one study. On the other hand, there are no studies demonstrating conclusively that hypertension is associated with adverse outcome. Tachycardia has not been definitely shown to be associated with PCE, although studies suggest a relationship.

The easiest technique for myocardial ischemia monitoring in the anesthetized patient is with a multiple-lead ECG. Monitoring precordial chest leads V_4 and V_5 detects greater than 90% of ischemic events that would be seen on a 12-lead ECG, but it has been reported to have as low as a 9% sensitivity compared with the gold standard (myocardial lactate extraction). ST-segment depressions and T-wave morphology changes are most commonly seen. However, there are patients in whom the ECG is not an effective intraoperative monitor of myocardial ischemia, such as those with LV hypertrophy, conduction abnormalities, and ventricular pacemaker dependence.

The development of V waves on the pulmonary artery wedge pressure waveform may be an indication of myocardial ischemia, but it is not sensitive or specific enough to be regarded as a reliable monitor for this purpose (Figure 3.1).

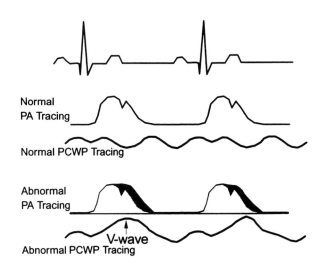

FIGURE 3.1 The relationship between the ECG, pulmonary artery (PA) waveform, and pulmonary capillary wedge pressure (PCWP) waveform is illustrated in the normal situation and in the presence of V waves. Note the widening of the pulmonary artery waveform and the loss of the dicrotic notch in the presence of V waves. Also note that the peak of the V wave occurs about the same time as the T wave on the ECG.

The utility of the PAC, however, extends beyond its questionable ability to detect ischemia. It provides information about the patient's intravascular volume status, a quantitative estimate of myocardial compliance, and allows for calculation of cardiac output and other hemodynamic measurements, such as systemic vascular resistance and stroke volume. A PAC would be mandatory if this patient showed signs of CHF preoperatively.

The TEE is the most sensitive detector of intraoperative ischemia, and it is capable of detecting ischemia earlier than any other modality. However, studies have questioned its specificity. Specifically, it is not clear what TEE changes are predictive of ischemia and PCE. In the largest study of patients with or at-risk for CAD who were scheduled for noncardiac surgery, Mangano and Goldman (1995) did not find that LV wall motion abnormalities were predictive of ischemia or PCE. The TEE also provides physiologic information, such as estimates of LV ejection fraction and intravascular volume status, which may help with intraoperative management in patients with ventricular dysfunction.

5. What additional drugs would you have prepared?

Intravenous nitroglycerin, esmolol, and vasopressors should be immediately available to treat ischemia and hemodynamic aberrations. Phenylephrine is particularly useful in restoring myocardial blood flow in hypotensive

Monitoring

Electrocardiogram
  Multiple lead (V_4, V_5)
    ST segment depression
    T-wave morphology changes

Intra-arterial line
  Beat-to-beat blood pressure

Pulmonary artery catheter
  V wave on pulmonary capillary wedge pressure
    tracing
    Nonspecific, nonsensitive
  Intravascular volume status
  Quantitative estimate of myocardial
    compliance
  Calculation of hemodynamic parameters

Transesophageal echocardiography
  Left ventricular wall motion changes
  Calculate left ventricular ejection fraction
  Intravascular volume status

patients without causing major increases in myocardial oxygen consumption due to tachycardia.

6. What anesthetic technique would you use?

The anesthetic technique has not been shown to be a predictor of PCE. Thus, the anesthetic technique used should be based on the patient assessment and the best technique for maintaining stable intraoperative hemodynamics and adequate postoperative analgesia. There is no definitive evidence that one anesthetic technique is safer than another. Tachycardia should be avoided in patients with CAD, thus, agents such as ketamine and pancuronium are probably best avoided. There is some preliminary evidence that epidural analgesia in the postoperative period is associated with a lower incidence of PCE.

7. How would you manage this patient postoperatively?

Ideally, the patient should be monitored in an intensive care setting postoperatively. Furthermore, the results of the study by Rao et al. (1983) suggest that patients may benefit from a more prolonged stay (at least 3 days) in the intensive care unit with intensive hemodynamic monitoring.

SUGGESTED READINGS

American Society of Regional Anesthesia: recommendations for neuraxial anesthesia and anticoagulation. http://www.asra.com/items_of_interest/consensus_statements/

Eagle KA, Berger PB, Calkins H, et al.: ACC/AHA guideline update for perioperative cardiovascular evaluation for noncardiac surgery – executive summary: a report of the ACC/AHA task force on practice guidelines (Committee to Update the 1996 Guidelines on Perioperative Cardiovascular Evaluation for Noncardiac Surgery). Circulation 105:1257, 2002

Fleisher LA, Barash PG: Preoperative cardiac evaluation for noncardiac surgery: a functional approach. Anesth Analg 74:586, 1992

Goldman L, Caldera DL, Nussbaum SR, et al.: Multifactorial index of cardiac risk in noncardiac surgical procedures. N Engl J Med 297:845, 1978

Kaluza GL, Joseph J, Lee JR, et al.: Catastrophic outcome of noncardiac surgery soon after coronary stenting. J Am Coll Cardiol 35:1288, 2000

Lee TH, Marcantonio RE, Mangione CM, et al.: Derivation and prospective validation of a simple index for prediction of cardiac risk of major noncardiac surgery. Circulation 100:1043, 1999

Mangano DT: Perioperative cardiac morbidity. Anesthesiology 72:153, 1990

Mangano DT, Goldman L: Preoperative assessment of patients with known or suspected coronary disease. N Engl J Med 333:1750, 1995

Park KW, Lee J, Breen P, et al.: The risk of perioperative cardiac complications is high in major vascular surgery performed within a month of coronary artery bypass graft surgery. Anesth Analg 94:S63, 2002

Posner KL, Van Norman GA, Chan V: Adverse outcomes after noncardiac surgery in patients with prior percutaneous transluminal coronary angioplasty. Anesthesiology 89:553, 1999

Rao TLK, Jacobs KH, Eletr AA: Reinfarction following anesthesia in patients with myocardial infarction. Anesthesiology 59:499, 1983

Van Norman GA, Posner K: Coronary stenting or percutaneous transluminal coronary angioplasty prior to noncardiac surgery increases adverse perioperative cardiac events: the evidence is mounting. J Am Coll Cardiol 36:2351, 2000

Vicenzi MN, Ribitsch D, Luha O, et al.: Coronary artery stenting before noncardiac surgery: more threat than safety? Anesthesiology 94:367, 2001

Wilson SH, Fasseas P, Orford JL, et al.: Clinical outcome of patients undergoing non-cardiac surgery in the two months following coronary stenting. J Am Coll Cardiol 42:234, 2003

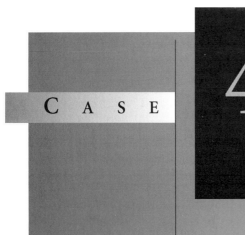

C A S E

4

CONGESTIVE HEART FAILURE

Alexander Mittnacht, MD

David L. Reich, MD

A 55-year-old man with a dilated cardiomyopathy presents for open reduction and internal fixation of a tibial fracture following a motor vehicle accident. The patient has a past medical history of alcohol abuse, orthopnea, dyspnea on exertion, and several episodes of pulmonary edema. The patient's medications include digoxin, furosemide, and captopril. Physical examination revealed bibasilar rales and an S_3 gallop. A gated blood pool scan showed a left ventricular ejection fraction of 15%. Cardiac catheterization indicated a left ventricular end-diastolic pressure of 25 mmHg, a cardiac index of 1.8 L/min/m², 2^+ mitral regurgitation, and no coronary artery disease.

QUESTIONS

1. What are possible etiologies for dilated cardiomyopathy?
2. What is the pathophysiology of dilated cardiomyopathy?
3. How would you monitor this patient during the perioperative period?
4. How would you anesthetize this patient?

1. What are possible etiologies for dilated cardiomyopathy?

Dilated (congestive) cardiomyopathies exist in both inflammatory and non-inflammatory forms. The inflammatory variety, or myocarditis, is usually the result of infection or parasitic infestation. Myocarditis presents with the clinical picture of fatigue, dyspnea, and palpitations usually in the first weeks of the infection, progressing to overt congestive heart failure (CHF) with cardiac dilatation, tachycardia, pulsus alternans (regular alternation of pressure pulse amplitude with a regular rhythm), and pulmonary edema. Complete recovery from infectious myocarditis is usually the case, but there are exceptions such as myocarditis associated with diphtheria or Chagas' disease. The non-inflammatory variety of dilated cardiomyopathy also presents with the picture of myocardial failure, but in this case secondary to idiopathic, toxic, degenerative, or infiltrative processes in the myocardium.

Alcoholic cardiomyopathy is a typical hypokinetic, non-inflammatory cardiomyopathy associated with tachycardia and premature ventricular contractions (PVC) that progresses to left ventricular failure with incompetent mitral and tricuspid valves. This cardiomyopathy is probably due to the direct toxic effect of ethanol or its metabolite, acetaldehyde, which releases and depletes cardiac norepinephrine. In chronic alcoholics, acute ingestion of ethanol produces decreases in contractility, elevations in ventricular end-diastolic pressure, and increases in systemic vascular resistance.

2. What is the pathophysiology of dilated cardiomyopathy?

The dilated cardiomyopathies are characterized by elevated filling pressures, failure of myocardial contractile strength, and a marked inverse relationship between arterial impedance and stroke volume. The dilated cardiomyopathies present a picture very similar to that of CHF produced by severe coronary artery disease (CAD).

The pathophysiologic considerations are familiar ones. As the ventricular muscle weakens, the ventricle dilates in order to take advantage of the increased force of contraction resulting from increasing myocardial fiber length. As the ventricular radius increases, however, ventricular wall tension rises, increasing both the oxygen consumption of the myocardium and the total internal work of the muscle. As the myocardium deteriorates further, the cardiac output

falls, and a compensatory increase in sympathetic activity occurs to maintain organ perfusion and cardiac output.

One feature of the failing myocardium is the loss of its ability to maintain stroke volume in the face of increased arterial impedance to ejection. As left ventricular dysfunction worsens, stroke volume becomes more dependent on arterial impedance (afterload). In the failing ventricle, stroke volume falls almost linearly with increases in afterload. The increased sympathetic outflow that accompanies left ventricular failure initiates a vicious cycle of increased resistance to forward flow, decreased stroke volume and cardiac output, and further sympathetic stimulation in an effort to maintain circulatory homeostasis (Figure 4.1).

There is some degree of mitral regurgitation in severe dilated cardiomyopathies due to stretching of the mitral annulus and distortion of the geometry of the chordae tendineae. The forward stroke volume improves with afterload reduction, even though there is no increase in ejection fraction. This suggests that reduction of mitral regurgitation is the mechanism of the improvement. Afterload reduction also decreases left ventricular filling pressure, which relieves

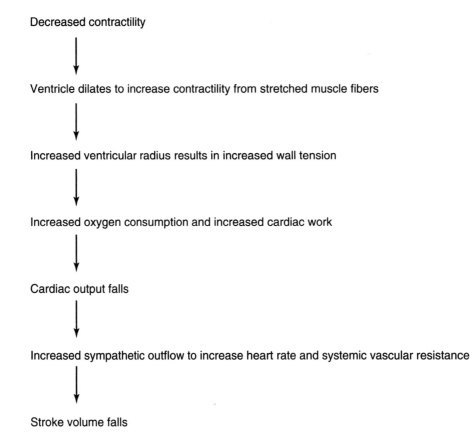

Decreased contractility

↓

Ventricle dilates to increase contractility from stretched muscle fibers

↓

Increased ventricular radius results in increased wall tension

↓

Increased oxygen consumption and increased cardiac work

↓

Cardiac output falls

↓

Increased sympathetic outflow to increase heart rate and systemic vascular resistance

↓

Stroke volume falls

FIGURE 4.1   Pathophysiology of dilated cardiomyopathy.

Manifestations of Ventricular Failure

"Forward": diminished cardiac output and organ
   perfusion
   Fatigue
   Hypotension
   Oliguria
   Activation of renin-angiotensin-aldosterone
      system

"Backward": elevated ventricular filling pressures
   and valvular regurgitation
   Left-sided
      Orthopnea
      Paroxysmal nocturnal dyspnea
      Pulmonary edema
   Right-sided
      Jugular venous distention
      Hepatomegaly
      Peripheral edema

pulmonary congestion and should preserve coronary perfusion pressure.

The clinical picture of the dilated cardiomyopathies falls into the two familiar categories of "forward" failure and "backward" failure. The features of "forward" failure, such as fatigue, hypotension, and oliguria, are due to diminished cardiac output and organ perfusion. Decreased renal perfusion results in activation of the renin-angiotensin-aldosterone system that increases the effective circulating blood volume through sodium and water retention. "Backward" failure is related to the elevated filling pressures required by the failing ventricle(s). As the left ventricle dilates, "secondary" mitral regurgitation occurs due to the mechanisms noted above. The manifestations of left-sided ventricular failure include orthopnea, paroxysmal nocturnal dyspnea, and pulmonary edema. The manifestations of right-sided ventricular failure include hepatomegaly, jugular venous distention, and peripheral edema.

3. How would you monitor this patient during the perioperative period?

Electrocardiographic monitoring is essential in the management of patients with dilated cardiomyopathies, particularly in those with myocarditis. Ventricular dysrhythmias are common, and the development of complete heart block requires rapid diagnosis and treatment. The electrocardiogram (ECG) is also useful for monitoring of ischemic changes when CAD is associated with the cardiomyopathy, as in amyloidosis. Direct intra-arterial blood

pressure monitoring during surgery provides continuous blood pressure information and a convenient route for obtaining arterial blood gases.

Any patient in CHF with a severely compromised myocardium who requires anesthesia and surgery should have central venous access for monitoring and vasoactive drug administration. The use of a pulmonary artery catheter is much more controversial, but is probably of value in patients with severely compromised left ventricular function. While there is no evidenced-based medicine to support outcome differences, left-sided filling pressures should be monitored, if at all possible. Monitoring right-sided filling pressures is of equal importance in patients with pulmonary hypertension or cor pulmonale. In addition to measuring filling pressures, a thermodilution pulmonary artery catheter can be used to obtain cardiac outputs and the calculation of systemic and pulmonary vascular resistances, which allow for serial evaluation of the patient's hemodynamic status. Additionally, there are pulmonary artery catheters with fiberoptic oximetry, and rapid-response thermistor catheters that calculate right ventricular ejection fraction. Pacing catheters and external pacemakers provide distinct advantages in managing the patient with myocarditis and associated heart block.

Two-dimensional transesophageal echocardiography provides useful data on the response of the impaired ventricle to anesthetic and surgical manipulations. The short-axis view of the left ventricle would provide real-time information on preload and ventricular performance that would be valuable in judging the need for inotropic support or vasodilator therapy. The degree of mitral regurgitation could also be followed intraoperatively.

4. How would you anesthetize this patient?

The avoidance of myocardial depression still remains the goal of anesthetic management for patients with dilated cardiomyopathy. All the potent volatile anesthetic agents are myocardial depressants. For this reason, these agents, especially in high concentrations, are probably best avoided in this group of patients. An anesthetic based on a combination of narcotics and sedative-hypnotics (with or without nitrous oxide) can be employed instead. Etomidate and ketamine are acceptable anesthetic induction agents, while thiopental and propofol are relatively contraindicated.

For the patient with a severely compromised myocardium, the synthetic piperidine opioids (fentanyl, sufentanil, remifentanil, and alfentanil) are useful, since myocardial contractility is not depressed. Chest wall rigidity associated with these medications is treated with muscle relaxants. Bradycardia associated with high-dose opioid anesthesia may be prevented by the use of pancuronium for muscle relaxation, anticholinergic drugs, or pacing. For peripheral or lower abdominal surgical procedures, the use of a regional anesthetic technique is a reasonable alternative, provided filling pressures are carefully controlled and the hemodynamic effects of the anesthetic are adequately monitored. Regional techniques may not be possible in many patients due to anticoagulation for associated atrial fibrillation or mural thrombus prevention.

In planning the anesthetic management of the patient with dilated cardiomyopathy, associated cardiovascular conditions, such as the presence of CAD, valvular abnormalities, outflow tract obstruction, and constrictive pericarditis, should also be considered. Patients with CHF often require circulatory support intra- and postoperatively. Inotropic drugs, such as dopamine or dobutamine, have been shown to be effective in low-output states, and produce modest changes in systemic vascular resistance at lower dosages. In severe failure, more potent drugs, such as epinephrine, may be required. The effects of β-adrenergic agents are limited, however, by the downregulation of β-adrenergic receptors that occurs in chronic CHF. Milrinone is a phosphodiesterase III inhibitor with inotropic and vasodilator properties that may improve hemodynamic performance. As noted above, stroke volume is inversely related to afterload in the failing ventricle, and reducing left ventricular afterload with vasodilating drugs, such as nitroprusside and milrinone, is also effective in increasing cardiac output. In patients with myocarditis, especially of the viral variety, transvenous or external pacing may be required should heart block occur. Intra-aortic balloon counterpulsation and left ventricular assist devices are further options to be considered in the case of the severely compromised ventricle.

There is a definite increase in the incidence of supraventricular and ventricular dysrhythmias in myocarditis and the dilated cardiomyopathies. These dysrhythmias often require extensive electrophysiologic investigation, and may be unresponsive to maximal medical therapy.

Anesthetic Management

Induction
  Etomidate or ketamine

Maintenance
  Opioids: fentanyl, sufentanil, alfentanil
  Sedative-hypnotics
  +/– Nitrous oxide

Monitoring
  Electrocardiogram for dysrhythmias
  Arterial line
  Pulmonary artery catheter
  Transesophageal echocardiography

Dysrhythmia management
  Esmolol
  Amiodarone
  Cardioversion
  Transvenous/external pacing

Inotropic support
  Dopamine
  Dobutamine
  Milrinone
  Epinephrine

Vasodilators
  Milrinone
  Nitroprusside

TABLE 4.1	Hemodynamic Goals in Congestive Heart Failure

Parameter	Goal	Indicated	Contraindicated
Heart rate	Normal to elevated	Dopamine Dobutamine	β-Adrenergic blockers (high doses)
Preload	Normal to high	Intravenous fluids	Nitroglycerin Thiopental
Afterload	Low	Angiotensin converting enzyme inhibitors Nitroprusside Milrinone	Phenylephrine
Contractility	Increased	Dopamine Dobutamine Epinephrine Milrinone	High-dose volatile anesthetics High-dose β-adrenergic blockers

Implantable cardioverter-defibrillators are often implanted in these patients, and must be turned off during surgery requiring electrocautery. Thus, proper ECG monitoring and access to a charged external cardioversion device are crucial in the management of these patients. Amiodarone is a long-acting antidysrhythmic medication with intrinsic myocardial depressant properties. Nevertheless, amiodarone seems to have an overall beneficial effect in patients with CHF, especially those who present with chronic atrial fibrillation. Furthermore, amiodarone is currently the antiarrhythmic medication of choice in persistent ventricular tachycardia/ventricular fibrillation, which may be encountered at any time in patients with severely impaired myocardial function (Table 4.1)

SUGGESTED READINGS

Ammar T, Reich DL, Kaplan JA: Uncommon cardiac diseases. pp. 70–122. In Katz J, Benumof J, Kadis L. (eds): Anesthesia and Uncommon Diseases, 4th edition. Philadelphia, WB Saunders, 1998

Cohen MC, Pierce ET, Bode RH, et al.: Types of anesthesia and cardiovascular outcomes in patients with congestive heart failure undergoing vascular surgery. Congest Heart Fail 5:248, 1999

Lake CL: Chronic treatment of congestive heart failure. p 131. In Kaplan JA, Konstadt S, Reich DL (eds): Cardiac Anesthesia, 4th edition. WB Saunders, Philadelphia, 1999

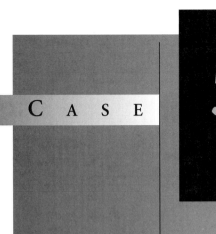

CASE 5

AORTIC STENOSIS

Alexander Mittnacht, MD
David L. Reich, MD

A 65-year-old woman presents for aortic valve replacement. The patient had an episode of congestive heart failure, which led to a recent hospital admission. A cardiac catheterization at that time showed a peak systolic gradient of 90 mmHg between the left ventricle and the aorta. During anesthetic induction with fentanyl and vecuronium, the patient develops a junctional rhythm and severe hypotension.

QUESTIONS

1. What are the symptoms and long-term prognosis of aortic stenosis?
2. What is the etiology of aortic stenosis?
3. How is the aortic valve area calculated?
4. Why is it important to maintain sinus rhythm?
5. What is the treatment for supraventricular tachy-dysrhythmias or bradydysrhythmias?
6. How is hypotension best treated in the patient with aortic stenosis?
7. How would you anesthetize this patient for cardiac or noncardiac surgery?

1. What are the symptoms and long-term prognosis of aortic stenosis?

The classic symptoms in patients with severe aortic stenosis (AS) are angina, syncope and congestive heart failure (CHF). Life expectancy in untreated cases is approximately 5 years after developing angina, 3 years after developing syncope, and 2 years after developing CHF. Angina is the initial symptom in 50–70% of patients, but only about 25–50% have coronary artery disease (CAD). Patients without CAD develop angina because of inadequate oxygen delivery to a hypertrophied myocardium.

Concentric hypertrophy occurs in AS as the left ventricular wall thickness increases in a symmetrical fashion. The advantage of the hypertrophied myocardium is that greater intraventricular pressures may be generated with lower wall tension. The relationship between intra-cavitary pressure (P), wall tension (T), left ventricular radius (R), and wall thickness (h) is described by the Law of Laplace:

$$T = P \times R/2h$$

Tension generation in the myocytes is the most inefficient way of performing cardiac work because it requires large amounts of oxygen. In addition, oxygen delivery is decreased because of the lower coronary perfusion pressure (CPP):

$$CPP = \text{diastolic aortic pressure} - \text{left ventricular end-diastolic pressure}$$

As the AS becomes more severe, a decrease in the diastolic aortic pressure compromises the CPP even more. The hypertrophied myocardium also results in decreased left ventricular compliance and higher left ventricular filling pressures. The neovascularization of the pressure-overloaded heart has also been shown to be inadequate for the degree of hypertrophy. Finally, the isovolumic phase of relaxation is inappropriately long, shortening diastole, and leaving less time for coronary perfusion. For all these reasons, patients with AS are prone to developing myocardial ischemia during anesthesia.

Syncope is the initial symptom of AS in 15–30% of patients. It is usually exertional, and is caused by exercise-induced vasodilation in the face of a fixed cardiac output. CHF portends the worst long-term prognosis. At this time, the heart has exceeded its ability to compensate for pressure work with myocardial hypertrophy. The heart then progressively dilates, and symptoms of left ventricular failure appear.

2. What is the etiology of aortic stenosis?

AS may be congenital or acquired. In adults, a congenitally bicuspid valve may become calcified and stenotic. Senile calcification of a tri-leaflet aortic valve is common in patients over 70 years of age. Rheumatic AS is almost always associated with rheumatic mitral valve disease. This etiology is becoming less common in developed countries because of the widespread use of antibiotic therapy.

3. How is the aortic valve area calculated?

The normal valve area is 2.5–3.5 cm^2 and a valve area less than 0.75 cm^2 is considered to be severe AS. In the cardiac catheterization laboratory, the aortic valve area is calculated using the Gorlin formula. The simplified version states that the valve area is proportional to the flow across the valve divided by the square root of the mean pressure gradient.

Knowing the pressure gradient in the absence of the cardiac output (flow) is not a reliable indicator of the severity of aortic disease. For example, a patient with extremely severe AS but with a very low cardiac output, would have a small measured transvalvular gradient because of the diminished flow across the valve. However, in most patients one can assume that a mean pressure gradient >50 mmHg or a peak pressure gradient >80 mmHg implies severe stenosis.

4. Why is it important to maintain sinus rhythm?

Atrial systole normally contributes about 15–20% to stroke volume. In AS, this increases to 40–50%. The atrial "kick" is crucial in preserving left ventricular filling (and stroke volume) since passive filling is decreased because of the noncompliant left ventricle. The onset of a non-sinus rhythm is often associated with marked hypotension because of the decrease in stroke volume. It is difficult for the patient with AS to compensate for the loss of sinus rhythm because marked increases in left atrial pressure would be required to maintain an adequate stroke volume.

5. What is the treatment for supraventricular tachydysrhythmias or bradydysrhythmias?

The treatment of dysrhythmias in patients with AS must be accomplished rapidly to prevent hemodynamic decompensation. Cardioversion should be considered as the first-line therapy in the unstable patient with supraventricular tachydysrhythmias. In the stable patient, a therapeutic diagnostic maneuver (vagal stimulation, adenosine) should be attempted. When the exact underlying rhythm is identified, treatment usually consists of β-adrenergic blockers (e.g., esmolol), amiodarone, or cardioversion depending upon the rhythm. In the patient with impaired cardiac function (ejection fraction < 40%, CHF), or when ventricular tachycardia cannot be ruled out, amiodarone is the preferred drug.

Bradydysrhythmias should be treated with anticholinergics, combined α- and β-adrenergic agonists, or atrioventricular sequential pacing. The ideal heart rate is probably between 70 and 80 beats per minute. This allows for adequate diastolic filling while providing sufficient cardiac output in a heart with a relatively fixed stroke volume.

6. How is hypotension best treated in the patient with aortic stenosis?

Patients with severe AS do not tolerate hypotension, and even brief episodes may lead to hemodynamic decompensation. The determinants of cardiac output are preload, afterload, heart rate, and contractility (Table 5.1). The priorities of treatment should be the following:

- preservation of blood pressure using vasoconstrictors to increase afterload
- restoration of sinus rhythm and intravenous fluids to maintain preload

Treatment of Supraventricular Dysrhythmias

Tachydysrhythmias
    Therapeutic diagnostic maneuvers
        Vagal maneuvers
        Adenosine
    Treatment
        β-Adrenergic blockers
        Amiodarone
        Cardioversion

Bradydysrhythmias
    Anticholinergics
    α- and β-adrenergic agonists
    Atrioventricular sequential pacing

- maintaining a heart rate in the normal range
- maintenance of myocardial contractility

If the etiology is not immediately obvious, then empiric treatment with an α-adrenergic receptor agonist (phenylephrine) should be attempted. The goal is to preserve CPP so that the heart does not enter a vicious cycle of irreversible ischemia. In general, pure α-adrenergic receptor agonists are the preferred vasoconstrictor agents because they do not cause tachycardia. In this way, the CPP is increased and diastolic filling time is maintained

7. How would you anesthetize this patient for cardiac or noncardiac surgery?

Premedication in patients with AS has to be carefully administered. Oversedation may lead to hypotension and decreased CPP, while undersedation may result in an anxious, tachycardic patient who is prone to myocardial ischemia. Patients with AS are critically sensitive to preload and an appropriate intravascular volume status has to be assured prior to anesthesia induction. Systemic vascular resistance (SVR) must be maintained at all times. Thus, neuraxial anesthesia with the risk of sympatholysis is relatively contraindicated in patients with AS. Dysrhythmias are poorly tolerated, making maintenance of a sinus rhythm imperative. A defibrillator should be readily available in the operating room.

Perioperative monitoring should be according to the recommendations of the American Society of Anesthesiologists. Patients with AS are at increased risk for ischemia and dysrhythmias and monitoring should include leads II and V_5. The sensitivity of this lead combination for detecting myocardial ischemia is approximately 80%. A pulmonary artery catheter is routinely used to estimate left-sided filling pressures in some centers, but this remains controversial.

The main goals for inducing anesthesia in patients with AS are to avoid major alterations in preload, afterload, heart rate, and contractility. Thus, etomidate opioids, and midazolam are reasonably good choices, but should be titrated to effect. Vecuronium and cisatracurium are neuromuscular blockers with favorable hemodynamic profiles. Drugs such as ketamine and pancuronium may increase heart rate and should be avoided. Thiopental may cause decreased preload and should probably be avoided. Similarly, propofol is associated with hypotension and should probably be avoided.

Anesthesia can be maintained with many different techniques so long as the preload, afterload, heart rate, and contractility are monitored to avoid adverse hemodynamic responses. Opioids, benzodiazepines, potent volatile anesthetics, and nitrous oxide should all be titrated, paying careful attention to maintaining perfusion pressure. Tachycardia, bradycardia, and loss of sinus rhythm are all problematic. Stroke volume across the stenotic aortic valve is relatively fixed and is lower than normal; thus, an

---

TABLE 5.1   **Hemodynamic Goals in Aortic Stenosis**

Parameter	Goal	Indicated	Contraindicated
Heart rate	Normal to slow sinus rhythm	Atrioventricular sequential pacing	Potent volatile agents (in high doses)
Preload	Normal to high	Intravenous fluids	Nitroglycerin
			Thiopental
Afterload	High	Phenylephrine	Nitroprusside
Contractility	Normal to increased	Dopamine	High-dose β-adrenergic blockers
		Dobutamine	
		Epinephrine	Potent volatile agents (in high doses)

α-agonist, such as phenylephrine, is the agent of choice for treating hypotension.

SUGGESTED READINGS

Kaplan JA, Reich DL, Konstadt SN (eds): Cardiac Anesthesia, 4th edition. WB Saunders, Philadelphia, 1999

Kertai MD, Bountioukos M, Boersma E, et al.: Aortic stenosis: an underestimated risk factor for perioperative complications in patients undergoing noncardiac surgery. Am J Med 116:8, 2004

Torsher LC, Shub C, Rettke SR, Brown DL: Risk of patients with severe aortic stenosis undergoing noncardiac surgery. Am J Cardiol 81:448, 1998

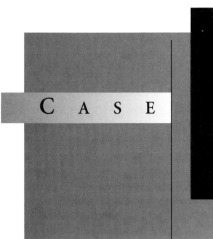

C A S E

6

MITRAL STENOSIS

Alexander Mittnacht, MD

David L. Reich, MD

A 77-year-old, 55-kg woman is admitted to the hospital with severe pulmonary edema and atrial fibrillation with a rapid ventricular response. Cardiac catheterization demonstrates severe mitral stenosis with pulmonary hypertension and tricuspid regurgitation. Mitral valve replacement with tricuspid valve annuloplasty is planned.

QUESTIONS

1. What is the etiology and pathophysiology of mitral stenosis?
2. How should preload, afterload, heart rate, and contractility be managed in a patient with mitral stenosis?
3. How would you optimize this patient's condition preoperatively?
4. What intraoperative monitoring would be appropriate?
5. How would you anesthetize this patient?
6. How should hypotension be treated in a patient with mitral stenosis?
7. What is the treatment for perioperative right ventricular failure?

1. What is the etiology and pathophysiology of mitral stenosis?

Mitral stenosis is frequently rheumatic in origin. In many patients, there is a latency period of 30–40 years between the episode of rheumatic fever and the onset of clinical symptoms. Dyspnea is the most common symptom. The initial presentation is often due to an episode of atrial fibrillation or to an unrelated condition, such as pregnancy, thyrotoxicosis, anemia, or sepsis. Other common symptoms include fatigue, palpitations, or hemoptysis.

In the normal adult, the mitral valve orifice is 4–6 cm². As the orifice narrows, to less than 2 cm², the pressure gradient between the left atrium and left ventricle must increase to maintain adequate flow. The high left atrial pressure causes pulmonary venous congestion, which eventually leads to pulmonary edema, particularly in the presence of tachycardia (Figure 6.1). Tachycardia shortens diastole and diminishes the time available for flow across the mitral valve. This, in turn, impairs left atrial emptying and left ventricular filling. Cardiac output decreases, pulmonary congestion increases, and decompensation ensues. A mitral valve area less than 1.0 cm² is considered critical. The decision to perform valve surgery, however, is usually based on the severity of symptoms (i.e., New York Heart Association Classification).

Although the left ventricle is "protected" from pressure or volume overload, left ventricular contractility may be

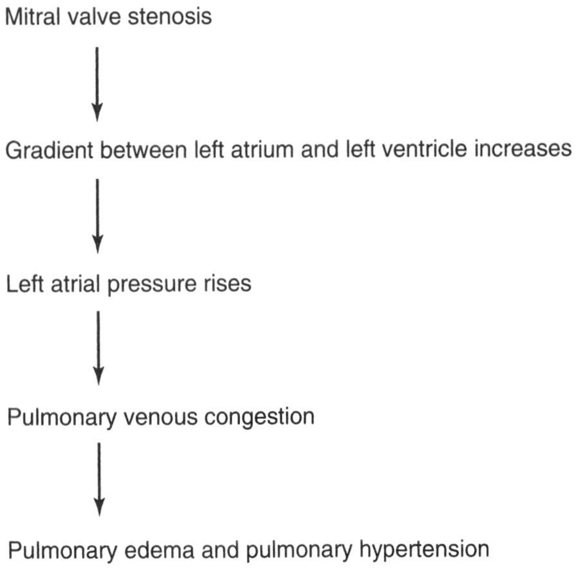

Mitral valve stenosis

↓

Gradient between left atrium and left ventricle increases

↓

Left atrial pressure rises

↓

Pulmonary venous congestion

↓

Pulmonary edema and pulmonary hypertension

FIGURE 6.1   Pathophysiology of mitral stenosis.

impaired by rheumatic involvement of the papillary muscles and mitral annulus. Left ventricular function might also be impaired by a shift of the interventricular septum due to right ventricular (RV) pressure overload. Pulmonary hypertension and RV failure are often observed in mitral stenosis.

2. How should preload, afterload, heart rate, and contractility be managed in a patient with mitral stenosis?

It is useful to consider the goals for preload, afterload, heart rate, and contractility as the major principles guiding intraoperative management in patients with mitral stenosis.

Left atrial pressure should remain high to maintain preload. Thus, hypovolemia and venodilating drugs should be avoided. Afterload (systemic vascular resistance) should be kept high to maintain perfusion pressure in the face of a relatively fixed cardiac output. Heart rate should be kept slow to maximize diastolic filling of the left ventricle. Contractility should not be diminished because the cardiac output is already low in these patients. The hemodynamic goals in mitral stenosis are summarized in Table 6.1.

3. How would you optimize this patient's condition preoperatively?

Before surgery, it is essential to optimize the physical condition in patients with mitral stenosis. The ventricular rate must be slow and, when atrial fibrillation is present, it should be controlled with drugs such as cardiac glycosides or β-adrenergic blockers. These drugs are continued until the time of surgery. Hypokalemia from diuretics is corrected to prevent digitalis toxicity and dysrhythmias. Although these patients are unusually sensitive to narcotics and central nervous system depressants, an adequate anesthetic premedication is important to prevent anxiety-induced tachycardia. Supplemental oxygen is indicated in transit to the operating room.

4. What intraoperative monitoring would be appropriate?

An intra-arterial catheter and pulmonary artery catheter (PAC) are clearly indicated in this patient and should be placed before the induction of anesthesia. The benefits of a PAC include the ability to gather information on left atrial filling pressure, pulmonary artery pressure, cardiac output, and pulmonary and systemic vascular resistances. Knowledge of pulmonary artery pressures is

TABLE 6.1   **Hemodynamic Goals in Mitral Stenosis**

Parameter	Goal	Indicated	Contraindicated
Heart rate	Slow	β-Adrenergic blockers Digoxin	Dopamine Dobutamine Ketamine Pancuronium
Preload	High	Intravenous fluids	Nitroglycerin Thiopental
Afterload	High	Phenylephrine	Angiotensin-converting enzyme inhibitors (except for RV failure) Nitroprusside
Contractility	Normal to increased	Norepinephrine	High-dose volatile anesthetics High-dose β-adrenergic blockers

particularly important in the presence of RV dysfunction because successful therapy includes manipulations of RV afterload.

Transesophageal echocardiography (TEE) also provides the opportunity to observe biventricular function, left atrial dimensions, and valvular function. TEE offers information on left ventricular filling, left ventricular contractility, RV function, interventricular septal shift and, following cardiopulmonary bypass, on the function of the repaired valve or the prosthetic valve.

5. How would you anesthetize this patient?

Phenylpiperidine opioids (fentanyl, sufentanil, remifentanil and alfentanil), benzodiazepines, and etomidate are all reasonable choices for anesthetic induction in patients with mitral stenosis (Table 6.2). Opioids also have the advantage of increasing vagal tone and slowing the heart rate, usually without associated hypotension. Short-acting barbiturates produce undesirable venodilation and myocardial depression. Ketamine is contraindicated on the basis of its tachycardic effects. Volatile agents produce both myocardial depression and vasodilation and should be used cautiously in low concentrations.

Theoretically, the most suitable neuromuscular blocking agents for mitral stenosis are succinylcholine, vecuronium, rocuronium and cisatracurium. For long cardiothoracic procedures continuous intravenous infusions are a good choice to maintain an adequate level of neuromuscular blockade, which decreases oxygen consumption during cardiopulmonary bypass. Pancuronium is relatively contraindicated since it produces tachycardia.

6. How should hypotension be treated in a patient with mitral stenosis?

Hypotension is best treated with an α-adrenergic agonist such as phenylephrine, which would increase arterial pressure and decrease heart rate via baroreceptor-mediated reflexes. Vasoconstriction is necessary in this case, because it is essential to preserve vital organ perfusion in the face of a fixed low cardiac output. β-Adrenergic agonists cause tachycardia and vasodilation, which are undesirable effects in mitral stenosis patients. Thus, ephedrine, dopamine, dobutamine, and epinephrine are relatively contraindicated before valvular repair.

7. What is the treatment for perioperative right ventricular failure?

Following mitral valve replacement, weaning from cardiopulmonary bypass is sometimes complicated by pulmonary hypertension and RV failure. Monitoring of the left atrial pressure is helpful in calculating the pulmonary

TABLE 6.2	Mitral Stenosis and Anesthesia	
Category	**Recommended**	**Not recommended**
Induction agents	Etomidate	Thiopental
	Opioids	Ketamine
	Benzodiazepines	
Maintenance agents	Opioids	Potent inhalation agents in high concentrations
Muscle relaxants	Succinylcholine	Pancuronium
	Vecuronium	
	Rocuronium	
	Cisatracurium	
Hypotension	Phenylephrine	β-Adrenergic agonists
		Ephedrine
		Epinephrine
		Dopamine
		Dobutamine
Right ventricular failure	Reverse pulmonary vasoconstriction: correct hypoxia, hypercarbia, acidosis, hypothermia	
	Dilate pulmonary vasculature: nitroglycerin, prostaglandin E_1, inhaled nitric oxide, inhaled prostacyclin (iloprost)	

vascular resistance, because a gradient is often present between the pulmonary capillary wedge and left atrial pressures. Factors that predispose to pulmonary vaso-constriction (e.g., hypoxia, hypercarbia, acidosis, and hypothermia) should be corrected.

The main goals in the anesthetic management of RV failure are to reduce RV afterload, optimize RV preload, maintain RV coronary perfusion, and support RV contractility. In the presence of pre-existing pulmonary hypertension and increased pulmonary vascular resistance, RV failure will respond favorably to pulmonary vasodilatation. Drugs with pulmonary vasodilating activity that are used after termination of cardiopulmonary bypass include nitroprusside, nitroglycerin, and prostaglandin E_1. However, none of these medications is selective for the pulmonary circulation and their use may be limited due to their systemic effects. Milrinone, a phosphodiesterase III inhibitor, increases RV contractility and has pulmonary vasodilating properties. This pharmacologic profile makes phosphodiesterase III inhibitors particularly appealing in the treatment of RV failure. Inhaled aerosolized milrinone is an experimental therapy that may be used for selective pulmonary vaso-dilatation if preliminary studies prove its effectiveness.

Inhaled nitric oxide (NO) is an established therapy for pulmonary hypertension and RV failure following mitral valve surgery. NO is an endothelium-derived vasodilator and when inhaled selectively causes pulmonary vascular relaxation. Prostacyclin acts via specific prostaglandin receptors and has also been shown to reduce pulmonary hypertension after cardiac surgery. However, the vasodilation is not selective for the pulmonary vasculature and systemic hypotension may ensue. Various newer prostacyclin analogs are now given for chronic pulmonary hypertension, and may be useful for intraoperative use in the future.

Vasopressin or norepinephrine is particularly effective for the treatment of systemic hypotension in patients with RV failure. Vasopressin (antidiuretic hormone) is a posterior pituitary hormone that causes dose-dependent vasoconstriction and antidiuretic effects. Epinephrine is the preferred catecholamine in patients with pulmonary hypertension and RV failure when RV contractility is suspected to be severely impaired.

SUGGESTED READINGS

Fischer LG, Van Aken H, Burkle H, et al.: Management of pulmonary hypertension: physiological and pharmacological considerations for anesthesiologists. Anesth Analg 96:1603, 2003

Mahoney PD, Loh E, Blitz LR, Herrmann HC: Hemodynamic effects of inhaled nitric oxide in women with mitral stenosis and pulmonary hypertension. Am J Cardiol 87:188, 2001

Steudel W, Hurford WE, Zapol WM: Inhaled nitric oxide. Basic biology and clinical applications. Anesthesiology 91:1090, 1999

7

EISENMENGER SYNDROME (SUBACUTE BACTERIAL ENDOCARDITIS PROPHYLAXIS)

Alexander Mittnacht, MD

David L. Reich, MD

A 25-year-old woman with an uncorrected ventricular septal defect presents for extraction of multiple impacted molar teeth. She has a history of palpitations, cyanosis since 5 years of age, and limited exercise tolerance. Her oxygen saturation on room air measured by pulse oximetry is 75%.

QUESTIONS

1. What are the anesthetic considerations for a patient with Eisenmenger syndrome?
2. What is the association between bacterial endocarditis and structural heart disease?
3. Which patients should receive endocarditis prophylaxis?
4. What are the most likely pathogens involved in subacute bacterial endocarditis, and what are the antibiotics of choice for its treatment?

1. What are the anesthetic considerations for a patient with Eisenmenger syndrome?

Eisenmenger syndrome occurs in patients with congenital heart disease (CHD) who have had prolonged shunting of blood to the lungs with excessive pulmonary blood flow and pressure. It occurs after several years in patients who have uncorrected cardiac lesions, such as atrial septal defects, ventricular septal defects, or patent ductus arteriosus, with pulmonary-to-systemic blood flow ratios greater than 2:1 (left-to-right shunting). As irreversible changes occur in the pulmonary vasculature, the pulmonary vascular resistance (PVR) rises to the point where there is reversal of flow across the cardiac defect resulting in cyanosis (right-to-left shunting).

Once right-to-left shunting occurs, the cardiac defect is no longer surgically correctable. In Eisenmenger syndrome, the PVR is so high that an attempted surgical closure of the defect would cause the right ventricle to fail due to the increased impedance to ejection. The only possible surgical treatment is heart-lung transplantation. Untreated Eisenmenger syndrome is associated with a poor long-term prognosis. These patients are at greatly increased risk for any elective procedure. They are usually anesthetized for emergency procedures as well as labor and delivery.

The anesthetic considerations are similar to those in any patient with CHD and right-to-left shunting. These concerns include managing a patient who could decompensate due to increased right-to-left shunting with worsened hypoxemia and/or myocardial dysfunction. Polycythemia is a major preoperative concern in these patients who are at risk of having thrombotic complications, especially if they are dehydrated. Preoperative phlebotomy or autologous blood donation should be considered if the hematocrit is >55–60%. These patients are also at high risk of paradoxical embolization and bacterial endocarditis.

The ratio of pulmonary-to-systemic blood flow depends on the ratio of PVR to systemic vascular resistance (SVR). A decrease in SVR or an increase in PVR will increase right-to-left shunting and increase cyanosis. PVR is increased with low inspired oxygen concentration, acidosis, hypercarbia, hypothermia, high lung inflation pressures or positive end-expiratory pressures, endobronchial intubation, and high catecholamine levels.

The goal is to maintain the baseline PVR:SVR ratio. Preoperatively, the patient should be well hydrated. These patients may receive anesthetic premedication, but do not tolerate respiratory depression well. Supplemental oxygen may be helpful following sedative medications. Monitoring should be tailored to the procedure, but an intra-arterial line is indicated in all but the most minor procedures, such as monitored cases performed under local anesthesia. The indications for a pulmonary artery catheter are controversial. It may be impossible to enter the pulmonary artery, and the placement and maintenance of the pulmonary artery catheter may result in significant morbidity and mortality. A central line can often serve as an indicator of right ventricular function and allows for central administration of medications.

The anesthetic should be designed to minimize myocardial depression and PVR. To avoid enlarging any inadvertent air emboli, it is probably wisest to avoid nitrous oxide. Regional and general anesthetics have been used successfully but require judicious management, invasive monitoring, and appropriate hemodynamic interventions. For prophylaxis against endocarditis, antibiotics must be administered early enough so that therapeutic tissue levels are achieved at the time of skin incision, and postoperative doses must be

---

Factors that Increase Pulmonary Vascular Resistance

Low partial pressure of alveolar oxygen
Acidosis
Hypercarbia
Hypothermia
High inspiratory pressures
Positive end-expiratory pressure
Endobronchial intubation
Elevated catecholamine levels

---

ordered (Tables 7.1, 7.2). Arrangements should be made to closely monitor the patient postoperatively.

2. What is the association between bacterial endocarditis and structural heart disease?

Known structural heart disease is present in only approximately 50% of patients who develop bacterial endocarditis. In patients with known cardiac disease, fewer than 25% present with streptococcal endocarditis of oral origin and only about 40% of patients with enterococcal endocarditis develop endocarditis in association with a procedure for which prophylaxis could have been given. Unfortunately, this implies that even if prophylaxis were always effective, it is impossible to identify the time of exposure in the majority of cases.

TABLE 7.1		Antibiotic Prophylactic Regimen for Dental, Oral, Respiratory Tract, or Esophageal Procedures
Standard regimen:	Adult:	Amoxicillin 2 g po 1 hour pre-procedure (no second dose)
	Children:	Amoxicillin 50 mg/kg po (maximum 2 g) 1 hour pre-procedure
Penicillin-allergic:	Adult:	Clindamycin 600 mg; cephalexin[a] or cefadroxil[a] 2 g; azithromycin 500 mg po 1 hour pre-procedure
	Children:	Clindamycin 10 mg/kg; Cephalexin[a] or Cefadroxil[a] 50 mg/kg; azithromycin 15 mg/kg po 1 hour pre-procedure
Unable to take po:	Adult:	Ampicillin 2 g IV or IM 30 minutes pre-procedure
	Children:	Ampicillin 50 mg/kg IV or IM 30 minutes pre-procedure
Penicillin-allergic and unable to take po:	Adult:	Clindamycin 600 mg IV; cefazolin[a] 1 g IV 30 minutes pre-procedure
	Children:	Clindamycin 10 mg/kg IV; cefazolin[a] 25 mg/kg IV 30 minutes pre-procedure

po, per os; IV, intravenous; IM, intramuscular.
Total dose for children should not exceed adult doses.
[a]Should not be administered if the patient has immediate-type hypersensitivity reaction to penicillin.
(From Dajani AS, Taubert KA, Wilson W, et al.: Prevention of bacterial endocarditis: recommendations by the American Heart Association. Circulation 96:358, 1997.)

TABLE 7.2	Antibiotic Prophylactic Regimen for Genitourinary or Gastrointestinal Procedures

High-Risk Patients

Adult:
Ampicillin 2 g IV or IM 30 minutes pre-procedure
AND
Gentamicin 1.5 mg/kg IV or IM (maximum 120 mg) 30 minutes pre-procedure
THEN
Ampicillin 1 g IV or IM or amoxicillin 1 g po 6 hours later

Children:
Ampicillin 50 mg/kg IV or IM (maximum 2 g) 30 minutes pre-procedure
AND
Gentamicin 1.5 mg/kg IV or IM 30 minutes pre-procedure
THEN
Ampicillin 25 mg/kg IV or IM or amoxicillin 25 mg/kg po 6 hours later

Penicillin-allergic:

Adult:
Vancomycin 1 g IV over 1–2 hours (complete within 30 minutes of procedure)
AND
Gentamicin 1.5 mg/kg IV or IM (maximum 120 mg) 30 minutes pre-procedure

Children:
Vancomycin 20 mg/kg IV over 1–2 hours (complete within 30 minutes of procedure)
AND
Gentamicin 1.5 mg/kg IV or IM 30 minutes pre-procedure

Moderate-Risk Patients

Adult:
Amoxicillin 2 g po 1 hour pre-procedure or ampicillin 2 g IV or IM 30 minutes pre-procedure

Children:
Amoxicillin 50 mg/kg po 1 hour pre-procedure or ampicillin 50 mg/kg IV or IM 30 minutes pre-procedure

Penicillin-allergic:

Adult:
Vancomycin 1 g IV over 1–2 hours (complete within 30 minutes of procedure)

Children:
Vancomycin 20 mg/kg IV over 1–2 hours (complete within 30 minutes of procedure)

po, per os; IV, intravenous; IM, intramuscular.
Total doses for children should not exceed adult doses.
(From Dajani AS, Taubert KA, Wilson W, et al.: Prevention of bacterial endocarditis: recommendations by the American Heart Association. Circulation 96:358, 1997)

3. Which patients should receive endocarditis prophylaxis?

Prophylaxis against endocarditis is recommended for patients with abnormal or prosthetic heart valves, patients with a history of endocarditis, even in the absence of heart disease, surgically constructed systemic-pulmonary shunts, most congenital cardiac malformations, hypertrophic cardiomyopathy, and mitral valve prolapse (MVP) with valvular regurgitation (Tables 7.1, 7.2). Prophylaxis in certain classes of patients is controversial. Some patients with MVP have dynamic regurgitation that disappears with certain maneuvers. Also, echocardiography occasionally detects regurgitation when auscultation does not. Some have recommended that such patients do not require prophylaxis unless they are found to have thickening of mitral valve leaflets and redundancy on echocardiography.

Patients with prosthetic heart valves, a previous history of endocarditis, or surgically constructed shunts are considered to be at high risk for developing endocarditis. Infection in these patients is associated with significant morbidity and mortality. In the past, only parenteral prophylaxis was recommended. Currently, oral prophylaxis regimens are acceptable.

Prophylaxis is not recommended for patients who have had coronary artery bypass surgery, innocent murmurs, previous rheumatic heart disease without valvular disease, cardiac pacemakers, implantable defibrillators, and surgical repair of secundum atrial septal defects, or patent ductus arteriosus ligation.

4. What are the most likely pathogens involved in subacute bacterial endocarditis and what are the antibiotics of choice for its treatment?

The most common organism depends on the site of surgery. α-Hemolytic streptococci are the most common cause of endocarditis following dental procedures. Other procedures around the oropharynx and airway, such as tonsillectomy and rigid bronchoscopy, also expose the patient to the same flora. The recommended antibiotic regimen is outlined in Table 7.1.

Prophylaxis for genitourinary and gastrointestinal procedures is directed against enterococci. The recommended antibiotic regimen is outlined in Table 7.2.

Patients at risk for endocarditis who are scheduled for cardiac surgery should receive prophylaxis against *Staphylococcus aureus*, staphylococcal coagulase-negative microbes, and diphtheroids. A first-generation cephalosporin is most often used; however, the choice must depend on the pathogen's susceptibility pattern at each hospital. To reduce the risk of developing resistant organisms, patients should not be treated for more than 24 hours.

SUGGESTED READINGS

Ammash NM, Connolly HM, Abel MD, et al.: Noncardiac surgery in Eisenmenger syndrome. J Am Coll Cardiol 33:222, 1999

Dajani AS, Taubert KA, Wilson W, et al.: Prevention of bacterial endocarditis: recommendations by the American Heart Association. JAMA 277:1794, 1997

Dajani AS, Taubert KA, Wilson W, et al.: Prevention of bacterial endocarditis: recommendations by the American Heart Association. Circulation 96:358, 1997

Delahaye F, Hoen B, McFadden E, et al.: Treatment and prevention of infective endocarditis. Expert Opin Pharmacother 3:131, 2002

Martin JT, Tautz TJ, Antognini JF: Safety of regional anesthesia in Eisenmenger syndrome. Reg Anesth Pain Med 27:509, 2002

Pollack KL, Chestnut DH, Wenstrom KD: Anesthetic management of a parturient with Eisenmenger syndrome. Anesth Analg 70:212, 1990

Raines DE, Liberthson RR, Murray JR: Anesthetic management and outcome following noncardiac surgery in nonparturients with Eisenmenger's physiology. J Clin Anesth 8:341, 1996

8 HYPERTROPHIC OBSTRUCTIVE CARDIOMYOPATHY

Alexander Mittnacht, MD
David L Reich, MD

A 28-year-old woman with hypertrophic obstructive cardiomyopathy (HOCM) presents for labor and delivery. She is initially managed by the obstetrician with intravenous meperidine, but becomes progressively more uncomfortable. The anesthesiologist is then consulted for further management.

QUESTIONS

1. Describe the anatomic abnormalities in HOCM.
2. What changes in preload, afterload, heart rate, and contractility will optimize hemodynamic performance in a patient with HOCM?
3. What are the treatment options for HOCM?
4. What monitoring would be required in HOCM patients?
5. What considerations should be given in planning the anesthetic management of a patient with HOCM?
6. What are the special considerations for anesthetic management of labor and delivery in a patient with HOCM?

1. Describe the anatomic abnormalities in HOCM.

Hypertrophic cardiomyopathies usually result from asymmetric hypertrophy of the basal ventricular septum, and occur in either obstructive or nonobstructive forms. A dynamic pressure gradient is present in the obstructive forms. Other conditions can also produce the picture of an obstructive cardiomyopathy due to massive infiltration of the ventricular wall, as in Pompe's disease, where a massive accumulation of cardiac glycogen in the ventricular wall produces obstruction to ventricular outflow. The following discussion concentrates on the obstructive form.

HOCM, asymmetric septal hypertrophy (ASH), and idiopathic hypertrophic subaortic stenosis (IHSS), are all terms applied to the same disease process. The main anatomic feature of HOCM is hypertrophied ventricular muscle at the base of the septum in the outflow tract of the left ventricle. Histologically, this is a disorganized mass of hypertrophied myocardial cells extending from the left ventricular septal wall and may involve the papillary muscles. Intramural ("small vessel") coronary artery disease has been identified in autopsy specimens, especially in areas of myocardial fibrosis. This may play some role in the etiology of myocardial ischemia in these patients.

Obstruction to left ventricular outflow is caused by the hypertrophic muscle mass of the interventricular septum and systolic anterior motion (SAM) of the mitral valve's anterior leaflet. It was thought that SAM is caused by a Venturi effect of the rapidly flowing blood in the left ventricular outflow tract (LVOT). Recently, echocardiographic data has revealed that a different mechanism might be the cause of SAM and consequently LVOT obstruction. The hypertrophied ventricular septum causes the mitral valve to be positioned more anteriorly in the left ventricular cavity. This brings the leaflet coaptation point closer to the interventricular septum than normal. Excessive anterior mitral valve tissue in combination with the more anterior position of the mitral valve causes the anterior mitral valve leaflet to protrude into the LVOT. Additionally, the hypertrophied ventricular septum changes blood flow in the LVOT, redirecting it behind and lateral to the enlarged anterior mitral valve leaflet, and thus also pushing it into the septum.

Consequently, a dynamic subaortic pressure gradient is present. The outflow tract obstruction can result in hypertrophy of the remainder of the ventricular muscle, secondary to increased pressures in the ventricular chamber. As the ventricle hypertrophies, ventricular compliance decreases, and passive filling of the ventricle during diastole is limited. Therefore, the ventricle increasingly depends on atrial systole ("kick") to maintain ventricular end-diastolic volume. Furthermore, most patients with HOCM and dynamic LVOT obstruction present with some degree of mitral regurgitation. Occasionally, HOCM is associated with right ventricular outflow tract obstruction as well.

2. What changes in preload, afterload, heart rate, and contractility will optimize hemodynamic performance in a patient with HOCM?

Determinants of the severity of the ventricular obstruction in HOCM are:

- systolic volume of the ventricle
- force of ventricular contraction
- transmural pressure distending the outflow tract

Large systolic volumes in the ventricle distend the outflow tract and reduce the obstruction. Paradoxically, when ventricular contractility is increased, the outflow tract is narrowed, which increases the obstruction and decreases cardiac output. When aortic pressure (afterload) is elevated, there is an increased transmural pressure distending the LVOT during systole and this reduces the degree of obstruction. However, during periods of systemic vasodilation the outflow tract is narrowed. This results in marked decreases in cardiac output and even mitral regurgitation as the mitral valve becomes the relief point for ventricular pressure (Table 8.1).

3. What are the treatment options for HOCM?

Medical therapy of HOCM is based on β-blockers (Table 8.1). Their beneficial effects are likely due to a depression of systolic function and an improvement in diastolic filling and relaxation. However, it is still not clear whether life expectancy is prolonged by this treatment. Amiodarone is a commonly used agent for the control of supraventricular and ventricular dysrhythmias.

Nonmedical treatment options are surgical myotomy/ myomectomy, percutaneous transluminal septal myocardial ablation, alcohol septal ablation, mitral valve replacement/valvuloplasty, or a combination of the former. The potential complications of surgical correction of the LVOT obstruction include complete heart block and late formation of a ventricular septal defect due to septal infarction.

Controlled studies did not confirm earlier reports that atrioventricular sequential (DDD) pacing is beneficial for

TABLE 8.1	Hemodynamic Goals in Hypertrophic Obstructive Cardiomyopathy		
Parameter	**Goal**	**Indicated**	**Contraindicated**
Heart rate	Slow	β-Adrenergic blockers Verapamil	Dopamine Dobutamine Ephedrine
Preload	Normal to high	Intravenous fluids	Nitroglycerin Thiopental
Afterload	High	Phenylephrine	Angiotensin-converting enzyme inhibitors Nitroprusside Milrinone
Contractility	Decreased	Halothane High-dose β-adrenergic blockers	Dopamine Dobutamine Epinephrine Milrinone
Heart rhythm	Normal sinus	Atrial pacing	

patients with HOCM. Dual-chamber pacing can currently be recommended only in selected patients. The reported annual mortality rate is 1–3%, mostly due to ventricular dysrhythmias, sudden death, progressive heart failure, and atrial fibrillation with embolic stroke. There is accumulating evidence that implantable automated defibrillator devices are highly effective in terminating malignant ventricular dysrhythmias in HOCM patients and, thus, decreasing the incidence of sudden death.

4. What monitoring would be required in HOCM patients?

Patients with HOCM may be extremely sensitive to slight changes in ventricular volume, blood pressure, heart rate, and rhythm. Accordingly, monitoring should allow for continuous assessment of these parameters, particularly in patients with severe obstruction. In patients with HOCM coming to surgery for septal myomectomy, the electrocardiogram (ECG), an intra-arterial catheter, and a central venous catheter are necessary. Many anesthetists would also use a pulmonary artery catheter. Two-dimensional transesophageal echocardiography (TEE) provides useful data on ventricular performance, the dynamic mechanism of the LVOT obstruction, and the accompanying mitral regurgitation. After septal myomectomy, TEE provides invaluable information about residual obstruction and mitral regurgitation. It can also be useful for the detection of surgical complications, such as ventricular septal perforation. TEE should certainly be employed if the equipment and trained personnel are available.

In patients with HOCM coming for other procedures, monitoring should provide some indication of ventricular volume, force of ventricular contraction, and transmural pressure distending the outflow tract. Central venous pressure should be an adequate indicator of ventricular volume in procedures that do not result in major volume shifts or alterations in ventricular function. An intra-arterial catheter is almost always indicated for beat-to-beat observation of ventricular ejection during major regional or general anesthesia in patients with symptomatic HOCM. Intraoperative TEE is the most accurate monitor of ventricular loading conditions and performance in HOCM and its use will certainly increase as more centers have the means to employ this type of monitoring.

5. What considerations should be given in planning the anesthetic management of a patient with HOCM?

Anesthetic management of patients with HOCM revolves around alterations in intravascular volume, ventricular contractility, and transmural distending pressure of the outflow tract (see Table 8.1). Blood loss, sympathectomy secondary to spinal or epidural anesthesia,

nitroglycerin, or postural changes can decrease preload. Sympathetic stimulation caused by tracheal intubation or surgical manipulation results in an increase in contractility and tachycardia, both of which may worsen LVOT obstruction. Inotropes, β-adrenergic agonists and calcium are contraindicated for the same reason. Transmural distending pressure can be decreased by hypotension secondary to anesthetic drugs, hypovolemia, or positive-pressure ventilation. Tachycardia is poorly tolerated in patients with HOCM because it decreases systolic ventricular volume thereby narrowing the outflow tract. As noted, atrial contraction is extremely important to filling of the hypertrophied ventricle. Therefore, nodal rhythms should be aggressively treated, using atrial pacing if necessary.

Anesthesia can be induced intravenously or by inhalation of a potent anesthetic agent. Ketamine and pancuronium are best avoided because of their sympathomimetic effects. Halothane is probably the most efficacious choice if a potent volatile agent is used. Halothane decreases heart rate and myocardial contractility, has the least effect on systemic vascular resistance (SVR), and tends to minimize the severity of the obstruction when volume replacement is adequate. Isoflurane and desflurane cause pronounced peripheral vasodilation and therefore are less desirable. Sevoflurane decreases SVR to a lesser extent, and may thus be preferable. Agents that release histamine, such as morphine and d-tubocurarine, are not recommended due to the venodilation and hypovolemia they produce. High-dose opioid anesthesia causes minimal cardiovascular side-effects along with bradycardia, and thus may be a useful anesthetic technique in these patients. Preoperative β-adrenergic blockade or calcium channel blocker therapy should be continued. Intravenous propranolol, metoprolol, esmolol, or verapamil may be administered intraoperatively to improve hemodynamic performance (Table 8.2).

6. What are the special considerations for anesthetic management of labor and delivery in a patient with HOCM?

Anesthesia management for labor and delivery in the parturient with HOCM is quite complex. β-Adrenergic blocker therapy may have been discontinued during pregnancy because of the association with fetal bradycardia and intrauterine growth retardation. Spinal and epidural anesthesia are relatively contraindicated because of the associated vasodilation. If hypotension occurs during anesthesia, the use of β-adrenergic agonists, such as ephedrine, may result in worsening outflow tract obstruction, whereas α-adrenergic agonists, such as phenylephrine, may result in uterine vasoconstriction and fetal asphyxia. The successful management of cesarean section with both general and epidural anesthetics has been reported. However, careful titration of anesthetic agents

TABLE 8.2	Anesthetic Agents and HOCM	

Anesthetic Agent	Advantage	Disadvantage
Halothane	Decreases heart rate Decreases contractility Minimal decrease in SVR	
Sevoflurane		More peripheral vasodilation than halothane but less than isoflurane and desflurane Increases heart rate
Isoflurane		More peripheral vasodilation than halothane Increases heart rate
Desflurane		More peripheral vasodilation than halothane Increases heart rate
Fentanyl	Slows heart rate	
Morphine		Histamine release, predisposing to peripheral vasodilation
Ketamine		Sympathomimetic
Pancuronium		Increases heart rate
d-Tubocurarine		Histamine release, predisposing to peripheral vasodilation

and adequate volume-loading (guided by invasive monitoring) is essential to the safe conduct of anesthesia in this clinical setting.

SUGGESTED READINGS

Ammar T, Reich DL, Kaplan JA: Uncommon cardiac diseases. pp. 70–122. In Katz J, et al. (eds): Anesthesia and Uncommon Diseases, 4th edition. WB Saunders, Philadelphia, 1998

Fananapazir L, Cannon RO 3d, Tripodi D, Panza JA: Impact of dual-chamber permanent pacing in patients with obstructive hypertrophic cardiomyopathy with symptoms refractory to verapamil and beta-adrenergic blocker therapy. Circulation 85:2149, 1992

Freedman RA: Use of implantable pacemakers and implantable defibrillators in hypertrophic cardiomyopathy. Curr Opin Cardiol 16:58, 2001

Kaplan JA, Reich DL, Konstadt SN (eds): pp. 743–749. Cardiac Anesthesia, 4th edition. WB Saunders, Philadelphia, 1999

Kovacic JC, Muller D: Hypertrophic cardiomyopathy: state-of-the-art review, with focus on the management of outflow obstruction. Intern Med J 33:521, 2003

Maron BJ: Hypertrophic cardiomyopathy: a systematic review. JAMA 287:1308, 2002

Maron BJ, Shen WK, Link MS, Epstein AE: Efficacy of implantable cardioverter-defibrillators for the prevention of sudden death in patients with hypertrophic cardiomyopathy. N Engl J Med 342:365, 2000

Sherrid MV, Chaudhry FA, Swistel DG: Obstructive hypertrophic cardiomyopathy: echocardiography, pathophysiology, and the continuing evolution of surgery for obstruction. Ann Thorac Surg 75:620, 2003

van der Lee C, Kofflard MJ, van Herwerden LA: Sustained improvement after combined anterior mitral leaflet extension and myectomy in hypertrophic obstructive cardiomyopathy. Circulation 108:2088, 2003

9

CARDIAC PACEMAKERS AND DEFIBRILLATORS

Alexander Mittnacht, MD
David L Reich, MD

An 85-year-old man with a VVI pacemaker presents for repair of an abdominal incisional hernia. He refuses spinal anesthesia. Induction of anesthesia with propofol, fentanyl, and succinylcholine results in muscle fasciculations and asystole.

QUESTIONS

1. What do the first three letters of the pacemaker code represent?
2. What is the difference between a demand and an asynchronous pacemaker?
3. What is the difference between ventricular (single-chamber) and dual-chamber pacemakers?
4. Is a unipolar or bipolar pacemaker more sensitive to electrocautery interference?
5. How is pacemaker interference by electrocautery prevented?
6. What is pacemaker hysteresis?
7. What causes myopotential inhibition of a pacemaker?
8. What is an automatic implantable cardioverter-defibrillator (AICD)?
9. How is the patient with an AICD managed in the perioperative period?

1. What do the first three letters of the pacemaker code represent?

There are five letters to the complete pacemaker code of which only the first three are commonly used. The first letter represents the cardiac chamber paced (A for atrium, V for ventricle, D for dual). The second letter represents the chamber sensed (A for atrium, V for ventricle, D for Dual, and O for none). The third letter represents the mode of the pacemaker, which could be described as the response of the pacemaker to the chamber it senses (I for inhibited, T for triggered, D for dual, O for none). The fourth letter indicates programmability and the fifth letter indicates anti-dysrhythmia functions. Codes for commonly used pacemakers are listed in Table 9.1.

2. What is the difference between a demand and an asynchronous pacemaker?

A demand pacemaker discharges in the absence of intrinsic electrical activity. For example, a demand ventricular pacemaker (VVI) will only pace when it does not sense R waves from the ventricular electrode. This is advantageous because it does not interfere with intrinsic cardiac rhythm when the ventricular rate is adequate and will not stimulate the ventricle during the vulnerable repolarization interval (and potentially induce a dysrhythmia). Extraneous electrical activity may interfere, however, by

TABLE 9.1   Pacemaker Codes

Pacemaker Code	Pacemaker Function
VOO	Asynchronous ventricular
VVI	Demand ventricular
VVIR	Demand ventricular rate-responsive (increases rate during physical activity)
VDD	Atrially triggered ventricular
AOO	Asynchronous atrial
AAI	Demand atrial
VAT	Atrially triggered ventricular
DVI	Atrioventricular sequential, ventricularly inhibited
DDD	Atrioventricular sequential (full function)

inhibiting the pacemaker when, in fact, no intrinsic cardiac activity is present. A classic example of this is electrocautery inhibition of a ventricular pacemaker which is set to sense ventricular activity. In this situation, the pacemaker will remain inhibited despite bradycardia or asystole.

An asynchronous pacemaker discharges continuously regardless of the heart's intrinsic rhythm. Almost all cardiac pacemakers will convert to the asynchronous mode (at least temporarily) during the placement of a magnet on the skin overlying the pacemaker generator. Asynchronous pacemaker modes are generally not used in patients outside the operating room. The operating room is unique, however, in that there are multiple potential sources of electrical interference which may prevent normal functioning of demand pacemakers.

3. What is the difference between ventricular (single-chamber) and dual-chamber pacemakers?

Single-chamber ventricular pacemakers are capable of ensuring adequate ventricular rates but are not capable of synchronizing atrial and ventricular contractions. Dissociation between atrial and ventricular contractions decreases ventricular filling and reduces stroke volume. Patients with cardiovascular diseases that reduce ventricular compliance (e.g., aortic stenosis, hypertrophic obstructive cardiomyopathy) may depend upon atrial systole for up to 50% of ventricular stroke volume. Dual-chamber pacemakers are preferable for almost all patients, except those with chronic atrial fibrillation.

4. Is a unipolar or bipolar pacemaker more sensitive to electrocautery interference?

A unipolar pacemaker lead system positions the negative electrode (cathode) in the heart and the positive electrode (anode) in the casing of the subcutaneously placed pacemaker generator. It is unipolar in the sense that only one pole of the electrical circuit is physically in the myocardium. A bipolar pacemaker lead system has two electrodes: the negative (distal) electrode is in the myocardium, and the positive (proximal) electrode is several millimeters proximal but still within the paced cardiac chamber.

Unipolar electrodes are differentiated from bipolar electrodes in several ways. Unipolar electrodes produce a larger "spike" on the surface electrocardiogram because of the greater distance between the positive and negative electrodes. This distance between electrodes produces a large electrical field change on the body surface. The bipolar pacemaker lead often appears as a coaxial cable and has a characteristic ridge between the two electrical poles near the end of the lead. This can be seen on the chest radiograph.

Electrocautery induces voltage (potential) differences across tissues. Pacemakers can be inhibited by these voltage changes, which mimic QRS complexes within the pacemaker circuitry. A unipolar pacemaker lead system is more likely to have this problem because the greater distance between the positive and negative poles will sense voltage changes from electrocautery. Conversely, bipolar lead systems are less likely to be effected by electrocautery, because it is difficult to induce a large enough voltage change over the small space between the poles of the pacemaker leads to simulate QRS complexes within the pacemaker circuitry.

5. How is pacemaker interference by electrocautery prevented?

Electrocautery interference can be prevented by electively reprogramming the pacemaker to asynchronous ventricular pacing in the preoperative period. In an emergency, a magnet placed over the pacemaker generator will (at least temporarily) convert the pacemaker to an asynchronous pacing mode. It is important to recognize that differences exist between manufacturers and devices, such that not all pacemakers will convert with magnet application to a stable asynchronous mode for the duration of surgery. It is possible that the magnet response may have been turned off or other responses may have been programmed that do not protect from electrocautery interference.

The use of bipolar electrocautery, where the current enters and leaves the patient at the cauterization site through a forceps-like device, may also prevent electrocautery interference. (In standard unipolar electrocautery, the current enters the patient through the cautery instrument tip and returns to the cautery machine through a return pad, which is often inaccurately referred to as a "grounding" pad.)

6. What is pacemaker hysteresis?

It is generally desirable to preserve intrinsic cardiac rhythm if the rate and rhythm are adequate to maintain an acceptable cardiac output. If the heart rate transiently decreases below that to which the pacemaker is set, it may not be necessary for the pacemaker to discharge. This is especially important for patients whose intrinsic cardiac rhythm is normal sinus and who have ventricular pacemakers. Considering the contribution of the atrial "kick" to cardiac output, the patient may have a better cardiac output in a slow sinus rhythm than would be created by single-chamber pacing. The additional delay that the pacemaker allows before initiating discharge after an intrinsic beat is known as *hysteresis*.

For example, if the pacemaker is set to pace at a rate of 60 beats per minute, then the pacing interval is 1,000 msec (1 second) between each paced beat. If we wish to program the pacemaker to wait until the intrinsic heart rate is less than 50 per minute (1,200 msec between beats) before firing, then the hysteresis is considered to be 200 msec. Once 1,200 msec have elapsed since the last intrinsic beat, the pacemaker will begin pacing every 1,000 msec. For the intrinsic rhythm to inhibit the pacemaker, an intrinsic beat will have to occur within the 1,000 msec interval following the last paced beat.

7. What causes myopotential inhibition of a pacemaker?

In addition to electrocautery, other forms of electrical activity may also interfere with pacemaker function. Succinylcholine causes diffuse muscle fasciculations in many patients, and these fasciculations are only partially prevented by defasciculating doses of nondepolarizing muscle relaxants. During muscle fasciculations, depolarizing membranes produce electrical discharges, which may inhibit a pacemaker. A unipolar pacemaking system's positive pole (anode) is in the generator case, which is usually located in close proximity to the pectoralis major muscle. This can result in myopotential inhibition.

Asystole following the administration of succinylcholine is best treated by placing a magnet over the pacemaker generator to temporarily convert the pacemaker to an asynchronous mode. Alternate means of pacing include external pacemakers and temporary transvenous pacemakers (including specially designed pulmonary artery catheters).

8. What is an automatic implantable cardioverter-defibrillator (AICD)?

An AICD is an implantable device capable of detecting ventricular tachycardia or fibrillation and terminating these dysrhythmias by antitachycardia pacing or cardioversion/defibrillation. AICDs also have pacing functions incorporated as a back-up for bradydysrhythmias following defibrillation or in patients who are pacemaker-dependent and also need to have a defibrillator implanted. Patients presenting with AICDs usually have significant cardiovascular disease and are at high risk of sudden cardiac death due to ventricular tachydysrhythmias. The list of indications for implanting AICDs is rapidly growing and subject to ongoing studies.

9. How is the patient with an AICD managed in the perioperative period?

There are two major concerns with the patient presenting for surgery who has an AICD implanted. First, the reason why the patient had the device implanted should be thoroughly evaluated and anesthetic management planned accordingly. For example, patients with severe left ventricular dysfunction require more intensive monitoring and altered anesthetic technique. Second, factors that may interfere with proper function of the device must be anticipated and measures taken to prevent malfunction. In the perioperative period, the most likely source of interference with AICD function stems from high-frequency electromagnetic signals caused by surgical electrocautery. The AICD software may interpret these signals as ventricular fibrillation or tachycardia and the AICD device may respond with inappropriate shock delivery or antitachycardia pacing. This, in turn, could potentially cause severe dysrhythmias. Therefore, the current recommendation for patients with an AICD undergoing elective surgery is to reprogram the device prior to surgery in order to deactivate dysrhythmia-sensing and defibrillator functions, and to set the pacemaker function to an asynchronous mode if possible. Preoperative assessment should include determining the details of the manufacturer, the model, the programmed settings, and when the device was last checked for proper function and battery charge. Once the device is deactivated, an external defibrillator must be readily available at any time and external defibrillator pads may be placed on the patient. In emergency cases only, a magnet can be placed over the device to deactivate the dysrhythmia detection and defibrillator functions of the AICD. Various models and manufacturers might differ in details as to how the pacing mode or the defibrillator mode is altered when a magnet is placed over the device or after the magnet has been removed. After any procedure, elective or emergency, the proper function of the AICD device has to be evaluated by qualified personnel.

SUGGESTED READINGS

Atlee JL, Bernstein AD: Cardiac rhythm management devices. Part I. Indications, device selection, and function. Anesthesiology 95:1265, 2001

Atlee JL, Bernstein AD: Cardiac rhythm management devices. Part II. Perioperative management. Anesthesiology 95:1492, 2001

Kaplan JA, Reich DL, Konstadt SN (eds): Cardiac Anesthesia, 4th edition. WB Saunders, Philadelphia, 1999

Senthuran S, Toff WD, Vuylsteke A: Implanted cardiac pacemakers and defibrillators in anaesthetic practice. Br J Anaesth 88:627, 2002

Stone ME, Weiss M: Anesthetic management of the patient with significantly decreased cardiac function who presents for noncardiac surgery: the patient with a pacemaker and/or implantable cardioverter defibrillator (ICD). Prog Anesthesiol 7:279, 2003

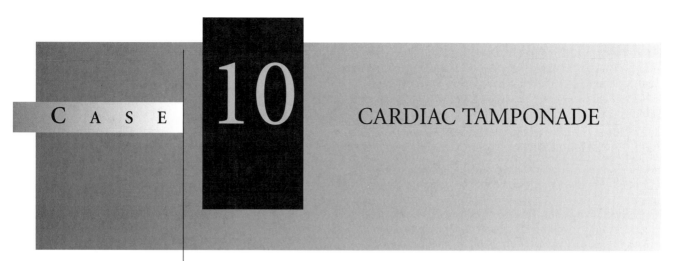

Michael Ostrovsky, MD

Linda J. Shore-Lesserson, MD

A 46-year-old woman with systemic lupus erythematosus (SLE) and mild renal insufficiency presents with shortness of breath and orthopnea of 5 days' duration. Her medications include tacrolimus, prednisone, and furosemide. On presentation to the emergency room, she has systemic hypotension, and distended neck veins which distend further upon inspiration. Transthoracic echocardiography reveals a large amount of pericardial fluid and echocardiographic signs of cardiac tamponade.

QUESTIONS

1. What is the pathophysiology of cardiac tamponade?
2. What are the clinical signs and symptoms of cardiac tamponade?
3. What is the initial management of this patient's condition?
4. What intraoperative monitoring techniques should be used?
5. Describe the implications for the conduct of general anesthesia in this patient.

1. What is the pathophysiology of cardiac tamponade?

The accumulation of pericardial fluid of virtually any etiology leads to cardiac tamponade when rising intra-pericardial pressure impedes atrial and ventricular filling. Rapid fluid accumulation of less than 200–250 mL in the pericardial space of an average adult will raise the central venous pressure by 10–12 cm H_2O. Increased impedance to ventricular filling results in a reduced stroke volume. The sympathetic response to rising intra-pericardial pressure leads to an increase in heart rate and constriction of the peripheral vasculature. Initially, when stroke volume is reduced and heart rate is increased, cardiac output can be maintained. With the further accumulation of pericardial fluid, rapid deterioration may ensue, owing to the fact that the parietal pericardium has a limited ability to stretch acutely. When the pericardial effusion is a chronic condition, the parietal pericardium can accumulate significant amounts of fluid without significant rises in intra-pericardial pressures.

In order for venous return to reach the right ventricle, systemic venous pressure should be equal to or greater than intra-pericardial pressure. Since right ventricular pressure is lowest in diastole and right atrial pressure is lowest in systole, these chambers tend to collapse when intra-pericardial pressure exceeds the chamber pressure. Echocardiographic studies have illustrated these findings. Echocardiographic signs of cardiac tamponade include right ventricular diastolic collapse and right atrial late systolic collapse.

Cardiac tamponade is defined by elevation and equalization of all diastolic pressures within the heart. With spontaneous inspiration, blood enters the right atrium and right ventricle. This causes interventricular septal shift into the left ventricle causing a partially obliterated left ventricular cavity. The resultant reduction in left ventricular output and blood pressure upon inspiration is typical. When pericardial effusion makes the pericardium tense, the leftward shift of the interventricular septum is more pronounced and the reduction in blood pressure is excessive. When the systolic pressure decreases by 10 mmHg or greater, the term "pulsus paradoxus" is used.

2. What are the clinical signs and symptoms of cardiac tamponade?

Cardiac tamponade can present in a variety of different scenarios. Patients can describe malaise and weakness. Often signs of right ventricular failure and left ventricular failure are seen. The chest radiograph can show a large cardiac silhouette. The electrocardiogram (ECG) shows low voltage in all leads with nonspecific ST-T wave changes. Electrical alternans is a hallmark of cardiac tamponade and relates to shifting of the position of the heart due to pericardial fluid.

Cardiac echocardiography reveals pericardial fluid and its impact on cardiac hemodynamics. Right atrial systolic collapse (for longer than one third of systole) and right ventricular diastolic collapse have high sensitivity and specificity for cardiac tamponade. A large prospective study demonstrated that any chamber collapse had a 92% negative predictive value but only a 58% positive predictive value. It is not uncommon to see variable ventricular septal motion with respiration as well as inferior vena cava plethora. Doppler studies in tamponade indicate respiratory variation in trans-mitral and trans-tricuspid flow patterns. These are inspiratory increases in right ventricular filling accompanied by concomitant inspiratory decreases in left ventricular filling.

Beck's triad is the other classic constellation of signs and symptoms of cardiac tamponade: distant heart sounds, hypotension, and elevated central venous pressure. Of note, the postoperative cardiac surgical patient can present with small loculated pericardial effusions that mimic tamponade physiology.

Kussmaul's sign may also be present. This sign is present in many different forms of right ventricular failure. It is marked by an increase in central venous pressure upon inspiration that results from inability of the right heart to fill.

Signs and Symptoms of Cardiac Tamponade

Malaise

Weakness

Right ventricular failure: ascites, peripheral edema, prerenal azotemia, hepatomegaly, jugular vein distention

Left ventricular failure: orthopnea, dyspnea, hypotension, decreased urine output

Chest radiograph: large cardiac silhouette

ECG: low voltage, electrical alternans

Echocardiogram: pericardial fluid, right atrial systolic collapse and right ventricular diastolic collapse

Beck's triad: distant heart sounds, hypotension, elevated central venous pressure

Kussmaul's sign

---

3. What is the initial management of this patient's condition?

Temporizing measures include volume infusion to increase central venous pressure to promote right ventricular filling. Vasoconstrictor and inotropic medications might not be fully efficacious, but can occasionally provide temporary benefit. Dobutamine has been used for its positive inotropic effects. α-Agonists may improve coronary perfusion and protect the heart from ischemia. Heart rate is critical to the maintenance of cardiac output because of the fixed stroke volume. Therefore, β-blockade would be contraindicated. Vagal reflexes should be treated with atropine. It is also important to maintain spontaneous respiration because positive pressure ventilation will further reduce right ventricular filling.

Pericardiocentesis is therapeutic and should be performed as soon as possible. Pericardiocentesis is often performed with local anesthesia through a sub-xiphoid approach using electrocardiographic guidance. This is accomplished by connecting the needle to the V lead of the ECG and looking for ST segment elevation (the current of injury) when the needle contacts the epicardial surface. Echocardiographic guidance has also increased the safety and decreased the complication rate of pericardiocentesis. Complications include pneumothorax, right ventricular puncture, left ventricular puncture, coronary artery laceration, and dysrhythmias.

Treatment for Cardiac Tamponade

Definitive
    Pericardiocentesis

Temporizing
    Volume expansion
    Vasoconstrictors
    Inotrope
    Atropine

---

4. What intraoperative monitoring techniques should be used?

Standard American Society of Anesthesiologists (ASA) monitors are a minimum requirement for intraoperative monitoring. Invasive monitoring, such as an intra-arterial line and a pulmonary artery catheter, can be used to enhance patient management in the perioperative period. Post-pericardiocentesis pulmonary edema, right and left ventricular dysfunction, and circulatory collapse have been described. Intraoperative echocardiography is extremely useful in the management of the above-mentioned complications.

5. Describe the implications for the conduct of general anesthesia in this patient.

With the surgeon present in the operating room, general anesthesia is induced only after the skin has been prepared and the surgical drapes placed. This is to ensure that if further hemodynamic compromise ensues upon induction of general anesthesia, rapid and immediate pericardiocentesis can be performed. The venodilatation and hypotension that occur upon induction of general anesthesia can cause devastating hypotension in the patient with cardiac tamponade. In addition, it is important to minimize the time from induction of anesthesia to relief of the tamponade. Strong consideration should be given to performing pericardiocentesis under local anesthesia, as this would maintain hemodynamic stability prior to drainage.

The hemodynamic goals to be achieved on induction of anesthesia are:

- Adequate inotropic state
- Increased heart rate
- Increased filling pressures
- Avoidance of vasodilatation
- Avoidance of myocardial depression

Induction of general anesthesia is often achieved with the use of ketamine or etomidate. Ketamine can cause myocardial depression at high doses or in the patient who is in a chronic state of myocardial failure. Potent inotropic and vasoconstrictive medication should be available to treat hemodynamic decompensation. There is a risk of circulatory collapse and/or pulmonary edema following relief of the tamponade.

SUGGESTED READINGS

Callahan JA, Seward JB, Nishimura RA, et al.: Two-dimensional echocardiographically guided pericardiocentesis: experience in 117 consecutive patients. Am J Cardiol 55:476–479, 1985

Hamaya Y, Dohi S, Ueda N, Akamatsu S: Severe circulatory collapse immediately after pericardiocentesis in a patient with chronic cardiac tamponade. Anesth Analg 77:1278–1281, 1993

Merce J, Sagrista-Sauleda J, Permanyer-Miralda G, et al.: Correlation between clinical and Doppler echocardiographic findings in patients with moderate and large pericardial effusion: implications for the diagnosis of cardiac tamponade. Am Heart J. 138:759–764, 1999

Wolfe MW, Edelman ER: Transient systolic dysfunction after relief of cardiac tamponade. Ann Intern Med 119:42–44, 1993

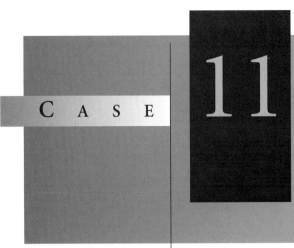

CARDIOMYOPATHY MANAGED WITH A LEFT VENTRICULAR ASSIST DEVICE

Marc E. Stone, MD

A 52-year-old man with ischemic bowel presents for urgent exploratory laparotomy. He has end-stage idiopathic dilated cardiomyopathy, and is listed for cardiac transplantation. While awaiting availability of a donor heart, he is managed at home with a long-term implanted left ventricular assist device (LVAD). A dual-chamber pacemaker (DDD mode) and implanted cardioverter-defibrillator (ICD) were also present.

QUESTIONS

1. What is a cardiomyopathy?
2. Distinguish dilated cardiomyopathy from other cardiomyopathies.
3. Explain the treatment options for dilated cardiomyopathies.
4. What is an LVAD?
5. What are the important anesthetic considerations for patients supported by LVADs?
6. What intra-anesthetic monitoring might be required for patients with LVADs?

1. What is a cardiomyopathy?

Cardiac failure is the heart's inability to deliver sufficient blood flow for metabolic demands. Cardiomyopathy is a myocardial abnormality that may lead to cardiac failure

(Table 11.1). Cardiomyopathy may result from a primary abnormality of the myocardium, or may be secondary to valvular, hypertensive, ischemic, infiltrative, structural, or pericardial disease processes. Regardless of the underlying etiology, compensatory changes (e.g., dilation and/or hypertrophy of the heart chambers) represent a final common outcome of adverse myocardial remodeling. A thorough evaluation of the patient presenting with typical signs and symptoms of heart failure (e.g., fatigue, shortness of breath, impaired exercise tolerance, peripheral edema, pulmonary rales, and renal insufficiency) is often required to establish the true underlying etiology. In addition to history, physical examination and focused laboratory testing, evaluation often requires both noninvasive and invasive modalities, including echocardiography, cardiac catheterization, and endomyocardial biopsies.

2. Distinguish dilated cardiomyopathy from other cardiomyopathies.

Dilated cardiomyopathy (DCM) is characterized by impaired systolic function and dilation of the left ventricle (LV) or sometimes both ventricles. The ejection fraction is moderately-to-severely depressed, and both tricuspid and mitral regurgitation generally result from stretching of their respective annuli. Diastolic dysfunction typically develops as the disease progresses, and pulmonary artery (PA) pressures are elevated secondary to chronically high left atrial (LA) pressures. Of the three predominant primary cardiomyopathies (dilated, restrictive, and hypertrophic), DCM is the most common. DCM may result

TABLE 11.1   Terms

Cardiomyopathy is a primary heart abnormality that may lead to cardiac failure.

Cardiac failure is the heart's inability to deliver sufficient blood flow for metabolic demands.

from infectious entities, cytotoxic substances, metabolic errors, endocrinopathies, familial inheritance, or immunologic mechanisms. Where no specific etiology can be identified, the term *idiopathic* dilated cardiomyopathy is applied. An excellent review of DCMs was recently published by Felker et al. (1999) (Table 11.2). It should be understood, however, that dilation of the heart chambers

is a final, common outcome of many pathophysiologic processes, not all of which represent primary DCM. While a dilated cardiomyopathy is not always DCM, per se, the anesthetic considerations and management are the same.

Severe LV dysfunction resulting from recurrent myocardial infarctions is commonly termed ischemic cardiomyopathy (ICM). ICM is not a primary cardiomyopathy because the primary underlying etiology is coronary artery disease. ICM presents with a similar pattern of impairment as DCM. ICM is characterized by LA and LV enlargement, LV segmental wall motion abnormalities, LV wall thinning, severely depressed ejection fraction, mitral regurgitation due to stretching of the mitral annulus, and elevated pulmonary artery pressures. Diastolic dysfunction is often present. In the absence of right ventricular (RV) infarction, RV size and function can be normal. While ICM frequently

TABLE 11.2   Characteristics of Four Cardiomyopathies

	Dilated	Ischemic	Restrictive	Hypertrophic
Pathophysiology	Moderately to severely depressed ejection fraction Dilated LV (or both LV and RV) Mitral regurgitation Tricuspid regurgitation Increased LA pressures Increased PA pressures Often left-sided, but right side frequently involved	Severely depressed ejection fraction LV and LA enlargement LV segmental wall motion abnormalities LV wall thinning Mitral regurgitation Increased PA pressures Usually left-sided	Systolic ventricular function usually normal, but impaired diastolic ventricular filling depresses cardiac output Stiff ventricle with normal wall thickness Chronically elevated end-diastolic pressures Signs of right heart failure	Asymmetric septal hypertrophy (ASH) Systolic anterior motion (SAM) of the anterior mitral valve leaflet Midsystolic LV outflow obstruction
Etiologies	Infectious Cytotoxic Metabolic Endocrine Inherited Immunologic Idiopathic	Myocardial ischemia Repeated myocardial infarction	Infiltration of myocardium Inflammation of myocardium	Autosomal dominant inheritance with variable penetrance

LV, left ventricle; RV, right ventricle; LA, left atrium; PA, pulmonary artery.

causes cardiac chamber dilation, a history of repeated myocardial infarctions and predominantly left-sided dilation and dysfunction helps to distinguish ICM from DCM.

Restrictive cardiomyopathy (RCM) usually results from infiltration or inflammation of the myocardium. The result is a stiff ventricle with an abnormally restrictive pattern of diastolic filling, and chronically elevated end-diastolic pressures are characteristic of this disease. While systolic ventricular function and wall thickness are usually normal, impairment of diastolic filling results in depressed cardiac output. Many patients with RCM present with signs of right-sided heart failure (peripheral edema, jugular venous distention, ascites, and hepatomegaly without shortness of breath or pulmonary rales). True RCM is relatively uncommon.

Hypertrophic cardiomyopathy (HCM) generally develops from asymmetric hypertrophy of the ventricular septum. Some patients with HCM have an obstructive form, hypertrophic obstructive cardiomyopathy (HOCM). In HOCM, systolic anterior motion (SAM) of the anterior mitral valve leaflet contacts the hypertrophied basal septum, producing mid-systolic obstruction of the left ventricular outflow tract. Those afflicted with HOCM are at risk for sudden death. Nonobstructive forms of hypertrophic cardiomyopathy also exist. HCM is an autosomal dominant disease with variable penetrance. Long-standing hypertension can also produce significant LV hypertrophy (often termed hypertensive heart disease, HHD). While diastolic dysfunction due to hypertrophied myocardium, and therefore some degree of pulmonary hypertension, tend to be present in both diseases, their characteristics and management are different. LV hypertrophy is asymmetric in HCM, but is concentric in HHD. Systolic function in HCM tends to be normal, while cardiac output tends to decline as HHD progresses. Systolic obstruction to LV outflow is a dynamic, subaortic process in HOCM and in HHD there is midventricular cavitary obliteration.

3. Explain the treatment options for dilated cardiomyopathies.

The treatment of DCM is essentially the symptomatic management of left-sided heart failure (Table 11.3). Four stages of heart failure are described: initial cardiac injury; neurohormonal activation and cardiac remodeling; fluid retention and peripheral vasoconstriction; and ultimate contractile failure. Mild to moderate heart failure is treated with preventative measures (dietary manipulations, blood pressure control, lowering of serum lipids, weight loss, and cessation of smoking) in combination with progressive pharmacologic interventions. Medications are aimed at antagonizing specific neurohormonal mechanisms of injury and controlling fluid retention. Beneficial classes of drugs include angiotensin-converting enzyme inhibitors

TABLE 11.3	Management of End-Stage Cardiomyopathy

Preventative measures
- Dietary
- Blood pressure control
- Reduction of serum lipids
- Weight loss
- Cessation of smoking

Medications
- Angiotensin-converting enzyme inhibitors – enalapril, captopril
- Angiotensin II receptor blocking agents – losartan
- β-Blockers – metoprolol, carvedilol
- Diuretics – furosemide
- Aldosterone antagonists – spironolactone
- Cardiac glycosides – digoxin
- Antiarrhythmics – amiodarone

Devices
- Dual-chamber pacemakers
- Automatic implantable cardioverter-defibrillator (AICD)
- Intra-aortic balloon pump (IABP)
- Left ventricular assist device (LVAD)

Surgery
- Heart transplantation

(e.g., enalapril, captopril), angiotensin II receptor blocking agents (e.g., losartan), β-blockers (e.g., carvedilol, metoprolol), diuretics (e.g., furosemide), aldosterone antagonists (spironolactone), and digoxin.

Diastolic dysfunction tends to develop as myocardial function deteriorates, resulting in chronically elevated LA pressures and, often, atrial fibrillation. In the patient with severe DCM, the maintenance of sinus rhythm becomes a key factor in maintaining forward cardiac output, so this population is often placed on antiarrhythmic agents, commonly amiodarone. When pharmacologic interventions fail to maintain sinus rhythm, dual-chamber (atrioventricular sequential) pacemakers are often implanted, for maintenance of the atrial contribution to diastolic ventricular filling.

Ventricular dysrhythmias cause severe decompensation and are potentially fatal. To prevent this, an automatic implantable cardioverter-defibrillator (AICD) is often implanted. As ventricular failure progresses, symptoms become refractory to outpatient medical therapy. Patients may require hospitalization for careful fluid management and administration of positive inotropic, as well as vasoactive agents. At this point, cardiac transplantation is frequently considered. In the interim, maintenance of adequate tissue perfusion may require temporary support with an intra-aortic balloon pump (IABP) or implantation of a left ventricular assist device (LVAD). The use of implantable LVADs has become common management for intractable cardiac failure in patients with end-stage cardiomyopathy who are awaiting transplantation.

A number of experimental surgical procedures (LV reconstruction, dynamic cardiomyoplasty, and others) have been developed to treat end-stage cardiomyopathy, but results to date have been variable. A comprehensive review of surgical treatments for heart failure was recently published by Kumpati et al. (2001).

4. What is an LVAD?

An LVAD replaces the LV's pumping function and potentially provides adequate systemic perfusion to prevent multi-system organ failure. Blood is drained through a conduit from the LV apex and is diverted to a pump implanted in the pre-peritoneal space or posterior rectus sheath. Output from the device is directed through a conduit into the ascending aorta. Current models have a percutaneous power cable/driveline that exits the abdominal wall in the right lower abdomen to connect with an external power pack and system controller. Currently available LVADs do not provide oxygenation/ventilation of the blood, nor dialysis.

The Novacor LVAS® (World Heart, Ottawa, Canada) and the Heartmate LVAS® (Thoratec Corporation, Woburn, MA) are fully implantable LVADs approved for long-term mechanical circulatory assistance as bridges to transplantation for patients with end-stage cardiomyopathy. A new indication, "destination therapy," refers to intentionally permanent implantation of an LVAD, in a non-transplant-eligible patient with cardiac failure. At the time of writing, the Heartmate is FDA-approved for destination therapy in the United States. Trials to establish efficacy of the Novacor for this indication are ongoing.

Although the two devices are conceptually similar, differences exist in engineering, durability, and the need for anticoagulation. Both the Novacor and the Heartmate are implanted similarly, both can operate in either fixed-rate or automatic "full-to-empty" modes (explained below), and both will provide flows on the order of 5–8 L/min as long as intravascular volume status is adequate. Filling of both devices relies on gravity drainage augmented by residual ventricular contractions. Ejection is accomplished in both by mechanical compression of a blood chamber. Ejection from the LVAD occurs asynchronously with respect to any underlying cardiac rhythm.

Following perioperative recovery and rehabilitation, LVAD patients are often discharged home to await transplantation. Implantable LVADs provide sophisticated control algorithms enabling device outputs to change as physiologic needs are altered. Some LVAD patients are confined to bed or remain limited to activities of daily living, but many experience a return to activities they had not enjoyed for years.

5. What are the important anesthetic considerations for patients supported by LVADs?

Preoperative Considerations

The preoperative clinical status of LVAD-supported patients depends on multiple issues, such as the amount of end-organ damage sustained during low-output states prior to ventricular assist device (VAD) implantation, post-implantation complications, and underlying surgical problems. Many LVAD recipients are ambulatory and otherwise uncompromised. Others experience varying degrees of renal, hepatic, pulmonary, and/or central nervous system insufficiency. Preoperative evaluation of neurologic dysfunction and other major organ system problems is essential. Any further deterioration in the perioperative period may preclude full recovery or disqualify a patient from later heart transplantation.

One of the most serious complications of extracorporeal circulation is thromboembolism, and LVADs are no exception. The Heartmate's blood chamber is designed with an antithrombogenic surface and requires no formal anticoagulation; however, the Novacor's polyurethane-lined blood chamber mandates anticoagulation. Initially heparin is used and then long-term warfarin therapy is commenced. International normalized ratios (INRs) are maintained at 2.5–3.5 times normal. In elective situations, Novacor patients may discontinue warfarin therapy preoperatively and convert to carefully monitored heparin infusions. **In most cases, heparin infusions should not be discontinued preoperatively.** The majority of surgical procedures (except for neurosurgical cases) can proceed safely in the presence of anticoagulation; however, scrupulous attention to hemostasis is required intraoperatively. Fresh frozen plasma or cryoprecipitate may be infused to decrease the level of anticoagulation toward the lower limit of manufacturer's recommendations. Frequent partial thromboplastin time (PTT) measurements are important to balance the dual potential complications of hemorrhage and thromboembolism. Anesthesiologists must determine (perhaps in consultation with the surgeon) a safe anticoagulation regimen for the perioperative period.

Adherence to strict aseptic technique is mandatory for all invasive procedures and prophylactic perioperative antibiotics are routinely employed. Infection of an LVAD is a catastrophic complication. They are very large foreign bodies that cannot be sterilized.

As with all critical life-support equipment in the operating room, an LVAD must be connected to a reliable power supply. Its battery life is limited.

Preoperative considerations and practices regarding pacemakers and AICDs are much the same in LVAD-supported patients as in other patients. The pre-set pacemaker mode is ascertained and it is interrogated for proper functioning. Usually, atrioventricular sequential pacing will be in use (DDD or DOO mode), because this frequently preserves RV output (and therefore LV filling) in these patients. Magnets should be available in case of pacemaker malfunction. Modern pacemakers will usually convert to an asynchronous mode (e.g., AOO, VOO, or DOO) when a magnet is applied, and should revert to their prior programming when the magnet is removed. In any event, pacemaker-dependent patients should have their device interrogated postoperatively to assure proper functioning. Many, but not all LVAD patients will have an AICD. Unipolar electrocautery emits a high-frequency signal that could potentially be interpreted as ventricular fibrillation, resulting in unnecessary defibrillatory discharges. Consequently, AICDs are usually deactivated in the immediate preoperative setting, assuming that a defibrillator is immediately available. Where possible, bipolar electrocautery should be preferentially used. In an emergency situation, a magnet may be used to deactivate the AICD. Most AICDs (Medtronics, St. Jude, Biotronik) will remain deactivated as long as the magnet remains in place; however, a Guidant AICD is permanently deactivated by application of a magnet. Removal and subsequent reapplication of the magnet is required to reactivate a Guidant AICD.

Cardiovascular collapse in LVAD patients is treated with standard advanced cardiac life support (ACLS) protocols. However, **one should never perform chest compressions on a ventricular assist device (VAD)-supported patient. Dislodgment of intracardiac cannulae will result in immediate exsanguination and certain death.** The Novacor is very well shielded, and will not be affected by defibrillation or electrocautery. Unfortunately, the Heartmate may be reset to a fixed-rate mode by electrocautery and potentially damaged by external defibrillation. For Heartmate patients, preoperative consultation with the physician managing the LVAD is advisable to discuss the implications of electrocautery and external defibrillation.

Intraoperative considerations

Novacor's requisite anticoagulation contraindicates major conduction anesthesia, which relegates most patients to general anesthesia. In some cases, sedation with local skin infiltration, or a regional intravenous technique (Bier block) is appropriate. Heartmate patients are not anticoagulated and remain potential candidates for major conduction anesthesia. Unfortunately, no specific recommendations exist regarding this issue at the time of writing.

The pump's pre-peritoneal location places the LVAD-supported patient at increased risk for aspiration pneumonitis. Consequently, "full stomach" precautions (e.g., gastric

acid prophylaxis and rapid sequence induction with cricoid pressure) should be considered. Extubation criteria of the LVAD-supported patient are the same as in any other patient.

The anesthetic drugs used should be appropriate for the planned operation, and should take into account any alterations of physiology resulting from insufficiency of, or prior injury to, major organ systems. For example, it may be disadvantageous to use pancuronium or vecuronium in the patient with renal insufficiency or biliary obstruction, respectively. Succinylcholine may be contraindicated in patients with recent cerebrovascular accidents. VADs do not specifically contraindicate any particular anesthetic agents, but the anesthetic plan should consider the potentially dysfunctional unassisted RV. Consequently, particular attention should be paid to optimizing RV preload, afterload, and inotropic support as required.

Long-term, implanted LVADs are typically set to automatically eject as soon as the blood chamber is full. The faster the device fills, the faster it pumps and the higher the pump output. Hypovolemia results in slow pump filling, decreased LVAD output, and hypotension. Consequently, the goal of fluid management is to maintain normal or slightly elevated intravascular volume. Markedly increased systemic vascular resistance (SVR) impairs forward flow, resulting in incomplete pump emptying, which leads to stagnation of blood in the pump and increased risk of thrombosis. Therefore, maintenance of normal or slightly low systemic vascular resistance is desirable. Management must be individualized. Inotropes, vasodilators, and vasopressors are administered to achieve optimal hemodynamics. LVADs generally function well as long as there is sufficient intravascular volume to fill the pump.

Depth of anesthesia is judged, in part, by hemodynamic parameters. However, LVAD-supported patients may not manifest increased pulse rates, a classic sign of light anesthesia. As previously discussed, LVADs eject as soon as the blood chamber fills, and it is this rate of ejection which constitutes the LVAD-supported patient's pulse rate. Therefore, the pulse rate is rarely the same as the ECG-derived heart rate. For this reason, intraoperative tachycardia, as measured by the pulse rate, is reflective only of the speed of LVAD filling, and not of light anesthesia. However, while relative hypertension is reflective of relative volume overload and higher pump outputs, it could also reflect heightened adrenergic activity with increased SVR (Table 11.4). Nevertheless, lack of an acutely increased blood pressure with surgical stimulation is not always a reliable indicator of adequate depth of anesthesia in an LVAD-supported patient.

6. What intra-anesthetic monitoring might be required for patients with LVADs?

Electrocardiography, pulse oximetry, end-tidal carbon dioxide, temperature, and blood pressure are standard for patients undergoing general anesthesia, and the

TABLE 11.4	Anesthetic Considerations for LVAD-Supported Patients

Preoperative considerations:

- Pre-existing end-organ impairment—renal, hepatic, pulmonary, central nervous system
- Post-LVAD implant complications
- Underlying surgical problems
- Anticoagulation
  Novaor LVAD – required, FFP may be needed to reduce levels of anticoagulation towards manufacturer's lower limits
  Heartmate LVAD – not required
- Prophylactic antibiotics
- Pacemaker – functions properly (if present)
- Deactivate AICD
- Never perform chest compressions on LVAD-supported patients

Intraoperative considerations:

- Novacor LVAD – continue intraoperative anticoagulation for most cases, major conduction anesthesia contra-indicated, frequent PTT measurements, shielded from electrocautery and defibrillation
- Heartmate LVAD – major conduction anesthesia acceptable, adversely affected by electrocautery and defibrillation
- Maintain normal or slightly expanded intravascular volume
- Aspiration prophylaxis
- Maintain normal or slightly low SVR
- Elevated pulse rate does not necessarily indicate light anesthesia
- Hypertension could result from expanded intravascular volume or increased adrenergic activity (which could be a sign of light anesthesia)
- Reliable electric power supply required
- Defibrillator should be readily available
- Optimize RV preload, afterload, and contractility

PTT, partial thromboplastin time; LVAD, left ventricular assist device; AICD, automatic implantable cardiovecter-defibrillator; SVR, systematic vascular resistance; FFP, fresh frozen plasma.

LVAD-supported patient is no exception. LVAD command consoles offer continuous digital readouts of the effective cardiac output (VAD-output). Invasive hemodynamic pressure monitoring is not mandatory for all procedures. Blood pressure can be monitored noninvasively, at the anesthesiologist's discretion. Arterial pressure monitoring catheters are generally inserted for procedures anticipated to produce large swings in blood pressure or for frequent arterial blood sampling.

Central venous pressure (CVP) monitoring is used when large fluid shifts are anticipated. As explained above, optimal LVAD function depends on adequate intravascular volume. However, LVADs increase the risk of RV failure. High output from an LVAD will increase RV preload. Sometimes, this alone is enough to cause RV failure in patients with moderate-to-severe RV dysfunction. Decompression of the LV by an LVAD causes a leftward shift of the interventricular septum, resulting in altered RV geometry, increased RV compliance, and decreased RV contractility. While an optimally functioning LVAD will reduce RV afterload and often improve RV function in patients with normal pulmonary vascular resistance (PVR), patients with fixed, elevated PVR may actually experience an increased RV afterload, due to increased right-sided and PA flows. Finally, moderate-to-severe tricuspid regurgitation occasionally results from dilation of the tricuspid annulus during LVAD support. In addition to monitoring CVP to detect developing RV failure and guide fluid management, central access is useful for drug infusions and the potential introduction of a transvenous pacing wire. Additionally, one can calculate SVR in the LVAD-supported patient with an indwelling CVP monitor by substituting the VAD output for the cardiac output in the hemodynamic formula. The calculation would then be as follows:

$$SVR = [(MAP - CVP)/LVAD\ output] \times 80\ dynes\text{-}sec/cm^5$$

Central catheters are a potential source of sepsis, and should be avoided when not absolutely necessary.

Pulmonary artery catheters (PACs) are a "double edged sword." Generally, they provide no useful information in LVAD-supported patients. The LVAD console offers a continuous cardiac output display. PACs pose an increased risk of PA rupture in the patient with pulmonary hypertension. PACs can be of some help in the pharmacologic management of pulmonary hypertension. If the patient has a CVP catheter, SVR can be calculated without a PAC as outlined above. Further, though it is not quantitative, one can tell that the SVR has abruptly increased in the LVAD-supported patient when the residual volume in the pump abruptly increases. Transesophageal echocardiography (TEE) is the intraoperative monitor of choice if there is concern about failure of an unassisted ventricle.

SUGGESTED READINGS

Felker GM, Hu W, Hare JM, Hruban RH, et al.: The spectrum of dilated cardiomyopathy: the Johns Hopkins experience with 1,278 patients. Medicine 78:270, 1999

Kumpati GS, McCarthy PM, Hoercher KJ: Surgical treatments for heart failure. Cardiol Clin 19:669–681, 2001

Massie BM: Pathophysiology of heart failure and diagnosis. Chapter 55. In Goldman L, Ausiello D (eds): Cecil Textbook of Medicine, 22nd edition. WB Saunders, Philadelphia, 2003

Packer M: Management and prognosis of heart failure. Chapter 56. In Goldman L, Ausiello D (eds): Cecil Textbook of Medicine, 22nd edition. WB Saunders, Philadelphia, 2003

Pavie A, Leger P: Physiology of univentricular versus biventricular support. Ann Thorac Surg 61:347, 1996

Santamore WP, Gray LA: Left ventricular contributions to right ventricular systolic function during LVAD support. Ann Thorac Surg 61:350, 1996

Wynne J, Braunwald E: The cardiomyopathies and myocarditides. Chapter 48. In Braunwald E (ed): Heart Disease: A Textbook of Cardiovascular Medicine, 6th edition. WB Saunders, Philadelphia, 2001

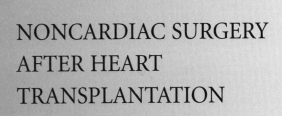

CASE 12

NONCARDIAC SURGERY AFTER HEART TRANSPLANTATION

Marc E. Stone, MD

A 57-year-old man with hypertension, elevated serum cholesterol, and mild renal insufficiency presents for laparoscopic cholecystectomy. His past medical history is significant for idiopathic dilated cardiomyopathy followed by cardiac transplantation at age 55 years. His medications include nifedipine, tacrolimus, azathioprine, prednisone, atorvastatin, and omeprazole.

QUESTIONS

1. Describe the physiology of transplanted hearts.
2. Is reinnervation of the transplanted heart a concern?
3. Which immunosuppressive medications are typically used following cardiac transplantation?
4. Explain the pre-anesthetic concerns for patients with a transplanted heart.
5. What anesthetic techniques are applicable to patients with cardiac transplants?
6. Which intraoperative monitors are recommended for patients with a transplanted heart?
7. What emergency drugs are likely to be effective in the patient with a transplanted heart?
8. For patients with a transplanted heart, is it necessary to administer anticholinergics when antagonizing neuromuscular blockade?

1. Describe the physiology of transplanted hearts.

The donor heart is denervated during harvesting. Consequently, the recipient lacks efferent and afferent innervation. The transplanted heart does not receive autonomic or somatic input. Although denervation prevents responses to extrinsic neural signals, intrinsic myocardial mechanisms and reflexes remain intact. While transplanted hearts function in isolation from the nervous system, they respond to humoral factors (e.g., catecholamines) circulating in blood.

The results of cardiac denervation are:

- Relative tachycardia from absent vagal input to the transplanted heart. Heart rates approximate 90–100 beats per minute.
- Loss of rapid heart rate responses to autonomic reflexes. Heart rates remain unchanged with carotid massage, acute hyper- or hypotension, and from Valsalva maneuvers.
- Absence of many pharmacologic effects. Drugs which alter the heart rate indirectly, via the autonomic nervous system, will not have their usual effects on the transplanted heart. Vagolytic drugs, such as atropine, pancuronium, and meperidine, will not increase heart rate. Vagotonic drugs, such as acetylcholinesterase inhibitors and opioids, will not decrease heart rate. Medications with both direct and indirect cardiac actions will maintain their direct effects on the denervated heart. Digoxin, for

example, maintains its positive inotropic effects on the graft, but will not slow heart rate through its parasympathetically mediated effects on the atrioventricular (AV) node.

- Delayed and attenuated responses to laryngoscopy, intubation, painful stimuli, and light anesthesia because direct sympathetic innervation of the heart no longer occurs. However, prolonged stimulation results in rising levels of circulating catecholamines that will eventually induce an increase in heart rate, or even an exaggerated one, directly through myocardial adrenergic receptors.
- Inability to perceive angina. Despite sporadic case reports to the contrary, which have been touted as evidence of reinnervation, the majority of post-transplantation patients do not perceive angina.

Despite denervation, intrinsic myocardial mechanisms remain intact in the transplanted heart:

- The denervated myocardium responds normally to circulating or administered catecholamines (e.g., epinephrine, norepinephrine) and direct-acting sympathomimetic agents (e.g., isoproterenol, dobutamine) directly through myocardial adrenergic receptors. In this regard, denervation appears to induce downregulation of β_1 receptors, so most β-adrenergic receptors on the denervated myocardium will be β_2 subtypes.
- The Frank-Starling mechanism (increased preload results in increased stroke volume) remains intact, and is the primary mechanism for increased cardiac output during exercise or stress. For this reason, it is important to maintain adequate preload in post-transplantation patients. Since they already have elevated heart rates, the only way a post-transplant patients can initially increase cardiac output is through the Frank-Starling mechanism. Any further increases in heart rate and cardiac output with prolonged exercise or stress are the result of increased levels of circulating catecholamines, and are therefore slightly delayed in onset (and in resolution).
- Metabolic autoregulation of coronary blood flow in response to changes in pH and pCO_2 remains intact.
- Normal electrical impulse formation and conductivity along the usual pathways is maintained in the transplanted heart. Classic orthotopic heart transplantation techniques leave cuffs of native right and left atrial tissue behind in the recipient, to facilitate surgical anastomoses. The native sinoatrial (SA) node is contained in the right atrial cuff. Impulses continue to emanate from the native SA node, but these can not cross atrial suture lines and do not depolarize the transplanted heart. Frequently, two independent p-waves are discernible on the post-transplant electrocardiogram (ECG) (Fig. 12.1).

Physiology of the Transplanted Heart

Cardiac denervation
  Resting tachycardia of 90–100 beats/min
    Due to vagus nerve denervation
  Absence of autonomic reflexes
    No change in heart rate to:
      carotid massage
      Valsalva maneuver
      atropine
      pancuronium
      meperidine
      acetylcholinesterase inhibitors
      opioids
      digoxin
    Delayed tachycardic response to:
      hypotension
      painful stimuli
      light anesthesia (mediated through catecholamine release)
    Phenomenon of reinnervation remains speculative

Intrinsic myocardial mechanisms
  Normal response to:
    Circulating catecholamines (epinephrine, norepinephrine)
    Direct-acting sympathomimetics (isoproterenol, dobutamine)
  Frank-Starling mechanism remains intact:
    Primary mechanism to increase cardiac output
    Important to maintain adequate preload
  Metabolic autoregulation of coronary blood flow:
    Responds to local pH and pCO_2
  Normal electrical impulse formation and conduction:
    Action potentials from native SA node do not cross suture line and are not propagated to donor heart

2. Is reinnervation of the transplanted heart a concern?

Whether or not significant reinnervation occurs in transplanted human hearts remains to be determined. Laboratory evidence of functional reinnervation exists in non-human cardiac transplantation, and there are some reports supporting sympathetic reinnervation late in the post-transplantation period (>5 years postoperatively) in human patients. However, reinnervation appears to be incomplete in human grafts, and in the first few years

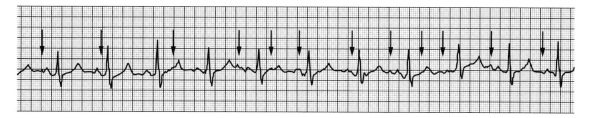

FIGURE 12.1 ECG strip of Lead II from a cardiac transplantation patient in sinus rhythm. While the graft SA node is depolarizing the transplanted heart at approximately 80 beats per minute, there is another, smaller p-wave marching through this strip at an independent rate, reflecting depolarization of the retained native SA node. Several native p-waves are indicated by the arrows; however others may be present, buried within the complexes, giving the appearance of an irregular rate of native SA node discharge.

following transplantation, there is currently no evidence that reinnervation of transplanted human hearts is a clinically important phenomenon.

3. Which immunosuppressive medications are typically used following cardiac transplantation?

Frequently, immunosuppressive regimens consist of selective T-cell inhibitors such as cyclosporine or tacrolimus; nonspecific purine antimetabolites, such as azathioprine; and corticosteroids, such as prednisone. Characteristics of these medications are summarized in Table 12.1. Classic regimens based on high-dose steroids

and multiple immunosuppressive agents are falling out of favor, and may soon be replaced by regimens based on rapidly tapered steroids and tacrolimus. Other agents, including mycophenolate mofetil (CellCept) and sirolimus (Rapamune), are approved for use following cardiac transplantation, and are becoming part of typical immunosuppressive maintenance regimens.

While immunosuppressive agents are the key to survival following cardiac transplantation, they also have detrimental side-effects. Cyclosporine and tacrolimus tend to cause renal insufficiency, hepatotoxicity, hypertension, and neurotoxicity. Neurotoxicity manifests as seizures, which result from lowering the seizure threshold. Azathioprine primarily

TABLE 12.1   Characteristics of the Immunosuppressives Commonly Used Following Cardiac Transplantation

Agent	Mechanism of Action	Main Side-Effects
Cyclosporine (*Neoral, Sandimmune, SangCya*)	Selective T-cell inhibitor	Nephrotoxicity Hypertension Hepatotoxicity Neurotoxicity (seizures)
Tacrolimus (*Prograf, FK-506*)	Selective T-cell inhibitor with 10× potency of cyclosporine	Same as cyclosporine
Azathioprine (*Imuran*)	Purine antimetabolite	Thrombocytopenia Anemia Leukopenia Hepatotoxicity
Corticosteroids (*prednisone*)	Decreased circulating lymphocytes Impairment of antigen presentation Interference with cytokine production Impairment of phagocytosis Inhibition of T-cell proliferation Impaired lymphocyte adhesion Impaired lymphocyte margination	Hypertension Diabetes mellitus Pancreatitis Potential adrenal insufficiency Psychiatric disturbances

causes hematologic toxicity, producing thrombocytopenia and anemia, but also causes hepatotoxicity. Steroids can cause hypertension, diabetes mellitus, adrenal insufficiency, pancreatitis, and psychiatric disturbances.

While side-effects such as those listed in Table 12.1 may require medical management, some others mandate surgical management. These side-effects will constitute some of the most frequent indications for non-cardiac surgery in the post-transplantation period.

Steroids predispose to peptic ulceration, aseptic bone necrosis, and cataracts. Consequently, patients receiving chronic high-dose steroids may present for drainage of abscesses; orthopedic procedures on the hips, knees, elbows, or shoulders; bowel resection for perforated viscus and diverticulitis; as well as ophthalmologic procedures related to cataracts and retinal detachments.

Cyclosporine, tacrolimus, and azathioprine tend to cause biliary stasis, so patients on these agents often present for cholecystectomy. Their nonspecific gastrointestinal toxicities can also cause severe symptoms (e.g., nausea, vomiting, diarrhea, anorexia, and abdominal pain) mimicking an intra-abdominal process that occasionally prompts exploratory laparotomy.

Immunosuppression predisposes to malignancies. Some of these patients may present for lymphoma staging, node sampling, and resection of gynecologic or skin malignancies.

4. Explain the pre-anesthetic concerns for patients with a transplanted heart.

Preoperatively, the primary concern is the transplanted heart's function. Without rejection, the post-transplantation patient generally does not perceive any functional limitations and is classified as a New York Heart Association (NYHA) class I or II. However, ventricular function must be assessed preoperatively. Information regarding prior episodes of rejection (if any) and ventricular function is usually available from the managing cardiologist. This is especially important in patients who are a few years out from their transplant, because the post-cardiac transplantation patient is subject to accelerated atherosclerotic coronary disease (possibly the result of a vasculitis from low-level, subclinical rejection). The likelihood of significant coronary occlusion increases directly with time from transplantation. Post-transplant coronary occlusion is reported to occur at a rate of 10–20% incidence at 1 year, 25–45% incidence at 3 years, and a 50% incidence at 5 years.

While some benign dysrhythmias are common following transplantation (e.g., incomplete right bundle branch block, premature atrial contractions, occasional premature ventricular contractions, and first-degree AV block), more ominous rhythms may be signs of acute rejection. Given the propensity toward accelerated atherosclerotic disease, one should always consider that new perioperative dysrhythmias accompanied by hypotension may be a sign of ischemia.

Pre-anesthetic Concerns for Patients With a Transplanted Heart

Histories of rejection and ventricular function from the managing cardiologist

Anticipated accelerated atherosclerosis

Dysrhythmias
  Common benign dysrhythmias:
    incomplete right bundle branch block
    premature atrial contractions
    occasional premature ventricular
      contractions
    first-degree AV block
  Other malignant dysrhythmias may represent
    rejection
  New dysrhythmias and hypotension may be
    due to ischemia

Impaired renal and hepatic function
  Secondary to cyclosporine and tacrolimus

Anemia and thrombocytopenia
  Secondary to azathioprine

Immunosuppression
  Aseptic technique for all intravenous and
    intra-arterial catheter placements
  Prophylactic antibiotics

Corticosteroids
  Consider stress dose steroid replacement

Preinduction intravascular volume repletion

During the preoperative evaluation, special attention should be paid to renal and hepatic function because impairment of these organs is a major side-effect of the immunosuppressive medications cyclosporine and tacrolimus. Renal and/or hepatic impairment may predispose to acid-base and electrolyte derangements. A complete blood count should be reviewed for anemia and thrombocytopenia, as hematologic toxicity is a major side-effect of azathioprine.

Infection is a major source of morbidity and mortality for the immunosuppressed post-transplant patient, so aseptic technique is mandatory for all invasive procedures, including intravenous catheter placement. Prophylactic antibiotics are routinely employed where appropriate.

Many immunosuppressive regimens include fairly high dose corticosteroids, and unless the patient has recently been tapered off steroids, the issue of a preoperative "stress dose" should be discussed with the primary managing physician.

Finally, given the dependence of the graft on the Frank-Starling mechanism (discussed above), one must assure an adequate intravascular volume status prior to anesthetic induction.

5. What anesthetic techniques are applicable to patients with cardiac transplants?

General anesthesia, spinal anesthesia, epidural anesthesia, regional blockade (axillary, wrist, ankle, and Bier blocks), and local infiltration have all been used successfully in this population. The choice of agents for general anesthesia is not crucial. Multiple small doses titrated to effect frequently works out best. Induction agents, benzodiazepines, opioids, and potent inhalation agents are usually well tolerated. All the usual caveats apply in the presence of renal or hepatic dysfunction. Early (if not immediate) postoperative extubation is preferable, because prolonged intubation increases the risk of pulmonary infection.

Plasma levels of various anesthetic agents which depend on P450 metabolism may be increased or decreased by immunosuppressive and anticonvulsant medications, and can themselves alter immunosuppressant blood levels. Increased blood levels of immunosuppressants result in undesirable side-effects (e.g., nephrotoxicity of cyclosporine and tacrolimus). Administered agents which compete for P450 metabolism (e.g., furosemide) can decrease cyclosporine elimination and increase blood levels. Agents which increase cyclosporine metabolism (e.g., barbiturates) can lower blood levels.

It is believed that neuromuscular blockade is augmented by cyclosporine, and can be antagonized by anticonvulsants (e.g., phenytoin) often given to patients on immunosuppressants with seizures. However, this should not pose a problem if close monitoring of neuromuscular blockade is used.

Regardless of technique, volume depletion and acute vasodilation (e.g., as may occur with spinal anesthesia) will be poorly tolerated because the transplanted heart initially depends on the Frank-Starling mechanism to maintain cardiac output. Sudden vasodilation will not result in a reflex tachycardia. One certainly can perform a spinal anesthetic in the post-transplantation patient, but one must be prepared to augment preload and prevent sudden decreases in systemic vascular resistance. It is often said that an epidural technique with a level brought up gradually results in better hemodynamic stability.

6. What intraoperative monitors should be used in the patient with a transplanted heart?

In the absence of rejection, graft function is usually fairly good and a noninvasive blood pressure (NIBP) cuff and routine monitors are usually sufficient. Invasive arterial and central venous pressure monitoring are generally only employed if there is hemodynamic instability (e.g., from bleeding, sepsis, myocardial dysfunction, during acute rejection) or if indicated by the planned procedure (e.g., for frequent arterial blood gas sampling during one-lung ventilation, or when one needs to follow and/or optimize filling pressures and indices of cardiac function). It must be remembered that requisite endomyocardial biopsies to monitor rejection are preferentially performed via the right internal jugular (IJ) vein, and one should use the left IJ or subclavian veins for central access if possible. Where available, transesophageal echocardiography (TEE) may be preferable to invasive central monitoring.

7. What emergency drugs are likely to be effective in the patient with a transplanted heart?

Only direct-acting inotropes, chronotropes, and vasoconstrictors will be immediately effective. Epinephrine is usually the direct-acting inotrope of choice. Direct-acting chronotropes include epinephrine, isoproterenol, and dobutamine. Pacing (via external pacing pads or a transvenous pacing wire) is also an option to increase heart rate. For reasons previously discussed, atropine is not likely to increase heart rate in a denervated graft. Direct-acting vasoconstrictors include phenylephrine and perhaps vasopressin. For the majority of situations, small bolus doses of epinephrine and phenylephrine are effective and are used as first-line agents when necessary.

Ephedrine is a noncatecholamine sympathomimetic agent with both direct and indirect actions on α- and β-adrenergic receptors. The indirect actions of ephedrine come from enhanced release of norepinephrine. While ephedrine can be used advantageously in the patient with a transplanted heart, it is not usually considered a first-line emergency drug because at least part of its desired action must await the subsequent release of norepinephrine.

Dopamine, a drug which also has both direct and indirect effects, is the immediate precursor of, and causes the release of, norepinephrine. In the cardiac transplantation patient, dopamine would initially be expected to exert only its direct dopaminergic effects (e.g., coronary and splanchnic vasodilatation) through dopaminergic receptors. The vasoconstrictive α-effects and the desired β-adrenergic effects on heart rate and contractility are only going to come from subsequently released norepinephrine. When all this is taken into account, dopamine may not be the optimal first-line choice when inotropy or chronotropy is urgently needed.

8. For patients with a transplanted heart, is it necessary to administer anticholinergics when antagonizing neuromuscular blockade?

While bradycardia is unlikely following the administration of an acetylcholinesterase inhibitor (e.g., neostigmine) to a

Intra-anesthetic Concerns for Patients With a Transplanted Heart

Anesthetic technique
    No specific method is indicated or
        contraindicated
    Early extubation is preferable to avoid
        ventilator-associated pneumonias
    Vasodilation is poorly tolerated and must be
        aggressively treated with intravascular
        volume repletion and/or vasoconstrictors

Monitors
    In the absence of rejection, graft function
        generally good
        Noninvasive monitors are usually adequate
        Invasive monitors are chosen for their usual
            indications
        Left internal jugular vein is used preferentially
            to allow for future heart biopsies via the
            right internal jugular vein

Emergency medications
    Inotropes
        Epinephrine
    Chronotropes
        Epinephrine
        Isoproterenol
        Dobutamine
        Pacing—external pads or internal wire
    Vasoconstrictors
        Phenylephrine
        Vasopressin

Antagonism of neuromuscular blockade
    Neostigmine
    Glycopyrrolate

post-cardiac transplantation patient, the usual muscarinic blockers (e.g., glycopyrrolate) should be given concurrently to prevent noncardiac cholinergic side-effects (e.g., bronchospasm). Another reason to provide an anticholinergic is that significantly increased levels of acetylcholine can cause coronary vasospasm in the denervated heart. While there is some evidence that neostigmine has direct effects on the myocardium, and there are a few case reports of bradycardia following neostigmine administration in this population, it should not deter one from reversing neuromuscular blockade when appropriate because prolonged intubation may predispose to pulmonary infection.

SUGGESTED READINGS

Backman SB, Ralley FE, Fox GS: Neostigmine produces bradycardia in a heart transplant patient. Anesthesiology 78:777, 1993

Borkon AM: Morbidity following heart transplantation. p. 249. In Baumgartner WA (ed): Heart and Heart-Lung Transplantation. WB Saunders, Philadelphia, 1990

Cameron DE, Traill TA: Complications of immunosuppressive therapy. p. 237. In Baumgartner WA (ed): Heart and Heart-Lung Transplantation. WB Saunders, Philadelphia, 1990

Diasio RB, LoBuglio AF: Immunomodulators: immunosuppressive agents and immunostimulants. p. 1291. In Hardman JG, Limbird LE, Molinoff PB, Ruddon RW, et al. (eds): Goodman and Gilman's The Pharmacologic Basis of Therapeutics, 9th edition. McGraw-Hill, New York, 1996

Kostopanagiotou G, Smyrniotis V, Arkadopoulos N, Theodoraki K, et al.: Anesthetic and perioperative management of adult transplant recipients in nontransplant surgery (review). Anesth Analg 89:613, 1999

Stark RP, McGinn AL, Wilson RF: Chest pain in cardiac transplant recipients: evidence of sensory reinnervation after cardiac transplantation. N Engl J Med 324(25):1791, 1991

13

CORONARY ARTERY BYPASS GRAFTING

Linda J. Shore-Lesserson, MD

A 64-year-old man with hypertension, non-insulin-requiring diabetes mellitus, elevated serum cholesterol, and mild renal insufficiency presents for coronary artery bypass grafting. His recent cardiac catheterization results indicate 75% stenosis of his left main coronary artery and 70% stenosis of his right coronary artery. Left ventricular function is normal. His medications include metoprolol, nitroglycerin patch, aspirin, clopidogrel, and omeprazole.

QUESTIONS

1. What are the major determinants of myocardial oxygen supply and demand?
2. What types of medications are used to treat coronary artery disease?
3. What are the pre-anesthetic concerns in the patient with coronary artery disease?
4. What intraoperative monitoring techniques can be used for the patient undergoing cardiac surgery using cardiopulmonary bypass (CPB)?
5. What are the common intraoperative monitors for myocardial ischemia?
6. What are the effects of CPB on the lungs, the brain, and the kidneys?
7. What are the effects of CPB on hemostasis?

1. What are the major determinants of myocardial oxygen supply and demand?

The major determinants of myocardial oxygen supply include:

- Coronary anatomy
- Diastolic filling time↑
- Aortic diastolic pressure (ADP)↑
- Left ventricular end-diastolic pressure (LVEDP)↓
- Coronary perfusion pressure↑ (CPP).

  $$CPP = ADP - LVEDP$$

The major determinants of myocardial oxygen demand in decreasing order include:

- Left ventricular wall tension

  $$Tension = (pressure \times radius)/2 \times wall\ thickness$$

- Heart rate
- Contractility
- Afterload.

2. What types of medications are used to treat coronary artery disease?

The medications used to treat coronary artery disease are employed to either augment the supply or reduce the demand for myocardial oxygen. In order to overcome possible anatomic obstructions to coronary artery blood flow by thrombus, anticoagulants or antiplatelet agents are used, especially in the acute coronary setting. Medications that will augment diastolic filling time include drugs that lower heart rate: β-adrenergic blockers and Ca^{2+} channel blockers. Increases in ADP, and hence the driving pressure behind coronary perfusion, can be achieved by using vasopressors. Reductions in LVEDP can be achieved using nitrates, diuretics, and other venodilators (e.g., morphine). A single intervention which augments aortic diastolic pressure and reduces LVEDP is intra-aortic balloon counterpulsation (Table 13.1).

3. What are the pre-anesthetic concerns in the patient with coronary artery disease?

Pre-anesthetic anxiety will cause patients to develop tachycardia. Patients with coronary artery disease should have adequate anxiolysis, in the form of either pharmacology or counseling, so that they do not have a dramatic increase in oxygen consumption.

Patients with coronary artery disease also have concomitant diseases such as hypertension and diabetes. Patients with severe diabetes mellitus may be at risk for autonomic and peripheral neuropathy. That is the reason why silent ischemia is so prevalent in the diabetic patient. Diabetic patients may also have delayed gastric emptying if autonomic neuropathy is present. Appropriate prophylaxis for a full stomach should be considered.

Patients with hypertension have intravascular hypovolemia and may present with hypotension upon induction of anesthesia. It is important to ascertain the volume status of the patient prior to induction and to volume-load the patient to prevent hypotension. The response to laryngoscopy may include tachycardia, which increases oxygen consumption. Medication (narcotics, β-blockers, lidocaine) must be administered to patients with coronary artery disease to ensure that they have a blunted catecholamine release in response to intubation.

4. What intraoperative monitoring techniques can be used for the patient undergoing cardiac surgery using cardiopulmonary bypass (CPB)?

Intraoperative monitoring should include intra-arterial blood pressure monitoring. This is necessary due to the nature of the disease, the nature of the surgery, the need for frequent arterial blood gas sampling, and the necessity of monitoring mean arterial blood pressure directly while on CPB. Additional monitors include a central venous catheter, which is needed to administer vasoactive medications directly into the central circulation. If patients have severe left ventricular dysfunction or valvular heart disease, a pulmonary artery catheter would be preferable. Pulmonary arterial catheterization allows for the direct measure of pulmonary capillary wedge pressure (PCWP), which is often directly related to LVEDP. Monitoring the PCWP gives the anesthesiologist a close approximation of intravascular volume status assuming that the left ventricular compliance is normal. Intravascular volume is more sensitively measured using transesophageal echocardiography (TEE) because the end-diastolic area of the left ventricle can be directly visualized.

The CPB pump uses nonpulsatile flow and the heat exchanger system is sometimes used to lower the patient's body temperature. Vasoconstriction and vasodilation are common and do not represent an alteration in the anesthetic depth of the patient. Also, the addition of crystalloid fluid to

TABLE 13.1	Drugs Useful to Treat or Prevent Myocardial Ischemia	
Drug Class	**Mechanism of Action**	**Treating Ischemia**
β-Blockers	Antagonize effects at β-receptors	Reduce heart rate, contractility
Ca^{2+} channel blockers	Prevent calcium influx	Reduce heart rate, contractility
Nitrates	Smooth muscle relaxation	Reduce preload, augment epicardial coronary artery flow
Diuretics	Proximal tubule, distal tubule, or loop promotes diuresis	Reduce preload
Morphine	Arterial and venodilation	Reduce preload
Phosphodiesterase inhibitors	Increase cAMP, smooth muscle relaxation	Reduce preload, improve relaxation, increase contractility
α_1-Agonist (phenylephrine)	Systemic vasoconstriction	Augment coronary perfusion pressure
Intra-aortic balloon counterpulsation	Inflate during diastole, deflate during systole	Reduce afterload, augment coronary perfusion pressure

the pump prime increases the blood volume of the patient thereby diluting the blood concentrations of anesthetic agents and other drugs. For these reasons, many practitioners choose to use a monitor of anesthetic depth during and after CPB.

The heat exchanger as a part of CPB helps to lower and to raise the patient's body temperature to facilitate the conduct of CPB. The rate or speed of temperature change should be small, and the gradient between body temperature and blood temperature should not be excessive. For these reasons, it is important to monitor at least two temperatures during CPB: one temperature reflects blood temperature (esophageal), and a second reflects core body temperature (rectal or bladder).

5. What are the common intraoperative monitors for myocardial ischemia?

The most common monitor of intraoperative ischemia is electrocardiography. At least two leads should be monitored in order to diagnose more than 95% of ischemic episodes. The pulmonary artery catheter can also be used to diagnose ischemia when the PCWP or the pulmonary artery diastolic pressure increases. This can also be referred to as a "v wave" of the PCWP tracing. The PCWP is not as sensitive as the electrocardiogram for detecting ischemia. The most sensitive monitor for ischemia is TEE, in which regional wall motion abnormalities occur very early in the course of reduced coronary perfusion. TEE is probably too sensitive; PCWP is probably not sensitive enough; thereby leaving electrocardiography as the most accurate monitor of coronary ischemia.

6. What are the effects of CPB on the lungs, the brain, and the kidneys?

CPB causes a total body inflammatory reaction that results in the release of vasoactive substances, cytokine mediators, and endotoxins into the bloodstream. All major organs are affected and the degree of the response is dependent on the length of CPB, the extent of tissue trauma, and patient genetic factors. As a result, major organs such as the lungs, brain, and kidneys suffer. Factors that lead to organ dysfunction include edema, reduced perfusion, and nonpulsatile perfusion. Mild renal dysfunction is common after CPB and is often reversible. The lungs are often dysfunctional after CPB due to atelectasis and inflammation. The brain suffers similar effects in that edema and reduced perfusion may occur. However, the brain suffers additional potential insults during CPB. Cerebral dysfunction is the major morbidity that occurs after cardiac surgery. Most of this dysfunction is the result of atheroemboli that dislodge from the aorta during procedures such as aortic cross-clamping, cannulation, and proximal vein graft anastomosis. Some of these atheroemboli can be seen using epiaortic ultrasound before cannulation of the aorta. However, the majority of cerebral dysfunction probably results from microemboli that can be neither detected nor prevented. A large portion of the neuropsychological dysfunction seen after CPB resolves within the first year after surgery.

7. What are the effects of CPB on hemostasis?

Patients undergoing CPB have a variety of hemostatic defects that lead to bleeding and the frequent need for transfusions. Dilution of the patient's blood volume by the extracorporeal circuit priming solution causes depletion of platelets and a lowering of coagulation factor levels. Contact of blood with the extracorporeal circuit causes activation of many systems. Contact activation causes intrinsic coagulation to begin, subsequently leading to the formation of thrombin and fibrin. Then fibrinolysis ensues creating a subclinical disseminated intravascular coagulation (DIC) to occur. Sometimes this DIC is clinically evident and hemorrhage and thrombosis occurs. The formation of kallikrein, bradykinin, and complement leads to a "whole-body inflammatory reaction." Platelet dysfunction also occurs and is due to the effects of the extracorporeal circuit on platelet membrane integrity and the effects of circulating platelet inhibitors. Heparin causes platelet activation and dysfunction. Protamine, given to reverse heparin's effects, has antiplatelet properties and anticoagulant effects when given in excess.

SUGGESTED READINGS

Despotis GJ, Joist JH: Anticoagulation and anticoagulation reversal with cardiac surgery involving cardiopulmonary bypass: an update. J Cardiothorac Vasc Anesth 1999; 13:18–29

Hindman B: Cerebral physiology during cardiopulmonary bypass: pulsatile versus nonpulsatile flow. Adv Pharmacol 1994; 31:607–616

Hirsh J, Raschke R, Warkentin TE, Dalen JE, Deykin D, Poller L: Heparin: mechanism of action, pharmacokinetics, dosing considerations, monitoring, efficacy, and safety. Chest 1995; 108:258S–275S

Murkin JM, Martzke JS, Buchan AM, Bentley C, Wong CJ: A randomized study of the influence of perfusion technique and pH management strategy in 316 patients undergoing coronary artery bypass surgery. II. Neurologic and cognitive outcomes. J Thorac Cardiovasc Surg 1995; 110:349–362

Song Z, Wang C, Stammers AH: Clinical comparison of pulsatile and nonpulsatile perfusion during cardiopulmonary bypass. J Extracorpor Technol 1997; 29:170–175

Svennevig JL, Lindberg H, Geiran O, Semb BK, Abdelnor M, Ottesen S, Vatne K: Should the lungs be ventilated during cardiopulmonary bypass? Clinical, hemodynamic, and metabolic changes in patients undergoing elective coronary artery surgery. Ann Thorac Surg 1984; 37:295–300

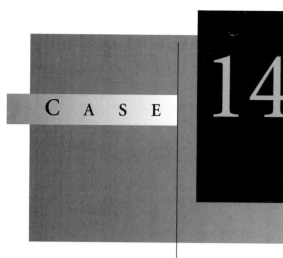

Linda J. Shore-Lesserson, MD

An 84-year-old man has metastatic small cell carcinoma of the lung. He presents with hoarseness and a 2 kg weight loss. An investigation reveals tumor in the mediastinal lymph nodes and two 1 cm lesions in the liver, which are currently asymptomatic. The patient has prepared a living will stating that he does not want any heroic measures such as intubation and cardiopulmonary resuscitation in the event that he should suffer a cardiac arrest. He will accept a feeding tube if he should become unable to feed himself. The patient presents to the operating room for placement of a tunneled central venous catheter for chemotherapy. While the surgeon is infiltrating the surgical site with local anesthetic, it becomes apparent that an excessive dose of local anesthetic has been injected. The patient suffers a grand mal seizure.

QUESTIONS

1. What is meant by temporary revocation of do-not-resuscitate (DNR) orders in the operating room?
2. What did you discuss with the patient prior to surgery regarding resuscitation efforts in the operating room?
3. What options are available to the patient and clinician in order to more fully define a patient's DNR wishes?
4. What would you do in this case, if the patient could not be adequately ventilated with a mask?
5. If this patient were intubated for the resuscitation but did not regain consciousness for 48 hours, is it ethical to withdraw mechanical ventilation at this time?

1. What is meant by temporary revocation of do-not-resuscitate (DNR) orders in the operating room?

Prior to the early 1990s, it was generally felt that DNR orders were to be automatically revoked while a patient was in the operating room. The prevailing opinion was that surgery and anesthesia represented *temporary* alterations in the patient's medical condition and, thus, interventions such as intubation and cardiopulmonary resuscitation should be able to be instituted without it being felt that one was violating a patient's wishes to *not* be resuscitated. In 1993–1994, ethical guidelines for managing DNR patients undergoing anesthesia care were established by the American Society of Anesthesiologists.

2. What did you discuss with the patient prior to surgery regarding resuscitation efforts in the operating room?

It is critical to discuss with the patient what options are available. It is also imperative that the physician understands the patient's perspective so that in an ambiguous clinical situation the physician can act with the patient's interest in mind. Patients should be given the option of either "full" resuscitative efforts or "partial" resuscitative efforts. Full efforts are relatively simple to exercise. Partial efforts are more difficult because patients may choose to accept certain procedures which are medically inconsistent with other procedures they have chosen to refuse. For example, a patient may state that they would accept emergency surgery but refuse intubation. It may be necessary, however, to perform intubation in order for the emergent surgery to proceed.

The physician should have the patient sign a consent form that explicitly documents their wishes with regard to the DNR in the operating room. This informed consent is an important document and is explained in the next section.

3. What options are available to the patient and clinician in order to more fully define a patient's DNR wishes?

The following are four choices for informed consent for DNR. The patient should be asked to choose an option and sign the consent.

- Option 1: full resuscitation. This option assures the patient that no efforts will be overlooked or spared in order to assist with full resuscitative efforts. It is not inappropriate for a patient to revoke the DNR for the operative setting. This option works well for patients who will accept any intervention in exchange for the possibility of benefit.
- Option 2: limited resuscitation, procedure-directed. Patients select which interventions they accept and reject. This works well for the patient who wants complete control over what procedures they will receive. However, it does not allow for the "clinical license" of the physician to interpret wishes when the patient's desires may be ambiguous or inconsistent with clinical conditions.
- Option 3: limited resuscitation, goal-directed (temporary and reversible). This allows the physician to make a clinical judgment that the adverse clinical events present are both temporary AND reversible. If this is the case, then interventions to temporize the patient during the adverse event are acceptable to the patient. An example of this could be the need to intubate the trachea of a patient undergoing general anesthesia for surgery which is planned and elective.
- Option 4: limited resuscitation, goal-directed (patient's wishes known). This option allows the physician to make a clinical judgment to treat a patient based upon the known preferences and goals of the patient. This option is ideal in that it allows decision-making to take place based upon outcomes, rather than procedures. It is not

necessarily contingent upon the outcome of the events being obviously temporary and reversible. Rather it allows a physician to make a decision about the care of a patient after that patient communicates a desired outcome. This is a more ambiguous statement for the patient but is more consistent with the practice of medicine, in which clinical situations are very dynamic. An example of this might be the case of an arterial injection of local anesthetic resulting in a grand mal seizure. The outcome of the grand mal seizure is not known, yet the physician knows that the event was accidental, the event is unrelated to the reason that the patient has elected to be "DNR", and the symptoms are treatable. In this case, the physician may elect to control the airway and intubate the trachea until the outcome is known.

4. What would you do in this case, if the patient could not be adequately ventilated with a mask?

This clinical situation of local anesthetic overdose and seizure resulting in respiratory insufficiency is likely temporary and reversible. It is not related to the patient's underlying disease state directly. It would be imperative to secure the patient's airway and begin ventilation with either a mask or an endotracheal tube until baseline mental status is restored. This would be consistent with honoring the patient's wishes rather than just procedure-directed therapy.

Many patients choose procedure-directed therapy (list of procedures they will and will not accept). This works well to alleviate anxieties but is often inconsistent or impossible to reconcile medically. Goal-directed therapy is preferable in circumstances such as this.

5. If this patient were intubated for the resuscitation but did not regain consciousness for 48 hours, is it ethical to withdraw mechanical ventilation at this time?

It is considered appropriate to withdraw care in the postoperative period if continued care is unlikely to achieve the desired goals of the patient. Since it is more ethically challenging to withhold therapy not knowing if an event is temporary, it is suggested that therapy be initiated. Once a trial and assessment are performed, an evaluation at a later time may determine that withdrawal of that therapy would be more in line with the patient's wishes.

Despite the published guidelines suggesting the re-evaluation of DNR for the perioperative period, many practitioners still feel uncomfortable doing so for ethical and personal reasons. Others may find it too difficult to re-evaluate and customize a DNR order for the perioperative period, especially if the anesthesiologist is not comfortable interpreting the patient's wishes.

SUGGESTED READINGS

Bastron RD: Ethical concerns in anesthetic care for patients with do-not-resuscitate orders. Anesthesiology 85:1190–1193, 1996

Cohen CB, Cohen PJ: Do-not-resuscitate orders in the operating room. N Engl J Med 325:1879–1882, 1991

Margolis JO, McGrath BJ, Kussin PS, Schwinn DA: Do not resuscitate (DNR) orders during surgery: ethical foundations for institutional policies in the United States. Anesth Analg 80:806–809, 1995

Truog RD: Do-not-resuscitate orders during anesthesia and surgery. Anesthesiology 74:606–608, 1991

Truog RD, Waisel DB, Burns JP: DNR in the OR: a goal-directed approach. Anesthesiology 90:289–295, 1999

www.asahq.org/Standards/09.html: American Society of Anesthesiologists. Ethical guidelines for the anesthesia care of patients with do-not-resuscitate orders or other directives that limit care. 2001

15

ONE-LUNG ANESTHESIA

Steven M. Neustein, MD
James B. Eisenkraft, MD

A 70-year-old man with a long history of cigarette smoking presents for resection of a left upper lobe tumor.

QUESTIONS

1. Describe the anesthetic evaluation before lung resection.
2. How are ventilation and oxygenation monitored noninvasively during surgery, and how do these monitors work?
3. What are the indications for one-lung ventilation?
4. Describe the use of single-lumen endotracheal tubes for one-lung ventilation.
5. Which sided double-lumen endobronchial tube should be used for this patient?
6. Describe the proper technique for placing a double-lumen endobronchial tube.
7. How is correct positioning of the double-lumen endobronchial tube assessed?
8. What clinical problems are associated with the placement and use of double-lumen endobronchial tubes?
9. What complications are related to placing the patient in the lateral decubitus position?
10. How are pulmonary perfusion and ventilation altered during one-lung ventilation?

11. What is the treatment for hypoxemia during one-lung ventilation?
12. Describe the role of a thoracostomy tube following pulmonary resection, and describe the system used for pleural drainage.
13. Describe a commonly used pleural drainage system.
14. Discuss potential post-thoracotomy complications.

1. Describe the anesthetic evaluation before lung resection.

Preoperative evaluations begin with basic information required before all anesthetics. A determination is then made as to whether the patient is in optimal condition for the planned procedure or whether further preoperative preparation is indicated. Finally, an assessment is formulated to predict lung function following resection. The specific pulmonary evaluation will include history of cough, sputum production, chest pain (possibly pleuritic), dyspnea, wheezing, arm pain (resulting from Pancoast tumor involving the brachial plexus), weakness (resulting from myasthenic syndrome), other endocrine syndromes (caused by tumors secreting hormones), and weight loss (hypoproteinemia). Physical examination includes auscultation for wheezing, rales, and rhonchi. Wheezing may require treatment with bronchodilators, and infected sputum indicates antibiotic treatment. Chest radiograph, tomography, computed tomography (CT), and magnetic resonance imaging (MRI) provide further information on the tumor site, structures involved, and possible airway compromise.

Lung function tests are indicated to predict the risk of respiratory failure, right heart failure (cor pulmonale), or atelectasis, as well as to guide bronchodilator therapy. Spirometry is a noninvasive test that provides data on lung volumes and gas flow rates. Flows are tested without, and then following bronchodilator therapy, such as albuterol by inhaler, to determine reversible obstructive airway disease. Improved flows following bronchodilator therapy indicate preoperative adjustments in the bronchodilator regimen.

Pulmonary function tests that may correlate with outcome include forced expiratory volume in 1 second (FEV_1), forced vital capacity (FVC), maximum voluntary ventilation (MVV), and ratio of residual volume to total lung capacity (RV/TLC). Based on how much lung tissue is to be resected, a predicted postoperative (PPO) function can be calculated. A PPO FEV_1 greater than 40% predicted has been correlated with improved outcome. An FVC less than 50% predicted, or RV/TLC greater than 50% predicted may indicate higher risk.

Whereas spirometry reflects respiratory mechanics, gas exchange correlates with diffusing capacity for carbon monoxide (DLCO). A PPO DLCO less than 40% predicted indicates reduced lung parenchymal function, and correlates with increased risk.

Cardiopulmonary reserve can be evaluated by measuring the maximal oxygen consumption ($\dot{V}O_2max$). A $\dot{V}O_2max$ less than 10 mL/kg/min indicates very high risk, and a $\dot{V}O_2max$ greater than 20 mL/kg/min indicates reduced risk. Other tests of cardiopulmonary reserve include exercise oximetry, and a fall in oxygen saturation by pulse oximetry (SpO_2) of 4% during exercise may indicate increased risk.

If lung function results are poor, split lung function testing (ventilation–perfusion radiospirometric studies) and even unilateral pulmonary artery occlusion studies (to temporarily exclude blood flow to the ipsilateral lung) may be indicated. Ultimately, the operative decision to perform pneumonectomy versus lobectomy versus wedge resection is a clinical one in which the patient's overall condition is considered.

2. How are ventilation and oxygenation monitored noninvasively during surgery, and how do these monitors work?

The purpose of ventilation is to remove carbon dioxide (CO_2) from the lungs. The average 70-kg man produces approximately 220 mL/min of CO_2 and normally maintains an arterial CO_2 ($PaCO_2$) of 40 mmHg. If removal of CO_2 is impaired, or if production increases, and ventilation does not increase, the $PaCO_2$ rises. Arterial blood gas analysis provides the ultimate monitor of ventilation: $PaCO_2$. In the

lungs, CO_2 diffuses into alveoli, and in those areas where ventilation and perfusion are well matched, alveolar CO_2 ($PACO_2$) approximates $PaCO_2$. $PACO_2$ may be sampled as end-tidal ($PE'CO_2$) and analyzed by various technologies to provide a noninvasive estimation of $PACO_2$ and thereby, $PaCO_2$. Overall, $PE'CO_2$ is normally 4–6 mmHg less than $PaCO_2$. Increases in dead space (VD/VT) or a decrease in alveolar ventilation result in increased $PaCO_2$.

Capnography is the science whereby CO_2 is measured and displayed as a concentration plotted against time (the capnogram). CO_2 in gas mixtures may be measured using the following technologies: mass spectrometry, infrared light spectroscopy, infrared acoustic spectroscopy, and Raman scattering. The principle of mass spectrometry is ionization of molecules in a high vacuum chamber and separation on the basis of mass-to-charge ratio. CO_2 has a mass/charge ratio of 44 (m.w. 44/charge of +1) and is indistinguishable from N_2O. Mass spectrometers therefore usually measure the presence of carbon ions from fragmented CO_2 molecules. Carbon ions are present in fixed ratio to CO_2. The mass spectrometer is a proportioning system and provides true readings of percentage composition. If the computer is programmed such that 100% is equivalent to 713 mmHg, percentages can be expressed in mmHg.

Infrared (IR) light spectroscopy is based on 4.3 μm (4300 nm) wavelength IR radiation absorbance by intermolecular bonds in the CO_2 molecule. The greater the number of CO_2 molecules present, the greater the radiation absorbance. Gas is drawn through a sample cell (cuvette). IR light of 4.3 μm is passed through the cell. Transmission of light through the gas sample to a photodetector is inversely proportional to the PCO_2 in the gas sample. Such systems are in widespread use and sampling may be of the sidestream or mainstream (in the airway) design.

In photoacoustic IR spectrometry units, IR beams are pulsed through the cuvette. Pulsed beams cause heating and pulsatile expansion of the gas in proportion to the number of CO_2 molecules present. The pulsatile expansions are detected as sound waves by a sensitive microphone. The amplitude of the waves ("volume") is proportional to PCO_2.

In Raman spectroscopy (Rascal II, Datex-Ohmeda, Boulder, CO), a helium–neon laser generates monochromatic light of wavelength 633 nm, which is transmitted through a sampling cuvette. CO_2 molecules absorb this light and re-emit it at a different and characteristic wavelength. The light re-emitted at the new wavelength is specific for CO_2, and its intensity is related to PCO_2.

By continuously following the percentage (mass spectrometer) or tension (other methods) of CO_2 against time, the highest value is designated *end-tidal* and defines exhalation, whereas the lowest value is designated *inspiratory* and defines inspiration. Continuous capnography is considered the standard of care because it provides a continuous monitor of ventilation and can, with certain limitations, provide a noninvasive *estimate* of $PaCO_2$.

Oxygenation is monitored best by sampling arterial blood and analyzing it for tension (PaO_2), hemoglobin saturation with oxygen (fractional saturation, i.e., O_2Hb/total Hb), and total hemoglobin. The oxygen content of arterial blood (CaO_2) is then given by the equation:

$$CaO_2 = [(Hb \times 1.34 \times SaO_2) + (PaO_2 \times 0.003)]$$

Normal arterial oxygen content can be calculated by substituting variables as shown:

$$CaO_2 = [(15 \times 1.34 \times 0.95) + (95 \times 0.003)]$$
$$= 19.1 + 0.29$$
$$= 20 \text{ mL oxygen/100 mL blood}$$

This, however, requires invasion of an artery for blood sampling.

Noninvasive monitoring of oxygenation is most commonly achieved using a pulse oximeter, which has also become the standard of care. The principle of operation of the pulse oximeter is based on two technologies: (1) spectrophotometry of oxygenated and deoxygenated Hb and (2) optical plethysmography. The latter detects pulsatile components of changes in light transmitted through a fingertip. Each pulse oximeter probe has two light-emitting diodes (LEDs), which emit light at 660 nm and 940 nm, and one photodetector. The ratio of the pulse-added absorbance of light at 660 nm to that at 940 nm is related through an empirically derived algorithm, to a saturation reading which is designated SpO_2. Pulse oximeter readings have a standard deviation of approximately 2% in the saturation range of 70–100%. At lower SpO_2 levels, their accuracy decreases. Nevertheless, the pulse oximeter is valuable as a saturation trend monitor. Pulse oximeters are inaccurate or may fail in the presence of poor perfusion (vasoconstriction from low cardiac output or cold extremities), venous pulsations, severe peripheral vascular disease, intravascular dyes, dyshemoglobins, certain nail polishes, and certain pigmentations. If doubt exists as to the validity of a pulse oximeter reading, an arterial blood gas sample should be drawn for blood gas tension analysis and saturation analysis in a laboratory co-oximeter.

3. What are the indications for one-lung ventilation?

Indications for double-lumen tubes revolve around the requirements to isolate one lung from the other. Reasons for separating the lungs include prevention of blood or pus spillage; control of ventilation distribution, and improved surgical exposure. Situations in which hemorrhage or infectious material might affect the contralateral lung include bronchiectasis, lung abscess, and hemoptysis. Positive pressure ventilation through a single-lumen tube risks losing large segments of tidal volume through a bronchopleural fistula or pneumothorax in the case of giant unilateral lung cyst. Surgical exposure is improved during pneumonectomy, descending thoracic-abdominal aortic aneurysm repair, and resection of mid-esophageal as well as upper esophageal lesions. Video-assisted thoracoscopy is a high priority for one-lung ventilation.

4. Describe the use of single-lumen endotracheal tubes for one-lung ventilation.

Although one-lung ventilation using a single-lumen endotracheal tube is accomplished by advancing the tube into one of the mainstem bronchi, refinements of this technique exist. A combined single-lumen endotracheal tube and bronchial blocker serve this purpose even better. The single-lumen tube is equipped with a narrow internal lumen through which a balloon-tipped bronchial blocker is advanced into the right or left mainstem bronchus. With the bronchial blocker retracted and deflated, the tube is positioned by standard techniques into the trachea. The tube is then turned 90° toward the side to be blocked, and the blocker is advanced blindly or under flexible fiberoptic bronchoscopic guidance into the appropriate bronchus. The balloon is inflated, and lung separation is confirmed by auscultation of breath sounds. This system provides a larger lumen for more efficient suctioning of blood and obviates the need for changing tubes at the completion of surgery for patients who require postoperative intubation and ventilation. Lung deflation through the small blocker lumen is time-consuming. More rapid collapse of the lung follows deflation of the blocker balloon and disconnection from the anesthesia breathing circuit to allow for lung deflation. After successful collapse, reinflation of the blocker balloon and connection to the anesthesia breathing circuit allows for ventilation of one lung and collapse of the other.

5. Which sided double-lumen endobronchial tube should be used for this patient?

There is no one correct answer to this question. Different approaches to the choice of double-lumen endobronchial tube depend on the side of thoracotomy. In this case of a left thoracotomy, either a left- or right-sided tube can be selected. These authors agree that left-sided tube placement is more prudent in this situation. In the adult, the left mainstem bronchus is 4–5 cm in length, compared with 2–3 cm for the right mainstem bronchus. The right upper lobe bronchus is more likely to be accidentally occluded by the endobronchial tube than is the left upper lobe bronchus. Resection of the left lung will necessitate continuous ventilation of the right lung. Obstruction of the right upper lobe bronchus would likely lead to hypoxemia during one-lung ventilation. For this reason, some anesthesiologists routinely place a left-sided double-lumen tube, regardless of the side of thoracotomy, unless this is specifically contraindicated by the presence of a diseased left mainstem bronchus, or if the bronchus will likely become part of the surgical field.

Some anesthesiologists routinely place the endo-bronchial tube on the side ipsilateral to pulmonary resection. With this arrangement, obstruction of the upper lobe bronchus by the endobronchial tube is not as likely to cause hypoxemia because this is the lung to be deflated during one-lung ventilation. Also, before chest closure, reinflation of the remaining lung ipsilateral to the tube can be verified by direct inspection. Failure to reinflate the upper lobe is treated by deflation of the bronchial cuff so that it can be ventilated from the tracheal lumen. Alternatively, the double-lumen tube can be withdrawn until the distal end of the endobronchial tube is proximal to the upper lobe bronchial orifice. In the case of a pneumonectomy, the tube must be withdrawn to a position where the distal end of the tube is in the trachea before division of the main bronchus. Withdrawal may also become necessary if the intubated bronchus is involved in the surgery.

A different approach used by a smaller percentage of anesthesiologists is to routinely place the double-lumen tube into the nonoperative side. This strategy prevents damage from placing the tube into a diseased bronchus. Placement of a right-sided tube for a left thoracotomy, however, may lead to hypoxemia during one-lung ventilation, as discussed.

Our approach is to place a left-sided double-lumen tube for both left and right thoracotomies, unless contraindicated by anatomy or pathology. However, during a right thoracotomy performed under this arrangement, misplacement of the endobronchial tube too distal in the left bronchus will occlude the left upper lobe, predisposing the patient to hypoxemia during one-lung ventilation. This is because only the left lower lobe will be ventilated during right lung deflation.

6. Describe the proper technique for placing a double-lumen endobronchial tube.

The largest size Robertshaw-type double-lumen tube that can easily pass the glottis is chosen. The larger the tube size, the less air that is required for endobronchial tube cuff inflation; the larger the lumen for suctioning; and the less likelihood of tube malposition distally in the bronchus. Clear polyvinylchloride disposable Robertshaw-type endo-bronchial tubes are available in sizes 41, 39, 37, 35, and 28 French (French size = external diameter of tube in mm ×3). Sizes 39 and 37 French fit most adults.

Curved laryngoscope blades usually provide more space in the mouth than straight blades for passage of double-lumen tubes, which are bulky compared with single-lumen tubes. In some patients, however, a straight blade may be required.

Induction agents are selected based on the patient's medical condition. Nondepolarizing muscle relaxants offer the advantage of longer duration of action than succinylcholine. This allows for prolonged duration of muscle relaxation, which facilitates double-lumen tube placement without repeat doses of nondepolarizing agent.

This double-lumen tube is placed through the mouth with its distal concave curve pointed anteriorly. After the endobronchial cuff passes the vocal cords, an assistant removes the stylette. The tube is rotated 90° toward the side of intended intubation and advanced until resistance is encountered. Alternatively, the endobronchial lumen can be advanced over a flexible fiberoptic laryngoscope into the appropriate bronchus. Air is injected into the tracheal cuff, and the tube's position is checked.

7. How is correct positioning of the double-lumen endobronchial tube assessed?

Correct placement of the endobronchial tube must be confirmed immediately after intubation and after turning the patient into the lateral decubitus position. The patient's lungs are initially ventilated through both lumens with the tracheal cuff inflated. Bilateral breath sounds, bilateral chest excursion, and bilateral fogging of endobronchial tube lumens should be present. Gas should not leak around the cuff. The capnogram should be examined for excretion of CO_2. Successful response to these maneuvers ensures that the distal end of the tracheal lumen is in the trachea and is above the carina. Unilateral breath sounds and chest movement indicate that the tube has been inserted too far, and the tracheal lumen is in the bronchus, ipsilateral to the side on which breath sounds are present. In this case, the tracheal cuff should be deflated and the tube withdrawn until bilateral ventilation is established.

Next, the bronchial balloon is inflated with less than 2 mL of air (Figure 15.1). The tracheal lumen is clamped and the access cap opened. Ventilation should result in chest movement and breath sounds on the endobronchial side. The presence of bilateral breath sounds and chest movement indicates that the bronchial lumen's orifice is proximal to the carina (Figure 15.2). Unilateral breath sounds and chest movement of the side opposite the bronchus intended for intubation indicate that the tube has been placed in the wrong side (Figure 15.3). If this has happened, both cuffs should be deflated and the tube withdrawn to a point where the distal end of the endobronchial tube is in the trachea. The tube is then rotated and advanced again until there is resistance to further movement. An alternative method is to insert a fiberscope through the bronchial lumen, visualize the carina, pass the fiberscope down the bronchus intended for intubation, and then slide the tube distally using the fiberscope as a guide until resistance is met. If the trachea was easy to intubate, instead of remanipulating the tube within the patient, the tube can be removed from the patient entirely, and the procedure repeated. A right-sided tube will almost always go to the right side, but a left-sided tube will sometimes pass to the right side. A left-sided tube should not be allowed to remain in the right side, because there is no opening for the right upper lobe bronchus on a left-sided tube. Rotating

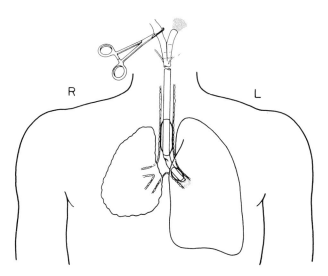

FIGURE 15.1 Left endobronchial tube properly placed. Separation of lungs achieved.

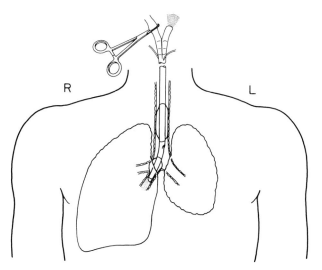

FIGURE 15.3 Left endobronchial tube inserted into the right bronchus.

the patient's head to the right, as is performed for left endobronchial rigid bronchoscopy, may facilitate passage of the tube to the left side.

Ventilation of the lung while the endobronchial lumen is clamped should provide breath sounds and chest movement only on the side opposite the bronchus intended for intubation, provided the tube has been placed in the appropriate bronchus (Figure 15.4). Inability to ventilate during this maneuver indicates that the tube has been malpositioned and is either too deep in the bronchus or too shallow in the trachea. Deflation of the endobronchial cuff while keeping the endobronchial lumen clamped will allow

ventilation of only one lung if the tube is too deep in the bronchus (Figures 15.5 and 15.6), or bilateral lung ventilation if the tube is too shallow in the trachea (Figures 15.7 and 15.8). Ventilation of the lung contralateral to the position of the endobronchial lumen and only the upper lobe of the side ipsilateral to endobronchial tube placement indicates that the cuff of the endobronchial tube is distal to the upper lobe bronchus and that the tube needs to be withdrawn.

The precise positioning of the tube can be evaluated with the use of a flexible fiberoptic bronchoscope. Passage down the tracheal lumen should reveal the carina and just the proximal tip of the blue cuff of the bronchial lumen at

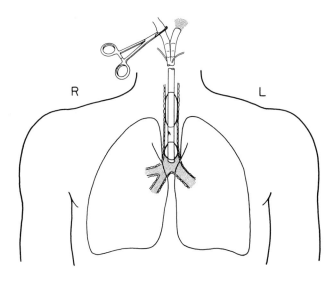

FIGURE 15.2 Left endobronchial tube placed too shallow.

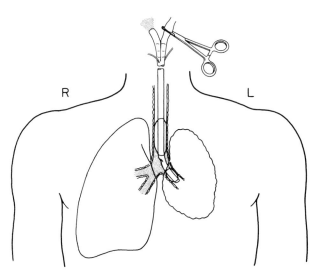

FIGURE 15.4 Left endobronchial tube inserted correctly for right lung ventilation

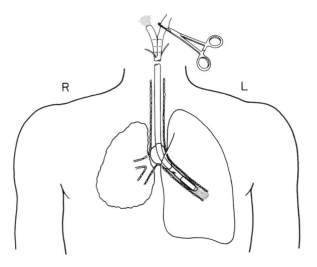

FIGURE 15.5   Left endobronchial tube placed too deeply into the bronchus (both cuffs inflated).

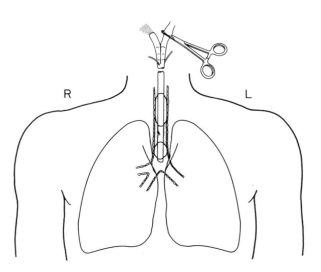

FIGURE 15.7   Left endobronchial tube placed too shallow (both cuffs inflated).

the entrance to the mainstem bronchus. Visualization of the tube passing into the bronchus beyond the carina without observation of the blue bronchial cuff indicates that the tube is positioned too deep into the bronchus. Inspection via the bronchial side should reveal a patent bronchial lumen that is not occluded internally by the cuff. If the tube's distal opening opposes the bronchial wall, ventilation of that lung becomes difficult because double-lumen tubes lack Murphy eyes. Visualization of the bronchial carina indicates that the tube is not placed too deeply. If the tube is right-sided, visualization through the side opening should allow proper alignment with

the right upper lobe bronchus. If, after placing a fiberscope through the tracheal lumen, the carina is not visualized, the tube is probably too shallow, too deep, or located in the unintended bronchus. If the tube is too shallow, then deflation of the bronchial balloon should provide a view of the carina. If the tube is down the contralateral bronchus, then deflation of the bronchial cuff will not demonstrate tracheal carina, but opposite side anatomy will be observed. For example, if a left-sided tube lodges in the right bronchus, then deflation of the bronchial cuff will demonstrate bronchus intermedius (right upper lobe, right middle lobe, and right lower lobe bronchi).

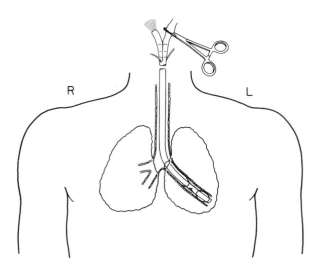

FIGURE 15.6   Left endobronchial tube placed too deeply into the bronchus (endobronchial cuff deflated).

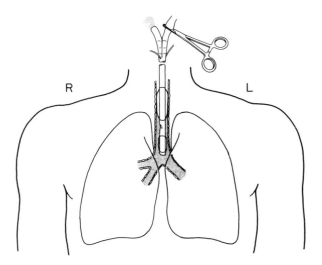

FIGURE 15.8   Left endobronchial tube placed too shallow (endobronchial cuff deflated).

8. What clinical problems are associated with the placement and use of double-lumen endobronchial tubes?

Depending on the type of tube malposition, and the side of surgery, hypoxemia or poor surgical exposure may result. In the case of a bronchopleural fistula, poor separation of the lungs may lead to loss of tidal volume, hypercarbia, and hypoxemia. Poor isolation in the case of hemorrhage or empyema may lead to contamination of the uninvolved lung, which is in the dependent portion during the surgical procedure and thus is prone to contamination that is due to gravity.

Forcing the endobronchial tube too distal or using an excessive volume of air in the bronchial cuff may lead to bronchial hemorrhage and perforation. Rupture may be more likely if the bronchus has been weakened by disease such as a mediastinal tumor. A descending thoracic aortic aneurysm may impinge on the left mainstem bronchus and could possibly be ruptured if an endobronchial tube is forced past this point of resistance. Movement of the tube without deflating the cuff may lead to airway trauma, especially by the endobronchial cuff.

9. What complications are related to placing the patient in the lateral decubitus position?

Pulmonary resection is usually performed with the patient in the lateral decubitus position. The operative lung is placed in the nondependent location. Cardiopulmonary complications of the lateral decubitus position depend mostly on the patient's preoperative condition.

The patient should be well anesthetized and paralyzed before turning them on their side, to prevent coughing, hypertension, and tachycardia. Blood pooling in the dependent portion of the body may lead to hypotension. Flexing the table exacerbates pooling and hypotension. The dependent lung is well perfused, and the nondependent lung is poorly perfused, which is due to gravitational effects on the distribution of pulmonary blood flow.

In an awake spontaneously breathing patient the dependent lung is better ventilated than the nondependent lung, which is due to more efficient contraction of the dependent hemidiaphragm. Greater curve (stretch) is present in the dependent diaphragm, which is due to abdominal contents pushing cephalad. In the anesthetized and paralyzed patient, most of the ventilation is distributed to the nondependent lung, while perfusion remains preferentially diverted to the dependent lung, creating a ventilation–perfusion mismatch. Reduction of lung volume that is due to induction of anesthesia moves the nondependent lung to a more compliant portion of the pressure–volume curve. With paralysis of the diaphragm, the abdominal contents impede movement of the dependent lung to a greater extent than the nondependent lung. Opening the chest further improves the compliance of the nondependent lung, thereby improving its

> ## Complications Associated with the Lateral Decubitus Position for Thoracic Surgery
>
> Coughing, tachycardia, and hypertension during turn into lateral decubitus position
>
> Hypotension from blood pooling in dependent portions
>
> $\dot{V}/\dot{Q}$ mismatching leading to hypoxemia
>
> Interstitial pulmonary edema of the dependent lung (down-lung syndrome)
>
> Brachial plexus and peroneal nerve injuries
>
> Monocular blindness
>
> Outer ear ischemia
>
> Axillary artery compression

ventilation. Downward pressure from the mediastinum, and pressure from lying on the lateral chest wall, exacerbate impaired dependent lung compliance and ventilation. Rolls beneath the hips and lower axilla lift the chest wall off the table and improve dependent lung ventilation.

Maintaining the lateral decubitus position for a long time leads to transudation of fluid in the dependent lung, causing interstitial pulmonary edema. This is called *down-lung syndrome*. Administrations of large amounts of intravenous fluid increase left atrial pressure and leads to further transudation of fluid.

Peripheral nerve injuries from pressure or stretching may also occur. Padding the lower extremities and placing a low axillary roll help prevent injury to the peroneal nerve and brachial plexus. The dependent eye should remain clear of head supports, and the dependent ear pinna should not be folded over. An arterial catheter in the dependent arm allows for constant monitoring for excessive pressure on the dependent axillary artery.

10. How are pulmonary perfusion and ventilation altered during one-lung ventilation?

During two-lung ventilation in the lateral decubitus position, ventilation is preferentially diverted to the nondependent lung and perfusion is primarily directed to the dependent lung. Once the nondependent lung is collapsed,

'Ventilation and Perfusion Effects During One-Lung Anesthesia

Lateral decubitus position

Two-lung ventilation
  Ventilation best in nondependent areas
  Perfusion best in dependent areas

Nondependent lung collapsed
  Ventilation eliminated in nondependent lung
    and best in dependent areas
  Perfusion best in dependent area, but residual
    nondependent perfusion results in shunt
  Alveolar hypoxia and other factors initiate HPV
  CO_2 exchange minimally affected

Factors Affecting Hypoxic Pulmonary Vasoconstriction

Factors inhibiting HPV
  High $P\bar{v}O_2$
  Potent inhaled anesthetics (controversial in
    humans)
  Vasodilators (nitroglycerin, nitroprusside)
  β_2-Agonists (isoproterenol)
  Vasoconstrictors (phenylephrine, epinephrine,
    dopamine)
  Pulmonary artery hypertension
  Increased cardiac output
  Calcium channel blockers
  Hypocarbia
  Surgical manipulations
  Cold
  PEEP

Factors that do not appear to alter HPV
  Ketamine
  Opioids
  Benzodiazepines

ventilation to that side is eliminated, but some perfusion persists. Blood passing through the deflated lung does not exchange gas with alveoli and is called *shunted blood*. This unoxygenated (shunted) blood mixes with oxygenated blood from the dependent lung in the pulmonary vein and left atrium. Shunted blood dilutes oxygenated blood, resulting in a significant overall reduction in oxygen tension. In cases where the nondependent lung was mostly healthy preoperatively, its contribution to overall oxygenation is important and loss of its function produces major reductions in oxygenation. When the nondependent lung was significantly impaired preoperatively, its contribution to overall oxygenation is not as great. When its contribution to oxygenation is lost during one-lung anesthesia, expected falls in oxygen tension are not as great. Consequently, one might expect greatest hypoxemia associated with one-lung anesthesia in patients without pulmonary disease, such as during esophageal surgery.

CO_2 exchange is not affected by one-lung ventilation to the same extent as oxygenation.

Fortunately, there is a reduction in pulmonary blood flow to the nondependent lung during one-lung anesthesia, which tends to decrease the shunt fraction. Gravity, surgical compression, and ligation of nondependent pulmonary vessels decrease blood flow to the nondependent lung. Alveolar hypoxia in the nondependent lung from atelectasis stimulates hypoxic pulmonary vasoconstriction (HPV), which leads to further diversion of blood to the dependent (ventilated) lung.

HPV is a local mechanism that constricts pulmonary vessels and diverts blood flow to the better-oxygenated (ventilated) portions of the lung. Continued blood flow to hypoxic lung constitutes true shunt. The stimulus for HPV appears to be related to PO_2 in the mixed venous ($P\bar{v}$) blood, and the alveolar PO_2 (PAO_2). Active HPV can decrease blood flow to hypoxic lung by 50%, thereby decreasing shunt and improving PaO_2.

In numerous in vitro and in vivo animal studies, HPV has been shown to be inhibited by potent inhaled anesthetics; vasodilators (nitroglycerin, nitroprusside, and β_2-agonists such as isoproterenol); surgical manipulation; calcium channel blockers; cold; positive end-expiratory pressure (PEEP); vasoconstrictors (phenylephrine, epinephrine, and dopamine); high $P\bar{v}O_2$; increased cardiac output; hypocarbia; and certain granulomatous infections.

Intravenous agents such as ketamine, opioids, and benzodiazepines do not appear to inhibit HPV. These effects on HPV are difficult to demonstrate in the clinical situation because of the many confounding variables present in patients undergoing surgery. Thus, whether inhaled anesthetics inhibit HPV in humans remains controversial. Cyclo-oxygenase inhibitors (aspirin, ibuprofen, etc.) appear to potentiate HPV in some animal studies, but they have not been evaluated for their possible side-effects on HPV in humans. A potential disadvantage of such agents in the clinical situation is their adverse effect on coagulation.

11. What is the treatment for hypoxemia during one-lung anesthesia?

Ventilation of the dependent lung with large tidal volumes (10–12 mL/kg) is recommended during one-lung anesthesia to prevent atelectasis in the dependent lung.

Treatment of Hypoxemia During One-Lung Ventilation

Ventilate the dependent lung with 10–12 mL/kg tidal volume

Use 100% oxygen

Periodically reinflate nondependent lung with 100% oxygen

Search for causes of hypoxemia
    Double-lumen tube malposition
    Double-lumen tube kinking
    Secretions
    Pneumothorax
    Bronchospasm
    Low cardiac output
    Low FIO_2
    Hypoventilation

Apply CPAP 5–10 cm H_2O to nondependent lung

Apply PEEP 5–10 cm H_2O to dependent lung

Clamp the nondependent pulmonary artery

Increased airway pressures also reduce transudation of fluid from pulmonary capillaries. However, too much of an increase in airway pressure may increase dependent lung pulmonary vascular resistance (PVR) and divert blood flow to the nondependent lung.

Ventilatory rate is adjusted to maintain the $PaCO_2$ near 40 mmHg. This is usually achieved with a rate similar to that employed during two-lung ventilation. One hundred percent oxygen is administered during one-lung ventilation. Large tidal volumes can prevent absorption atelectasis, which tends to occur with the use of high FIO_2 levels. The benefits of 100% oxygen generally outweigh the possible risks of its use. Patients at risk for oxygen toxicity should receieve the lowest FIO_2 compatible with adequate oxygenation.

Temporarily reinflating and ventilating the nondependent lung with 100% oxygen rapidly corrects sudden and precipitous drops in arterial saturation. Possible causes for hypoxia should be sought and corrected. These etiologies include malposition of the double-lumen endobronchial tube, kinking of the tube, secretions, pneumothorax of the dependent lung, bronchospasm, low cardiac output, low FIO_2, and hypoventilation.

In the absence of an identifiable cause for hypoxemia, shunting of blood through the nondependent lung is likely to be responsible. Therefore, 5–10 cm H_2O of continuous positive airway pressure (CPAP) should be applied to the nondependent lung. This maneuver has been shown to increase PaO_2 during one-lung ventilation. CPAP to the nondependent lung opens alveoli so that they can participate in gas exchange and allows oxygenation of blood passing through the nondependent lung. Ten centimeters of water pressure expands the lung by only 100 mL, a relatively small volume. Insufflation of oxygen at zero airway pressure does not improve PaO_2, and using greater than 10 cm H_2O CPAP may lead to interference with surgical exposure. CPAP is usually effective in restoring the PaO_2 to a safe level.

If functional residual capacity (FRC) is low, PEEP to the dependent lung may improve oxygenation by returning FRC toward normal and by lowering PVR in the dependent lung. Further increase of FRC, however, may increase dependent lung PVR and decrease blood flow to the dependent lung. If CPAP to the nondependent lung is ineffective in improving PaO_2, 5–10 cm H_2O of PEEP to the dependent lung can be used in addition.

Other treatment modalities include intermittent ventilation of the nondependent lung with oxygen and clamping the nondependent pulmonary artery to eliminate shunting.

12. Describe the role of a thoracostomy tube following pulmonary resection, and describe the system used for pleural drainage.

Before chest closure, thoracostomy tubes are placed to drain air and fluid as well as to keep remaining lung tissue expanded. One tube is placed anteriorly at the apex for air drainage, and another is placed posteriorly for fluid drainage. The chest tubes are connected to underwater seals with negative 15–20 cm H_2O pressure (suction). Inadequate suction may lead to tension pneumothorax if the rate of air removal from the pleural space is less than the rate of air leakage into the pleural space. In this case, an underwater seal without suction would be safer. Thoracostomy tubes are usually not placed following pneumonectomy because there is no remaining lung tissue to re-expand.

13. Describe a commonly used pleural drainage system.

Different drainage systems are in use. The most commonly employed disposable system is a modification of the three-bottle system. It consists of a water seal, a low-negative-pressure water limiter bottle, and a dry trap. The low-negative-pressure water limiter bottle prevents application of excess pressure by allowing entrainment of atmospheric air. Use of only a dry trap bottle (single-bottle system) allows for reversal of air flow into the pleural space and for contamination of the suction source.

Clamping the chest tube is dangerous because it may lead to accumulation of air and fluid in the chest. Elevation of the underwater seal bottle above the patient allows water to flow into the pleural space. Patency of the chest tube is maintained by "milking" and "stripping" (squeezing the tube toward and away from the chest, respectively).

14. Discuss potential post-thoracotomy complications.

Respiratory failure may occur following thoracic surgery. Atelectasis is the most common cause for a decrease in oxygenation postoperatively, and respiratory failure is the most common serious complication. Patients presenting for thoracic surgery typically have a history of cigarette smoking and preoperative lung disease, which is a risk factor.

Respiratory failure may be due to pulmonary edema, which can be cardiogenic or noncardiogenic in origin. Re-expansion pulmonary edema is usually unilateral, and may occur after removal of large amounts of fluid or air from the pleural space. The etiology may be related to increased capillary permeability occurring with atelectasis in conjunction with rapid re-expansion.

There is a high incidence of dysrhythmias following thoracic surgery. Sinus tachycardia, atrial fibrillation, and supraventricular tachycardia are the most common dysrhythmias. Possible etiologies include cardiac manipulation, right atrial distention from pulmonary hypertension, or hypoxemia, especially in the setting of pre-existing cardiac disease.

Right heart failure may occur following pneumonectomy. This can be due to an increase in right ventricular afterload and/or decrease in right ventricular contractility. If the pulmonary vasculature is normal and distensible, the remaining lung can accommodate all of the pulmonary blood flow, with only a small increase in pulmonary artery pressure. If there is a large increase in pressure, the right ventricle is prone to failure due to its relatively thin wall. Traditional treatment includes vasodilation and inotropic support, including catecholamines and phosphodiesterase inhibitors. Nitric oxide is beneficial in treating pulmonary hypertension following pneumonectomy. Nitric oxide does not have a systemic effect.

Cardiac herniation is a rare complication, but may occur following intrapericardial pneumonectomy. The heart may herniate through the pericardial defect into the empty thoracic cavity. Torsion may then impede blood flow and lead to cardiovascular collapse. Torsion usually occurs if there is a right intrapericardial pneumonectomy. The torsion can obstruct the superior vena cava and produce a superior vena cava syndrome. Left-sided cardiac herniation may occur following a left intrapericardial pneumonectomy. The apex of the heart herniates through the defect, and the portion of the ventricle that herniates becomes edematous. This may result in obstruction to flow and ischemia, which can lead to infarction and cardiac arrest.

Following an intrapericardial pneumonectomy, the patient should not be positioned on the side with the operative side dependent. Gravity may pull the heart down through the pericardial defect into the empty hemithorax. If cardiac herniation does occur, the patient should be positioned in the lateral position, with the operative side nondependent, which may improve cardiac function. Surgical treatment is almost always necessary.

Significant postoperative bleeding may occur and is usually diagnosed by quantifying the collection of blood from drainage tubes. Blood loss continuing at a rate greater than 100 mL/h may warrant surgical re-exploration. If bleeding is significant, the blood from the tubes may have a hematocrit above 20%. It is possible for there to be significant blood loss in the absence of drainage of blood from the tubes, if the tubes are clotted. In that case, a tension hemothorax or pneumothorax can occur.

Lobar torsion may occur following thoracic surgery. The chest radiograph may reveal a lobe that is collapsed or

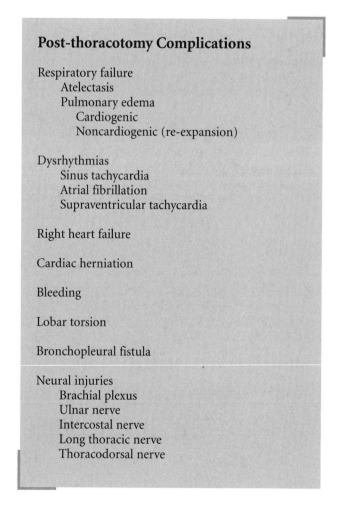

Post-thoracotomy Complications

Respiratory failure
    Atelectasis
    Pulmonary edema
        Cardiogenic
        Noncardiogenic (re-expansion)

Dysrhythmias
    Sinus tachycardia
    Atrial fibrillation
    Supraventricular tachycardia

Right heart failure

Cardiac herniation

Bleeding

Lobar torsion

Bronchopleural fistula

Neural injuries
    Brachial plexus
    Ulnar nerve
    Intercostal nerve
    Long thoracic nerve
    Thoracodorsal nerve

consolidated and in an abnormal position. Immediate surgical correction is necessary. Following rotation of the lobe or lung into the normal position, serosanguinous fluid may then drain into the nonaffected lung portion, which needs to be suctioned. A late diagnosis may result in further lung resection and may lead to death.

There may be an air leak following lung resection. This can be detected by air bubbles in the water seal chamber of the chest tube drainage. A bronchopleural fistula (BPF) is a serious complication which can develop in the first 2 weeks after surgery or, less commonly, may be delayed. A chest tube is necessary to provide adequate drainage, and may also facilitate closure of the BPF. The majority of patients with BPF need surgery during which a double-lumen tube and lung isolation are required.

Neural injuries may occur following thoracic surgery. These can result from positioning, or surgical trauma. There can be brachial plexus or ulnar nerve injury from compression due to positioning. Surgery can lead to trauma to the intercostal, long thoracic, or thoracodorsal nerves. Most nerve injuries due to positioning typically resolve, but may take 3–6 months for complete resolution.

SUGGESTED READINGS

Alvarez JM, Panda RK, Newman MA, Slinger P, Deslauriers J, Ferguson M: Postpneumonectomy pulmonary edema. J Cardiothorac Vasc Anesth 17:388, 2003

Benumof JL: Isoflurane anesthesia and arterial oxygenation during one-lung ventilation. Anesthesiology 64:419, 1986

Benumof JL: One-lung ventilation and hypoxic pulmonary vasoconstriction: implications for anesthetic management. Anesth Analg 64:821, 1985

Benumof JL, Augustine SD, Gibbons JA: Halothane and isoflurane only slightly impair arterial oxygenation during one-lung ventilation in patients undergoing thoracotomy. Anesthesiology 67:910, 1987

Benumof JL, Partridge BL, Salvatiena C, et al.: Margin of safety in positioning modern double lumen endobronchial tubes. Anesthesiology 67:729, 1987

Brodsky JB, Adkins MO, Gaba DM: Bronchial cuff pressures of double-lumen tubes. Anesth Analg 69:608, 1989

Brodsky JB, Mark JBD: A simple technique for accurate placement of double-lumen endobronchial tubes. Anesth Rev 1:26, 1983

Brodsky JB, Shulman MS, Mark JBD: Malposition of left-sided double-lumen endobronchial tubes. Anesthesiology 62:667, 1985

Buniva P, Aluffi A, Rescigno G, Rademacher J, Nazari S: Cardiac herniation and torsion after partial pericardiectomy during right pneumonectomy. Tex Heart Inst J 28:73, 2001

Cable DG, Deschamps C, Allen MS, et al.: Lobar torsion after pulmonary resection: presentation and outcome. J Thorac Cardiovasc Surg 122:1091, 2001

Campos JH: Lung separation techniques. pp. 159–173. In Kaplan JA, Slinger PD (eds): Thoracic Anesthesia, 3rd edition. Churchill Livingstone, Philadelphia 2003.

Cohen JA, Denesio RA, Richards TS, et al.: Hazardous placement of a Robertshaw-type endobronchial tube. Anesth Analg 65:100, 1986

Eisenkraft JB: Effects of anesthetics on the pulmonary circulation. Br J Anaesth 65:63, 1990

Eisenkraft JB, Cohen E, Neustein SM: Anesthesia for thoracic surgical procedures. pp. 813–851. In Barash PG, Cullen BF, Stoelting RR (eds): Clinical Anesthesia, 4th edition. JB Lippincott, Philadelphia, 2001

Eisenkraft JB, Raemer DB: Monitoring gases in the anesthesia delivery system. pp. 201–220. In Ehrenwerth J, Eisenkraft JB (eds): Anesthesia Equipment: Principles and Applications. Mosby Year Book, St. Louis, 1993

Felson B: Lung torsion: radiographic findings in nine cases. Radiology 162:631, 1987

Fujiwara M, Abe K, Mashimo T: The effect of positive end-expiratory pressure and continuous positive airway pressure on the oxygenation and shunt fraction during one-lung ventilation with propofol anesthesia. J Clin Anesth 13: 473, 2001

Good ML, Gravenstein N: Capnography. pp. 237–248. In Ehrenwerth J, Eisenkraft JB (eds): Anesthesia Equipment: Principles and Applications. Mosby Year Book, St. Louis, 1993

Grichnik KP, McLvor W, Slinger PD: Intraoperative Management of thoracotomy. pp. 132–158. In Kaplan JA, Slinger PD (eds): Thoracic Anesthesia, 3rd edition, Churchill Livingstone, Philadelphia, 2003

Hansen M, Hoyt J: Postoperative complications. pp. 384–422. In Cohen E (ed): The Practice of Thoracic Anesthesia. JB Lippincott, Philadelphia, 1995

Hastori N, Takeshima S, Aoki T, et al.: Effectiveness of prostaglandin E_1 on pulmonary hypertension and right cardiac function induced by single-lung ventilation and hypoventilation. Ann Thorac Cardiovasc Surg 6:236, 2000

Igbal M, Multz AS, Rossoff LJ, Lackner RP: Reexpansion pulmonary edema after VATS successfully treated with continuous positive airway pressure. Ann Thorac Surg 70:669, 2000

Katz JA, Laverne RG, Fairley HB, et al.: Pulmonary oxygen exchange during endobronchial anesthesia: effect of tidal volume and PEEP. Anesthesiology 56:164, 1982

Kim EA, Lee KS, Shim YM, et al.: Radiographic and CT findings in complications following pulmonary resection. Radiographics 22:67, 2002

Lindberg LG, Lennmarken C, Vegfors M: Pulse oximetry – clinical implications and recent technical developments. Acta Anaesthesiologica Scand 39:279–287, 1995

Neustein SM, Cohen E: Preoperative evaluation of thoracic surgical patients. pp. 181. In Cohen E (ed): The Practice of Thoracic Anesthesia. JB Lippincott, Philadelphia, 1995

Neustein SM, Kahn P, Krellenstein D, Cohen E: Incidence of arrhythmias after thoracic surgery: thoracotomy versus video-assisted thoracoscopy. J Cardiothorac Vasc Anesth 12:659, 1998

Nurozler F, Argenziano M, Ginsburg ME: Nitric oxide usage after posttraumatic pneumonectomy. Ann Thorac Surg 71:364, 2001

Schamaun M: Postoperative pulmonary torsion: report of a case and survey of the literature including spontaneous and post-traumatic torsion. Thorac Cardiovasc Surg 42:116, 1994

Slinger P, Johnston M: Preoperative assessment for pulmonary resection. J Cardiothorac Vasc Anesth 14:202, 2000

Thompson DS, Read RC: Rupture of the trachea following endotracheal intubation. JAMA 204:995, 1968

Tornvall SS, Jackson KH, Oyanedel TEO: Tracheal rupture, complication of cuffed endotracheal tube. Chest 59:237, 1971

Triantafillov AN, Benumof JL, Lecamwasam, HS. Physiology of the lateral decubitus position. pp. 71–94. In: Kaplan JA, Slinger PD (eds): Thoracic Anesthesia, 3rd edition. Churchill Livingstone, Phildelphia, 2003

Yanagidate F, Dohi S, Hamaya T, Tsujito T: Reexpansion pulmonary edema after thoracoscopic mediastinal tumor resection. Anesth Analg 92:1416, 2001

Yokota K, Yasukawa T, Kimura M, et al.: Right heart failure in the setting of hemorrhagic shock after pneumonectomy: successful treatment with percutaneous cardiopulmonary bypass. Anesth Analg 85:1268, 1997

THORACOSCOPY

Steven M. Neustein, MD

James B. Eisenkraft, MD

A 60-year-old man with a long history of cigarette smoking presents for video-assisted thoracoscopy (VAT) and wedge resection of a mass in the upper lobe of the right lung.

QUESTIONS

1. What types of operations can be done with VAT?
2. What are the advantages of performing the surgery utilizing VAT in comparison with traditional thoracotomy?
3. What anesthetic techniques can be utilized for VAT?
4. How can hypoxemia due to shunting during one-lung ventilation be treated?
5. What complications can occur with VAT?

1. What types of operations can be done with VAT?

Minimally invasive thoracic surgery can be achieved with video-assisted thoracoscopy (VAT). Typically, three to five small incisions (portals) are created to allow entry of instruments, including the camera, which is connected to a monitor, into the thoracic cavity.

VAT can be used for biopsy of intrathoracic structures, such as lung masses, pleura, and mediastinal masses. If the biopsy of the lung nodule is positive for cancer, the surgeon can then proceed with an open thoracotomy for a more extensive resection, such as a pneumonectomy. A lung lobectomy can also be performed via VAT. Other lung surgery that can be performed with VAT includes resection of bullae, treatment of pneumothorax or empyema, and diagnosis and treatment of thoracic trauma.

Esophageal surgery can be performed with VAT. This includes esophagomyotomy for achalasia, although this can be performed from the abdominal approach with laparoscopy and thoracoscopy. Traditionally, the Ivor Lewis esophagectomy was accomplished through the use of laparotomy and right thoracotomy incisions.

Pericardial surgery can be done with VAT. This includes pericardiectomy as treatment for pericardial effusion. Excision of a pericardial cyst and "takedown" of the internal mammary artery for coronary artery bypass grafting can also be accomplished with VAT.

2. What are the advantages of performing the surgery utilizing VAT in comparison with traditional thoracotomy?

VAT entails small incisions, compared with a much larger thoracotomy incision. Surgery via thoracotomy incision also requires cutting across chest wall muscles. The ribs are usually spread apart, allowing access to the thoracic cavity. In some thoracotomy cases, however, it is necessary to resect a rib to achieve adequate access. This is sutured back together prior to chest closure.

VAT is followed by less pain and respiratory impairment than open thoracotomy. Therefore, patients are discharged home earlier following VAT surgery. There is also a high incidence of dysrhythmias following thoracic surgery, which may be partially related to postoperative pain. The use of epidural analgesia is very effective for postoperative pain treatment, and may lead to a lower incidence of dysrhythmias.

3. What anesthetic techniques can be utilized for VAT?

VAT is usually performed under general anesthesia. It is essential to provide excellent lung deflation and maintain oxygenation using one-lung ventilation. With a thoracotomy incision, the surgeon can manually retract the lung if necessary, and has greater access and exposure. Under VAT, if the lung is not fully deflated, it is difficult for the surgeon to operate on the lung using the thoracoscopic instruments and it may be difficult to locate the lung nodule. If the pneumothorax is inadequate, the surgeon will have too small a working space. Inadequate surgical exposure may then necessitate a thoracotomy incision, which is associated with a higher incidence of morbidity and mortality.

One-lung ventilation can most reliably be achieved with a double-lumen endobronchial tube, which allows for lung deflation by egress of gas through the lumen of the tube. As soon as the patient is turned to the lateral decubitus position, and the position of the tube is rechecked, the lung to be operated on is deflated, and one-lung ventilation is instituted.

An alternative to the double-lumen tube is a single-lumen tube, with a bronchial blocker, or a Univent® tube, which is a single-lumen tube that incorporates a blocker and a channel for the blocker. Prior to inflating the blocker, the breathing circuit should be disconnected, and the tracheal tube suctioned to facilitate deflation of the lungs. If the lung is not allowed to deflate prior to inflation of the bronchial blocker, it will take a long time for lung deflation to occur. Next the blocker is inflated, and ventilation is resumed. If a Fogarty embolectomy catheter is used as the blocker, the pathway for gas egress from the operated lung is completely occluded.

An alternative to the Fogarty embolectomy catheter is the Arndt blocker, which is a blocker specifically designed for use in the bronchi. The Arndt blocker has a lumen, which passes through the balloon to the tip of the catheter. There is a wire through the lumen, which protrudes beyond the distal tip, and ends in a loop. A fiberscope is passed through the loop and positioned in the bronchus to be blocked. The blocker is then advanced. Once the wire is removed from the catheter, it cannot be reinserted.

A blocker that has been recently introduced into practice is the Cohen blocker. This blocker contains a wheel at the proximal end that bends the tip of the blocker when it is turned. This blocker also contains a lumen. However, the lumens of the Arndt and the Cohen blockers are much smaller than the lumen of a double-lumen tube, resulting in a much slower lung deflation.

VAT may be performed to evaluate and/or treat pleural disease, such as in a patient with a pneumothorax or a pleural effusion. A pleural biopsy and pleurodesis may be planned. In these cases, it may be possible to perform the surgery under epidural anesthesia or intercostal blocks; a general anesthetic may not be necessary. If surgery is performed under a regional block in a spontaneously breathing patient, the lung will collapse when the chest (pleural cavity) is opened.

4. How can hypoxemia due to shunting during one-lung ventilation be treated?

During an open thoracotomy, the most effective treatment for hypoxemia during one-lung ventilation is the administration of continuous positive airways pressure (CPAP) with oxygen to the nondependent (collapsed) lung. The CPAP does lead to some distention of the lung, which is not usually a problem during an open thoracotomy if the amount of CPAP is small (e.g., 5 cm H_2O). However, during VAT, even a small amount of CPAP can make it difficult for the surgeon to operate.

An alternative to the application of CPAP to the nondependent lung is positive end-expiratory pressure (PEEP) to the dependent ventilated lung. PEEP will help to prevent atelectasis that may worsen shunting.

During one-lung ventilation, 100% oxygen is administered. In some cases, the patient may have received chemotherapeutic agents, such as bleomycin, which may predispose them to pulmonary oxygen toxicity. In these

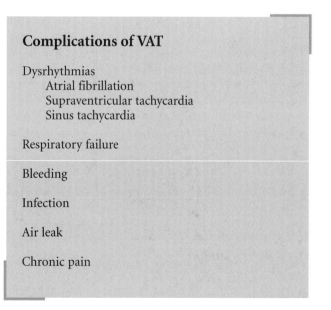

Complications of VAT

Dysrhythmias
    Atrial fibrillation
    Supraventricular tachycardia
    Sinus tachycardia

Respiratory failure

Bleeding

Infection

Air leak

Chronic pain

cases, 100% oxygen should still be administered at the onset of one-lung ventilation, and then the FIO_2 may be reduced, as tolerated, according to pulse oximetry (SpO_2) monitoring.

It may be necessary to accept a lower SpO_2 during VAT, due to the reduced ability to provide treatment. Thus, a balance must be struck between the surgical need for a deflated lung and the oxygenation needs of the patient.

5. What complications can occur with VAT?

There is a high incidence of dysrhythmias following thoracic surgery via open thoracotomy. Dysrhythmias may also occur following VAT, and may include atrial fibrillation, supraventricular tachycardia (SVT), and sinus tachycardia. Elderly patients and patients who are receiving digoxin preoperatively may be at greater risk. Risk factors for postoperative SVT are significant surgical bleeding and increased tricuspid valve regurgitation as seen on echocardiography. The use of epidural analgesia for postoperative pain treatment may be associated with a decrease in the incidence of dysrhythmias.

Patients may also experience respiratory failure after VAT, although this is usually more common following thoracotomy with more extensive resection. Patients with significant pre-existing pulmonary dysfunction, which can be identified with preoperative pulmonary function testing, are particularly at risk. The pain following VAT is usually minimal, which produces less respiratory impairment than would a thoracotomy incision.

Other potential complications include bleeding, infection, and air leak. Although not as common as following thoracotomy, there may be chronic pain following VAT.

SUGGESTED READINGS

Ali A, Pellegrini CA: Laparoscopic myotomy: technique and efficacy in treating achalasia. Gastrointest Endosc Clin North Am 11:347–358, 2001

Amar D, Roistacher N, Burt M, et al.: Clinical and echocardiographic correlates of symptomatic tachydysrhythmias after noncardiac thoracic surgery. Chest 108:349–354, 1995

Bauer C, Winter C, Hentz JG, Ducrocq X, Steib A, Dupeyron JP: Bronchial blocker compared to double-lumen tube for one-lung ventilation during thoracoscopy. Acta Anaesthesiol Scand 45:250–254, 2001

Bolotin G, Lazarovici H, Uretzky G, Zlotnick AY, Tamir A, Saute M: The efficacy of intraoperative internal intercostal nerve block during video-assisted thoracic surgery on postoperative pain. Ann Thorac Surg 70:1872–1875, 2000

Luketich JD, Fernando HC, Christie NA, Buenaventura PO, Keenan RJ, Ikramuddin S, Schauer PR: Outcomes after minimally invasive esophagomyotomy. Ann Thorac Surg 72:1909–1912, 2001

Neustein SM, Kahn P, Krellenstein DJ, Cohen E: Incidence of arrhythmias after thoracic surgery: thoracotomy versus video-assisted thoracoscopy. J Cardiothor Vasc Anesth 12:659–661, 1998

Nguyen NT, Follette DM, Lemoine PH, Roberts PF, Goodnight JE Jr: Minimally invasive Ivor Lewis esophagectomy. Ann Thorac Surg 72:593–596, 2001

Shah JS, Bready LL: Anesthesia for thoracoscopy. Anesthesiol Clin North Am 19:153–171, 2001

Yim AP, Lee TW, Issat MG, Wan S: Place of video-thoracoscopy in thoracic surgical practice. World J Surg 25:157–161, 2001

17

INTRACRANIAL MASS, INTRACRANIAL PRESSURE, VENOUS AIR EMBOLISM, AND AUTOREGULATION

Irene P. Osborn, MD

A 63-year-old woman with a brain tumor presents for bifrontal craniotomy in the supine position. She is neurologically intact but has had a recent onset of headaches, nausea, and blurred vision. The magnetic resonance imaging (MRI) scan has revealed a large meningioma near the sagittal sinus. Following induction of anesthesia and the start of surgery, the end-tidal carbon dioxide (ETCO$_2$) starts to decrease and the patient becomes hypotensive.

QUESTIONS

1. What is cerebral autoregulation?
2. What factors contribute to increased intracranial pressure (ICP)?
3. How do anesthetic agents and vasoactive drugs affect cerebral blood flow (CBF) and ICP?
4. What are the signs and symptoms of increased ICP?
5. How is ICP monitored?
6. How is increased ICP treated?
7. How is venous air embolism (VAE) detected and treated?
8. What are the contraindications to the sitting position?
9. How would you induce and maintain anesthesia in this patient?

1. What is cerebral autoregulation?

Cerebral autoregulation is the control process by which cerebral blood flow (CBF) is maintained constant over a wide range of cerebral perfusion pressures (CPP) (Figure 17.1). CPP represents the difference between mean arterial pressure (MAP) and ICP. Autoregulation adjusts cerebral vessel caliber as CPP changes. Normal CBF is 45–65 ml/100 g of brain tissue per minute. It is coupled to alterations in cerebral metabolic rate, which is linked to oxygen consumption (CMRO$_2$). CBF parallels the changes in CMRO$_2$. Several parameters affect CBF.

Autoregulation maintains CBF between a CPP of 50 and 150 mmHg. Below 50 mmHg, cerebral blood vessels achieve maximal dilation; resistance to flow is low; and CBF falls in direct proportion to CPP. Chronically hypertensive patients undergo an upward shift of autoregulation to higher perfusion pressures. Consequently, these patients require higher CPP to maintain normal CBF. At the upper level of autoregulation, cerebral blood vessels are maximally constricted, and CBF will rise linearly with increasing CPP. Integrity of the blood–brain barrier (BBB) is lost at these high pressures; transudation of fluid occurs; and cerebral edema forms. Autoregulatory compensation generally occurs over 1–3 minutes.

The second parameter affecting CBF is arterial carbon dioxide tension (PaCO$_2$). Increasing levels of PaCO$_2$

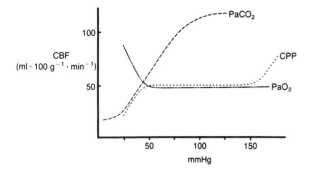

FIGURE 17.1   Effects of $PaCO_2$, PaO_2, and cerebral perfusion pressure (CPP) on cerebral blood flow (CBF). (From Bode, 1990, by permission of Mayo Foundation.)

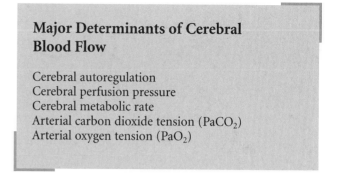

produce elevated levels of extracellular hydrogen ion concentrations, which induce cerebral vessel smooth muscle relaxation and vasodilation. Consequently, cerebral vascular resistance falls, increasing CBF by as much as twofold. This effect plateaus at a $PaCO_2$ of approximately 80 mmHg. Conversely, decreasing $PaCO_2$ increases cerebral vasoconstriction and CBF decreases. At a $PaCO_2$ of 20 mmHg, cerebral vasoconstriction is maximal and CBF decreases by 50%. Further decreases in $PaCO_2$ have no greater vacoconstricting influence. These physiologic principles remain in effect for several hours, after which cerebral spinal fluid (CSF) bicarbonate levels drop to compensate for the induced CSF alkalosis. Once CSF pH returns toward normal, respiratory alkalosis no longer provokes cerebral vasoconstriction. The $PaCO_2$ response at the limits of autoregulation can be blunted. If CPP is low and cerebral vessels are maximally dilated, lowering $PaCO_2$ will have little beneficial effect on cerebral vascular resistance.

The third parameter affecting CBF is arterial oxygen tension (PaO_2). At a PaO_2 below 50 mmHg, CBF rises linearly with falling PaO_2. Local accumulation of acidic metabolites such as lactate results in cerebral vasodilation. In contradistinction, hyperoxia has no effect on cerebral vascular tone.

2. What factors contribute to increased intracranial pressure (ICP)?

The cranial vault contains brain tissue, blood, and CSF. It has a fixed volume with one exit, the foramen magnum. A small increase in its contents alters ICP minimally, because compensation occurs by decreasing CSF and blood volumes. Once compensatory mechanisms have been exhausted, however, intracranial compliance falls dramatically and ICP rises above its normal range of 5–13 mmHg. At this point, any increase in the volume of the three intracranial components has a profound effect on increasing ICP.

Brain tissue volume increases by two mechanisms. Tumors enlarge the parenchymal tissue volume, and surrounding edema increases brain water content. Both contribute to expanding total intracranial mass, which can be compounded by hemorrhage into or around the neoplasm.

CSF is contained in the subarachnoid space of the central nervous system and in the ventricles within the brain. In adults, total CSF volume approximates 150 ml, and daily production is approximately 600 ml. Enough CSF is synthesized to replace itself three to four times a day. CSF is formed in the choroid plexus and the ventricles within the brain. Production is reduced by decreased CPP and increased ICP, but the latter effect is minimal. Absorption of CSF occurs at the microscopic villi of the subarachnoid membrane. The rate of absorption is a balance between two interrelated factors: CSF pressure and resistance to absorption. Resistance to absorption decreases dramatically as CSF pressure rises above 30 mmHg. This appears to represent a closed loop venting mechanism to prevent excessive increases in ICP. Therefore, the amount of CSF present is determined by the balance between production and reabsorption.

Changes in cerebral blood volume usually have little effect on ICP. When intracranial compliance is low, however, and intracranial volume has increased to critical levels, then these changes may have dramatic consequences.

3. How do anesthetic agents and vasoactive drugs affect cerebral blood flow (CBF) and ICP?

The effects of anesthetic agents and vasoactive drugs are multifactorial (Table 17.1). They are described assuming normal brain anatomy and physiology, which is not commonly the situation for the neurosurgical patient. The potent inhaled anesthetics are generally cerebral vasodilators, which attenuate cerebral autoregulation. Inhalation anesthetics produce increases in CBF in a dose-dependent manner while producing progressive depression of cerebral metabolism. The mechanism by which inhalation anesthetics produce vasodilation is not clearly understood. Mechanisms that partially explain the vasodilation include effects on nitric oxide (NO) and ATP-dependent potassium channels.

| TABLE 17.1 | Some Central Nervous System Effects of Anesthetic Agents and Adjuvants |

Agent	Effect	Agent	Effect
Potent inhalation agents	Lowers $CMRO_2$ Increases cerebral blood flow by vasodilatation; this effect is prevented by prior hyperventilation	Curare	Decreases MAP Cerebral vasodilator
		Pancuronium	Increases heart rate Increases MAP
Desflurane	Similar to isoflurane, rapid uptake	Vecuronium[a]	No significant effects
Enflurane	Increases CSF production Decreases CSF reabsorption	Atracurium	Large bolus doses may release histamine, predispoing to decreased MAP and cerebral vasodilatation
Halothane	Decreases CSF production Decreases CSF reabsorption	Alfentanil	Decreases MAP Decreases CPP
Isoflurane[a]	No effect on CSF production Increases CSF reabsorption May protect from ischemia	Fentanyl[a]	With normal or low $PaCO_2$ plus N_2O, decreases $CMRO_2$, decreases CBF With increased $PaCO_2$, cerebral vasodilator
Sevoflurane	Autoregulation maintained at 1.5 MAC		
Nitrous oxide[a]	No change in $CMRO_2$, CSF production, or CSF reabsorption Cerebral vasodilating effects inhibited by hyperventilation Expands intradural air Expands venous air emboli	Remifentanil	Decrease in MAP, no change in ICP, very short-acting Increases CSF reabsorption
		Sufentanil	Decreases CVR Increases CBF
Barbiturates[a]	Decreases $CMRO_2$ Decreases CBF Cerebral vasoconstrictor Decreases CSF production Increases CSF reabsorption	Lidocaine	Low dose: Decreases CBF, and decreases $CMRO_2$ High dose: Increases CBF, and increases $CMRO_2$
Ketamine	Increases ICP Increases CBF Increases MAP No change in $CMRO_2$ No change in CSF production Decreases CSF reabsorption	Sodium nitroprusside	No effect on CBF despite cerebral vasodilation Decreases MAP Increases CBV
		Nitroglycerin	Increases CBF Increases CBV Decreases MAP
Etomidate[a]	Similar to barbiturates Myoclonus indistinguishable from seizures	Hydralazine	Increases CBF Increases CBV Decreases MAP Onset 10–20 minutes
Benzodiazepines[a]	Decreases CBF Decreases $CMRO_2$	Labetalol[a]	Decreases MAP No effect on CBV
Propofol	Decreases MAP		
Succinylcholine	Increases $CMRO_2$ Increases CBF Increases muscle spindle activity diminished by pretreatment with a nondepolarizing neuromuscular blocker		

Abbreviations: CBF, cerebral blood flow; CBV, cerebral blood volume; $CMRO_2$, cerebral metabolic rate of oxygen consumption; CPP, cerebral perfusion pressure; CVR, cerebral vascular resistance; CSF, cerebrospinal fluid; ICP, intracranial pressure; MAP, mean arterial pressure.
[a]Recommended for patients with increased ICP.

Isoflurane increases CBF in a dose-dependent fashion, but increases in subcortical CBF are greater than neo-cortical. CO_2 reactivity is maintained but is greater in the awake state. Autoregulation is adequately maintained at 1 MAC (minimal alveolar concentration) but is progressively impaired by higher concentrations. Sevoflurane has very similar CBF effects to isoflurane, although it appears to produce slightly less vasodilation and autoregulation in humans is maintained up to 1.5 MAC. Desflurane produces an increase in CBF similar to that seen with isoflurane but greater than that seen with sevoflurane at >1 MAC. Autoregulation is progressively abolished as the dose increases. Nitrous oxide (N_2O) is used in many neurosurgical anesthetics. Although it is a cerebral vasodilator, this effect is diminished by hyperventilation, barbiturates, and moderate concentrations of potent inhalation agents. When administered on its own, N_2O increases both CBF and metabolism. However, when added to the background of another anesthetic, it increases CBF without changing metabolism.

Most of the intravenous anesthetics are cerebral vaso-constrictors and maintain the relationship between $CMRO_2$ and CBF. Barbiturates, notably thiopental, reduce $CMRO_2$ primarily and CBF secondarily. Thiopental acts as a cerebral vasoconstrictor. CO_2 reactivity is maintained but is quantitatively reduced compared with the awake state. Cerebral autoregulation is also maintained intact. Thiopental is an excellent drug to acutely lower ICP; however, amounts sufficient to induce an isoelectric electroencephalogram (EEG) can produce significant hemodynamic side-effects.

Ketamine causes a significant rise in CBF without an important effect on metabolic rate. It is not considered a wise choice in the neurosurgical setting. However, small to moderate doses in a background of volatile anesthetic or intravenous infusion have not been shown to be significantly harmful. The trauma patient with hypovolemia and concurrent injuries may be a suitable candidate for ketamine as blood pressure and CPP may be more easily maintained. Etomidate behaves similarly to thiopental and is an appropriate induction agent for patients who cannot tolerate the hemodynamic effects seen with thiopental. Myoclonus, which occurs after etomidate administration, may be difficult to differentiate from seizure activity. Benzodiazepines offer beneficial effects on elevated ICP by lowering CBF and diminishing $CMRO_2$, without meaningful effects on CSF dynamics.

Propofol is a short-acting intravenous agent used for induction and maintenance of anesthesia. It appears to maintain the relationship between CBF and $CMRO_2$. Propofol does not cause cerebral vasodilation and does not interfere with the normal response to $PaCO_2$. It can be used to supplement anesthesia during long operations or as part of a total intravenous technique. It is particularly useful for, and may be a good choice for, neurodiagnostic procedures, keeping in mind that it produces dose-dependent decreases in blood pressure.

Muscle relaxants have no direct intracerebral effects because they do not cross the BBB. Nevertheless, they possess indirect effects because of their actions in the periphery, which are sometimes significant. There is clear evidence from both experimental animals and humans that succinylcholine can increase ICP under conditions of intracranial hypertension. The magnitude of the increase is typically small and transient. It has been shown in humans that ICP changes caused by succinylcholine can be blocked by preadministration of a defasciculating dose of a non-depolarizing relaxant. A probable mechanism is the massive fasciculation-induced afferent barrage from muscle spindles to the brain that causes transient increases in metabolic rate and coupled increases in CBF. The decision to use this agent is determined by the need to rapidly secure the airway. Pretreatment with a small dose of a nondepolarizing agent is helpful and recommended.

The nondepolarizing agents such as vecuronium, rocuronium, and cisatracurium have no significant hemodynamic or ICP effects. There is clear evidence that the duration of action of nondepolarizing muscle relaxants is reduced by a variety of anticonvulsant medications. The mechanism remains unclear. Most patients requiring craniotomy are being treated with anticonvulsants and thus the nondepolarizing relaxant dosing regimen will require alteration. Atracurium and cisatracurium seem to be largely resistant to these effects, most likely because metabolism is achieved by Hoffman elimination.

Opioids are known to produce respiratory depression, which results in an increase in $PaCO_2$. Consequently, opioids are administered sparingly in the spontaneously breathing patient with cerebral disease. Opioids at low doses produce very little effect on CBF provided $PaCO_2$ is not allowed to rise. During controlled ventilation with normocapnia or hypocapnia, opioids provide significant advantages. Independently, fentanyl seems to have little effect on CBF or $CMRO_2$, but when combined with N_2O it decreases $CMRO_2$ and CBF, which is due to the hemodynamic changes caused by this combination of anesthetic agents. It increases the rate of CSF reabsorption without affecting its rate of production. There is much controversy about how and whether opioids, such as sufentanil and alfentanil, increase ICP. With cerebral autoregulation intact, a drop in blood pressure results in a compensatory vasodilation to maintain CBF. This increases cerebral blood volume and thus ICP. Remifentanil has become increasingly used in neurosurgery for its rapid onset and offset, and titratability to changing stimuli. However, the lack of residual analgesia requires a plan for postoperative pain relief as well as blood pressure control.

Sodium nitroprusside is a direct-acting smooth muscle relaxant that produces arteriolar and venous dilatation. It is sometimes used in neurosurgery for control of arterial blood pressure. Although it acts as a cerebral vasodilator and decreases MAP, there is little effect on CBF. However, cerebral blood volume is increased and ICP may be elevated. It is best avoided if ICP is high. Thiopental, lidocaine or labetalol should be used instead. Nitroglycerin is primarily a veno-dilator and coronary vasodilator that acts by relaxing smooth muscle and works on the intracerebral venous capacitance vessels. Hydralazine is a direct arteriolar vasodilator with an onset time of 10–20 minutes. It increases cerebral blood volume and may increase ICP when the dura is closed. Labetalol, a mixed α- and β-blocker, lowers MAP by lowering systemic vascular resistance and depressing cardiac output. It has no direct effect on cerebral blood vessels.

4. What are the signs and symptoms of increased ICP?

Gradual, chronic increases in ICP cause few signs and symptoms. Symptoms of acute intracranial hypertension are likely caused by decreased CPP resulting in cerebral ischemia and/or mechanical forces on the brainstem, which thrust intracranial contents through the foramen magnum. These may include headache, nausea or vomiting, and mental status changes. Acute increases in ICP can cause loss of consciousness, hypertension and bradycardia, absent brainstem reflexes, cranial nerve dysfunction, decerebrate posturing, apnea or irregular respiration, fixed and dilated pupils, as well as death due to impaired medullary perfusion.

5. How is ICP monitored?

Ventriculostomy is the most common method of measuring ICP. A catheter is placed through a burr hole and into the anterior horn of a lateral ventricle. Obliteration of

---

Signs and Symptoms of Increased Intracranial Pressure

Signs
    Vomiting
    Mental status changes (drowsiness progressing
      to coma)
    Hypertension
    Bradycardia
    Absent brainstem reflexes
    Cranial nerve dysfunction
    Decerebrate posturing
    Respiratory rhythm changes
    Fixed and dilated pupils

Symptoms
    Headache
    Nausea

---

the ventricle due to tumor or edema may create technical difficulties inserting the catheter. Subdural bolts also serve to measure ICP. These devices are placed via a twist drill hole in the calvarium and a small hole in the dura. They are less invasive than a ventriculostomy and provide only local pressure data instead of global information. Subdural bolts can become infected and lack the potential to withdraw CSF for lowering ICP. Proper positioning requires the bolt's head to be aligned in the same plane as underlying brain. Catheters or electronic transducers placed in the epidural space can also be used for ICP monitoring. Lumbar subarachnoid catheters are occasionally used. The accuracy of these devices is impaired by patient positioning other than horizontal. Abrupt withdrawal of CSF through lumbar subarachnoid catheters risks brain herniation.

6. How is increased ICP treated?

Treatment of increased ICP may begin by changing the patient's position. Recent studies have shown that a change to the reverse Trendelenburg position in anesthetized patients will rapidly reduce ICP. Head elevation promotes drainage of venous blood from the brain and is surprisingly effective at reducing brain bulk. Obstruction of this venous outflow (e.g., by improperly placed tape around the neck, improper positioning of the patient, positive end-expiratory pressure (PEEP), etc.) is often an overlooked cause of increased brain volume. Hyperventilation is the most common means of acutely reducing ICP. Acutely lowering ICP via hyperventilation ($PaCO_2$ reduction) is another method frequently employed in the intubated patient. Hyperventilation is simple to perform and results in rapid and dramatic decreases in ICP. Until recently it was implemented in all patients suspected of having raised ICP, but neuronal ischemia caused by hyperventilation has now been demonstrated in humans. Alteration of $PaCO_2$ within the range of approximately 20–80 mmHg causes parallel changes in CBF.

The two other intracranial compartments, CSF and brain parenchyma, are also amenable to volume reduction. CSF withdrawal can take place through a ventriculostomy, and its production reduced by acetazolamide, a carbonic anhydrase inhibitor. Brain edema may respond to osmotic or loop diuretics, such as mannitol and furosemide respectively. The resulting diuresis reduces intravascular volume and cerebral blood volume. Mannitol's onset of action is approximately 30 minutes and its effect is accelerated by furosemide. Use of osmotic agents requires a globally intact BBB with only minimal areas of disruption.

Struggling or coughing against a tracheal tube should be prevented and is best accomplished via administration of sedative agents such as benzodiazepines, barbiturates, propofol and opioids, as well as muscle relaxants. Prevention of hypertension, tachycardia and straining results in lowering of $CMRO_2$ and CBF.

7. How is venous air embolism (VAE) detected and treated?

VAE is a potentially life-threatening event which must be detected and treated promptly. It is often associated with cases performed in the sitting position but it can occur under certain physiologic circumstances. In neurosurgical procedures, air may enter the venous system via non-collapsible venous channels such as the dural sinuses and diploic veins. When the head is elevated above the heart a pressure gradient can exist which facilitates air entrainment. In the sitting position, the incidence of VAE is almost 4 times higher than the incidence in other positions (45% vs. 12%). Air can also be entrained from the pin sites during a stereotactic biopsy in the semi-sitting position.

Monitoring for VAE generally includes a precordial Doppler, capnometry, central venous pressure (CVP) catheter, pulse oximeter, and esophageal stethoscope. When placed properly, as determined by rapid bolus fluid injection through a CVP catheter, a precordial Doppler can detect 0.1 ml of air. Transesophageal echocardiography (TEE) is also sensitive for detecting and recognizing intracardiac air but is not generally used in this setting due to technical difficulty and cost. The CVP catheter is best located at the junction of the superior vena cava and the right atrium, where air collects after its entrainment into the venous system. It is a diagnostic device for detection or confirmation of VAE, rarely a therapeutic measure. It is of value when aspirating air from the right atrium in the rare instance of massive VAE creating an air lock. Multiorifice catheters are more efficacious for air aspiration than single-lumen catheters.

Treatment of Increased Intracranial Pressure

Reduce cerebral blood volume
  Raise head, change position
  Hyperventilate to $PaCO_2 = 23–27$ mmHg
  Prevent straining/coughing on the endotracheal tube with sedatives, narcotics, and/or muscle relaxants

Reduce CSF volume
  Drain through ventriculostomy or lumbar sub-arachnoid catheter

Reduce brain water
  Osmotic diuretics (mannitol)
  Loop diuretics (furosemide)
  Steroids (dexamethasone)

Pulmonary artery catheters may provide valuable information because pulmonary artery pressures rise during VAE. Unfortunately, pulmonary artery catheters are less efficient for air aspiration than CVP catheters. Continuous end-tidal carbon dioxide ($ETCO_2$) monitoring demonstrates a rapid decline as VAE ensues. Arterial $PaCO_2$ rises simultaneously, increasing the gradients between these two measurements. The difference rises as alveolar dead space increases. If minute ventilation remains constant, the divergence between $PaCO_2$ and $ETCO_2$ may represent a useful marker for the severity of VAE. Classically, the "mill wheel" murmur heard through an esophageal stethoscope is associated with intracardiac air. Once detected, VAE requires rapid treatment.

Surgeons must be alerted immediately when VAE is detected so that open sinuses may be identified and flooded with saline or closed surgically to halt the entrainment of air. In the absence of an obvious source of air entrainment, venous pressure in the head should be raised in an attempt to force blood through the concealed opening. This is accomplished by lowering the head relative to the heart, manipulating the table's position, or occluding venous outflow from the head with jugular compression. N_2O administration should cease immediately. Rapid diffusion of N_2O into air bubbles will expand their volume, creating mechanical obstruction to flow, and hemodynamic compromise may ensue. Volume, inotropes, and vasopressor administration contribute to hemodynamic support, churning large air pockets into smaller ones to be carried out to the pulmonary blood vessels.

The application of PEEP in an attempt to increase CVP and decrease the magnitude of VAE is controversial. High levels of PEEP greatly increase the risk of hypotension in patients who are already intravascularly depleted. Furthermore, right atrial pressure may be increased in the face of lowered left atrial pressure, predisposing the patient to paradoxical air embolism through a patent foramen ovale. Application of PEEP should probably be limited to situations in which all other attempts at preventing continuous VAE have failed. Even moderate amounts of VAE may result in decreased PaO_2. Initial treatment should be supportive with enhanced inspired oxygen concentrations guided by pulse oximetry and arterial blood gas determinations. Postoperatively, patients may develop an interstitial pulmonary process that usually resolves in 24–48 hours.

8. What are the contraindications to the sitting position?

There are no strict contraindications; however, each patient requires careful evaluation to determine the feasibility of positioning and risks for complications. Specific contraindications involve the presence of a patent foramen ovale or suspected intracardiac shunt. Other conditions which may predispose to development of complications are hemodynamic instability or noted cerebral compromise

Monitors for Detection of Venous Air Embolism

Precordial Doppler
Transesophageal echocardiography
Mass spectrometry (end-tidal N_2)
Capnography ($ETCO_2$)
Pulse oximetry (SpO_2)
Central venous pressure
Pulmonary artery pressure
Esophageal stethoscope

when sitting upright preoperatively. Other concerns involve positioning of the neck, which may compromise spinal cord perfusion in the patient with severe cervical arthritis. The sitting position is being used less frequently today as neurosurgeons attempt to avoid the inherent problems associated with its use. Many surgeons now employ the lateral, prone, or supine position with the head turned.

9. How would you induce and maintain anesthesia in this patient?

The preoperative assessment of this patient includes an evaluation of mental status and determination of acute increased ICP. Co-existing diseases should be optimally treated before arrival in the operating room. The MRI examination reveals a large mass which has slowly increased in size. This patient can be induced in the typical manner with caution to avoid additional increases in ICP. Intravenous anesthetic induction is followed by moderate hyperventilation until neuromuscular blockade is achieved. Thiopental or propofol are commonly used for induction with an opioid, such as fentanyl, to blunt the hemodynamic response to laryngoscopy and intubation. Moderate hyperventilation is achieved to an $ETCO_2$ of 28–30 mmHg. A radial artery catheter and additional intravenous lines may be placed after endotracheal intubation. A CVP catheter is useful but not essential for this case unless required for intravenous access. The potential for blood loss may be considerable and, thus, large-bore intravenous catheters are needed. Mannitol is commonly started at a dose of 0.5–1.0 g/kg.

Maintenance of anesthesia may proceed with low doses of volatile agent (less than 1 MAC), continuous infusion or bolus doses of an opioid and muscle relaxant. N_2O may be administered at a concentration of 50%, if surgical conditions do not indicate a "tight brain". Intravenous fluid administration generally requires isotonic crystalloid solutions; colloids are also useful for maintenance of intravascular volume. Extensive blood loss is replaced with packed red blood cells. Hypotonic solutions exacerbate cerebral edema and are generally contraindicated, while glucose-containing solutions are avoided unless truly necessary.

Neurosurgery is characterized by periods of intense stimulation followed by minimal pain during brain resection. Hypertension may occur and is treated promptly to prevent bleeding and potential cerebral swelling. The use of β-blockers in addition to adequate anesthesia is recommended throughout. Upon closure and emergence, blood pressure control is especially important. Patients who have had an uneventful procedure are expected to emerge promptly at the end of surgery for neurologic evaluation. Extubation is managed carefully, after assurance of airway reflexes and stable hemodynamics. Postoperative respiratory insufficiency adversely affects cerebral physiology.

Acute Treatment of Venous Air Embolism

Notify surgeons to identify open sinuses

Close sinuses surgically or flood field with saline

Increase venous pressure in the head
    Lower head relative to heart
    Place table in Trendelenburg position
    Jugular vein compression
    Positive end-expiratory pressure
      – controversial

Discontinue N_2O administration

Support cardiovascular system
    Volume
    Inotropes
    Vasopressors

SUGGESTED READINGS

Artru A: CSF dynamics, cerebral edema, and intracranial pressure. pp. 61–116. In Albin MS (ed): Textbook of Neuroanesthesia: With Neurosurgical and Neuroscience Perspectives. McGraw-Hill, New York, 1997

Bendo AA, Luba K: Recent changes in the management of intracranial hypertension. Int Anesthesiol Clin 38:69–86, 2000

Bode ET: Neurointensive care. p. 438. In Cuchiara RF, Michenfelder JD: Clinical Neuroanesthesia. Churchill Livingstone, New York, 1990

Smith DS, Osborn IP: Posterior fossa: anesthetic considerations. pp. 340–347. In Cottrell JE, Smith DS (eds): Anesthesia and Neurosurgery, 4th edition. Mosby, St Louis, 2001

Warner DA: Anesthesia for craniotomy. IARS Review Courses, 2004

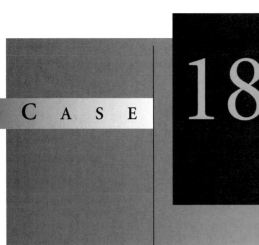

Arthur E. Schwartz, MD

A 55-year-old woman is admitted with severe headache and decreased consciousness, and found to have a subarachnoid hemorrhage from a ruptured intracranial aneurysm.

QUESTIONS

1. How are patients graded following subarachnoid hemorrhage from a ruptured aneurysm?
2. What are the most serious complications following subarachnoid hemorrhage from aneurysm rupture?
3. What are the treatment options?
4. What monitoring is indicated for patients undergoing craniotomy for clipping of intracranial aneurysms?
5. How is arterial blood pressure controlled?
6. What is cerebral vasospasm, and how is it treated?
7. How is aneurysm rupture during aneurysm clipping managed?

1. How are patients graded following subarachnoid hemorrhage from a ruptured aneurysm?

The incidence of subarachnoid hemorrhage is about 10–15 per 100,000 person-years. Angiography shows an intracranial aneurysm as the cause of subarachnoid hemorrhage in 80–85% of patients. Cerebral aneurysms are most often found at bifurcations near the circle of Willis, and the risk of rupture is increased with increasing size. Subarachnoid hemorrhage almost always presents with rapid onset of severe headache. The presence of other signs and symptoms is used to clinically grade these patients. The Hunt–Hess Clinical Grade classification is most widely used (Table 18.1).

2. What are the most serious complications following subarachnoid hemorrhage from aneurysm rupture?

The most serious sequela of subarachnoid hemorrhage is re-bleeding. The incidence of re-bleeding following aneurysm rupture is approximately 15% in the first week, and approximately 10% in the second week. Morbidity and mortality following re-bleed is very great and has motivated the trend towards early intervention following aneurysm rupture.

Cerebral vasospasm is also a major cause of morbidity and mortality following subarachnoid hemorrhage. Symptomatic brain ischemia from vasospasm occurs in 15–35% of patients. Angiographic evidence of vasospasm occurs in as many as 70% of patients. Vasospasm may lead to cerebral infarction.

Subarachnoid hemorrhage often also leads to hydrocephalus and may result in dangerously elevated intracranial pressure.

TABLE 18.1	Hunt–Hess Clinical Grade Classification

Grade	Clinical Manifestations
0	Unruptured
I	Minimal headache or nuchal rigidity
II	Moderate to severe headache
	Nuchal rigidity with or without cranial nerve palsy
III	Drowsiness
	Confusion or mild focal deficit
IV	Stupor
	Hemiparesis
	Early decerebrate rigidity
	Moribund

3. What are the treatment options?

After the diagnosis of an intracranial aneurysm, treatment is either by craniotomy or by endovascular therapy. After angiography, endovascular treatment most often consists of packing the aneurysm with detachable coils. In many centers endovascular embolization is the preferred treatment. The most common complication of endovascular treatment is ischemic injury. The second most common complication is vascular perforation. Aneurysms without a sufficiently narrow neck cannot be treated successfully by endovascular embolization. In some cases, a stent is initially placed in the artery whose lumen feeds the aneurysm. Thereafter, coils are introduced across the stent wall into the aneurysm cavity.

Classical treatment consists of craniotomy and clipping of the aneurysm. Most centers attempt early clipping following subarachnoid hemorrhage to prevent re-bleeding and permit safe induction of hypertension and hypervolemia as treatment of vasospasm. The worst time for craniotomy is considered to be at 7–10 days post-rupture, when the risk of ischemic vasospasm is greatest.

4. What monitoring is indicated for patients undergoing craniotomy for clipping of intracranial aneurysm?

In addition to routine monitoring for general anesthesia, aneurysm patients should have intra-arterial measurement of blood pressure. Most will agree that the intra-arterial catheter is best inserted prior to anesthetic induction, as hypertension associated with laryngoscopy increases the risk of rupture. A urinary catheter is also indicated as in all craniotomies. Central venous pressure monitoring may be helpful in assessing fluid status, especially if mannitol is administered.

Many centers use electrophysiologic monitoring for aneurysm surgery when temporary arterial occlusion is anticipated during surgical dissection of the aneurysm. In these cases, arterial branches feeding the aneurysm may be temporarily occluded with surgical clips to reduce the risk of rupture. However, temporary arterial occlusion may lead to cerebral ischemia. This ischemic risk depends on the duration of arterial occlusion, collateral cerebral circulation, and brain temperature. Electroencephalogram (EEG) electrodes may be placed directly on the cerebral cortex over regions supplied by the arteries in question. Routine scalp electrodes for EEG may also be placed. In some centers somatosensory evoked potentials are monitored for detection of ischemia. Motor evoked potentials are highly sensitive to ischemia, but are probably still investigational for aneurysm surgery. Although hypothermia is believed to improve the safety of temporary arterial occlusion in these patients, a recent large randomized trial of mild hypothermia for aneurysm surgery demonstrated no clinical benefit over normothermia.

5. How is arterial blood pressure controlled?

Careful control of arterial blood pressure is critical in the management of these patients. Aneurysmal re-bleed and its consequent high morbidity and mortality may be triggered by arterial hypertension. This has been reported to occur commonly during tracheal intubation. Risk of aneurysm rupture is also great during surgical manipulation of tissue adjoining the aneurysm sac. For this reason, it is often advisable to decrease systemic arterial pressure during aneurysm dissection. However, this will depend on whether temporary arterial clips are effectively placed. In this case, mild induced hypertension may be indicated to reduce cerebral ischemia. The absence of normal cerebral blood flow autoregulation following subarachnoid hemorrhage makes these interventions highly critical. Therefore, induced hypotension should be limited in duration and magnitude. The effect on intracranial dynamics of agents used to decrease arterial pressure should be taken into account.

6. What is cerebral vasospasm, and how is it treated?

Cerebral vasospasm is arterial narrowing and decreased blood flow following subarachnoid hemorrhage. The incidence of vasospasm following surgical treatment of ruptured aneurysms is approximately 30%, with the overall incidence of severe cerebral infarct being approximately 10%. The occurrence of vasospasm following endovascular coiling may be higher, and is presumed to be due to the continued presence of subarachnoid blood, which is normally evacuated during craniotomy. The mechanism leading to vasospasm is poorly understood, but appears to result from the presence of blood degradation products in

Treatment Options for Cerebral Vasospasm

Calcium channel blockers

"Triple H therapy"
   Hypertension
   Hypervolemia
   Hemodilution

the subarachnoid space. Therapy usually consists of calcium channel blockers, such as nimodipine, and "triple H therapy". This consists of deliberate hypertension, hypervolemia, and hemodilution. However, hemodilution is rarely employed. Angioplasty and injection of endovascular papaverine have more recently gained popularity. Papaverine is usually applied on day 8 after subarachnoid hemorrhage. Its effect persists for less than 24 hours and the magnitude of its effect is greater when vasospasm is severe. Angioplasty, by balloon dilation of the arterial narrowing, has a longer-lasting effect than papaverine but presents a greater risk of vessel rupture. In some patients, multiple interventions of papaverine or angioplasty are performed, as guided by repeat angiography. Of course, the patient's clinical condition will also guide therapy

7. How is aneurysm rupture during aneurysm clipping managed?

Intraoperative aneurysm rupture may be catastrophic if not properly managed by the surgeon and anesthesiologist in a coordinated effort. Unless bleeding is controlled, the outcome is inevitably fatal. Therefore, the first priority is to permit the surgeon to visualize the rupture site and clip it.

If the arteries feeding the aneurysm have been previously dissected and exposed, the surgeon may need only apply temporary clips to these vessels. Thereafter, he can place a permanent aneurysm clip and then remove the temporary clips.

Under challenging circumstances, the anesthesiologist will be required to induce hypotension very rapidly and profoundly to permit surgical visualization of the ruptured aneurysm. Typically, a large bolus of intravenous thiopental is administered. Usually mean arterial blood pressure will need to be lowered well below 50 mmHg before adequate reduction in hemorrhage is achieved. A bolus of propofol may also suffice. With aneurysms of the anterior circulation it may be helpful to manually occlude both carotid arteries by reaching under the drapes and applying direct pressure on the patient's neck. At our institution we have also administered intravenous adenosine to induce reversible complete circulatory arrest following aneurysm rupture. As one would expect, this provides a completely bloodless field until cardiac activity resumes. In these situations one must balance the risks of cerebral ischemia against the surgical need to visualize the cerebrovascular anatomy.

SUGGESTED READINGS

Hijkra A, van Gijn J, Stefanko S, et al.: Delayed cerebral ischemia after aneurysmal subarachnoid hemorrhage: clinicoanatomic correlations. Neurology 36:329, 1986

Vanninen R, Koivisto T, Saari T, et al.: Ruptured intracranial aneurysms: acute endovascular treatment with electrolytically detachable coils. A prospective randomized study. Radiology 211:325, 1999

Zhman J, Heikanen O: Timing of operation for ruptured supratentorial aneurysms: a prospective randomized study. J Neurosurg 70:55,1989

CAROTID ENDARTERECTOMY

Arthur E. Schwartz, MD

A 68-year-old man with a history of a transient ischemic attack presents for carotid endarterectomy.

QUESTIONS

1. What are the indications for surgical carotid endarterectomy (CEA)?
2. What are the alternatives to surgical CEA?
3. What are the most serious perioperative complications?
4. How is the patient's neurologic status monitored?
5. What interventions may reduce the risk of neurological injury?

1. What are the indications for surgical carotid endarterectomy (CEA)?

Several studies involving large numbers of patients demonstrate that CEA reduces the risk of stroke in patients with critical carotid artery stenosis. Two large-scale studies show that symptomatic patients with greater than 70% luminal narrowing of the carotid artery had improved outcome after surgery when compared with patients receiving medical treatment alone. Symptoms included transient ischemic attack (TIA), reversible ischemic neurologic deficit, and nondisabling stroke.

For asymptomatic patients with greater than 60% luminal narrowing, CEA decreased the incidence of stroke at 5 years compared with patients treated medically.

2. What are the alternatives to surgical CEA?

Carotid artery angioplasty with or without placement of an arterial stent is a possible alternative treatment for carotid artery stenosis. This technique involves the endovascular placement of a catheter, usually from the femoral artery, with fluoroscopic guidance through the great arteries and heart to the carotid artery. A balloon is positioned in the area of the stenosis and inflated to dilate the artery. A filter or other device may be temporarily positioned distal to the lesion in order to limit embolization of material to the brain. After angioplasty, a stent may be positioned at the site to maintain the patency of the artery. The safety and preference of angioplasty compared with surgical treatment is uncertain and controversial. It may be the only practical treatment for cases of high-grade carotid stenosis where the lesion is located distally near the cranium and, therefore, poorly accessible to surgery.

3. What are the most serious perioperative complications?

The most serious perioperative complications of carotid surgery are neurologic or cardiac. Neurologic complications include cerebral infarction, transient ischemia, and cognitive dysfunction. Ischemic cerebral injury may result

Complications

Neurologic
    Infarction
    Transient ischemia
    Cognitive dysfunction

Cardiac
    Myocardial infarction

from embolization of thrombus or air during surgical manipulation. It may also result from decreased cerebral perfusion during temporary carotid artery occlusion during surgery. Arterial stenosis or occlusion after CEA may also produce an ischemic insult. A stroke-related morbidity of 2–3% for CEA is considered acceptable.

Patients with atherosclerotic disease of the carotid arteries often also have similar pathology of the coronary vessels. A perioperative incidence of myocardial infarction of 5% is considered acceptable.

4. How is the patient's neurologic status monitored?

The assessment of neurologic status depends on whether regional or general anesthesia is used. With regional anesthesia, intermittent evaluation of motor strength, sensation, and language is performed. This should be timed to coincide with interventions of relatively high risk. These include manipulation of the carotid artery, arterial occlusion, and reperfusion. The choice and timing of sedative may markedly interfere with proper evaluation. For example, administration of a benzodiazepine may elicit re-emergence of a focal deficit following recovery from a recent TIA.

With general anesthesia, neurologic status is most often assessed by electroencephalogram (EEG), somatosensory evoked potential (SSEP), or transcranial Doppler (TCD). EEG is the most widely used and considered the "gold standard" for monitoring neurologic function during general anesthesia. It is the most sensitive method for detecting cerebral ischemia in the unconscious patient. The sensitivity of the EEG will depend on the number of electrode channels monitored and the experience of the person evaluating the EEG. EEG changes indicative of ischemia are most likely to be observed from electrodes positioned near the anatomic site of brain suffering from ischemia. Furthermore, unilateral changes especially observed in regions dependent on the operative artery are more likely to reflect ischemic insult. EEG changes most indicative

of ischemia are decreased amplitude (voltage), slowing (decreased frequency), or burst suppression. It is useful to maintain a steady state of anesthetic agent during monitoring in order to best appreciate EEG changes not confounded by altered anesthetic dose.

SSEP depend on processing of signals from stimulation of a peripheral nerve. Since the response is described by latency and amplitude alone, analysis of SSEP requires less experience or training than does EEG. SSEP is probably less sensitive than EEG for detecting ischemia. Ischemia is indicated by an increase in latency or a decrease in amplitude of the SSEP waveform. This is of greatest concern when it is unilateral and on the operative side.

TCD is used to measure the middle cerebral artery blood flow velocity on the ipsilateral operative side. It does so by assessing the Doppler shift of sound waves reflected by moving red blood cells in the artery. It is also extremely sensitive for the detection of embolic material. Embolization is quite common during carotid surgery and depends on surgical technique and the presence of atherosclerotic plaque or entrained air. Positioning of the detector probes may be quite cumbersome and the readings will markedly depend on the probe direction (angle of insonation). Therefore, any movement of the Doppler probe may result in diminished or lost waveforms.

Less common, but useful monitors include motor evoked potential (exquisitely sensitive to ischemia) and cerebral blood flow measurement by washout of intra-arterial or intravenous xenon-133.

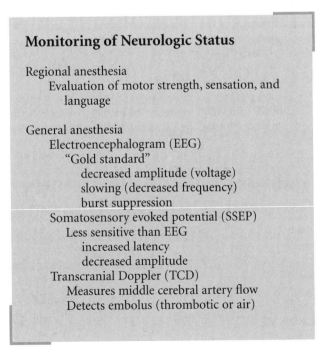

Monitoring of Neurologic Status

Regional anesthesia
    Evaluation of motor strength, sensation, and
        language

General anesthesia
    Electroencephalogram (EEG)
        "Gold standard"
            decreased amplitude (voltage)
            slowing (decreased frequency)
            burst suppression
    Somatosensory evoked potential (SSEP)
        Less sensitive than EEG
            increased latency
            decreased amplitude
    Transcranial Doppler (TCD)
        Measures middle cerebral artery flow
        Detects embolus (thrombotic or air)

5. What interventions may reduce the risk of neurologic injury?

Ischemic neurologic insult from carotid artery surgery may result from arterial embolization during surgical manipulation, decreased cerebral perfusion during temporary arterial occlusion, reperfusion injury, or unintentional arterial occlusion following surgery. Arterial embolization during surgery is very common and often depends on surgical technique and the preoperative presence of atherosclerosis. Surgical placement of a shunt may increase the incidence of embolization. Therefore, in many centers shunts are inserted only if indicated by EEG ischemic changes following carotid occlusion or other evidence of poor cerebral collateral circulation. Although thiopental may improve outcome following focal ischemia, it is not widely employed for maintenance of general anesthesia. This may be due to dose-dependent delayed awakening or its hemodynamic effects. Hypothermia also improves outcome following focal cerebral ischemia. However, it has not gained wide acceptance for carotid artery surgery. This may be due to the deleterious effects of hypothermia on cardiac function.

Decreased cerebral perfusion during temporary arterial occlusion is most often treated by deliberate hypertension. In many centers, systemic arterial pressure is increased by 10–20% during temporary arterial occlusion. Intravenous phenylephrine is most often employed for this purpose because of extensive evidence of improved outcome in animal models of focal cerebral ischemia. Surgical placement of a temporary vascular shunt during carotid artery occlusion will also improve cerebral blood flow. This may, however, prolong surgical time, obscure surgical exposure, and promote embolization.

Following reperfusion, ischemic or infarcted brain may be at risk for reperfusion injury. Usually arterial blood pressure is reduced to near normal prior to reperfusion.

The choice of anesthetic agent for CEA remains controversial. In a randomized study comparing potent inhalation anesthetics, EEG evidence of ischemia occurred at higher cerebral blood flow values in patients anesthetized with halothane compared with isoflurane. This supports the use of isoflurane in these patients. There is no widely accepted preference for either a primarily opioid-based or inhalation anesthetic technique. In any case, rapid emergence from general anesthesia permitting timely assessment of neurologic function will facilitate diagnosis of neurologic deficit resulting from cerebrovascular occlusion. This will allow for a more rapid intervention such as therapeutic surgical re-exploration, cerebral thrombolysis, or angioplasty, if indicated.

Interventions to Reduce Neurologic Injury

Embolization
    Insert shunt only when necessary

Decreased cerebral perfusion
    Deliberate hypertension (phenylephrine) during carotid artery occlusion
    Shunt (but may promote embolization)

Reperfusion injury
    Return blood pressure to normal levels prior to reperfusion

Emergence from general anesthesia at end of the procedure
    Earlier recognition of neurologic insult and institution of treatment

---

Control of arterial carbon dioxide tension also remains somewhat controversial. Mild hypocapnea may reduce cerebral blood flow, but may also preferentially shunt blood from normal brain to ischemic brain. Most practitioners maintain arterial carbon dioxide tension near normal.

SUGGESTED READINGS

Brott T, Toole JF: Medical compared with surgical treatment of asymptomatic carotid artery stenosis. Ann Intern Med 123:720, 1995

European Carotid Surgery Trialists Collaborative Group: MRC European carotid surgery trial: interim results for symptomatic patients with severe (70–90%) or with mild (0–29%) carotid stenosis. Lancet 337:1245, 1991

Lazar RM, Fitzsimmons BF, Marshall RS, Mohr JP, Berman MF: Midazolam challenge reinduces neurological deficits after transient ischemic attack. Stroke 34:794, 2003

North American Symptomatic Carotid Endarterectomy Trial Collaborators: Beneficial effect of carotid endarterectomy in symptomatic patients with high-grade stenosis. N Engl J Med 325:445, 1991

ELECTROCONVULSIVE THERAPY

David C. Kramer, MD

Michael E. Bilenker, DO

A 34-year-old woman with major depression presents for electroconvulsive therapy (ECT). Her condition has not responded to traditional medical treatments. She is on multiple psychotropic medications including amitriptyline and citalopram. In addition to her major depression, she has a long-standing history of gastroesophageal reflux disease (GERD) treated with omeprazole.

QUESTIONS

1. What are the physiologic effects of ECT?
2. What are the anesthetic agents of choice for ECT?
3. Describe the preanesthetic evaluation of ECT patients.
4. What are the anesthetic implications of psychotropic agents used in patients receiving ECT?
5. How would you anesthetize this particular patient for ECT?
6. What are the contraindications to ECT?

1. What are the physiologic effects of ECT?

The goal of ECT is the generation of a generalized seizure. This is accomplished by the placement of cutaneous electrodes over various points on the scalp through which an electric current is produced. There is a direct relationship between seizure duration and the success of ECT treatment. Successful treatments provide seizure activity of between 15 and 120 seconds. In addition to the local contraction of the facial muscles, there is a dramatic systemic hormonal response. Initially a parasympathetic discharge resulting in bradycardia, heart block, or asystole may occur. This is typically followed by a sympathetic discharge, which manifests as tachycardia, hypertension, and increased secretions. As a result, there are increases in cerebral blood flow, cerebral metabolic rate and oxygen demand, intracranial pressure, cardiac output, and myocardial oxygen demand. Patients with questionable myocardial reserve as well as organic brain lesions are at significant risk for ischemic sequelae, cardiac dysrhythmias, and cerebral hemorrhage. Along with these circulatory effects, there are violent muscular contractions. The seizures generated by ECT are self-limited, and these derangements subside within minutes of seizure termination. It is the goal of the anesthesiologist to limit the physical manifestations of these physiologic responses and prevent the sequelae associated with them.

2. What are the anesthetic agents of choice for ECT?

Short-acting intravenous anesthetic agents and muscle relaxation are used to facilitate ECT. As previously mentioned, the goal of ECT is to produce a generalized seizure;

Physiologic Effects of ECT

Central nervous system
  Generalized motor seizure

Initial parasympathetic discharge
  Bradycardia, heart block, or asystole

Secondary sympathetic discharge
  Tachycardia
  Hypertension
  Increased secretions

Secondary effects
  Increased cerebral blood flow
  Increased cerebral metabolic rate
  Increased intracranial pressure
  Increased myocardial oxygen demand
  Increased cardiac output

however, anesthetic agents have inherent anticonvulsant properties. Therefore, the most appropriate agent and dose should be selected for this short procedure.

Of the barbiturates, the most commonly used induction agent for ECT is methohexital. It is short-acting and has the least effect on seizure duration of all the intravenous induction agents. Thiopental has also been used but its duration of action and side-effect profile is not as favorable as methohexital.

Ketamine has also been used for ECT, but its utility is limited by subsequent increases in heart rate and blood pressure. Etomidate has been shown to increase the seizure duration when compared with methohexital. However, the usefulness of etomidate is limited by pain on injection, postprocedural confusion, and emesis. Its use may be appropriate, however, for patients with limited cardiac reserve.

There has been a long-standing debate over the role of propofol in ECT. Propofol has a greater anticonvulsant effect on ECT than other intravenous anesthetics, although propofol may itself be associated with the induction of seizures when used in higher doses. Propofol has been shown to be beneficial in patients with a history of prolonged ECT-induced seizure, as well as those with a history of post-ECT nausea and vomiting. Emergence from propofol is marginally faster than from other intravenous anesthetics when given in equipotent doses.

Remifentanil has recently been demonstrated to effectively attenuate the sympathetic response to ECT without affecting seizure duration or prolonging recovery time. Induction doses of benzodiazepines raise the seizure

threshold and may prolong emergence. Some authors have described the use of volatile agents, particularly sevoflurane, for ECT. Sevoflurane may be used in the pregnant patient to prevent preterm labor. If sevoflurane is used for induction of the pregnant patient beyond 12 weeks gestation, the airway must be secured with an endotracheal tube to prevent aspiration. The major disadvantage of sevoflurane is the requirement for an anesthesia machine.

The muscle relaxant of choice for ECT is succinylcholine because of its quick onset and short duration of action. If there are any contraindications to using succinylcholine, any of the short to moderate duration nondepolarizing muscle relaxants can be substituted. The short duration of action of mivacurium makes it the most commonly used muscle relaxant when succinylcholine is contraindicated. However, it should not be used in the patient with pseudocholinesterase deficiency.

A variety of medications have been used to control the cardiovascular responses associated with ECT. Anticholinergics, such as glycopyrrolate and atropine, have been administered as premedications to block the initial parasympathetic response (bradycardia) of ECT. To control the tachycardia and hypertension associated with the sympathetic response, β-blockers, calcium channel blockers, α_2 agonists and antagonists, vasodilators, ganglionic blockers, local anesthetics, and opioids have been used alone or in combination with mixed results. Short-acting drugs seem to be most appropriate for ECT.

3. Describe the preanesthetic evaluation of ECT patients.

The preanesthetic evaluation for ECT patients is the same as that for any patient about to undergo anesthetic care. However, the profound psychological disorder may make the preanesthetic history more difficult to obtain. Thus, ECT patients may be poor historians or may be completely nonverbal. In these cases, a history by medical records, family or other caregivers may be the best way to evaluate the anesthetic risk in these select patients. Patients about to undergo ECT may be receiving psychotropic agents that can interact with commonly used anesthetic agents.

Premedications may include an anticholinergic to prevent the ECT-induced bradycardia, aspiration prophylaxis for patients at risk for aspiration, and acetaminophen or nonsteroidal anti-inflammatory drugs to lessen the myalgias associated with ECT.

4. What are the anesthetic implications of psychotropic agents used in patients receiving ECT?

Patients undergoing ECT are usually taking multiple psychotropic medications. These medications may include tricyclic antidepressants (TCAs), lithium carbonate, monoamine oxidase inhibitors (MAOIs), selective serotonin reuptake inhibitors (SSRIs), antipsychotics, benzodiazepines,

Effects of Psychotropic Agents

Tricyclic antidepressants (TCAs)	■ Block the reuptake of norepinephrine at the postganglionic sympathetic nerve endings ■ Drug levels of certain SSRI (fluoxetine) may increase 2–5× when used with TCAs
Monoamine oxidase inhibitors (MAOIs)	■ Block the metabolism of catecholamines ■ Increased baseline sympathetic tone ■ Interaction with meperidine or indirect-acting sympathomimetic agents may lead to hypertensive crises, seizures, and hyperpyrexia
Selective serotonin reuptake inhibitors (SSRI)	■ Block serotonin reuptake pump via the $5HT_{1A}$ receptor, inhibit the rate of firing of serotonin neurons, and inhibit the release of serotonin ■ Long-term use may lead to down-regulation of $5HT_{1A}$ receptors ■ Little effect on norepinephrine reuptake ■ May be associated with "serotonin syndrome": restlessness, chills, ataxia, and insomnia (in combination with lithium or carbamazepine, may be fatal)
Lithium carbonate	■ Prolongs neuromuscular blockade
Benzodiazepines	■ May increase resistance to ECT by raising the seizure threshold

or miscellaneous second-generation antidepressants such as bupropion.

TCAs (amitriptyline, amoxapine, clomipramine, desipramine, doxepin, imipramine, nortriptyline, protriptyline, trimipramine) block the reuptake of norepinephrine at the postganglionic sympathetic nerve endings. As a result, the patient's baseline sympathetic tone is increased. Direct-acting sympathetic agents are therefore preferred to indirect-acting agents that will increase the release of norepinephrine.

Several categories of drugs must be used with caution with TCAs. These include: opioids (such as meperidine), antihypertensives, potent volatile agents, and anticholinergics. TCAs bind to albumin and therefore increase plasma levels of medications that bind to albumin, such as thiopental, diazepam, phenytoin, and propranolol.

MAOIs (phenelzine, tranylcypromine) block the metabolism of catecholamines, increasing baseline sympathetic tone as well. The interaction between MAOIs and meperidine or indirect-acting sympathomimetic agents has been shown to lead to hypertensive crises, seizures, and hyperpyrexia.

SSRIs (citalopram, fluoxetine, fluvoxamine, paroxetine, and sertraline) may be associated with "serotonin syndrome", which is characterized by restlessness, chills, ataxia, and insomnia. Fatal serotonin syndrome may develop when an SSRI is combined with lithium or carbamazepine. Certain SSRIs are inhibitors of the hepatic cytochrome P-450 system and may increase drug levels of TCAs and β-blockers to toxic levels. Extreme caution must be taken when prescribing SSRIs (particularly fluoxetine) to patients on these medications.

Lithium carbonate may prolong the neuromuscular blockade achieved by muscle relaxants. Patients taking long-acting benzodiazepines may be resistant to ECT. These patients may require higher energy levels in order to overcome their seizure threshold.

5. How would you anesthetize this particular patient for ECT?

This patient is at risk for aspiration because of the presence of GERD. Therefore, the patient should have nothing by mouth for 8 hours and receive aspiration prophylaxis with an H_2-blocker, promotility agent, and a non-particulate antacid. Her routine medications should be taken as prescribed. In the past, it was suggested that TCAs be discontinued 2 weeks before general anesthesia to reduce the risk of drug interactions. However, many anesthetics have been performed without incident and the benefit of antidepressants in this patient population outweighs the risk.

Normally, anesthesia for ECT is performed via mask ventilation. In this particular case, because of the increased risk of aspiration, a rapid sequence induction with succinylcholine followed by endotracheal intubation should be performed. Indirect-acting sympathomimetics should be avoided, and hypotension should be treated with intravenous fluids or direct-acting medications, if necessary. Standard American Society of Anesthesiologists monitoring should be employed. The patient should be awake and

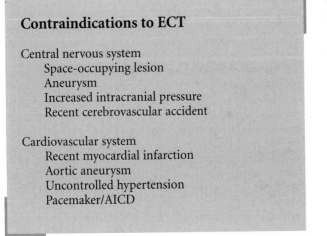

Contraindications to ECT

Central nervous system
    Space-occupying lesion
    Aneurysm
    Increased intracranial pressure
    Recent cerebrovascular accident

Cardiovascular system
    Recent myocardial infarction
    Aortic aneurysm
    Uncontrolled hypertension
    Pacemaker/AICD

alert prior to tracheal extubation in order to ensure adequate airway reflexes.

6. What are the contraindications to ECT?

Major risks of ECT involve the central nervous and cardiovascular systems. Central nervous system contraindications include space-occupying lesions, aneurysm, increased intracranial pressure, and recent cerebrovascular accident.

Cardiovascular system contraindications include recent myocardial infarction and aortic aneurysm. Scattered reports of successful ECT treatments in such patients do exist; therefore, each should be considered on an individual basis as to whether to proceed with ECT or not.

ECT current could interfere with permanent pacemaker activity. There is large variation in models of cardiac pacemakers and a consultation with a cardiologist is necessary to ascertain the best management for each patient.

SUGGESTED READINGS

Ding Z, White PF: Anesthesia for electroconvulsive therapy. Anesth Analg 94:1351–1364, 2002

Nishihara F, Ohkawa M, Hiraoka H, Yuki N, Saito S: Benefits of the laryngeal mask for airway management during electroconvulsive therapy. J ECT 19:211–216, 2003

Recart A, Rawal S, White PF, Byerly S, Thornton L: The effect of remifentanil on seizure duration and acute hemodynamic responses to electroconvulsive therapy. Anesth Analg 96: 1047–1050, 2003

Stoelting RK (ed): Drugs used for psychopharmacologic therapy. pp. 357–376.

In Stoelting RK (ed): Pharmacology and Physiology in Anesthetic Practice, 3rd Edition, Lippincott-Raven, Philadelphia

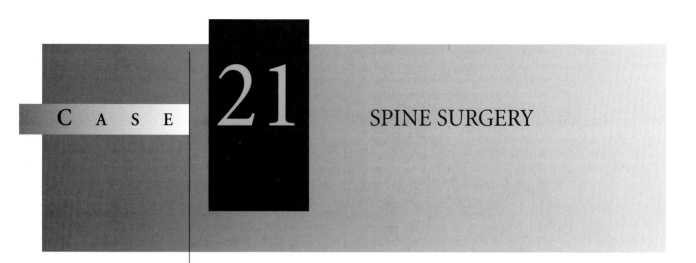

CASE 21

SPINE SURGERY

Irene P. Osborn, MD

A 54-year-old man is scheduled for lumbar laminectomy and spine fusion. He suffered a back injury 6 years previously and has undergone two previous operations without pain relief. The patient takes oxycodone daily and is limited in his activities. He reports increased numbness in the left leg and the surgeon requests monitoring of somatosensory evoked potentials.

QUESTIONS

1. What are the considerations for surgery in the prone position?
2. What monitors will you use for this case?
3. What are somatosensory and motor evoked potentials?
4. Describe the effects of anesthetics on somatosensory and motor evoked potentials.
5. What is a "wake-up" test?
6. What is the bispectral index state (BIS)? Is monitoring the BIS useful in this case?
7. Is this patient at risk for postoperative vision loss?
8. What modalities exist for pain relief after spine surgery?

1. What are the considerations for surgery in the prone position?

Induction of anesthesia normally occurs in the supine position using standard agents for hypnosis, analgesia, and muscle relaxation. Following tracheal intubation, patients are placed in the prone position. As with any position change, care must be taken to prevent dislodgment of intravenous lines, an intra-arterial line if placed, and the endotracheal tube. Positioning of the head and extremities requires attention to avoid hyperextension or flexion of the neck. A variety of bolstering devices allow optimal access and positioning while reducing intrathoracic and intra-abdominal pressure (Table 21.1).

2. What monitors will you use for this case?

Standard monitoring is used for all spine surgery with the addition of a urinary catheter for longer cases and consideration for fluid replacement. Arterial monitoring may be appropriate if the patient is significantly hypertensive and has associated disease processes. It is also useful when there is potential for significant blood loss or cuff pressure measurements are difficult to obtain. Central venous pressure monitoring is beneficial when it provides intravascular access and allows monitoring of fluid status. Lumbar fusions may involve numerous segments and anterior as well

TABLE 21.1	Anesthetic Considerations for Surgery in the Prone Position

Airway
    Endotracheal tube (ETT) secured
    Avoid excessive neck flexion, tongue swelling or ETT
        kinking
    Potential for ETT bronchial migration
    Avoid increased airway pressures
    Support the head
        Avoid ocular pressure
        Avoid pinching of the ears
Positioning
    Head neutral with padding or gently turned lateral
        with pillows
    Arms not abducted beyond 90°
    Padding over ulnar nerves
    Bolsters for chest/abdomen
    Avoid abdominal or thoracic compression
        Prevent venous engorgement
    Knees bent to avoid stretch on sciatic nerves
Physiologic
    Decreased sympathetic tone
        Potential for hypotension during positioning
    Increased intra-abdominal pressure
        May restrict venous return
        May increase venous pressure
    Increased peak airway pressure
        Potential for worsening of ventilation/perfusion
           matching

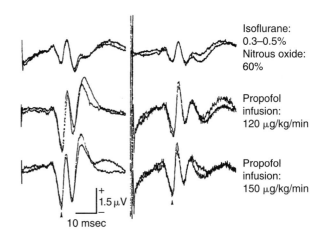

Isoflurane:
0.3–0.5%
Nitrous oxide:
60%

Propofol
infusion:
120 μg/kg/min

Propofol
infusion:
150 μg/kg/min

+
1.5 μV
−
10 msec

FIGURE 21.1 SSEPs: A characteristic pattern of peaks and valleys is obtained which can be used to follow the response at various points along the stimulated track.

as posterior exposure of the spine. Blood loss may be extensive and induced hypotension is often requested to decrease intraoperative bleeding. The adequacy of end-organ perfusion can be estimated with invasive monitoring, urine output of 0.5–1 cc/kg/hr, and periodic arterial blood gas analysis monitoring for evidence of metabolic acidosis. Neurophysiologic monitoring is often utilized when the spinal cord is at risk during surgery.

3. What are somatosensory and motor evoked potentials?

The electroencephalogram (EEG) is the measurement of the spontaneous activity of the brain. Evoked potentials are a measurement of the electrical responses "evoked" by a stimulus to the nervous system. Evoked potential monitoring is utilized in patients felt to be at high risk for spinal cord injury from surgical trauma, operative position, or impairment of blood supply.

The most commonly utilized evoked potentials are those produced by stimulation of the sensory system: somatosensory evoked potentials (SSEPs). In this technique a peripheral nerve (e.g., posterior tibial or median) is stimulated and the neural response measured. A characteristic pattern of peaks and valleys is obtained which can be used to follow the response at various points along the stimulated tract (Figure 21.1). This technology intermittently determines the integrity of the posterior spinal sensory pathways and large peripheral nerves. Significant changes in the SSEPs may consist of alterations in amplitude, latency, and/or morphology compared with baseline waveforms. Changes in SSEP waves that indicate possible disruption of the sensory pathway include a decrease in the amplitude of the waveform and an increase in the latency of those waves.

Motor evoked potentials (MEPs) are electrical impulses measured in the peripheral nerves and muscles in response to stimulation of the cortex or spinal cord. MEPs may be used in conjunction with SSEPs when there is a possibility of injury to the motor pathways in the anterior spinal cord. Two basic techniques for stimulating the cerebral motor cortex are direct transcutaneous electrical stimulation and transcutaneous magnetic stimulation. Addition of MEPs to SSEP monitoring may increase detection of potential injury by as much as 10%. MEPs may also be useful in the detection of spinal cord ischemia during aortic cross-clamping for thoraco-abdominal aneurysm repair.

4. Describe the effects of anesthetics on somatosensory and motor evoked potentials.

The EEG is sensitive to all anesthetics and becomes markedly depressed at the upper end of the clinically relevant dosage range, hence its use in monitoring depth of anesthesia. The anesthetic technique that provides for hemodynamic stability and effective recording of SSEPs and/or MEPs is obviously preferred. Inhalational agents

	SSEP		VER		BAER	
	Amp	Lat	Amp	Lat	Amp	Lat
N₂O	↓	X	↓	↑	X	X
Hal		↑	X		X	↑
Enf					X	
Iso	↓		↓		X	↑
Barbs	X	X	↓		X	X
Narcotic	X	X	X	X	X	X
Etomidate	↑	↑	X	X	X	X
Propofol	↓		X	X	↓	↑
Benzos	↓	X	X	X	X	X
Ketamine	X	↑	X	X	X	X

FIGURE 21.2 Effects of anesthetics on SSEPs. Amp, amplitude; Lat, latitude; N₂O, nitrous oxide; Hal, halothane; Enf, enflurane; Iso, isoflurane; Barbs, barbiturates; Benzos, benzodiazepines.

and bolus intravenous drugs can affect SSEPs (Figure 21.2). The inhalation response is generally dose-related; therefore a low concentration with or without nitrous oxide and a continuous opioid infusion is frequently utilized with success. Muscle relaxants do not interfere with SSEP recording and may facilitate anesthetic management. If the potentials remain difficult to obtain, changing to a total intravenous anesthesia (TIVA) technique may be necessary. It is important to note that SSEPs are also affected by ischemia, hypothermia, hypoxia, hypotension, and anemia.

While SSEPs are easily obtained using a low concentration of volatile agents and muscle relaxants, MEPs are more challenging and often require the use of TIVA with minimal or **no muscle relaxants**. The inhalational agents, including nitrous oxide, have been shown to depress MEPs in a variety of circumstances. Intravenous anesthetic agents, such as propofol, midazolam, droperidol, and sodium thiopental by infusion or bolus, may cause a significant decrease in the amplitude or latency of MEPs. Ketamine and opioid analgesics, such as fentanyl, produce less prominent changes. An opioid infusion with low concentrations of propofol is a frequently successful technique for monitoring MEPs. Remifentanil is particularly useful because of its potency and titratability. An intraoperative "wake-up test" may be requested if monitoring is unavailable or inadequate.

5. What is a "wake-up" test?

The "wake-up" test is the classic means of assessing motor function in the intraoperative and immediate postoperative period. Essentially it entails decreasing the anesthetic to a plane where the patient can respond to simple commands ("Move your toes", "Squeeze my fingers"). This demonstrates that the patient is without motor deficit from the procedure. It is considered the best way to assess the integrity of the spinal anterior motor tracts during spinal surgery. The anesthetic is then resumed for surgical completion or reversal of instrumentation. This monitoring technique has proven very effective in preventing postoperative paraplegia.

If a "wake-up" test is planned during the anesthetic regimen, the patient should be informed in advance of what to expect. Typically an opioid-based anesthetic with nitrous oxide and low-dose inhalational agent is utilized. The patient should be reassured that he or she will be comfortable for the procedure and unlikely to remember it. It is important to awaken the patient carefully and slowly to avoid inadvertent endotracheal extubation or injury with an overzealous response. This test is particularly useful in cases such as Harrington rod placement where the spinal cord is manipulated.

6. What is the bispectral index state (BIS)? Is monitoring the BIS useful in this case?

BIS is a processed EEG parameter that was developed to measure patient response during the administration of anesthetics and sedatives. In natural or drug-induced sleep states there are more harmonic and phase relationships between component waves of the EEG. This so-called bicoherence can be measured by bispectral analysis, not by power spectral analysis. Applying stepwise regression analysis to EEGs from anesthetized subjects in known awake/asleep states led to derivation of the BIS. The regression equation was transformed into a scale from 0 to 100, where 0 represents isoelectric and 100 represents awake. Therefore BIS uses bispectral analysis of the EEG waveform and other features of the EEG to detect subtle changes in levels of sedation, loss of consciousness, and recall. Clinical use of BIS monitoring demonstrates patient variability and response to anesthetic agents. It can be helpful in maintaining the patient at lower concentrations of volatile or hypnotic intravenous agent to obtain useful evoked potentials. BIS can assist in determining which anesthetic component is necessary in hypertensive patients for treatment of increased blood pressure. Patients with a potential narcotic tolerance and/or risk of awareness may be monitored to provide appropriate therapy and avoid complications. Clinical studies have demonstrated its usefulness in monitoring anesthetic depth, titrating agents for a "wake-up" test, and providing for a potentially faster emergence from anesthesia.

7. Is this patient at risk for postoperative vision loss?

Several techniques have been employed to reduce blood loss and limit the need for homologous transfusions: positioning that reduces intra-abdominal pressure; surgical hemostasis; deliberate controlled hypotensive anesthesia; reinfusion of salvaged blood; normovolemic hemodilution. A devastating complication of these procedures is the development of ischemic optic neuropathy (ION). This has been reported with increasing frequency over the last decade. Postoperative vision loss is most often due to anterior or posterior ischemic optic neuropathy (AION, PION) and rarely due to less common perioperative complications such as central retinal artery or vein occlusion and occipital lobe infarcts. Causes of ION include:

- decreased perfusion pressure due to systemic hypotension, increased venous pressure, or large vessel occlusive disease
- increased resistance to blood flow due to increased blood viscosity, local arterial disease, or increased external pressure
- decreased oxygen carrying capacity.

There are no identified effective treatments for ION and the vision loss is most often permanent. Prolonged surgery, large intraoperative blood loss, and large-volume fluid replacement have been reported to be associated with increased risk of ION. Patient risks are also noted in Table 21.2.

Maintenance of spinal cord perfusion is essential and must be maintained. Multiple-level surgery and fusion requires strict attention to replacement of intraoperative fluid losses and careful assessment before extubation of the trachea. This patient is relatively healthy but should be warned preoperatively of this potential complication.

8. What modalities exist for pain relief after spine surgery?

Postoperatively, patients are expected to emerge from anesthesia for neurologic evaluation. Adequate pain management is required to prevent hypoventilation or atelectasis and allow for early movement and rehabilitation. Opioid administration begins in the operating room, prior to emergence. Postoperative care is administered along clinical pathways and individualized for each patient. Patient-controlled analgesia (PCA) pumps are routinely used for 1–3 days, after which patients are switched to oral agents. Epidural or intrathecal administration of opioids is also an alternative, particularly in patients with high opioid tolerance. The epidural catheter may be placed by the anesthesiologist preoperatively or by the surgeon intraoperatively under direct vision. Communication with staff and the pain service consultant is essential to assure a safe postoperative course. Multimodal therapy involving opioids and nonsteroidal anti-inflammatory agents is an option for certain patients.

SUGGESTED READINGS

Black S. Anesthesia for Spine Surgery. ASA Refresher Course Lectures, 2003

Cheng MA, Sigurdson W, Templehoff R, Lauryssen C: Visual loss after spine surgery: a survey. Neurosurgery 46:625–630, 2000

Hagberg C, Welch W, Bowman-Howard M: Anesthesia and surgery for spine and spinal cord procedures. Pp.1059–1071. In Albin MS (ed) Textbook of Neuroanesthesia with Neurosurgical and Neuroscience Perspectives. McGraw-Hill, New York, 1997

Nuttall GA, Horlocker TT, et al.: Predictors of blood transfusions in spinal instrumentation and fusion surgery. Spine 25:596–601, 2000

TABLE 21.2	Risk Factors for Postoperative Vision Loss

Atherosclerotic disease
Hypotension
Anemia
Excessive blood loss
Long duration of surgery
Head-dependent position

22

TRANSSPHENOIDAL HYPOPHYSECTOMY

Irene P. Osborn, MD

A 44-year-old man presents for transsphenoidal hypophysectomy with marked features of acromegaly. The patient reports increasing shoe size, glove size, and worsening sleep apnea. Magnetic resonance imaging (MRI) revealed a pituitary mass. Laboratory findings are within normal limits with the exception of serum glucose of 170 mg/dL. The patient denies any allergies or medications. Past surgical history includes carpal tunnel release bilaterally. He denies other medical problems.

QUESTIONS

1. What is acromegaly?
2. What symptoms are typical of the disease?
3. How is the disease treated?
4. What are the anesthetic considerations of acromegaly?
5. How would you approach the airway management in this patient?
6. What structures lie within the transsphenoidal surgical field?
7. What is diabetes insipidus?
8. What are the postoperative concerns for this patient?

1. What is acromegaly?

The pituitary gland is anatomically and functionally separated into the anterior pituitary (adenohypophysis)

and posterior pituitary (neurohypophysis). Table 22.1 lists the hormones found in the pituitary gland.

Acromegaly is a rare disease caused by growth hormone (GH)-secreting tumors of the pituitary. In children, GH-secreting tumors cause gigantism, whereas acromegaly occurs in adults whose epiphyses have fused. Acromegaly is most common in patients 20–60 years of age, with equal distribution between the sexes. Diagnosis generally occurs 10–15 years after the onset of pathologic growth hormone (GH) secretion. There is a twofold to fourfold increase in mortality versus the general population. If untreated, 50% of acromegalic patients die before the age of 50 years. The most common cause of death is cardiac and may be the result of hypertension, coronary artery disease, compensatory hypertrophy as a result of generalized somatomegaly or the direct effects of GH on the heart.

Acromegaly results from excess secretion of GH and subsequent elevation of circulating and locally produced insulin-like growth factor I (IGF-I). GH and IGF-I levels are controlled via several interactions rather than stimulating growth directly. GH induces the release of IGF-I, which promotes DNA, RNA, and protein synthesis, as well as cell and tissue growth.

2. What symptoms are typical of the disease?

The structural changes that occur with acromegaly cause chronic pain and discomfort and reduce quality of life and life expectancy. These changes include skeletal

TABLE 22.1	Pituitary Hormone Products

Anterior pituitary
  Growth hormone
  Prolactin
  Corticotropin
  β-Lipotropin
  Follicle-stimulating hormone
  Luteinizing hormone
  Thyrotropin
Posterior pituitary
  Antidiuretic hormone
  Oxytocin

overgrowth deformities (particularly of the hands, feet, and face), cardiovascular disease (hypertension, enlarged heart), arthropathy, neuropathy, and respiratory obstruction (Tables 22.2 and 22.3).

3. How is the disease treated?

Surgical therapy is the primary treatment for most symptomatic adenomas. There are several surgical approaches to pituitary masses, but the majority can be removed adequately via the transsphenoidal approach. This approach offers less morbidity (hypopituitarism, diabetes insipidus) and mortality than radiation or transcranial resection. Some of the larger lesions with extensive

TABLE 22.2	Peripheral Effects of Excess Growth Hormone

Skeletal overgrowth
  Distortion of facial features
  Prognathism
  Enlarged hands and feet
  Gigantism
Soft tissue overgrowth
  Enlarged lips, tongue, epiglottis, vocal cords
  Visceromegaly
Connective tissue overgrowth
  Recurrent laryngeal nerve paralysis
Peripheral neuropathy
  Carpal tunnel syndrome
Glucose intolerance
Hypertension
Osteoarthritis
Osteoporosis
Skeletal muscle weakness

TABLE 22.3	Airway Changes in Acromegaly

Anatomic
Hypertrophy
  Facial bones – large bulbous nose
  Nasal turbinates
  Soft palate
  Tonsils
  Epiglottis
  Glottic stenosis
  Impaired mobility of the cricoarytenoid joints
  Compression of recurrent laryngeal nerves
  Limitation in head and neck mobility
Physiologic
  Development or exacerbation of sleep apnea
  Hoarseness
  Dyspnea

growth outside the sella are best approached through a craniotomy. Bromocriptine and L-dopa suppress GH levels and tumor size after oral administration. Bromocriptine, a dopamine agonist, and L-dopa, a dopamine precursor, suppress hypothalamic-mediated GH secretion. These agents in addition to somatostatin analogs may offer alternatives to surgery in debilitated or elderly patients. The advantages and disadvantages of various treatment modalities must be weighed and prescribed according to the individual patient's circumstances.

4. What are the anesthetic considerations of acromegaly?

The constellation of physical manifestations, especially heart and lung disease, combined with upper airway involvement, make these patients a particular concern to the anesthesiologist. Cardiac complications in acromegalic patients have been described and cardiomegaly can occur with or without coexisting hypertension. Many typical acromegalic features are suggested to cause a difficult airway in these patients. An anesthetic technique that can be used in a majority of patients involves the use of opioids, volatile agent, nitrous oxide, and muscle relaxants. Many surgeons use intranasal epinephrine-containing local anesthetics and cocaine as part of their pre-surgical preparation. The use of these solutions reduces bleeding but also may lead to dysrhythmias in the presence or absence of volatile agents. Hypertension and bleeding during intrasellar exploration may be effectively controlled with appropriate anesthetic depth and intravenous administration of β-blockers or vasodilators. Practical considerations include difficulty in positioning of large extremities and the placement (if needed) of intra-arterial catheters.

5. How would you approach the airway management in this patient?

Airway assessment begins with careful history-taking and physical examination. A recent history of an uneventful intubation may be reassuring; however, anatomic and physiologic changes over the course of 1–5 years may affect one's ability to manage the airway successfully. Patients without hoarseness or dyspnea and with adequate mouth opening may be approached in the routine manner. Only oral intubation or tracheostomy can be considered for transsphenoidal surgery because a nasal endotracheal tube would obstruct the surgical field. Patients are instructed preoperatively that mouth-breathing will be required in the postoperative period because of bilateral nasal packs. Typical features such as large tongue, large epiglottis, distortion of the larynx, and soft tissue swelling complicate visualization of the larynx in acromegalic patients.

The American Society of Anesthesiologists' algorithm should be followed in the event of failed intubation and difficult ventilation. If difficulties with the airway are suspected after a careful evaluation, it may be prudent to secure the airway with the patient awake, either by fiberoptic-guided intubation or alternative techniques. Anticipation of the possible need to insert a smaller diameter tracheal tube and minimizing mechanical trauma to the upper airway and vocal cords are important considerations, as additional edema can result in airway obstruction after the tracheal tube is removed.

6. What structures lie within the transsphenoidal surgical field?

The sella turcica, within the body of the sphenoid, provides bony protection for the pituitary gland. The diaphragma sella is a roof of dura pierced by the pituitary stalk with its arachnoid, which extends to the hypothalamus. The cavernous sinus surrounds the walls of the sella and contains the cavernous portion of the internal carotid artery as well as cranial nerves III, IV, and VI. The optic nerves converge above the diaphragm to form the chiasm. Arterial bleeding during transsphenoidal hypophysectomy may be from the carotid artery or its branches and venous bleeding arises from the cavernous sinus. If excessive bleeding from the cavernous sinus occurs, it may be difficult to control. Temporary or permanent packing of the sinus may be necessary.

7. What is diabetes insipidus?

The most common endocrine dysfunction postoperatively is diabetes insipidus (DI). The dilute polyuria of central DI is caused by diminished or absent antidiuretic hormone (ADH) synthesis or release. Neurosurgical procedures in the region of the sella result in DI for a variety of reasons: direct hypothalamic injury or ischemia; stalk

---

Diabetes Insipidus

Etiology
- Direct hypothalamic injury
- Pituitary stalk edema
- High pituitary stalk dissection

Symptoms
- Polydipsia
- Poorly concentrated polyuria
- High serum osmolarity

Differential diagnosis
- Diuresis from mannitol, hyperglycemia, or excessive crystalloid administration

Treatment
- Increase oral intake
- Intravenous infusion if oral intake inadequate or not possible
- Desmopressin

---

edema; or high pituitary stalk dissection. DI may be permanent or transient and rarely occurs intraoperatively in previously asymptomatic patients. Classic manifestations of DI are polydipsia and a high output of poorly concentrated urine despite increased serum osmolarity. DI that develops during or immediately after pituitary surgery is generally due to reversible trauma to the posterior pituitary and is therefore transient.

The differential diagnosis includes diuresis from mannitol, glucose, or excessive crystalloid administration. Initial treatment of DI consists of intravenous infusion of electrolyte solutions if oral intake cannot offset polyuria. When urinary volumes are excessive and the patient is unable to drink water, the administration of exogenous vasopressin is indicated. Aqueous vasopressin, 5–10 U, can be given subcutaneously every 4 hours. Alternatively, desmopressin (DDAVP) can be administered intravenously while the nasal packing is in place, and intranasally once the nasal packing is removed. Desmopressin therapy can be prescribed in patients with permanent, partial or complete DI.

8. What are the postoperative concerns for this patient?

Surgical considerations include cerebrospinal fluid (CSF) rhinorrhea and bleeding. Intraoperatively, after tumor resection, the sinus is occasionally packed with autologous fat. If a CSF leak occurs intraoperatively, a lumbar drain can be placed postoperatively to potentially divert the leak until the diaphragma sella has healed. A rare complication is excessive bleeding from the carotid artery or cavernous sinus requiring excessive pressure and packing for control. Such pressure may result in partial or complete occlusion of the intracavernous portion of the internal carotid artery and pressure on cranial nerves III, IV, V, and VI. Postoperative ophthalmoplegia, facial anesthesia, and contralateral hemiparesis or hemiplegia may result from direct pressure or vasospasm.

While intact airway reflexes are essential before extubation, emergence from anesthesia should proceed smoothly to avoid excessive coughing, bucking, and hypertension. Suctioning of the oropharynx commonly reveals blood as the throat pack is removed. Adequate tidal volume is confirmed and the head should be elevated to facilitate ventilation. Facemask application must be gently performed as one or both of the nares will be packed. The patient is asked to breathe via the mouth and is evaluated for return of consciousness and assessment of vision. Prolonged mouth-breathing requires airway humidification, which improves oxygenation. Postoperative pain is generally mild and limited to headache or mild discomfort. Small doses of opioids may help, as well as oral analgesics with a sip of water as soon as tolerated.

SUGGESTED READINGS

Dougherty TB, Cronau LH: Anesthetic implications for surgical patients with endocrine tumors. Int Anesth Clinics 36:31–44, 1998

Majesko MJ: Anesthetic considerations in patients with neuro-endocrine disease, pp. 591–603. In Cottrell JE, Smith DS (eds): Anesthesia and Neurosurgery, 4th edition, CV Mosby, St. Louis, 2001

Schmitt H, Buchfelder M, et al.: Difficult intubation in acromegalic patients: incidence and predictability. Anesthesiology 93:110–114, 2000

Seidman PA, Kofke WA, Policare R, Young M: Anaesthetic complications of acromegaly. Br J Anaesth 84:179–182, 2000

23

DEPOLARIZING NEUROMUSCULAR BLOCKADE

Mark Abel, MD

A 33-year-old man in the medical intensive care unit with 30% body surface area third-degree burns to the neck and trunk develops dyspnea over 6 days as a result of adult respiratory distress syndrome. On 100% oxygen, his saturation is 91%. He is given ketamine 1 mg/kg and succinylcholine 1 mg/kg intravenously. He is easily intubated and ventilation is controlled. Within 1 minute, the patient became pulseless and a cardiac arrest is apparent on the electrocardiogram.

QUESTIONS

1. Describe the anatomy and physiology of normal neuromuscular transmission.
2. How does succinylcholine produce muscle relaxation?
3. What are extrajunctional receptors?
4. How is the action of succinylcholine terminated?
5. What factors may decrease the normal metabolism of succinylcholine?
6. Describe a phase II block.
7. What is the treatment of phase II blockade?
8. Describe other recognized side-effects of succinylcholine.
9. What are the contraindications to succinylcholine administration?

1. Describe the anatomy and physiology of normal neuromuscular transmission.

Neuromuscular transmission begins with depolarization down the axon of a motor nerve to the motor nerve terminal (Figure 23.1). The wave of depolarization is propagated by sequential opening of sodium channels. This allows sodium to enter the cell, increasing the intracellular concentration of positively charged ions. The transmembrane potential is altered from negative to positive in the area of the open sodium channel. This electrical event causes the next sodium channel to open and continues the process until the nerve terminal is reached. When the nerve terminal is thus depolarized, calcium channels open, allowing calcium to enter. The rise in intracellular calcium facilitates the binding of intracellular "packets" or quanta of acetylcholine to the cell wall bordering the neuromuscular junction. Acetylcholine molecules are then released into the junctional (synaptic) cleft.

Nicotinic acetylcholine receptors on the motor endplate of the muscle cell have binding sites for acetylcholine. This receptor is made up of five transmembrane protein chains, two of which are identical and contain one acetylcholine receptor site each. When two acetylcholine molecules bind to these two sites, the receptor is activated to respond as an ion channel for the rapid ingress of sodium. This movement of positively charged ions into the cell creates a small electrical current. When enough receptors are activated, the summation of these small electrical currents becomes sufficient to depolarize the endplate.

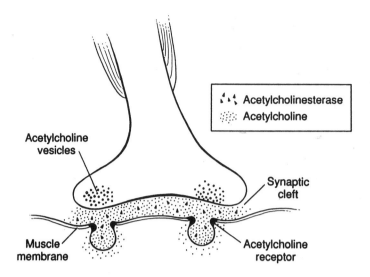

FIGURE 23.1   Anatomy of the neuromuscular junction.

Depolarization of the endplate stimulates the sodium channels in the perijunctional area to open, and thus the electrical current is propagated along the myocytes by sequential opening of sodium channels. When the myocytes are depolarized, stored calcium ions from the sarcoplasmic reticulum are released intracellularly. The free intracellular calcium ions activate myosin adenosine triphosphatase (ATPase), which precipitates excitation–contraction coupling of actin and myosin proteins to cause contraction.

At the same time, acetylcholine, which activated the receptors to initiate this process, is rapidly metabolized by acetylcholinesterase. Acetylcholinesterase is a protein on the muscle membrane in the junctional cleft that rapidly causes the hydrolysis of acetylcholine. Acetylcholine may alternatively be actively taken up into the nerve terminal from which it was released. This removal of acetylcholine from the neuromuscular junction allows for repolarization of the motor endplate. Subsequently, sodium channels along the muscle cell close, and the muscle cell repolarizes. Calcium is actively taken up into the sarcoplasmic reticulum and the actin-myosin fibers reset, allowing the muscle to relax.

2. How does succinylcholine produce muscle relaxation?

Succinylcholine is a depolarizing neuromuscular blocking drug that structurally consists of two acetylcholine molecules linked through acetate methyl groups. Because of its structural similarity to acetylcholine, it acts as an agonist at the nicotinic acetylcholine receptor. When two succinylcholine molecules bind to the α proteins of the receptor, it becomes activated as though two acetylcholine molecules were activating the receptors (agonism). The receptors

open for the ingress of sodium ions, and the endplate becomes depolarized, which leads to muscle contraction in the same fashion.

The activity that predominantly differentiates succinylcholine from acetylcholine agonism occurs after the initial depolarization. Whereas acetylcholine is hydrolyzed by acetylcholinesterase in milliseconds, succinylcholine is not. Succinylcholine remains active at the endplate for several minutes, maintaining endplate depolarization. The endplate cannot repolarize until succinylcholine leaves the neuromuscular junction. The sodium channels of the muscle cell, when activated by a depolarized endplate leading to the cell's depolarization, can remain in the activated (open) state for only 2 milliseconds. The sodium channels distal to the endplate return immediately to the ready (closed) state, while the sodium channels proximal to the endplate (perijunctional) remain influenced by the charge of the depolarized endplate. They cannot fully return to the ready (closed) state, nor are they able to remain activated (open), because sodium channels can activate for only 2 milliseconds. The perijunctional sodium channels are neither active nor ready to transmit a wave of depolarization to the myocytes, because they must fully close first before they can reopen (activate). Therefore, transmission is blocked with a depolarized endplate surrounded by a perijunctional area that has not fully repolarized and a repolarized (relaxed) myocyte.

3. What are extrajunctional receptors?

The ability of cells to make receptors is genetically encoded. The nicotinic receptor of the neuromuscular junction is made up of five proteins inserted into the cell membrane. Two of these five proteins are identical (referred to as α proteins). The extracellular projections of these two (of the five transmembrane proteins that form the receptor) are the binding sites for acetylcholine. Receptors, like most cellular proteins, turn over. The acetylcholine receptors turn over with half-lives of 1–10 days. They are inserted almost exclusively at the motor endplate near a nerve terminal. It is felt that the active nerve terminal must have some influence on receptor location, though the mechanism has not yet been determined. On removal of this neural influence, receptor density increases at the endplate and receptors begin appearing beyond the endplate.

These extrajunctional receptors occasionally have a minor structural difference from the normal acetylcholine receptor. One of the five protein chains may have a single different amino acid substitution. This structural difference can lead to a functional difference. When activated (e.g., by succinylcholine) they allow a greater exchange of ions across the cell membrane than the normal receptor. The ability to produce altered receptors also seems to be genetically encoded. Altered receptors are found in fetal tissue before neurologic development reaches a stage where it can influence muscle cells to insert adult nicotinic receptors at the neuromuscular junction.

Extrajunctional receptors are of significant clinical consequence. Interaction of succinylcholine with extrajunctional receptors results in massive efflux of potassium (K^+) from the cell, resulting in an acute rise in serum K^+.

4. How is the action of succinylcholine terminated?

Succinylcholine is rapidly metabolized by plasma cholinesterase (pseudocholinesterase) to succinylmonocholine and choline. When 1 mg/kg of succinylcholine is injected intravenously, about 90% is metabolized within 1 minute, so very little of the drug actually reaches the neuromuscular junction.

Plasma cholinesterase has no effect on succinylcholine once it has reached the neuromuscular junction. The action of succinylcholine at the neuromuscular junction is terminated when succinylcholine moves away from the neuromuscular junction, which occurs when its concentration gradient has reversed. When succinylcholine is first injected, its concentration is greatest in the plasma and lowest at the neuromuscular junction. As succinylcholine is metabolized in the serum and extracellular space, its concentration declines and succinylcholine diffuses away from the junction along this reversed gradient, and the clinical effect (block) of succinylcholine decreases. The onset of blockade from 1 mg/kg is typically 1 minute, while the normal duration of block is 5–8 minutes. Plasma cholinesterase is produced in the liver under genetic control. Its production is related to a pair of allelic genes E^U and E^U. The enzyme has a half-life of 5–12 days.

Pharmacology of Succinylcholine

Intubation dose: 1–2 mg/kg

Duration of action: 10–12 minutes

Metabolism: Plasma cholinesterase

Side-effects
  Hyperkalemia
  Fasciculations
  Myalgias
  Bradycardia to cardiac arrest
  Phase II block
  Slight increase in intraocular pressure
  Slight increase in intracranial pressure
  Allergy

5. What factors may decrease the normal metabolism of succinylcholine?

Succinylcholine is metabolized by plasma cholinesterase at an estimated rate of 0.1 mg/kg per minute. A decrease in enzyme concentration from many causes may decrease this rate. However, rarely does this have a significant clinical effect. A decrease in enzyme levels of 20% will prolong the duration of 1 mg/kg of succinylcholine by approximately 5 minutes.

During pregnancy, plasma cholinesterase activity can fall by 20–30%. It is lowest at 3 days postpartum and returns to normal by 2–6 weeks. The newborn has about 50% activity, reaching normal levels by 3–4 years of age.

Many pathologic states are associated with reduced plasma cholinesterase activity. They include hepatitis, cirrhosis, acute infections, carcinomas (particularly gastrointestinal), chronic debilitating disease, uremia, burns, renal failure, and others. Rarely do these cause clinically significant prolonged blockade.

Plasma cholinesterase may be inhibited by a number of drugs, both reversibly and irreversibly. Irreversible inhibition of the enzyme from echothiophate eye drops (used to treat glaucoma) has been reported to decrease plasma cholinesterase activity to nearly zero. Organophosphate pesticides and certain antineoplastic drugs (thiotepa and cyclophosphamide) may cause similar inhibition. Reversible inhibition decreases activity transiently and to a lesser degree. This is seen with neostigmine, pyridostigmine, and edrophonium. Other reversible inhibitors include monoamine oxidase inhibitors (MAOIs), oral contraceptives, local anesthetics, and pancuronium.

Variants of plasma cholinesterase have been recognized. Four alleles for the production of cholinesterase have been described; the normal gene E^U, the atypical gene E^A, the silent gene E^S, and the fluoride-resistant gene E^F. Abbreviations may be simplified by calling homozygotes UU, AA, SS, and FF, and heterozygotes can be abbreviated in a similar fashion (e.g., UA). These variants of the usual enzyme have an amino acid substitution that alters the hydrolytic activity of the protein. The homozygote abnormality will demonstrate prolonged apnea after succinylcholine that usually lasts from 1 to 2 hours. In the heterozygotes (UA, UF, and US), apnea is prolonged by only 10 or 15 minutes. The AF heterozygote may take 30 minutes to recover from succinylcholine.

The incidence of plasma cholinesterase variants differs among the population groups. The AA variant is found most commonly in Iranian Jews (1:175) and is rarest among Asians and Africans (1:25,000). The SS variant is most common in Alaskan Eskimos (1:58) and rare in Europeans (1:10,000). Incidence data are not available for the FF variant. The heterozygote state is common (estimated at 1:25), but the clinical response of these patients is rarely significant (or recognized). Variants are associated with quantitative decreases in enzymatic activity (H, J, and K), which are indistinguishable clinically in the heterozygote state. The H variant is extremely rare, found in only two families, and has a 90% decreased activity. The J variant is found in 1:150,000 and has a 66% decrease in activity. The K variant has a frequency of 1:100 and has a 33% decrease in activity.

When a patient has a prolonged response to succinylcholine, the plasma cholinesterase activity can be measured, and the qualitative function may be assessed in the presence of inhibitors. Inhibitors can be used to differentiate the responses of the qualitative variants A, F, and S. The usual (U) protein is markedly inhibited by dibucaine, while the atypical (A) is moderately inhibited, and the fluoride-resistant (F) and the silent (S) enzymes are mildly inhibited. Fluoride is used to differentiate the fluoride-resistant variant.

6. Describe a phase II block.

When succinylcholine is given to a patient for a prolonged period of time or in large doses, the nature of the block appears to change. The second form of block is referred to as a phase II, desensitization, or dual block. The recovery from succinylcholine in this circumstance generally is prolonged, and the character of the block is altered. Repeat nerve stimulation (train-of-four) following exposure to succinylcholine results in muscular response that is unchanged with repeated stimulation (no fade or decrement of response), and no fade occurs with tetanic stimulation (Figure 23.2). When a phase II block develops, fade is evident

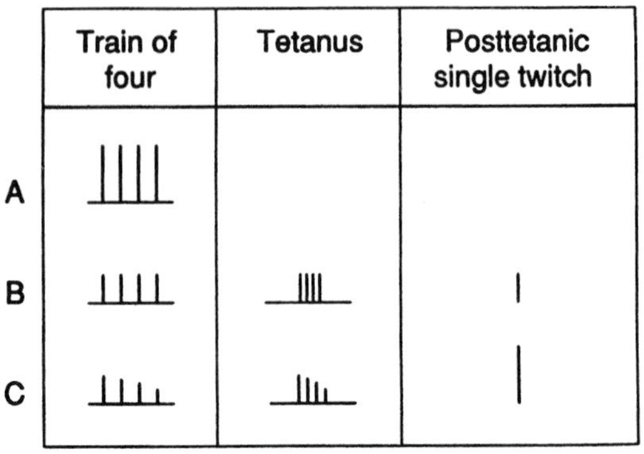

FIGURE 23.2 Train-of-four responses characteristic of (A) normal muscle, (B) phase I block, and (C) phase II block.

on train-of-four stimulation (T4/T1 less than 50%) and on tetanic stimulation. Post-tetanic potentiation may also be present. These patterns of response are typical of nondepolarizing muscle relaxants, not depolarizing drugs such as succinylcholine. The appearance of this block is related to the time and dose of succinylcholine administration. Reports of phase II blocks have been associated with 2–10 mg/kg administered over 1 hour. The onset may be accelerated by inhalation anesthetics.

Proposed mechanisms for phase II blockade include channel blockade of the receptor by succinylcholine, desensitization of the receptor in the presence of excessive agonists, and persistent ion flux causing distortion of the junctional membrane. *Channel blockade* refers to the interference with ion movements through the activated receptor by an obstructing molecule such as succinylcholine. When a receptor remains open (activated) for a prolonged period of time, such as during succinylcholine infusions, a molecule is more likely to enter the channel of the receptor and obstruct ion movements. Receptors are known to exist in at least three states: activated, receptive, and desensitized. The desensitized receptor is unable to respond to an agonist, even though the agonist may bind to the receptor. Prolonged agonist activity is thought to predispose to an increase in receptors in the desensitized state. If enough receptors are desensitized or have their channels blocked, they can no longer participate in the maintenance of endplate depolarization, which is responsible for succinylcholine's neuromuscular blockade.

Patients with atypical plasma cholinesterase are more likely to develop phase II blockade. This may be the result of excessive amounts of succinylcholine reaching the receptor and not being rapidly metabolized in the plasma before it reaches the neuromuscular junction. During the transition from phase I to phase II, a period of tachyphylaxis to succinylcholine has been noted by some authors.

7. What is the treatment of phase II blockade?

Treatment of weakness attributed to succinylcholine, regardless of its nature, is airway control and positive pressure ventilation until adequate strength returns to the muscles of respiration. Phase II block generally resolves spontaneously within 30–60 minutes. Some authors have noted an accelerated recovery from phase II block when neostigmine or edrophonium have been administered. The response is not predictable, and attention to clinical signs of neuromuscular strength must be followed during this period.

8. Describe other recognized side-effects of succinylcholine.

Succinylcholine administration is associated with a number of complications, ranging from benign to lethal. They include prolonged blockade (discussed above), myalgias, increased intraocular, intragastric, and intracranial pressures, dysrhythmias, masseter muscle spasm, anaphylactic and anaphylactoid reactions, and hyperkalemia.

Myalgias have been reported postoperatively in 5–83% of patients receiving succinylcholine. This complication is more common in ambulatory patients. It can be attenuated by pretreatment with a small dose of a nondepolarizing muscle relaxant or lidocaine. The mechanism of succinylcholine-induced myalgias is thought to be a result of a shift of calcium intracellularly, leading to damage of cellular structures via activation of phospholipase A_2. Patients who develop myalgias are reported to have a fall in serum calcium after succinylcholine. Alternatively, muscle spindle damage from asynchronous muscle contractions that is due to high intracellular calcium concentration has been proposed as a mechanism of myalgias following succinylcholine.

Succinylcholine causes a sustained increase in intraocular pressure of 5–15 mmHg for 10 minutes. This was attributed to extraocular muscle fasciculations. However, Kelly et al. (1993) demonstrated a rise in intraocular pressure after removal of extraocular muscles. Although it has been suggested that succinylcholine may aggravate open eye injuries, a 1985 report did not show worsening of eye injuries following succinylcholine administration. The use of succinylcholine in open eye injuries remains controversial.

Intragastric pressure is also reported to increase following succinylcholine. The increase is related to visible fasciculations and may be attenuated by a small dose of a nondepolarizing muscle relaxant before succinylcholine.

Intracranial pressure increases after succinylcholine administration to laboratory animals. The issue is more complicated in humans because it is difficult to separate succinylcholine's effect from those of other actions performed at the same period of time. Different views are expressed by different experts regarding the safety of succinylcholine in patients with raised intracranial pressure. Potential risks of brain stem herniation must be weighed against those of airway compromise from prolonged onset of profound muscle relaxation achieved in other ways.

Dysrhythmias are associated with succinylcholine administration. Tachydysrhythmias may occur but are less problematic than bradycardias. Bradycardia is more common in children but may occur in adults particularly after a second dose of succinylcholine. This problem can be attenuated by pretreatment with a vagolytic agent. Metabolic breakdown products of succinylcholine do not seem to play a part in causing dysrhythmias, because infusions of succinylcholine do not cause this problem.

Masseter muscle spasm (MMS) following succinylcholine presents a complicated problem. It has been suggested that MMS following succinylcholine is a harbinger of malignant hyperthermia (MH). Many of the patients who have demonstrated MMS have had positive muscle biopsies for MH susceptibility. Because succinylcholine is a triggering agent for MH, some authors have recommended aborting surgery and monitoring for MH. In a large retrospective series published by Littleford et al. (1991), patients who had MMS were allowed to continue with their anesthetic (often including inhaled agents) and surgery. None of their patients developed MH; however, some showed biochemical abnormalities associated with MH. VanDerSpeck et al. (1988) demonstrated in children that masseter muscle tone increases following succinylcholine while limb muscles are relaxed. This may represent a variant of the normal relaxant response to succinylcholine. However, it does not preclude the development of MH. Clinical management following succinylcholine-induced MMS is controversial.

Sustained generalized muscle contracture is associated with MH and must be considered in a different light from isolated MMS. Sustained muscle contracture may also occur in patients with myotonia and dermatomyositis. In these latter circumstances, laryngoscopy may prove difficult, but metabolic disturbances are unlikely.

Anaphylactic and anaphylactoid reactions may occur to many drugs used in anesthesia. Muscle relaxants are most often implicated (80% of cases), and succinylcholine is the most frequent relaxant responsible (54%).

Hyperkalemia is a serious complication of succinylcholine. Under certain conditions, upregulation (proliferation) of nicotinic receptors occurs. This increase in receptors is associated with the appearance of extrajunctional receptors. When exposed to succinylcholine, these receptors allow a massive egress of intracellular K^+, leading to hyperkalemia. Normal increases in serum K^+ following succinylcholine are 0.5–1.0 mEq/L. This rise usually lasts 10–15 minutes. The pathologic response may be far greater.

TABLE 23.1	Conditions Associated with a Hyperkalemic Response to Succinylcholine

Burns
Spinal cord injuries
Closed head injuries
Stroke
Subarachnoid hemorrhage
Intracranial tumors
Peripheral neuropathies
Tetanus
Guillain–Barré syndrome
Rhabdomyosarcoma
Intra-abdominal infections
Prolonged immobilization
Multiple trauma
Crush injuries
Renal failure

Hyperkalemia

Cardiac effects
    Bradycardia to cardiac arrest
    Ventricular fibrillation

Electrocardiogram (ECG) findings
    Peaked T waves
    ST segment depression
    Prolonged PR interval
    Loss of P waves
    Diminished R-wave amplitude
    QRS widening

Treatment
    Antagonism
    Calcium chloride 0.5–1.0 g intravenously; may
        repeat at 5 minute intervals as long as ECG
        changes persist

    Alkalosis
    Hyperventilation
    Sodium bicarbonate 50 mEq intravenously;
        may repeat every 10–15 minutes

    Intracellular shift
    Regular insulin 5–10 U and 25 mL 50%
        dextrose intravenously

    Elimination
    Sodium polystyrene sulfonate (Kayexalate) plus
        sorbital 50 g
    Dialysis

Increases of 7.0 mEq/L have been measured. Acute hyperkalemia may cause peaked T-waves, cardiac conduction block, ventricular dysrhythmias, or sine-wave cardiac arrest. Conditions associated with a hyperkalemic response to succinylcholine are listed in Table 23.1.

Many authors suggest that a safe period exists several months after injury. This is not well documented in the literature. The potential risk of hyperkalemia must be weighed against the benefits of succinylcholine administration.

The use of succinylcholine in renal failure is controversial. The increase in serum K^+ in these patients is no greater than in normal patients. Renal failure patients frequently have a higher initial K^+ level, and some authors suggest that even the small increase normally associated with succinylcholine may put these patients at risk for dysrhythmias. Obviously, the starting K^+ level is critical to the decision regarding succinylcholine's safety in these patients.

Hyperkalemic dysrhythmias following succinylcholine must be rapidly diagnosed and treated. Hyperkalemia may respond to induced alkalosis, which forces K^+ back into the cell. This may be accomplished by hyperventilation and bicarbonate administration. Calcium chloride, 15 mg/kg intravenously, antagonizes the cardiac conduction effects of hyperkalemia and may restore sinus rhythm. Insulin and glucose (10 U of regular insulin in 25 mL of 50% dextrose) also drive K^+ intracellularly.

9. What are the contraindications to succinylcholine administration?

Contraindications to succinylcholine administration follow logically from its known side-effects.

Denervation states leading to extrajunctional receptor upregulation generally contraindicate succinylcholine after 1–3 days following nerve interruption. Uncommon neuromuscular diseases, such as myotonia and dermatomyositis, react with sustained muscular contraction following succinylcholine administration. This defect appears to be intracellular and not at the neuromuscular junction. Such episodes can complicate ventilation and laryngoscopy.

Recently, recommendations for the use of succinylcholine in children have been revised. Several cases of hyperkalemic cardiac arrest in children have been attributed to previously undiagnosed neuromuscular disease, including the muscular dystrophies. Therefore, succinylcholine should only be used in children for rapid sequence induction or emergency control of the airway.

Contraindications to Succinylcholine

Muscle denervation states
  Spinal cord transection
  Cerebrovascular accident with resultant hemi-
    paresis or hemiplegia
  Major nerve plexus injury
  Prolonged immobilization
  Amyotrophic lateral sclerosis

Burns

Crush injury

Neuromuscular disease
  Rhabdomyosarcoma
  Myotonia
  Dermatomyositis
  Malignant hyperthermia

Renal failure?

Pseudocholinesterase deficiency

Suspected inability to intubate the trachea

Raised intracranial pressure?

Raised intraocular pressure?

Allergy

SUGGESTED READINGS

Bevan DR, Donati F: Muscle relaxants. pp. 419–447. In Barash PG, Cullen BF, Stoelting RK (eds): Clinical Anesthesia, 4th edition. Lippincott Williams & Wilkins, Philadelphia, 2001

Bevan DR, Donati F, Kopman AF: Reversal of neuromuscular blockade. Anesthesiology 77:785–805, 1992

Booij LH: Neuromuscular transmission and its pharmacological blockade. Part 2: Pharmacology of neuromuscular blocking agents. Pharmacy World Sci 19:13–34, 1997

Book WJ, Abel M, Eisenkraft JB: Adverse effects of depolarizing neuromuscular blocking agents: incidence, prevention, and management. Drug Safety 10:331–349, 1994

Fisher DM: Neuromuscular blocking agents in paediatric anaesthesia. Br J Anaesth 83:58–64, 1999

Gronert GA: Cardiac arrest after succinylcholine: mortality greater with rhabdomyolysis than receptor upregulation. Anesthesiology 94:523–529, 2001

Kelly RE, Dinner M, Turner LF, et al.: Succinylcholine increases IOP in the human eye with the extraocular muscles detached. Anesthesiology 79:948–952, 1993

Korvarick WD, Mayberg TS, Lam AM, et al.: Succinylcholine does not change intracranial pressure, cerebral blood flow velocity, or the electroencephalogram in patients with neurologic injury. Anesth Analg 78:469–473, 1994

Lando G, Mosca A, Bonora R, et al.: Frequency of butyrylcholinesterase gene mutations in individuals with abnormal inhibition numbers: an Italian population study. Pharmacogenetics 13:265–270, 2003

Littleford JA, Patel LR, Bose D, et al.: Masseter spasm in children: implications of continuing the triggering anesthetic. Anesth Analg 72:151–160, 1991

Martyn JAJ, White DA, Gronert GA, Jaffe RS, Ward JM: Up- and down regulation of skeletal muscle acetylcholine receptors' effects on neuromuscular blockers. Anesthesiology 76:822–843, 1992

Naguib M, Lien CA, Aker J, et al.: Posttetanic potentiation and fade in the response to tetanic and train-of-four stimulation during succinylcholine-induced block. Anesth Analg 98: 1686–1681, 2004

Pantuck EJ: Plasma cholinesterase: gene and variations. Anesth Analg 77:380–386, 1993

VanDerSpeck AFL, Fang WB, Ashton-Miller JA, et al.: Increased masticatory muscle stiffness during limb muscle flaccidity associated with succinylcholine administration. Anesthesiology 69:11–16, 1988

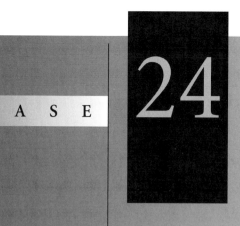

CASE 24

NONDEPOLARIZING NEUROMUSCULAR BLOCKADE

Mark Abel, MD

A 60-year-old, 60 kg woman with colon carcinoma, a history of temporal arteritis, and mitral valve prolapse presents for hemicolectomy. She is otherwise in good health. Her medications included prednisone 40 mg orally every day, ampicillin 2 g intravenously every 6 hours, and gentamicin 80 mg intravenously every 12 hours. She received pancuronium 4 mg intravenously at the beginning of the procedure. Two hours later, no twitches are visible on train-of-four monitoring.

QUESTIONS

1. Describe the mechanism by which nondepolarizing muscle relaxants produce neuromuscular blockade.
2. Differentiate between the commonly employed non-depolarizing muscle relaxants.
3. Briefly outline the mechanisms by which drugs other than neuromuscular muscle relaxants affect neuromuscular blockade.
4. What effects do antibiotics have on neuromuscular blockade?
5. How do drugs other than antibiotics affect neuromuscular blockade?
6. What are the metabolic factors that affect antagonism of neuromuscular blockade?

1. Describe the mechanism by which nondepolarizing neuromuscular blockers produce neuromuscular blockade.

Nondepolarizing muscle relaxants produce neuromuscular blockade by several mechanisms:

- They compete with acetylcholine for the α subunit of the acetylcholine receptor on the postjunctional membrane.
- They competitively inhibit acetylcholine from stimulating its receptor at the motor endplate.
- There is also evidence that they block prejunctional acetylcholine receptors, decreasing acetylcholine release in response to motor nerve stimulation.
- Noncompetitive blockade of open postjunctional acetylcholine channels plays a minor role as well.

2. Differentiate between the commonly employed non-depolarizing muscle relaxants.

All nondepolarizing muscle relaxants decrease striated muscle strength by competitive inhibition of postsynaptic acetylcholine receptors at the neuromuscular junction. Some muscle relaxants affect prejunctional acetylcholine receptors as well. Clinically important parameters that distinguish nondepolarizing muscle relaxants from one another include onset times, elimination times, routes of elimination, and potency (Table 24.1). Rocuronium is

TABLE 24.1   Pharmacology of Nondepolarizing Neuromuscular Blockers

Drug	ED$_{95}$ (mg/kg)	Clinical 75–25 RI (minutes)	Approximate Elimination Half-life (t$_{1/2}$B) (minutes)	Metabolism	Side-effects
Atracurium	0.2	11–23	20	Nonenyzmatic ester hydrolysis, Hoffman elimination	Skin flushing, hypotension, bronchospasm; histamine release after large doses
Cis-atracurium	0.05	11–23	20	Nonenzymatic ester hydrolysis, Hoffman elimination	
Doxacurium	0.025		99	Primarily renal elimination	
Mivacurium	0.07	6–8	18	Hydrolysis by plasma cholinesterase	Histamine release after large doses
Pancuronium	0.07	24	145	Primarily renal elimination, some hepatic degradation	Tachycardia, vagolysis
Pipecuronium	0.04	30–40	137	Primarily renal elimination, small degree of hepatic degradation	
Rocuronium	0.3	10–15	60–75	Primarily hepatic, some renal elimination	
d-Tubocurarine	0.5	25–35	80	Renal excretion, minimal hepatic degradation	Hypotension, autonomic ganglionic blockade, histamine release, prostacyclin release, skin flushing
Vecuronium	0.05	10–15	62	Primarily hepatic metabolism, some renal elimination	

ED$_{95}$, effective dose that produces 95% twitch height depression; RI, recovery index.

unique among the nondepolarizing muscle relaxants for its rapid onset of action. Intubating doses of 2–3 times the effective dose that produces 95% twitch height depression (ED$_{95}$) may provide intubating conditions in 60–90 seconds, which approaches but does not equal the onset time for succinylcholine.

3. Briefly outline the mechanisms by which drugs other than neuromuscular muscle relaxants affect neuromuscular blockade.

Most drugs that interact with neuromuscular muscle relaxants enhance the degree of block; however, some have the opposite effect. Some drugs have direct effects of their own on neuromuscular transmission, while some interact via alternate mechanisms at other sites. Sometimes, no single mechanism can account for the interaction. Sites of interference include motor nerves, nerve terminals, endplates, nicotinic receptors, postsynaptic muscle membrane, and interference with excitation–contraction coupling.

Non-neuromuscular components include the central nervous system and metabolic mechanisms.

4. What effects do antibiotics have on neuromuscular blockade?

Many antibiotics interact with neuromuscular transmission, enhancing the effect of neuromuscular muscle relaxants.

The aminoglycosides enhance nondepolarizing neuromuscular blockade by decreasing nerve terminal release of acetylcholine, a magnesium-like effect. Additionally, aminoglycosides decrease the sensitivity of the acetylcholine receptor to acetylcholine. Aminoglycosides may augment depolarizing neuromuscular blockade; however, this is less well studied.

Nonaminoglycoside antibiotics also augment neuromuscular blockade. Polymixin B augments blockade by decreasing acetylcholine release from nerve terminals and by decreasing endplate ion channel conductance. A local anesthetic-like effect may decrease the action potential of

Factors Potentiating Neuromuscular Blockade

Potentiate

Pre-existing neuromuscular pathology
    Myasthenia gravis
    Eaton Lambert syndrome

Acid–base alterations
    Respiratory acidosis
    Metabolic alkalosis

Electrolyte imbalance
    Hypocalcemia
    Hypokalemia
    Hyponatremia
    Hypermagnesemia

Potent inhalation agents
    Halothane
    Enflurane
    Isoflurane
    Sevoflurane
    Desflurane

Local anesthetics
    Lidocaine
    Procaine

Antibiotics
    Gentamicin
    Neomycin
    Clindamycin
    Polymixin B
    Tetracycline
    Streptomycin
    Lincomycin

Class IA anti-arrhythmics
    Quinidine
    Procainamide

Calcium-channel blockers
    Verapamil (case reports)

Dantrolene

Factors Inducing Resistance to Neuromuscular Blockade

Corticosteroids

Methylxanthines

Antiepileptics
    Phenytoin
    Carbamazepine

muscle as well. Both depolarizing and nondepolarizing neuromuscular blockades are affected. Clindamycin and lincomycin both enhance nondepolarizing neuromuscular blockade. They exert a nonmagnesium-like, prejunctional effect. Clindamycin but not lincomycin has a local anesthetic-like effect as well. The tetracyclines exert a prejunctional effect, increasing sensitivity to nondepolarizing neuromuscular blockade but not to succinylcholine.

5. How do drugs other than antibiotics affect neuromuscular blockade?

Local anesthetics and class IA anti–arrhythmic drugs block sodium channels and may decrease neuromuscular transmission throughout the neuromuscular chain of events, affecting axonal conduction and acetylcholine release. In larger concentrations, they may decrease endplate and muscle membrane ion conductance. Both succinylcholine and nondepolarizing muscle relaxants are affected. Calcium-channel blockers interfere with calcium conductance in the neuromuscular system and may potentiate depolarizing and nondepolarizing neuromuscular blockade. The effects of lithium are controversial, but it may potentiate both depolarizing and nondepolarizing neuromuscular blockade. High serum levels of magnesium, such as occur in pre-eclamptic and eclamptic patients, profoundly potentiate both depolarizing and nondepolarizing neuromuscular blockade by blocking calcium conductance in the nerve terminal and by stabilizing the postjunctional muscle fiber membrane. Calcium readily reverses the former effect, whereas it is less predictable for the latter effect. However, attempts to reverse the effects of magnesium and magnesium-like effects with calcium should be made. Dantrolene causes weakness by blocking excitation–contraction coupling, augmenting the effects of muscle relaxants. Echothiophate is a cholinesterase inhibitor used occasionally in the treatment of glaucoma. It significantly interferes with plasma cholinesterase, prolonging the duration of action of succinylcholine. The chemotherapeutic agent cyclophosphamide significantly decreases plasma cholinesterase concentrations, decreasing the metabolic rate of succinylcholine degradation. The immunosuppressant cyclosporine potentiates the effects of atracurium and vecuronium.

Thus far, the interactions discussed have focused on those that potentiate neuromuscular blockade. Several drugs induce resistance to neuromuscular muscle relaxants, such as corticosteroids, methylxanthines, and antiepileptic drugs. Corticosteroids may induce resistance to nondepolarizing muscle relaxants by increasing presynaptic acetylcholine levels. The clinical relevance of this effect remains controversial. Methylxanthines may induce resistance through a phosphodiesterase-dependent mechanism.

6. What are the metabolic factors that affect antagonism of neuromuscular blockade?

Respiratory acidosis and metabolic alkalosis increase the depth of neuromuscular blockade and make antagonism more difficult. Postoperative respiratory acidosis of some degree is common in patients following general anesthesia.

Hypothermia, hypokalemia, hypermagnesemia, and hypocalcemia may each decrease the likelihood of successfully antagonizing neuromuscular blockade.

SUGGESTED READINGS

Cammu G: Interactions of neuromuscular blocking drugs. Acta Anaesthesiol Belg 52:357–363, 2001

Feldman S, Karalliedde L: Drug interactions with neuromuscular blockers. Drug Safety 15:261–273, 1996

Magleby KL, Pallotta BS, Terrar DA: The effect of tubocurarine on neuromuscular transmission during repetitive stimulation in the rat, mouse, and hog. J Physiol (Lond) 312:97, 1981

Moore EW, Hunter JM: The new neuromuscular blocking agents: do they offer any advantages? Br J Anaesth 87:912–925, 2001

Ostergaard D, Engbaek J, Biby-Mogensen J: Adverse reactions and interactions of the neuromuscular blocking drugs. Med Toxicol Adverse Drug Experience 4: 351–368, 1989

ANTAGONISM OF NONDEPOLARIZING NEUROMUSCULAR BLOCKADE

Mark Abel, MD

A 50-year-old woman without significant medical history presents for total abdominal hysterectomy. Uneventful induction of anesthesia is achieved with thiopental and pancuronium. Ninety minutes later, the procedure ends. TOF monitoring demonstrates a single twitch, and you decide to antagonize the neuromuscular blockade.

QUESTIONS

1. Describe the overall strategy for terminating the action of nondepolarizing neuromuscular blockade.
2. List the clinically relevant acetylcholinesterase inhibitors.
3. What is the mechanism of acetylcholinesterase inhibition?
4. List the proper doses of muscle relaxant antagonists and their duration of action.
5. Explain the need for antimuscarinics used in conjunction with acetylcholinesterase inhibitors.
6. What is the onset of action for acetylcholinesterase inhibitors?
7. Describe the mechanism of muscle relaxant antagonism by cyclodextrins.
8. Explain the clinical indices of recovery from neuromuscular blockade.

1. Describe the overall strategy for terminating the action of nondepolarizing neuromuscular blockade.

Two strategies have traditionally existed for terminating the action of nondepolarizing neuromuscular blockade. Strength returns as neuromuscular muscle relaxants diffuse away from the receptor sites, so that spontaneous recovery occurs over time. Alternatively, drugs that inhibit the enzyme acetylcholinesterase can be administered. This inhibition causes a "flood" of acetylcholine at the neuromuscular junction, favoring competitive interaction of acetylcholine with its receptor. Depending on the relative amounts of acetylcholine and nondepolarizing muscle relaxant present, the block will be partially or completely antagonized.

A radical new approach for reversal of neuromuscular blockade is currently under investigation. Cyclodextrins are agents that encapsulate nondepolarizing muscle relaxants, effectively reducing their plasma concentration to zero.

2. List the clinically relevant acetylcholinesterase inhibitors.

The clinically relevant acetylcholinesterase inhibitors include neostigmine, pyridostigmine, and edrophonium (Table 25.1). They are all quaternary amines that do not cross the blood–brain barrier. Physostigmine, a tertiary amine, has profound central effects and, for this reason, is not used to antagonize neuromuscular blockade.

The active portion of acetylcholinesterase includes an anionic and an esteratic subsite. The anionic subsite

Commonly Used Acetylcholinesterase Inhibitors and Antimuscarinic Agents

Drug	Usual Dose (mg/kg)	Onset (min)	Duration (min)
Acetylcholinesterase inhibitors			
Neostigmine	0.06	6	60–120
Edrophonium	0.5–1.0	1–2	60–120
Pyridostigmine	0.2	15	60–120
Antimuscarinic agents			
Atropine	0.01 with edrophonium	1	30
	0.02 with neostigmine		
Glycopyrrolate	0.01 with neostigmine or pyridostigmine	2–3	60

interacts electrostatically with the quaternary nitrogen of either choline or the acetylcholinesterase inhibitors, while the esteratic subsite interacts with edrophonium by hydrogen bonding and with neostigmine by covalent bonding. The electrostatic and hydrogen bonds formed by edrophonium are rapidly reversible, while the covalent bond of neostigmine requires more time (a half-life of 30 minutes) to break, resulting in hydrolysis of the neostigmine molecule into two fragments. Conversely, edrophonium's interaction with acetylcholinesterase yields an intact edrophonium molecule, which is subsequently cleared by the kidney.

3. What is the mechanism of acetylcholinesterase inhibition?

The simple and widely accepted mechanism of acetylcholinesterase inhibition is the law of mass action. Large amounts of acetylcholine at the neuromuscular junction secondary to inhibition of acetylcholinesterase increase the interactions between acetylcholine and its postjunctional receptor. Excess acetylcholine effectively competes with nondepolarizing muscle relaxants for nicotinic receptor binding sites on the postjunctional membrane. Additionally, quaternary amines appear to exert a direct stimulatory action on skeletal muscle. Denervated muscle or muscle whose nerve terminals lack acetylcholine contract after exposure to quaternary acetylcholinesterase inhibitors, implying a direct action by these agents. Also, acetylcholinesterase inhibitors can convert a single action potential in a motor nerve into a pattern of repetitive firing. This repetitive firing may spread retrograde up the axon, causing other nerves in the same motor unit to fire. This results in increased muscular contraction.

4. List the proper doses of muscle relaxant antagonists and their duration of action.

Recommended "reversal" dosages depend on the depth of neuromuscular blockade and the particular muscle relaxant employed. Neostigmine is 5 times more potent than pyridostigmine and about 12 times more potent than edrophonium. Typical doses for neostigmine, pyridostigmine, and edrophonium are 0.04–0.06 mg/kg, 0.21 mg/kg, and 0.5 mg/kg, respectively (Table 25.1). These drugs offer differing onset times. Edrophonium has the most rapid onset time, exerting a peak effect in slightly over 1 minute. Neostigmine and pyridostigmine have slower onsets, exerting their peak effects in 6 and 15 minutes, respectively. All three commonly used acetylcholinesterase inhibitors are of sufficient duration to antagonize nondepolarizing neuromuscular blockade secondary to long- or intermediate-acting drugs provided the degree of residual blockade is moderate (detectable responses to train-of-four (TOF) stimulation).

Edrophonium, even when used in large doses (0.5–1 mg/kg), is an unreliable antagonist of deep neuromuscular blockade (T_1/T_C = 10–25%) induced by long-acting muscle relaxants (tubocurarine, pancuronium, pipecuronium, or doxacurium). When deep neuromuscular blockade is present, edrophonium should not be used as an antagonist.

5. Explain the need for antimuscarinics used in conjunction with acetylcholinesterase inhibitors.

Inhibitors of acetylcholinesterase cause a dramatic increase in the concentration of acetylcholine at all effector organs. While this improves neuromuscular transmission by acting on the nicotinic receptor of the neuromuscular junction, increased acetylcholine concentration has many undesirable effects on visceral end-organs. These effects are mediated by the muscarinic subset of acetylcholine receptors. Atropine and glycopyrrolate are used to prevent these muscarinic effects (Table 25.1).

The most dramatic and feared muscarinic effect is that on the heart. Acetylcholinesterase inhibitors may cause profound bradycardia, nodal or ventricular escape beats, or even asystole. Increased gastrointestinal motility with excess salivation and diarrhea are other undesirable effects.

Side Effects of Acetylcholinesterase Therapy

Vagal stimulation
    Sinus bradycardia
    Sinus arrest
    Slows atrial conduction
    Slows atrioventricular node conduction

Smooth muscle contraction
    Bronchoconstriction
    Increases gastrointestinal and urinary bladder
        tone
    Miosis

Increased secretions
    Saliva
    Tracheobronchial

Neuromuscular blockade
    Increase tetanic fade in the absence of prior
        nondepolarizing neuromuscular blockade
    ? Cholinergic crisis

The pulmonary system is profoundly affected as well, with increased airway secretions and bronchospasm causing wheezing and difficulty in ventilation.

To prevent these undesirable side-effects, acetylcholinesterase inhibitors are given with an antimuscarinic agent, either atropine or glycopyrrolate. Administration of these agents together with acetylcholinesterase inhibitors prevents life-threatening bradydysrhythmias and limits airway secretions, avoiding ventilatory problems.

Because the onset time of atropine is more rapid than that of glycopyrrolate, it is frequently used in combination with edrophonium. Atropine 0.01 mg/kg should precede the administration of edrophonium. Once a tachycardia occurs, appropriate doses of edrophonium may be given. This ensures that atropine's vagolytic effects precede the vagotonic (bradycardic) effects of edrophonium. Atropine, 0.02 mg/kg, may be combined with or precede the administration of neostigmine. This may result in tachycardia, however, because atropine has a more rapid onset than neostigmine. Glycopyrrolate, with a slower onset than atropine, is usually administered together with neostigmine, providing offsetting chronotropic stability. Neostigmine and glycopyrrolate may be given separately or combined in a single syringe. The latter approach, while generally safe, should not be used in patients with conduction defects or sick sinus syndrome, because life-threatening bradycardia may result. Occasionally, patients who do not demonstrate

a tachycardic response to antimuscarinics are encountered. These patients should not receive acetylcholinesterase inhibitors unless a functioning pacemaker is available. Alternatively, neuromuscular muscle relaxants may be allowed to wear off spontaneously.

6. What is the onset of action for acetylcholinesterase inhibitors?

When single twitch height exceeds 20% of control, neuromuscular blockade can be quickly antagonized by acetylcholinesterase inhibitors. Greater degrees of twitch height depression require more time, occasionally as much as 30–40 minutes. When twitches are absent on TOF stimulation, anticholinesterase therapy generally results in partial paralysis and unsafe extubation conditions.

7. Describe the mechanism of muscle relaxant antagonism by cyclodextrins.

Cyclodextrins are large doughnut-shaped molecules designed to encapsulate rocuronium. As rocuronium diffuses from the neuromuscular junction, it forms a guest–host complex with the cyclodextrin molecule. Neuromuscular recovery occurs rapidly as rocuronium diffuses from the neuromuscular junction. Cyclodextrins also have the potential to reverse other nondepolarizing muscle relaxants, although further study is indicated. Since cyclodextrins do not inhibit cholinesterases, they are free of autonomic side-effects, including cardiovascular and other muscarinic effects.

8. Explain the clinical indices of recovery from neuromuscular blockade.

Antagonism of neuromuscular blockade is undertaken to ensure adequate minute ventilation and satisfactory airway protection. Clinical predictors of the ability to accomplish these two goals include sustained head lift for 5 seconds and tongue protrusion. These tests, particularly head lift, are good predictors of clinical recovery. However, they require patient cooperation and will not be performed consistently by all patients.

Negative inspiratory force has been used as an indicator of strength. Adequate minute ventilation is associated with inspiratory forces of –25 cm H_2O. Until recently, this was felt to be sufficient for extubation; however, the ability to swallow and protect the airway do not return until inspiratory forces of –42 cm H_2O and –53 cm H_2O, respectively, are generated.

Neuromuscular transmission monitoring is frequently used to assess adequate recovery from neuromuscular blockade. A mechanomyograph T_4/T_1 ratio of 0.7 or an electromyograph T_4/T_1 ratio of 0.9 correlates well with clinical recovery from neuromuscular blockade. Visual observation

Extubation Criteria

Patient-dependent criteria
    Head lift for 5 seconds
    Tongue protrusion
    Vital capacity >15 mL/kg

Patient-independent criteria
    Inspiratory force >−53 cm H_2O
    PaO_2 >80 mmHg on 40% oxygen
    Gag reflex present
    Absence of fade for 5 seconds on 50 Hz tetanic
        stimulus

or manual palpation of standard twitch monitors tends to underestimate the degree of block. The trachea should not be extubated while the TOF fade is appreciable on these monitors.

SUGGESTED READINGS

Adam JM, Bennett DJ, Bom A, et al.: Cyclodextrin-derived host molecules as reversal agents for the neuromuscular blocker rocuronium bromide: synthesis and structure–activity relationships. J Med Chem 45:1806–1816, 2002

Bevan DR, Donati F, Kopman AF: Reversal of neuromuscular blockade. Anesthesiology 77:785, 1992

Cameron KS, Clark JK, Cooper A, et al.: Modified gamma-cyclodextrins and their rocuronium complexes. Org Lett 4: 3403–3406, 2002

Epemolu O, Bom A, Hope F, et al.: Reversal of neuromuscular blockade and simultaneous increase in plasma rocuronium concentration after the intravenous infusion of the novel reversal agent Org 25969. Anesthesiology 99:632–637, 2003

Kopman AF: Edrophonium antagonism of pancuronium-induced neuromuscular blockade in man: a reappraisal. Anesthesiology 51:139, 1979

Pavlin EG, Holle H, Schoene RB: Recovery of airway protection compared with ventilation in humans after paralysis with curare. Anesthesiology 70:381, 1989

Power SJ, Jones RM: Reversal of profound paralysis: use of large doses of edrophonium to antagonize vecuronium and pancuronium induced neuromuscular blockade. Acta Anaesthesiol Scand 33:478, 1989

Shorten GD, Ali HH, Goudsouzian NG: Neostigmine and edrophonium antagonism of moderate neuromuscular block induced by pancuronium or tubocurarine. Br J Anaesth 70:160, 1993

Weber S, Muravchick S: Electrical and mechanical train of four responses during depolarizing and non-depolarizing neuromuscular block. Anesth Analg 65:771, 1986

26

MONITORING THE NEUROMUSCULAR JUNCTION

Mark Abel, MD

Before purchasing a new nondepolarizing neuromuscular blocker, your hospital requests an evaluation. You decide to measure the median effective dose, ED_{50} (effective dose producing 50% twitch height depression) and ED_{95} (effective dose producing 95% twitch height depression) in 100 patients using electromyography.

QUESTIONS

1. Why is monitoring of neuromuscular function necessary in the practice of anesthesia?
2. What is the mechanomyograph (MMG)?
3. Describe the electromyograph (EMG).
4. What kind of nerve stimulator is in common clinical use?
5. Describe accelerography.
6. What is phonomyography?
7. Explain the different patterns of nerve stimulation and the relevance of pattern choice.

1. Why is monitoring of neuromuscular function necessary in the practice of anesthesia?

Muscle relaxants, by interfering with neuromuscular transmission, cause paralysis or clinical weakness. Because these drugs are frequently used as adjuncts to anesthetics, some means of monitoring depth of neuromuscular blockade and recovery are necessary to ensure adequate intubation conditions, sufficient surgical relaxation, and enough recovery of muscle strength to allow relaxant antagonism before tracheal extubation.

2. What is the mechanomyograph (MMG)?

The MMG is the historical standard for neuromuscular monitoring. Peripheral nerves are stimulated with a sufficient current to depolarize all axons of a motor nerve. This current is usually on the order of 50–60 milliamps and is called a *supramaximal stimulus*. Increasing the stimulus beyond supramaximal does not further increase the response. The current applied to a nerve causes a wave of depolarization, which results in acetylcholine release from nerve terminals with subsequent endplate and motor depolarization and muscle contraction. Mechanical twitch tension can then be measured using a force transducer. The force vector must be properly aligned with a transducer, or the measurement will not be accurate. Furthermore, the muscle must be preloaded with a specific tension (100–300 g) to ensure optimal contractile force. Clearly, MMG monitors must be carefully applied to ensure accurate and consistent measurements. MMGs are designed for preselected sites, usually ulnar nerve stimulation and adductor pollicis brevis force measurements.

3. Describe the electromyograph (EMG).

The EMG provides a more convenient means of measuring neuromuscular function. Like the MMG, a peripheral motor nerve is stimulated with a supramaximal current.

The electrical response of the muscle, the compound action potential, is then recorded. Stimulating electrodes are placed over a peripheral nerve, and recording electrodes are placed over an innervated muscle. A ground electrode is placed as well. Unlike the MMG, the EMG does not require a preloaded muscle or precise force vector measurements because the response is electrical rather than mechanical. A greater variety of muscles may be studied because the EMG is not specifically designed for a particular muscle, nor is direct, continuous access to the studied muscle required.

4. What kind of nerve stimulator is in common clinical use?

The peripheral nerve stimulator, which is used to subjectively observe or palpate the response, is most commonly used in practice. Although these stimulators provide subjective and potentially inaccurate results, they are compact, user-friendly, and inexpensive. In combination with sound clinical tests and judgment, they are usually adequate to evaluate the degree of neuromuscular responsiveness. Direct muscle stimulation may mimic a neuromuscular response. Care must be taken to evaluate a true neuromuscular response rather than direct muscle stimulation by the current. For example, the response to ulnar nerve stimulation should be observed or palpated in the adductor pollicis brevis of the thumb. This site, remote from the stimulating electrodes, eliminates the possibility of direct muscle stimulation. Other possible stimulation sites include facial, posterior tibial, and common peroneal nerves. Regardless of the site selected, quantitative evaluation of result is highly variable from one observer to another.

5. Describe accelerography.

A new method of monitoring neuromuscular response involves measuring acceleration. A supramaximal stimulus is applied to the ulnar nerve while a transducer affixed to the thumb measures its acceleration. Good correlation exists between the accelerograph and other monitoring modalities. Like the MMG and EEG, accelerography is useful in the quantitative measurement of neuromuscular blockade.

6. What is phonomyography?

Phonomyography is a new monitoring modality that employs the measurement of low-frequency sound waves. During muscle contraction, low-frequency sound waves are emitted. These can be detected using special microphones in order to measure the degree of neuromuscular blockade. Further study is needed prior to common usage of this modality.

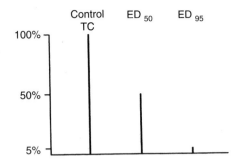

FIGURE 26.1 Schematic representation of single-twitch height measurement and depression following onset of neuromuscular blockade. Stimulus frequency is less than 0.15 Hz, and measured values are compared with control values (T_c) for ED_{50} and ED_{95} measurement.

7. Explain the different patterns of nerve stimulation and the relevance of pattern choice.

The simplest pattern is single-twitch stimulation (Figure 26.1). The stimulus should be a rectangular pulse of 0.1–0.3 millisecond duration. Stimulus frequencies of greater than 0.15 Hz may cause fade in single-twitch measurements; therefore, measurements are generally made at 0.1 Hz intervals. A supramaximal stimulus is required. A control (pre-neuromuscular blockade) single twitch (T_c) is measured and recorded. Subsequent single-twitch measurements are compared with the control value (T_1/T_c). This mode is primarily useful in research. Relative potencies of neuromuscular blocking agents are measured, and recovery rates are quantified. Single-twitch stimulation has its limitations. It requires recording of control values before administration of neuromuscular blockers. In addition, full return of single-twitch height to control levels does not guarantee normal function of the neuromuscular junction.

A clinically useful stimulation pattern (Figure 26.2) is the train-of-four (TOF). When a peripheral nerve is stimulated at a rate greater than 0.15 Hz, the muscular response will

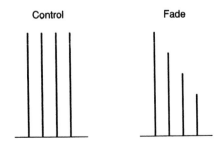

FIGURE 26.2 Schematic representation of train-of-four measurement. They must be separated by 10- to 12-second intervals.

show fade. The ratio of the fourth to the first twitch is measured (T_4/T_1), and called the T_4 ratio. Four stimuli applied at a frequency of 2 Hz are employed clinically. Multiple TOF stimuli are separated by 10- to 12-second intervals to ensure maximal twitch height. Fade on the TOF is a property of nondepolarizing muscle relaxants. It is a presynaptic phenomenon. Depolarizing muscle relaxants do not show fade on TOF unless a phase II block has occurred. An advantage of TOF monitoring compared with single-twitch monitoring is that a recorded control value is not required.

Furthermore, fade of the fourth twitch is still seen when the first twitch has fully recovered, making TOF measurements a more sensitive indicator of neuromuscular blockade than single-twitch measurements. A T_4 ratio of greater than 0.7 on MMG or 0.9 on EMG correlates well with clinical signs of recovery from nondepolarizing neuromuscular blockade. When TOF is measured by manual palpation or observation, as in most clinical situations, the degree of fade is generally underestimated. Therefore, the trachea should not be extubated when fade is visible or palpable.

The fourth twitch disappears completely when the first twitch height is 25% of control. This usually correlates well with adequate surgical relaxation. Disappearance of the third twitch occurs when the first twitch is 80% depressed, and at 90% first twitch height depression, the second twitch disappears. This is the degree of relaxation required to facilitate endotracheal intubation.

High-frequency (30–200 Hz) nerve stimulation is called tetanic stimulation and evokes a tetanic response without fade in the unrelaxed muscle (Figure 26.3). Physiologic frequencies of 50 Hz are most commonly employed in the operating room. Higher frequencies may produce fade even in the absence of neuromuscular blockade and are, therefore, overly sensitive for clinical situations. At a stimulus frequency of 50 Hz, tetanic fade is seen only in the presence of nondepolarizing or phase II neuromuscular blockade. As previously alluded to, fade is felt to be a presynaptic phenomenon resulting from a decrease in presynaptic

acetylcholine stores in the presence of a postsynaptic competitive blockade of acetylcholine receptors. Blockade of presynaptic acetylcholine receptors may play a role as well. A sustained response to a 50 Hz tetanic stimulus correlates very well with the ability to protect the airway.

Application of a tetanic stimulus elicits a phenomenon called *post-tetanic facilitation.* Following tetanic stimulation, responses to single-twitch or TOF stimulation are augmented. Tetanic stimulation at 50 Hz applied for 5 seconds requires a 2-minute recovery period to avoid post-tetanic facilitation. Care must therefore be taken not to apply a tetanic stimulus shortly before a TOF stimulus. When profound neuromuscular blockade is present and the TOF completely obliterated, the presence of TOF response following tetanic stimulation (post-tetanic facilitation) portends the return of TOF and eventual reversibility.

Another modality is double-burst stimulation. Two brief (0.2 milliseconds) tetanic stimuli are separated by 750 milliseconds. Consecutive double-burst stimulations must be separated by at least 15 seconds. Two palpable twitches are elicited. These twitches may exhibit fade, which correlates well with fade on the TOF. As previously mentioned, absence of palpable or visible fade on standard TOF monitoring may be associated with residual, measurable fade on TOF by MMG or EMG. The presence of two equivalent twitches following double-burst stimulation accurately indicates the absence of neuromuscular blockade and more sensitively indicates return of neuromuscular function than tetanus or TOF.

SUGGESTED READINGS

Bevan DR: Monitoring and reversal of neuromuscular block. Am J Health Syst Pharm 56:S10–13, 1999

Gill SS, Donati F, Bevan DR: Clinical evaluation of double-burst stimulation. Its relationship to train of four stimulation. Anaesthesia 45:543, 1990

Gorgias N, Maidatsi P, Zaralidou A, et al.: Monitoring the onset of neuromuscular blockade with double-burst stimulation (DBS). Methods Find Exp Clin Pharmacol 20:801, 1998

Hemmerling TM, Donati F: Neuromuscular blockade at the larynx, the diaphragm and the corrugator supercilii muscle: a review. Can J Anaesth 50:779, 2003

Sharpe MD: The use of muscle relaxants in the intensive care unit. Can J Anaesth 39:949, 1992

Suzuki T, Nagai H, Katsumata N, et al.: Investigation of fading responses induced by non-depolarising muscle relaxants in the evoked EMG of the gastrocnemius muscle of the cat. Acta Anaesthesiol Scand 43:658, 1999

Torda TA: Monitoring neuromuscular transmission. Anaesth Intensive Care 30:123, 2002

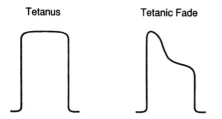

FIGURE 26.3 Schematic representation of tetanic stimulation. In the absence of neuromuscular blockade tetanic stimulation at 50 Hz does not evoke fade. During nondepolarizing neuromuscular blockade and phase II block from depolarizing muscle relaxants, tetanic stimulation at 50 Hz results in fade.

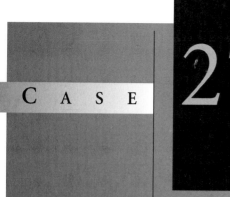

MYASTHENIA GRAVIS

Mark Abel, MD

A 56-year-old man with myasthenia gravis (MG) affecting extraocular and bulbar musculature presents for transcervical thymectomy. He is taking pyridostigmine 660 mg and prednisone 20 mg orally every day in divided doses. He is also taking metoclopramide 10 mg four times a day for reflux esophagitis. Spirometry reveals a vital capacity of 50% predicted and an FEV_1/FVC ratio of 80%. Maximum breathing capacity is 45% predicted. Following placement of monitors and while the patient is breathing 100% oxygen, rapid sequence induction with cricoid pressure is performed using thiopental 4 mg/kg and succinylcholine 1 mg/kg. After 60 seconds, twitch height is decreased by 60%, and the trachea is intubated with some difficulty. Anesthesia is maintained with nitrous oxide, oxygen, and sevoflurane as required. Ventilation is controlled. At return of twitch height to 100%, vecuronium 0.05 mg/kg is administered with resultant loss of twitch response to nerve stimulation. Surgery lasts 1½ hours. The anesthetic agents are discontinued, and the patient demonstrates four equal twitches to train-of-four (TOF) stimulation. Neostigmine 0.06 mg/kg and glycopyrrolate 0.01 mg/kg are administered. When the patient responds to command, the trachea is extubated, at which point the patient immediately becomes dyspneic.

QUESTIONS

1. What is the lesion of myasthenia gravis (MG)?
2. How is MG diagnosed?
3. Explain the treatment alternatives for MG.
4. Why are patients with MG sensitive to nondepolarizing muscle relaxants and resistant to depolarizing muscle relaxants?
5. How are patients with MG premedicated for surgery?
6. Describe a reasonable anesthetic technique for a patient with MG undergoing transcervical thymectomy.
7. Following emergence from anesthesia and before extubation, how is strength assessed?
8. What is cholinergic crisis?
9. Can preoperative evaluation predict the need for postoperative ventilation?

1. What is the lesion of myasthenia gravis (MG)?

MG is an autoimmune disease of the motor endplate. It presents with easy fatigability of voluntary muscles followed by recovery with rest. Its first manifestation is frequently diplopia. Often it is generalized and progressive. The incidence approximates 1:2,000 adults. MG is an antibody-mediated disorder. The amount of presynaptic acetylcholine released is normal or increased. Antibodies are produced to the acetylcholine receptor of the neuromuscular junction. In 10–15% of patients with MG, the presence of antibodies cannot be demonstrated. Antibodies are of the immunoglobulin G (IgG) class and are specific for the α subunit of the endplate receptor. Myasthenics are noted to have 70–80% fewer receptors on the motor endplate and fewer folds in the synaptic cleft. Reduction in the number of receptors is brought about by functional block, increased rate of receptor degradation, or complement-mediated lysis of the postsynaptic membrane. Under normal conditions, only 25–30% of receptors are required for neuromuscular transmission. The decrease in receptors represents a reduction in the margin of safety of neuromuscular transmission. These patients are extremely sensitive to any agent that interferes with neuromuscular transmission.

2. How is MG diagnosed?

The diagnosis of MG is made from a history of skeletal muscle weakness and easy fatigability that improves with rest. Any muscle group may be involved, but the ocular muscles are the most frequently affected. Bulbar muscle weakness predisposes to impaired breathing, swallowing, and airway control. Periods of exacerbation and remission are common.

Confirmatory tests include the following:

- *Edrophonium (Tensilon) test:* A small (2–5 mg) dose of edrophonium may elicit an improvement in strength in the myasthenic. Edrophonium is an acetylcholinesterase inhibitor. It increases the availability of acetylcholine to the receptor by inhibiting its degradation. The increased availability of acetylcholine enhances the likelihood of agonist–receptor interaction and therefore endplate depolarization, leading to improved neuromuscular transmission in the myasthenic. Strength will not improve in the normal patient. In fact, lingual fasciculations may be noted from an excess of acetylcholine.
- *Electromyography:* A motor nerve is stimulated three times per second, and the electrical activity of the muscle is recorded. A decrement of response of at least 10% (fade) by the fifth stimulation is usually present in the myasthenic.
- *Regional curare test:* A forearm tourniquet is applied and inflated. Curare 0.2–0.5 mg is then injected intravenously into the isolated forearm (distal to the tourniquet), and electromyography is performed on that limb. The myasthenic will show marked decrement of response to repeated stimuli, whereas no change should occur in the normal individual. This test is employed when the edrophonium test and simple electromyography are equivocal.
- *Acetylcholine receptor antibodies:* These antibodies are detectable in 85–90% of myasthenics and are diagnostic for MG. The titer of antibodies does not correlate with the severity of the disease.
- *Computed tomography (CT) scan or magnetic resonance imaging (MRI):* These radiologic tests may be used to confirm the presence of an abnormal thymus gland.

Once diagnosed, MG is clinically classified according to the Osserman Classification System:

- Osserman I: Confined to the extraocular muscles and presents with diplopia.
- Osserman II: Generalized weakness is present.
- Osserman III: Bulbar muscles and severe skeletal weakness are present along with respiratory compromise.
- Osserman IV: Late severe myasthenia, with severe disease developing 2 years after initial diagnosis. The response to therapy in stage IV is poor.

3. Explain the treatment alternatives for MG.

Historically, the similarity of symptoms between MG and curare poisoning led Jolly to propose in 1895 that physostigmine, a cholinesterase inhibitor that was known to antagonize curare, would be of therapeutic value in myasthenics. In 1934, this was first attempted by Walker and has since been the mainstay of therapy in MG. Anticholinesterase therapy is aimed at increasing the amount of acetylcholine available to the reduced number of active receptors, thus increasing the likelihood of agonist–receptor interaction and therefore neuromuscular transmission. Neostigmine, edrophonium, pyridostigmine, and ambenonium are all effective acetylcholinesterase inhibitors. Physostigmine crosses the blood–brain barrier, producing central nervous system symptoms, and is not used in myasthenics for this reason. Pyridostigmine is the most common acetylcholinesterase inhibitor employed because it has the fewest muscarinic side-effects and a 3–6 hour duration of action. Pyridostigmine is administered either intravenously 2 mg or orally 60 mg. A sustained-release preparation is available that is active over several hours. This sustained-release preparation is often used at night to ensure strength on awakening in the morning. Dose requirements vary from day to day. Patients usually learn to adjust doses appropriately.

Other medical treatments of MG are directed at decreasing the production of antibodies. Corticosteroids have been used for many years. Controlled studies reveal that corticosteroids promote clinical improvement in up to 80% of patients; however, prolonged therapy leads to a high incidence of unacceptable side-effects (cataracts, osteoporosis, hypertension, and peptic ulcers). Initiation of steroid therapy is often associated with an exacerbation of weakness that is due to a direct inhibitory effect on neuromuscular transmission. Diminished antibody production and its consequent beneficial effects are delayed. Other immunosuppressive agents have also been used, such as azathioprine and cyclosporine.

Plasmapheresis has been used to remove circulating antibodies and temporarily improve clinical symptoms in 45% of patients. Several treatments are required, and improvement may last only 4 days or as long as 12 weeks. It should be noted that plasmapheresis also decreases pseudocholinesterase levels, which results in a prolonged duration of action of succinylcholine.

Thymectomy has provided significant long-term improvement in most patients. It probably decreases production, or the stimulus for production, of antibodies directed at the nicotinic acetylcholine receptor. Because the thymus contains myoid cells with nicotinic receptors and a number of myasthenics have thymic abnormalities, the thymus may be responsible for the initial pathogenesis. It may also be the source of autoreactive helper T-cells. Thymectomy is the preferred treatment in patients under 55 years of age; however, there is no age limit for this surgery if the patient is otherwise medically stable.

Controversy exists as to the benefits of different surgical approaches to the thymus. The transcervical approach interferes less with respiratory mechanics compared with transsternal approaches. Sternal incision may offer a greater likelihood of complete thymectomy. Incomplete thymectomy results in suboptimal clinical improvement. Advocates of the transcervical approach feel that complete thymectomy is possible with this incision. Improvement after thymectomy may take months. When thymoma is present, removal of the thymus gland via sternotomy is required.

4. Why are patients with MG sensitive to nondepolarizing muscle relaxants and resistant to depolarizing muscle relaxants?

When an acetylcholine receptor is activated by two acetylcholine molecules, a small electrical current is established by the movement of ions through the channel of the open receptor. Endplate depolarization occurs when the summation of small currents from each open acetylcholine receptor reaches a threshold, which then results in membrane depolarization and muscle contraction. Because myasthenics have up to 80% fewer receptors available (decreased margin of safety) and 20% of receptors are required for neuromuscular transmission, a small amount of nondepolarizing muscle relaxant may block enough of the remaining receptors to inhibit endplate depolarization by acetylcholine. Similarly, any factor that minimally interferes with neuromuscular transmission and that may not cause clinical weakness in normal patients because of the large margin of safety may produce severe weakness in myasthenics because of the loss of excessive receptors.

Succinylcholine causes neuromuscular blockade by first depolarizing the motor endplate, then preventing rapid repolarization. Its agonist properties cause endplate depolarization by activating a sufficient number of acetylcholine receptors at the neuromuscular junction. With a decrease in the number of receptors available (downregulation), it would require an increase in the amount of agonist to increase the likelihood of sufficient agonist–receptor interactions for endplate depolarization. Thus, myasthenics are resistant to succinylcholine, and the ED_{95} in myasthenics is 2.6 times normal. The duration of succinylcholine may be prolonged in myasthenics for several reasons. Anticholinesterase drugs inhibit pseudocholinesterase, which is responsible for the metabolism of succinylcholine.

Plasmapheresis may decrease the amount of circulating pseudocholinesterase, which would also decrease the metabolism of succinylcholine.

5. How are patients with MG premedicated for surgery?

Optimization of the myasthenic patient's condition can markedly reduce the risk of surgery. Ideally, surgery is performed during a period of remission when all other medical problems are optimized. Careful preoperative evaluation of respiratory parameters and bulbar strength are necessary before prescribing premedication. Respiratory muscle strength may be quantified through pulmonary function tests (i.e., tidal volume, vital capacity, maximum breathing capacity, and inspiratory force). Premedication should be used with caution and avoided in patients with bulbar symptoms or respiratory difficulty. Anxiolysis may be achieved with small doses of benzodiazepines in those patients whose myasthenia is under good control. Opioid avoidance is sometimes recommended to prevent depressed respiratory drive from further interfering with the potential for respiratory failure based on myasthenic or cholinergic crisis.

Administration of anticholinesterases preoperatively remains controversial. Some authors advocate withholding anticholinesterases before surgical and anesthetic procedures that require muscle relaxation. The patient's baseline weakness facilitates muscle relaxation, requiring little or no exogenous neuromuscular blockade. Withholding anticholinesterases decreases the risk of drug interactions later. Such interactions include partial antagonism of nondepolarizing muscle relaxants and prolongation of the action of succinylcholine. Additionally, withholding anticholinesterases eliminates cholinergic crisis as a cause of postoperative respiratory failure. This approach does not work well for those patients who are physically or psychologically dependent on anticholinesterases. Other authors feel that these drugs may be given preoperatively without interfering significantly with anesthetic and postoperative management.

The relative immobility associated with hospitalization and surgery may produce a reduced requirement for anticholinesterases.

Steroids should be continued in the perioperative period for those patients on chronic therapy.

6. Describe a reasonable anesthetic technique for a patient with MG undergoing transcervical thymectomy.

All patients undergoing anesthetic care should have a continuous electrocardiogram, blood pressure, pulse oximeter, end-tidal carbon dioxide, peripheral nerve stimulation (when relaxants are used or weakness is anticipated), and inspired oxygen monitoring. In general, additional monitoring is dictated by surgical requirements

TABLE 27.1	Factors that Augment Nondepolarizing Neuromuscular Blockade

Acid-base alterations
  Respiratory acidosis
  Metabolic alkalosis
Electrolyte imbalance
  Hypocalcemia
  Hypokalemia
  Hyponatremia
  Hypermagnesemia
Residual potent inhalation agents
  Halothane
  Enflurane
  Isoflurane
  Sevoflurane
  Desflurane
Local anesthetics
  Lidocaine
  Procaine
Class IA antiarrhythmics
  Quinidine
  Procainamide
Antibiotics
  Gentamicin
  Neomycin
  Clindamycin
  Polymyxin B
  Tetracycline
  Streptomycin
  Lincomycin
Calcium-channel blockers
Dantrolene

and coexisting disease. Induction of anesthesia follows denitrogenation with 100% oxygen and proceeds with injection of a short-acting rapid-onset barbiturate, propofol, or etomidate.

Tracheal intubation and controlled ventilation are essential in these patients. Muscle relaxation for tracheal intubation is often not required but may be facilitated by ventilation with potent inhalation agents. If succinylcholine is used for rapid airway control, 2 mg/kg may be required and can have a prolonged duration of action. Despite the well-recognized resistance of myasthenics to succinylcholine, usual clinical doses, which exceed 5 times the ED_{95}, produce adequate relaxation for endotracheal intubation, making dosing unpredictable. Some authors feel that muscle relaxants are best avoided in these patients, recommending that potent inhaled agents will provide adequate relaxation for most procedures. Some patients may not tolerate the

cardiovascular depression associated with these agents and may require a balanced technique with muscle relaxants. Small incremental doses of intermediate-acting nondepolarizing muscle relaxants may be titrated with the assistance of peripheral nerve stimulation. Vecuronium, cisatracurium, and mivacurium have short elimination half-lives and may not require antagonism at the end of surgery.

Residual postoperative neuromuscular blockade presents another controversy. Some feel that continued ventilation until adequate strength has returned is the safest management for these patients. Others feel that anticholinesterases (with an antimuscarinic) may be titrated in small doses to nerve stimulation response. Administration of excessive amounts of an anticholinesterases risks cholinergic crisis. The decision to antagonize residual postoperative neuromuscular blockade must be individualized, and the risk of cholinesterase inhibitors (cholinergic crisis, bradydysrhythmias, and increased secretions) must be weighed against the risk of postoperative ventilation. Respiratory distress may be treated intravenously with 1/30th of the usual oral pyridostigmine dose.

Other factors with slight neuromuscular blocking properties can take on additional importance in the face of concomitant MG (Table 27.1).

Tracheal extubation is often predicated on a tidal volume of 6 mL/kg, negative inspiratory force of –25 cm H_2O, vital capacity of 15 mL/kg, and sustained head-lift for 5 seconds.

7. Following emergence from anesthesia and before extubation, how is strength assessed?

Neuromuscular transmission can be assessed in many ways. Patients can accomplish sustained head-lift for 5 seconds while 33% of receptors are still occupied or blocked. Sustained tetanus of 100 Hz for 5 seconds may be seen with 50% of receptors blocked. Negative inspiratory force of –20 cm H_2O also may be accomplished with 50% of receptors occupied. These measurements of neuromuscular strength suggest that patients can maintain adequate minute ventilation in the face of residual impairment of neuromuscular transmission. More recent data suggest that these parameters may not correspond with the ability to maintain control of the airway. Inspiratory forces of –40 cm H_2O may be required to ensure airway control. Other measures such as tidal volume of 6 mL/kg, TOF >70%, and vital capacity of 15 mL/kg are relatively insensitive measures of strength.

The myasthenic patient represents a special case where these numbers may not apply. Their disease, rather than residual neuromuscular blockade, may prevent myasthenics from reaching full strength. Consequently, preoperative measures of strength are important for postoperative comparisons. Such tests include negative inspiratory force, maximum breathing capacity, vital capacity, and tidal volume. Before the administration of an anesthetic drug that may interfere with neuromuscular transmission, a control electromyogram or TOF should be recorded. Response to tetanic stimulation should be assessed after induction of anesthesia and before administration of drugs that interfere with neuromuscular transmission.

Residual weakness on emergence from anesthesia must not automatically be assumed to represent residual muscle relaxant blockade. Inhaled anesthetics, antibiotics, local anesthetics, anticonvulsants, and β-blockers may interfere with neuromuscular transmission (Table 27.1).

Other extubation criteria are outlined in question 6.

Traditional Clinical Extubation Criteria

Tidal volume
≥6 ml/kg

Vital capacity
≥15 ml/kg

Negative inspiratory force
≥–25 cm of H_2O

Sustained head lift
>5 seconds

Sustained tetanus at 100 Hz
>5 seconds

Central nervous system
Awake, responsive

Respiratory system
Adequate oxygenation with an FiO_2<0.4
Sufficient ventilation
Respiratory rate <25 breaths per minute in adults

Cardiovascular system
Adequate blood pressure to perfuse vital organs
Freedom from serious new dysrhythmias

Metabolic
Normothermia
Normal glucose and electrolyte concentrations

Hematologic system
Adequate surgical hemostasis
Coagulopathy free

8. What is cholinergic crisis?

Cholinergic crisis results from an excess of acetylcholine at nicotinic and muscarinic receptor sites and usually occurs as a result of excess anticholinesterase administration. Manifestations of a cholinergic crisis include weakness, wheezing, increased secretions, fasciculations, nausea, vomiting, diarrhea, lacrimation, bradycardia, and hypotension. Respiratory muscle weakness may progress rapidly to respiratory failure. Dysphagia may impair swallowing of upper airway secretions, predisposing to upper airway obstruction and aspiration pneumonitis. Cholinergic crisis and myasthenic crisis can both present with muscle weakness and may be hard to differentiate (Table 27.2). Because their etiologies and treatment are the antithesis of each other, correct diagnosis is critical. Cholinergic crisis often presents with constricted pupils, and myasthenic crisis often presents with large dilated pupils. The edrophonium test usually helps to distinguish between the two entities. A small dose of edrophonium (2–10 mg) is administered. Myasthenic crisis (a relative dearth of acetylcholine) should show improved strength while a cholinergic crisis (a relative excess of acetylcholine) will demonstrate no change in strength or exacerbation of symptoms. Rapid progression to respiratory failure may necessitate emergent intubation and controlled ventilation. The muscarinic side-effects of a cholinergic crisis may be treated with atropine or glycopyrrolate.

9. Can preoperative evaluation predict the need for postoperative ventilation?

Many scoring systems have been proposed as predictors of postoperative ventilation. Factors involved include the severity and duration of disease, pyridostigmine dose requirements, and surgical approach. No single system has proven to be a reliable predictor in prospective analysis. Preoperative evaluation aims at quantifying the strength of respiratory muscles. Frequently used studies include pulmonary function tests and arterial blood gas analysis. These tests assist in evaluating the need for mechanical ventilation on an individual basis postoperatively.

Elective surgery should be scheduled to coincide with periods of remission. Coexisting diseases must be optimally treated.

TABLE 27.2	Differentiating Between Myasthenic and Cholinergic Crisis	
	Myasthenic Crisis	**Cholinergic Crisis**
Pupil size	Dilated	Constricted
Edrophonium	Improved strength	No improvement or exacerbation of symptoms

As of this writing, there are no reliable predictors of post-operative ventilatory requirements for myasthenic patients.

SUGGESTED READINGS

Barak A: Anesthesia and myasthenia gravis. Can J Anaesth 39:476–486, 1992

Barak A: Anesthesia and critical care of thymectomy for myasthenia gravis. Chest Surg Clin North Am 11:337–361, 2001

Busch C, Machens A, Pichlmeier U, et al.: Long-term outcome and quality of life after thymectomy for myasthenia gravis. Ann Surg 224:225–232, 1996

Eisenkraft JB: Myasthenia gravis and thymic surgery: anaesthetic considerations. Baillières Clin Anesthesiol 1:133–162, 1987

Hunt LA, Boyd GL: Superior laryngeal nerve block: a supplement to total intravenous anesthesia for rigid laser bronchoscopy in a patient with myasthènic syndrome. Anesth Analg 75:458–460, 1992

Newsom-Davis J: Therapy in myasthenia gravis and Lambert-Eaton myasthenic syndrome. Semin Neurol 23:191–198, 2003

Sharpe MD: The use of muscle relaxants in the intensive care unit. Can J Anaesth 39:949–962, 1992

28

MALIGNANT HYPERTHERMIA

Mark Abel, MD

A 20-year-old man without significant prior medical or surgical history presents for tonsillectomy. Induction of anesthesia is achieved with thiopental, fentanyl, and succinylcholine. Anesthesia is maintained with nitrous oxide 70%, oxygen 30%, and isoflurane 1%. Fifteen minutes into the procedure, his blood pressure rises to 190/100 mmHg, and the heart rate increases to 130 beats per minute. The mass spectrometer shows an end-tidal carbon dioxide ($ETCO_2$) concentration of 60 mmHg, despite a minute ventilation of 110 mL/kg/minute.

QUESTIONS

1. What is malignant hyperthermia (MH)?
2. How is susceptibility to MH inherited?
3. What is the pathophysiology of MH?
4. What characterizes a clinical episode of MH?
5. Outline the pharmacology of dantrolene.
6. How is MH treated?
7. How are patients with known MH susceptibility treated?
8. What are the recognized triggering agents?
9. What is the significance of masseter muscle rigidity (MMR)?
10. How is MH definitively diagnosed?
11. Describe the neurolept malignant syndrome.

1. What is malignant hyperthermia (MH)?

MH is a neuromuscular disorder that occurs following exposure to certain precipitants such as anesthetic agents. The reported incidence varies between 1:12,000 and 1:40,000. It is most common in children and young adults. After exposure to triggering agents, skeletal muscle metabolism increases dramatically. Skeletal muscle rigidity, metabolic and respiratory acidosis, tachycardia, hypoxemia, and hyperthermia follow. A full-blown episode may result in cardiac arrest unless promptly treated. A similar syndrome in susceptible swine may be initiated by stress, providing an animal model for MH.

2. How is susceptibility to MH inherited?

Susceptibility to MH is thought to be inherited by autosomal dominant pattern with mixed penetrance, although an autosomal recessive form exists as well. Multiple mutations for the ryanodine receptor of the sarcoplasmic reticulum are causative. Other genes may be involved as well. The identification of a single causative gene, therefore, is not possible. Siblings and children of MH-susceptible individuals experience a 50% risk of susceptibility.

3. What is the pathophysiology of MH?

An uncontrolled increase in intracellular calcium, usually due to an abnormal ryanodine receptor, results in sustained and forceful muscle contracture. This culminates in massive increases in both aerobic and anaerobic muscle metabolism, with subsequent production of heat, carbon dioxide (CO_2), and lactate. Eventually, muscle cell membrane integrity is lost, and spillage of intracellular contents into the circulation occurs. While the precise cellular events causing MH are not known, triggering agents cause an imbalance of calcium release and reuptake from sites of the sarcoplasmic reticulum. The resulting increase in intracellular calcium favors contraction and limits relaxation.

4. What characterizes a clinical episode of MH?

Typically, an episode is triggered by exposure to potent inhaled anesthetic agents and/or succinylcholine. The onset time may be immediate or delayed for as long as 24 hours. Exposure to desflurane frequently results in a delayed onset of MH. Fulminant MH occurs after a triggering agent causes massive skeletal muscle hyperexcitability. Hypercarbia manifesting as increasing $ETCO_2$ may be the initial sign. Other causes of hypercarbia are outlined in Table 28.1.

Metabolic acidosis occurs as well and may be profound. Sympathetic nervous system hyperactivity is demonstrated by tachycardia and hypertension. The differential diagnosis of sinus tachycardia is outlined in Table 28.2.

Cardiac dysrhythmias may occur as well. Elevations of serum potassium, creatine phosphokinase (CPK), myoglobin, and ionized calcium occur as result of increased skeletal muscle membrane permeability. Core temperature elevation, potentially exceeding 43°C, is a late sign. Death may follow. Fulminant episodes involving simultaneous occurrence of these signs are easily recognizable. Slow evolution of signs demonstrating certain features, but not others, complicates correct diagnosis. Confirmation may

TABLE 28.1	Differential Diagnosis of Hypercarbia

Medullary respiratory center depression
Muscle paresis
Inadequate ventilation
    Low minute volume
    Kinked breathing circuit or endotracheal tube
    Malfunctioning CO_2 absorber
Pneumoperitoneum with CO_2
Inadequate fresh gas flow
Increased dead space
    Pulmonary embolus
Increased CO_2 production
    Sepsis
    Fever
    Malignant hyperthermia
    Thyrotoxicosis

TABLE 28.2	Differential Diagnosis of Sinus Tachycardia

Hypoxia
Hypercarbia
Hypovolemia
Hypotension
Light anesthesia
Pheochromocytoma
Thyrotoxicosis
Sepsis
Fever
Myocardial infarction
Pulmonary embolus
Transfusion reaction
Pharmacologic agents
    Pancuronium
    Atropine
    Glycopyrrolate
    Ephedrine
    Epinephrine
    Isoproterenol
    Dopamine
    Theophylline
Malignant hyperthermia

require detection of myoglobin in the urine. Thyroid storm, pheochromocytoma, and neurolept malignant syndrome may be difficult to distinguish from MH.

5. Outline the pharmacology of dantrolene.

Dantrolene is an intracellular muscle relaxant. It works by reducing intracellular calcium concentrations. This may result from impaired release from the sarcoplasmic reticulum or inhibition of excitation–contraction coupling. As of this writing, dantrolene is the only mechanism-specific treatment for MH.

Dantrolene does not appear to possess cardiac toxicity but may alter other neuromuscular blocker requirements. After administration of dantrolene 2.5 mg/kg intravenously, therapeutic levels last 4–6 hours. Its half-life is almost 12 hours. Consequently, dantrolene is administered every 4 hours for the treatment of MH. Muscle weakness, nausea, hepatotoxicity, and phlebitis are the recognized side-effects of dantrolene treatment.

6. How is MH treated?

A suspected case of MH must be treated promptly, because full-blown episodes proceed rapidly to death.

Clinical Presentation of Malignant Hyperthermia

Onset
    Induction of anesthesia
    Intraoperatively
    Postanesthesia care unit
    Up to 24 hours postoperatively
    Re-emergence 24–36 hours later

Triggering agents
    Potent inhaled agents
    Succinylcholine

Respiratory
    Hypercarbia (both $ETCO_2$ and $PaCO_2$) despite
        increased minute ventilation
    Tachypnea – during spontaneous ventilation
    Hypoxemia

Cardiovascular
    Unexplained tachycardia
    Ventricular dysrhythmias
    Hypertension

Genitourinary
    Myoglobinuria
    Renal failure

Musculoskeletal
    Muscle rigidity
    Rhabdomyolysis

Hyperthermia

Hematologic
    Disseminated intravascular coagulation

Warm CO_2 absorber canister

Laboratory findings
    Hyperkalemia
    Respiratory and metabolic acidosis
    Hypercalcemia
    Creatine phosphokinase (CPK) >20,000 IU in
        12–24 hours

Triggering agents must be discontinued immediately. It is no longer recommended that the anesthesia machine be changed to a "clean" machine (one which has never been used to administer potent inhaled agents) nor does the breathing circuit have to be changed during an acute episode of MH. Dantrolene is the only drug that effectively treats MH. Each vial of dantrolene contains 20 mg of dantrolene and 3 g of mannitol, which must be dissolved in 60 mL of sterile water. The initial dose is 2.5 mg/kg intravenously, which may be repeated every 5 minutes until signs abate.

In addition to treating the cause of MH, its effects must be quickly dealt with. The increase in core temperature must be treated with cold intravenous fluids, cold irrigation fluids poured into open body cavities, as well as cold water lavage of the stomach and urinary bladder. Arterial blood gases should be monitored closely, preferably from an arterial catheter, and the patient should be vigorously ventilated with 100% oxygen to correct hypercarbia and hypoxemia. Sodium bicarbonate should be used to treat profound base deficits. Central venous catheters and urinary bladder drainage catheters help monitor intravascular volume and renal status. Maintaining renal blood flow is important to prevent renal damage. Intravenous sodium bicarbonate and acetazolamide alkalinize the urine and prevent precipitation of myoglobin in renal tubules. Diuretics should be given to maintain urine output, and examination of the urine for myoglobin should be carried out.

Hyperkalemia should be treated with insulin and 50% dextrose solutions, while cardiac dysrhythmias are treated according to standard protocols. *Calcium-channel blockers are contraindicated* because of their interaction with dantrolene, possibly resulting in significant hyperkalemia. Following an episode of proven or suspected MH, the patient should be monitored for 24–36 hours. Recognized complications of MH include re-emergence, disseminated intravascular coagulation, and myoglobinuric renal failure. Recommended treatments are given in Table 28.3.

7. How are patients with known MH susceptibility treated?

Anxiety may contribute to MH crises. Therefore, some anesthesiologists recommend premedication with anxiolytics such as benzodiazepines. Patients experiencing preoperative pain can receive opioids. Dantrolene premedication is no longer necessary and should be avoided in the pregnant patient because dantrolene crosses the placenta and produces uterine atony.

Either a "clean" machine or an anesthesia machine in which the oxygen flow has been on at 10 L flow for 20 minutes should be used. Iced saline solutions and dantrolene should be available. Regional anesthesia with either ester or amide local anesthetics may be preferable to general anesthesia when possible. General anesthesia may be induced

TABLE 28.3	Treatment of Malignant Hyperthermia

Acute
Discontinue all triggering agents
Hyperventilate with 100% oxygen
Administer 2.5 mg/kg of dantrolene, repeat as needed
    until tachycardia, muscle rigidity, increased $ETCO_2$,
    and fever are controlled
Administer sodium bicarbonate 1–2 mEq/kg or as
    guided by arterial blood gas analysis to correct
    metabolic acidosis
Cool the patient
    External ice packing and cooling blanket
    Irrigate body cavities: stomach, urinary bladder,
        rectum, and open cavities
    Infuse cold normal saline
Administer standard antidysrhythmic agents if no
    response to correction of acidosis and hyperkalemia;
    calcium-channel blockers are contraindicated
Manage hyperkalemia with hyperventilation, sodium
    bicarbonate, insulin and glucose, and calcium if
    hyperkalemia is life-threatening
Maintain urine output >2 mL/kg/hr
Send laboratory tests including arterial blood gas,
    serum K^+, electrolytes, calcium, PT/PTT, CPK
Monitor $ETCO_2$, electrocardiogram, temperature, urine
    output
Post-acute
Monitor vital signs and acid–base status for 36 hours
Follow acid–base status, K^+, CPK, urine and serum
    myoglobin, coagulation studies
Maintain urine output
Continue dantrolene 1–2 mg/kg intravenously every
    4 hours over a 36 hour period

TABLE 28.4	Nontriggering Agents

Benzodiazepines
Induction agents
    Barbiturates
    Propofol
    Ketamine
    Etomidate
Local anesthetics
Opioids
Nondepolarizing muscle relaxants
    Pipecuronium
    Doxacurium
    Tubocurarine
    Vecuronium
    Atracurium
    Mivacurium
    Pancuronium
    Cis-atracurium
Nitrous oxide
Droperidol
Vasoactive drugs
Propranolol
Antibiotics
Antipyretics
Antihistamines

with propofol, barbiturates, oxygen, and opioids. Muscle relaxation for tracheal intubation is achieved with nondepolarizing muscle relaxants such as vecuronium, mivacurium, and cis-atracurium. The advisability of administering curare is questionable. Anesthesia maintenance is accomplished with total intravenous anesthetics with or without nitrous oxide. Other acceptable agents include midazolam, diazepam, and droperidol. Antagonism of neuromuscular blockade may be achieved with acetylcholinesterase inhibitors and anticholinergics.

8. What are the recognized triggering agents?

Triggering agents include all the potent inhaled agents and succinylcholine. Although amide local anesthetics were previously classified as triggering agents, they are no longer believed to place patients at risk for MH. Nontriggering agents are listed in Table 28.4.

9. What is the significance of masseter muscle rigidity (MMR)?

MMR (trismus) has been reported to occur in 1% of children receiving halothane and succinylcholine for induction. It was previously thought to herald the onset of MH in 50% of cases as confirmed by skeletal muscle biopsy. Recent studies indicate that MMR may occur in otherwise normal patients. In the presence of MMR, whether to continue anesthesia for elective procedures and whether to discontinue triggering agents remains controversial. Some suggest that the anesthetic may be safely continued, while others suggest that all such episodes should be treated as MH until proven otherwise by skeletal muscle biopsy.

Other causes of MMR include temporomandibular joint dysfunction, myotonia, and rapid succinylcholine hydrolysis.

10. How is MH definitively diagnosed?

The search for a simple diagnostic blood test of MH continues. Genetic testing presently detects 50% of cases in families with known genetic mutations. Therefore, skeletal muscle biopsy remains the gold standard of MH diagnosis. Elevated serum CPK in a close relative of a patient with known MH is diagnostic of MH in 70–80% of cases. Normal values, however, do not rule out the diagnosis; consequently, such relatives must be tested.

A sizable muscle biopsy is taken under local anesthesia. The specimen is exposed to caffeine, halothane, or a combination of the two. Unfortunately, the caffeine–halothane contracture test is not standardized in centers around the world, and false-positives and to a lesser extent false-negatives occur.

11. Describe the neurolept malignant syndrome.

The clinical presentatipn of neurolept malignant syndrome (NMS) includes fever, tachycardia, hypertension, muscle rigidity, acidosis, rhabdomyolysis, and agitation. Its mortality rate approximates 20% and dantrolene is an effective treatment. It is easily confused with MH.

NMS is distinguished from MH by several features. NMS follows long-term exposure to phenothiazines or haloperidol. Sudden withdrawal of anti-parkinsonism drugs may precipitate NMS.

SUGGESTED READINGS

Ali SZ, Taguchi A, Rosenberg H: Malignant hyperthermia. Best Pract Res Clin Anaesthesiol 17:519–533, 2003

Ebadi M, Pfeiffer RF, Murrin LC: Pathogenesis and treatment of neurolept malignant syndrome. Gen Pharmacol 21:367, 1990

Girard T, Treves S, Voronkov E, et al.: Molecular genetic testing for malignant hyperthermia susceptibility. Anesthesiology 100:1076, 2004

Gurrera RJ: Is neuroleptic malignant syndrome a neurogenic form of malignant hyperthermia? Clin Neuropharmacol 25:183, 2002

Hoenemann CW, Halen-Holtgraeve TB, Booke M, et al.: Delayed onset of malignant hyperthermia in desflurane anesthesia. Anesth Analg 97:295, 2003

Iaizzo PA, Palahnuik RJ: Malignant hyperthermia diagnosis, treatment, genetics, and pathophysiology. Invest Radiol 26:1013, 1991

Johnson C, Edelman KJ: Malignant hyperthermia: a review. J Perinatol 12:61, 1991

Van Der Speck AFL, Fang WB, Ashton-Miller JA, et al.: The effects of succinylcholine on mouth opening. Anesthesiology 67:459, 1987

29

DIABETES MELLITUS

Leon K. Specthrie, MD

Allan P. Reed, MD

A 38-year-old woman is scheduled for an appendectomy. Blood chemistries include sodium 152 mEq/L, potassium 3.1 mEq/L, carbon dioxide 16 mEq/L, blood urea nitrogen (BUN) 67 mg/dL, and glucose 454.0 mg/dL.

QUESTIONS

1. Distinguish among the major types of diabetes mellitus (DM).
2. Summarize the physiologic effects of insulin.
3. Describe the oral hypoglycemic agents and insulin preparations available to treat DM.
4. How does DM affect perioperative morbidity and mortality?
5. What are the common causes and associated symptoms of hypoglycemia?
6. Outline perioperative management alternatives for the diabetic patient.
7. Explain the acute complications of DM.

1. Distinguish among the major types of diabetes mellitus (DM).

DM is the presence of elevated plasma glucose under fasting conditions. Type I, or insulin-dependent DM (IDDM), occurs in about 10% of all diabetics in the Western world (Table 29.1). Classically, this type of DM presents in childhood or early adolescence; however, it can manifest at any age. The presentation is usually abrupt, with onset of symptoms secondary to severe insulin insufficiency. Type I DM patients are prone to ketosis and are usually thin. The pathogenesis of IDDM is thought to involve certain histocompatibility locus antigens (HLA) on chromosome 6. In the most common form of IDDM (type IA), environmental factors, such as viral infections, are postulated to combine with genetic factors to cause cell-mediated autoimmune destruction of pancreatic beta cells. The second type of IDDM (type IB) is found in about 10% of all IDDM patients and is thought to involve primary autoimmune damage. This type of IDDM is associated with other autoimmune endocrinopathies such as Hashimoto's thyroiditis, Graves' disease, and other nonendocrine autoimmune disorders.

Type II DM, or non-insulin-dependent DM (NIDDM), occurs in 90% of all diabetics. However, the name may be misleading since some patients may require insulin to correct persistent fasting hyperglycemia if diet and oral agents fail to do so. The requirement of insulin for glucose control does not distinguish between IDDM and NIDDM. Although these patients are not ketosis prone, they still may develop ketosis under circumstances of severe stress. The pathogenesis of NIDDM is also thought to involve genetic factors as expressed by a strong familial pattern for NIDDM. There appears to be a difference between obese

TABLE 29.1	Characteristics of Insulin-Dependent and Non-Insulin-Dependent Diabetes Mellitus	
	Insulin Dependent (Type I)	**Non-Insulin Dependent (Type II)**
Incidence	10% of all diabetics	90% of all diabetics
Onset	Childhood or early adolescence	Middle age
Personal morphology	Usually not obese	Often obese
Pathogenesis	Pancreatic beta islet cell destruction	Pancreatic beta islet cells relatively normal
	Insulin deficiency	Insulin resistance
Usual therapy	Insulin	Diet
		Oral hypoglycemics
Metabolic complications	Ketosis	Hyperosmolar nonketotic state

and non-obese NIDDM patients. Sixty to eighty percent of NIDDM patients have insulin resistance resulting from weight gain and obesity. In most patients, a diagnosis of NIDDM is made during middle age. In a subclass of patients, DM presents during childhood or adolescence, which is known as maturity onset-type diabetes of the young (MODY). This has an established autosomal dominant inheritance pattern. Gestational DM (GDM) is defined as the onset of glucose intolerance during pregnancy. About 2% of all pregnancies are associated with GDM, which is related to an increase in perinatal morbidity and mortality. Although most patients return to a state of normal glucose tolerance following parturition, about 60% will develop DM within 15 years.

Other forms of DM include malnutrition-related DM, which is a non-ketosis-prone form associated with severe protein malnutrition and emaciation. Most cases require insulin for preservation of life. DM may also be secondary to other endocrine diseases (e.g., Cushing syndrome), drug administration (e.g., antihypertensive drugs, estrogens), and many genetic syndromes. DM may also result from severe pancreatic disease or resection of pancreatic tissue.

2. Summarize the physiologic effects of insulin.

Insulin is produced by the pancreatic beta islet cells as a prohormone, which is converted by proteolytic cleavage to insulin and C peptide. Its metabolism takes place in the liver and kidney. Normal insulin production approximates 40–50 U/day. Its half-life is measured in minutes.

Insulin release is stimulated primarily by glucose and amino acids. Its primary effect on carbohydrate homeostasis is to inhibit hepatic glucose production and drive glucose into skeletal muscle. Insulin does not affect the transport of glucose into brain or hepatic cells. Insulin stimulates hepatic glucose storage as glycogen and inhibits lipolysis. Because diabetics have depleted glycogen stores, proteins must be degraded to make glucose. Insulin also

assists the transport of amino acids into skeletal muscle. Consequently, insulin deficiency predisposes to protein catabolism. Insufficient insulin leads to fat breakdown, forming fatty acids and ketones. Amounts of insulin sufficient to prevent lipolysis may not be enough to prevent hyperglycemia. Therefore, severe hyperglycemia generally accompanies ketosis.

A 24-hour fast is associated with a mild insulin deficiency and a resultant decrease in peripheral glucose uptake. Glycogen, protein, and triglyceride synthesis decrease, while the breakdown of these storage molecules is accelerated. Counter-regulatory hormones play an important role in the breakdown of macromolecules. Decreased circulating insulin decreases glucose uptake in insulin-sensitive tissues to spare glucose for obligate use by the central nervous system (CNS). Hepatic glucose production is maintained for 12–24 hours by the breakdown of stored glycogen. Subsequent hepatic glucose production depends on breakdown of peripheral proteins and fat. In prolonged fasts, ketone bodies are produced from the breakdown of adipose tissue to provide a substrate that can be metabolized by the CNS.

Diabetic ketoacidosis (DKA) develops when severe insulin deficiency is present. It is marked by hyperglycemia, which is a result of increased hepatic glucose production and decreased peripheral uptake. Ketone body production occurs in the hepatocyte mitochondria from oxidation of fatty acids. In contrast to the euinsulinemic fed state, fatty acids freely enter the mitochondria while fatty acid and triglyceride synthesis are inhibited. The physiologic derangements of DKA (acidosis, ketonuria, osmotic diuresis, and hyperosmolarity) develop from the hyperglycemia and hyperketonemia.

3. Describe the oral hypoglycemic agents and insulin preparations available to treat DM.

Oral hypoglycemic agents fall into four broad classes depending on their mechanism of action. Table 29.2

TABLE 29.2   **Oral Hypoglycemic Agents and Their Duration of Action**

Class	Agent	Duration of Action (hours)
Sulfonylureas	Acetohexamide	12–18
	Chlorpropamide	Up to 60
	Tolazamide	12–24
	Tolbutamide	6–12
	Glipizide	Up to 24
	Glyburide	Up to 24
	Glimepiride	24
Biguanides	Metformin	12
Thiazolidinediones	Pioglitazone	24
	Rosiglitazone	12–24
α-Glucosidase inhibitors	Acarbose	3–4
	Miglitol	3–4

summarizes the commonly used agents and their anticipated duration of action. All these drugs are ineffective in IDDM.

- The sulfonylureas (tolbutamide, glyburide, glipizide, and glimepiride) and meglitinides (repaglinide and netaglinide) increase insulin secretion by the pancreas and reduce insulin resistance. Hypoglycemia is the major complication associated with sulfonylurea therapy. There has also been concern that some of the sulfonylureas increase the incidence of myocardial infarction.
- Biguanides (metformin) decrease gluconeogenesis in the liver. Other beneficial effects, which make metformin a popular treatment, include weight loss, a decrease in triglycerides and low-density lipoproteins, and an increase in high-density lipoproteins. Metformin has been shown to decrease the incidence of myocardial infarction in obese patients with type II DM.

- Thiazolidinediones (pioglitazone and rosiglitazone), the newest hypoglycemic agents, improve insulin sensitivity of muscle and fat cells.
- α-Glucosidase inhibitors (acarbose and miglitol) inhibit intestinal α-glucoside, thus the absorption of glucose is delayed in the intestine. Hypoglycemia does not occur if these drugs are used alone.

Insulin therapy is necessary for all IDDM patients, and NIDDM patients inadequately treated with oral hypoglycemics. Insulin comes in two concentrations: 100 U/mL and 500 U/mL (U-100 and U-500, respectively). Insulin preparations differ in their source (e.g., pork, recombinant human), degree of purity, and time course of action. Table 29.3 lists the characteristics of insulin preparations. The half-life of intravenous regular insulin is approximately 5 minutes; the effect lasts about 1 hour.

TABLE 29.3   **Properties of Various Insulin Preparations Administered Subcutaneously**

Class	Type	Onset (hr)	Peak Effect (hr)	Duration of Action (hr)
Rapid	Regular crystalline insulin	1	2–4	6–8
	Semilente	1.5	26	10–12
Intermediate	Neutral protamine (NPH)	3	6–12	18–24
	Lente	3	6–12	18–24
Long acting	Protamine zinc (PZI)	6	14–24	36
	Ultralente	6	18–24	36
	Insulin glargine	1	–	24–30

4. How does DM affect perioperative morbidity and mortality?

Early reports suggested that patients with DM have an increased risk for perioperative morbidity and mortality. Subsequent epidemiologic studies that segregated groups according to end-organ damage showed limited differences between diabetic and nondiabetic patients. In evaluating a diabetic patient, the focus should be on the end-organ dysfunction, which will influence the patient's perioperative course in addition to the degree of glycemic control. End-organ damage is probably responsible for the fivefold increase in perioperative mortality associated with DM.

Perioperative hyperglycemia increases mortality and major morbidity, such as renal failure and sepsis. This increased risk occurs even in patients not known to be diabetic, and is reduced by tight glucose control in the operating room and in the intensive care unit (ICU). Most of the intraoperative data come from the cardiac surgery population.

Healing of deep wounds that require collagen synthesis for healing is impaired by hyperglycemia. Purely epithelial wounds appear to heal well regardless of blood glucose levels. Diabetics have an increased incidence of infectious complications.

The relationship of blood glucose levels to neurologic recovery is the subject of ongoing research. The majority of available evidence supports a deleterious effect of hyperglycemia on neurologic recovery. Hyperglycemia appears to adversely affect recovery following global but not focal cerebral ischemia. Patients with diabetic autonomic neuropathy have a high incidence of both gastroparesis and painless myocardial ischemia. Gastroparesis is associated with an increased risk of aspiration; therefore, preoperative treatment with metoclopramide may be useful.

Responses to hypoxia may be impaired by autonomic neuropathy. Responses to the respiratory depressant effects of drugs may be accentuated. There is one report of the diabetic stiff joint syndrome leading to difficulty in endotracheal intubation. DM is associated with small-vessel problems such as coronary artery, cerebrovascular, and renal diseases.

5. What are the common causes and associated symptoms of hypoglycemia?

Hypoglycemia is a pathophysiologic state rather than a disease, and its presence warrants a search for the primary cause. Hypoglycemia is generally considered the glucose level below which symptoms appear, but in general, blood glucose determinations below 50 mg/dL are considered to reflect hypoglycemia. In the conscious patient, hypoglycemia may be well compensated with few symptoms or may be associated with diplopia, blurred vision, sweating, palpitations, or weakness. The clinical presentation of hypoglycemia is summarized in Table 29.4.

TABLE 29.4	Clinical Presentation of Hypoglycemia

Symptoms
CNS-related
  Tremulousness
  Agitation
  Headache
  Light-headedness
  Dizziness
Catecholamine-related
  Tremulousness
  Diaphoresis
  Palpitations
Signs
CNS-related
  Altered mental status
  Confusion
  Hypothermia
  Stupor
  Seizures
  Coma
Catecholamine-related
  Tachycardia
  Hypertension
  Dysrhythmias

During general anesthesia, the signs and symptoms of hypoglycemia are nonspecific. They may include sweating and hypotension or hypertension and tachydysrhythmias. Therefore, serum glucose assessment is needed to diagnose hypoglycemia during general anesthesia.

Common conditions associated with hypoglycemia include response to medications (oral hypoglycemic agents, insulin preparations); ethanol ingestion; tumors of the pancreas or liver; cirrhosis; hypopituitarism; and adrenal insufficiency. In the perioperative fasting period, infants, young children, and young adult women may become hypoglycemic without glucose supplementation. Patients receiving glucose-rich total parenteral nutrition (TPN) may become hypoglycemic if the infusion is abruptly discontinued, owing to the insulin levels it contains. Recent recommendations for patients receiving TPN are to continue the TPN in the operating room and reduce the infusion rates of other intravenous fluids appropriately. If TPN must be discontinued, a solution of 10% dextrose at a rate of approximately 75 mL/hr may be substituted. Glucose levels should be checked to ensure adequate glucose replacement.

CNS symptoms of hypoglycemia mimic those commonly seen in critically ill and sedated patients. Hypoglycemic signs related to catecholamine release resemble those associated with light anesthesia and may be misinterpreted. Treatment with β-adrenergic blockers and coexisting autonomic neuropathy may mask these signs.

Mild episodes of hypoglycemia can be treated with 5% dextrose boluses and infusions. More significant cases, manifested by mental status changes, are treated with 50 mL of 50% dextrose, which invariably causes hyperglycemia. Beneficial responses to glucose administration are both diagnostic and therapeutic. Continued dextrose administration may be necessary following initial treatment.

In the absence of intravenous access, hypoglycemia can be treated with intramuscular or subcutaneous glucagon. Diazoxide has been used for prolonged refractory cases such as sulfonylurea overdose and insulinoma.

6. Outline perioperative management alternatives for the diabetic patient.

The goals of perioperative management are to avoid hyperglycemia and hypoglycemia. Severe hyperglycemia predisposes patients to osmotic diuresis as well as ketosis or nonketotic hyperosmolar states. Hypoglycemia risks CNS damage. Recent studies from the ICU and cardiac surgery indicate that serum glucose concentrations above 120 mg/dL may significantly increase mortality and morbidity. Traditionally, the perioperative target for serum glucose was 120–200 mg/dL, to minimize the potential for hypoglycemia. This is probably still a reasonable goal for minor or moderately invasive procedures in noncritically ill patients. Patients who are critically ill or are having major procedures should have tighter glycemic control, in the range of 80–110 mg/dL. Protocols for tight glycemic control are still evolving, and several have been published (see Suggested Readings). This tighter control is more labor- and resource-intensive, and is currently not practical for all diabetic patients.

Oral hypoglycemic agents should be discontinued while patients are fasting. Residual hypoglycemic effects are opposed by administering 5% dextrose, if needed. The frequency of blood glucose measurements to monitor for hyperglycemia and hypoglycemia depends on the desired degree of control.

Because patients refrain from eating and drinking before surgery and anesthesia, insulin doses may be withheld or reduced, depending on the underlying physiology. Type I diabetics need insulin to avoid DKA. Type II diabetics with elevated fasting glucose concentrations also benefit from insulin therapy while fasting. Frequently, one half of the usual subcutaneous insulin dose is administered. Blood glucose concentrations determine the need for 5% dextrose infusion, typically started at 100 mL/hr. Insulin and dextrose infusions are adjusted based on blood glucose determinations at 1-hour intervals for major procedures or critically ill patients, and up to 4-hour intervals for minor

procedures. Intravenous administration is far more reliable than subcutaneous dosing during periods of hemodynamic instability, vasoconstrictor administration, and/or hypothermia.

Bolus intravenous insulin dosing results in rapid decline of glucose levels for short periods of time. In contrast, continuous intravenous administration of 0.01–0.02 U/kg/hr provides the optimal and easiest means of controlling serum glucose concentrations. The most reliable control is obtained with separate infusions of 5% dextrose and insulin mixed with half-normal saline to a concentration of 0.1 U/cc. Flushing the intravenous tubing with the insulin solution prevents significant loss of insulin to the plastic tubing. During periods of rapid glucose fluxes, blood glucose determinations are performed every hour. Measurements can be made every 4 hours after a steady state has been reached.

Autonomic dysfunction and/or severe cardiac disease may indicate invasive monitoring. Autonomic neuropathy predisposes patients to hypotension accompanying regional anesthesia and increases the risk of aspiration pneumonitis from gastroparesis. Aspiration prophylaxis and rapid sequence induction may be indicated. Peripheral neuropathies require particular care during positioning and moving to avoid traumatic injury. Hyperglycemia-induced osmotic diuresis indicates urinary bladder drainage.

Postoperatively, rapid resolution of sepsis and decreased levels of circulating catecholamines contribute to acute hypoglycemia.

7. Explain the acute complications of DM.

The acute complications of DM are metabolic in nature with extension to other systems secondarily. In the absence of adequate amounts of insulin, IDDM patients develop hyperglycemia, osmotic diuresis, and acidosis. Surgery, trauma, or infection frequently precipitates such episodes. Ketoacidosis may coexist with hyperglycemia of 1000 mg/dL or more. The various ketone bodies produce acidosis with a wide anion gap, as demonstrated in the case presented here. Ketones may rise to 30 mM/L from a normal level of 0.15 mM/L. Kussmaul's respirations develop in severe cases and are due to significant metabolic acidosis. Expired tidal volumes often emit an acetone odor. In the case of severe osmotic diuresis, lactic acidosis may exist on the basis of hypoperfusion. Acidosis from any source predisposes to depressed myocardial contractility and poor peripheral perfusion, thereby exacerbating lactic acidosis. Dehydration frequently results from osmotic diuresis and vomiting. Despite dehydration, oliguria generally does not manifest until late in the course of disease. Acidosis drives potassium extracellularly into the vascular space, where it is eliminated through the kidneys. As acidosis resolves and potassium moves intracellularly, serum hypokalemia manifests. Unless renal failure or anuria coexist, potassium replacement should start early. Hyponatremic sodium determinations are frequently found during periods of hyperglycemia, due to the increased serum osmolality. Hypothermia and mental status compromise may accompany DKA.

Treatment includes a bolus dose of 10 U of intravenous regular insulin, to rapidly suppress lipolysis and drive glucose intracellularly, followed by an infusion of regular insulin, 1–4 U/hr. Large amounts of normal saline will be needed for intravascular volume replacement. If there is adequate urine output and normal renal function, potassium supplementation should be administered to avoid the development of hypokalemia as the DKA resolves. Bicarbonate should be administered if the pH is less than 7.1 and there is hemodynamic instability.

NIDDM patients exposed to infection, surgery, or dehydration may develop hyperosmolar nonketotic states. Endogenous circulating insulin generally prevents ketosis but remains insufficient to avert hyperglycemia. Hyperglycemia in excess of 600 mg/dL results in extreme hyperosmolarity, producing osmotic diuresis, hypotension, acidosis, and mental status changes progressing to coma. Osmolarities of hyperglycemic nonketotic states may exceed 330 mOsm/L. Approximate serum osmolarity may be calculated from the following formula:

$$\text{Osmolarity} = 2[Na^+ + K^+] + \text{glucose}/18 + BUN/2.8$$

Hyperosmolar nonketotic states respond well to rehydration with normal saline and small doses of insulin. However, rapid correction of hyperosmolarity risks cerebral edema and worsening of mental processes.

Treatment Strategy

Diabetic ketoacidosis (DKA)
Regular insulin 10 U intravenously then 1–4 U/hr infusion
Rehydration with normal saline
Potassium supplement when
    Levels return to normal
    Adequate urine output
    Normal renal function

Hyperosmolar nonketotic states
    Rehydration
    Small doses of insulin

SUGGESTED READINGS

Carvalho G, Moore A, Qizilbash B, Lachapelle K, Schricker T: Maintenance of normoglycemia during cardiac surgery. Cardiovasc Anesth 99:319–324, 2004

Dale DC, ed: ACP Medicine (online version). www.acpmedicine.com

Drummond J, Moore S: The influence of dextrose administration on neurologic outcome after temporary spinal cord ischemia in the rabbit. Anesthesiology 70:64, 1989

Finney SJ, Zekveld C, Elia A, Evans TW: Glucose control and mortality in critically ill patients. JAMA 290:2041–2047, 2003

Foster WW, McGarry JD: The metabolic derangements and treatment of diabetic ketoacidosis. N Engl J Med 309:159, 1983

Furnary AP, Gao G, Grunkemeier GL, et al.: Continuous insulin infusion reduces mortality in patients with diabetes undergoing coronary artery bypass grafting. J Thorac Cardiovasc Surg 125:1007–1021, 2003

Pulsinelli W, Levy D, Sigsber B, et al.: Increased damage after ischemic stroke in patients with hyperglycemia with or without established diabetes mellitus. Am J Med Sci 74:540, 1983

Salzarulo HH, Taylor LA: Diabetic stiff joint syndrome as a cause of difficult endotracheal intubation. Anesthesiology 64:366–368, 1986

Van den Berghe G, Wouters P, Weekers F, et al.: Intensive insulin therapy in critically ill patients. N Engl J Med 345:1359–1367, 2001

Leon K. Specthrie, MD

A 28-year-old woman presents for an elective cesarean section for a breech presentation of a full-term fetus. An uneventful spinal anesthetic is administered. Soon after delivery of the baby, she develops a sinus tachycardia (heart rate 110–130 beats per minute) and hypertension (blood pressure 150–170/90–105 mmHg). These hemodynamic abnormalities persist during her first 30 minutes in the postanesthesia care unit. Upon questioning, the patient admits to a prior history of frequent palpitations and feeling jittery. She also claims that her husband is "always turning the heat too high." Her vital signs return to normal after treatment with a total dose of 25 mg of labetolol intravenously.

QUESTIONS

1. How does the thyroid affect vital organ function?
2. How is thyroid hormone synthesized and released?
3. How is thyroid hormone regulated?
4. How are thyroid disorders evaluated?
5. What other conditions are associated with thyroid disorders?
6. What is thyroid storm and how is it treated?
7. What are the causes of hyperthyroidism?
8. What are the causes of hypothyroidism?

9. What are the preoperative considerations in a patient with thyroid disease?
10. What are the appropriate preoperative tests for a patient with thyroid disease?
11. What are the intraoperative concerns with coexisting thyroid disease?
12. What are the postoperative concerns?

1. How does the thyroid affect vital organ function?

The thyroid gland secretes two active hormones: triiodothyronine (T_3) and thyroxine (T_4). These hormones increase the basal metabolic rate through unclear mechanisms and results in an increase in oxygen consumption and heat generation.

Thyroid hormones increase cardiac output by increasing heart rate, preload, and contractility. These changes occur because of the increase in oxygen demand. Excessive levels of thyroid hormones result in up-regulation of β-adrenergic receptors in all tissues. This change in β-receptors results in an exaggerated response to sympathetic stimulation and to the administration of exogenous catecholamines such as ephedrine or epinephrine. Decreased levels of thyroid hormones have the opposite effect, and can make the individual unresponsive to even large doses of β-agonists.

Hyperthyroidism can lead to angina, high-output cardiac failure, and atrial fibrillation. Hypothyroidism can lead to cardiomegaly and decreased cardiac output.

2. How is thyroid hormone synthesized and released?

■ **Step 1**: Iodine, essential for thyroid-hormone synthesis, is reduced to iodide in the stomach and absorbed into the bloodstream by the gastrointestinal tract. Iodide is then absorbed by thyroid follicular cells, which "trap" and concentrate it. *Inhibitors of iodide absorption* are: circulating iodide, thiocyanate, and perchlorate.

■ **Step 2**: Iodide combines with tyrosine residues on thyroglobulin to form monoiodotyrosine (MIT) and then diiodotyrosine (DIT). Iodinated tyrosines join to create T_3 (MIT + DIT) and T_4 (DIT + DIT) and bind to thyroglobulin. *Inhibitors of T_3 and T_4 synthesis* are: propylthiouracil (PTU) and methimazole.

■ **Step 3**: T_3 and T_4 are cleaved from thyroglobulin and secreted into the circulation. T_4 comprises 95% of released hormone. Approximately one third of secreted T_4 is converted to T_3 in the kidney and liver. *Inhibitor of conversion of T_4 to T_3* is: PTU but *not* methimazole.

3. How is thyroid hormone regulated?

The hypothalamus secretes thyrotropin-releasing hormone (TRH), which stimulates the release of thyroid-stimulating hormone (TSH) by the anterior pituitary gland. The thyroid gland, in response to TSH, releases T_3 and T_4 into the circulation. TSH also causes increased uptake of iodide and increased iodination of thyroglobulin. Both T_3 and T_4 have a negative-feedback effect on the hypothalamus and pituitary glands.

4. How are thyroid disorders evaluated?

Thyroid disorders can be suspected based on a patient's history, findings on physical examination, and/or abnormalities in routine laboratory tests. A thorough history and physical examination are essential for evaluation and will assist in determining whether the patient is clinically euthyroid, hypothyroid, or hyperthyroid. Symptoms associated with hyperthyroidism and hypothyroidism are shown in Table 30.1. The physical examination should focus on the signs of hyperthyroidism and hypothyroidism (shown in Table 30.2), as well as the size and position of the thyroid, palpable nodules, and tracheal position.

Standard laboratory evaluations of thyroid function include TSH and free serum T_4 levels. Initially, an ultrasensitive TSH level is obtained and, if abnormal, then a free T_4 level is obtained. Because greater than 99% of circulating thyroid hormone is bound to thyroxine binding globulin (TBG), total T_4 levels may be deceiving. Increases in TBG (pregnancy, estrogen therapy) or decreases in TBG (cirrhosis,

TABLE 30.1	Symptoms of Hyperthyroidism and Hypothyroidism
Hyperthyroidism	**Hypothyroidism**
Nervousness	Fatigue
Diaphoresis	Weakness
Heat sensitivity	Weight gain
Fatigue	Constipation
Palpitations/tachycardia	Cold intolerance
Weight loss	Hair loss
Dyspnea	Myalgias
Increased appetite	
Diarrhea	
Skeletal muscle weakness	

TABLE 30.2	Signs of Hyperthyroidism and Hypothyroidism
Hyperthyroidism	**Hypothyroidism**
Tachycardia	Bradycardia
Goiter	Hypotension
Skin changes	Delayed reflexes
Tremor	Lid lag
Exophthalmos	Hoarse voice
Atrial fibrillation	Dry coarse skin
Splenomegaly	Pleural effusions
Gynecomastia	

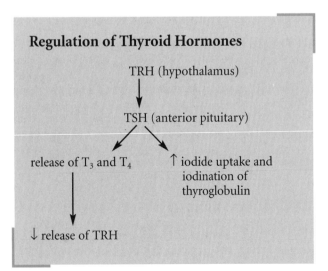

Regulation of Thyroid Hormones

TRH (hypothalamus)
↓
TSH (anterior pituitary)
↓   ↘
release of T_3 and T_4 ↑ iodide uptake and iodination of thyroglobulin
↓
↓ release of TRH

nephrotic syndrome) may result in abnormal levels of total T_4 but normal levels of free T_4.

In hyperthyroidism, the TSH levels will be low and the T_4 levels will be high. If the serum T_4 level is normal, a T_3 level should be obtained. In hypothyroidism, the TSH level is high in intrinsic thyroid gland abnormalities or low in hypothalamic or pituitary gland abnormalities.

Imaging studies can be helpful in evaluating thyroid disorders. Radioactive thyroid uptake scans are important for determining whether thyroid nodules are active ("hot") or inactive ("cold"). Hot nodules are rarely malignant. Ultrasound can be used to determine the size and number of thyroid nodules. CT scan or magnetic resonance imaging (MRI) will show the size of the thyroid, compression of neighboring structures, and the presence of lymphadenopathy.

5. What other conditions are associated with thyroid disorders?

Medullary thyroid carcinoma is one component of multiple endocrine neoplasia (MEN) type II. All patients with medullary carcinoma should be evaluated for the presence of a pheochromocytoma, hyperparathyroidism, and neuromas. Hashimoto's thyroiditis is associated with myasthenia gravis.

6. What is thyroid storm and how is it treated?

Thyroid storm is a hypermetabolic and sympathetic crisis caused by a sudden surge in thyroid hormones. Triggers of thyroid storm include infection, surgery, and pain. Thyroid storm presents with hypertension, tachycardia, and hyperthermia, and is easily confused with malignant hyperthermia and pheochromocytoma. However, the profound metabolic acidosis that occurs in malignant hyperthermia does not occur during thyroid storm and plays an important role in differentiating between the two disorders.

The immediate treatment of thyroid storm is the administration of β-blockade agents to alleviate the symptoms. Hyperthermic patients should be actively cooled. There are case reports of effective treatment of thyroid storm with dantrolene; however, this is not routinely recommended at this time. After initial control of the symptoms, the patient should receive PTU and potassium iodide.

7. What are the causes of hyperthyroidism?

Hyperthyroidism causing symptoms (thyrotoxicosis) can be primary, secondary, or tertiary.

In primary hyperthyroidism, the thyroid produces T_3 and T_4 independently of stimulation by TSH. The most common cause of hyperthyroidism is Graves' disease.

This typically occurs in women 20–40 years of age. In this disease, autoantibodies to thyroid TSH receptors result in stimulation of hormone production. Thyroiditis also causes release of thyroid hormones and may be either subacute (probably viral infection) or acute suppurative (bacterial infection). Toxic solitary nodules and toxic multinodular goiters may cause primary hyperthyroidism. A rare cause of primary hyperthyroidism is a molar pregnancy secreting chorionic gonadotropin, which has TSH-like activity. The laboratory abnormalities in primary hyperthyroidism are elevated levels of T_3 and T_4 and low levels of TSH.

In secondary hyperthyroidism, the pituitary produces excessive TSH, independent of stimulation by TRH. Pituitary

Causes of Hyperthyroidism and Their Laboratory Findings

Cause	Laboratory findings
Primary	
Graves' disease	TSH low
Thyroiditis	T_3 elevated
Toxic solitary nodule	T_4 elevated
Toxic multinodular goiter	
Molar pregnancy	
Secondary	
Pituitary adenoma	TSH elevated
	T_3 elevated
	T_4 elevated
	TRH low
Tertiary	
Excessive TRH secretion	TRH elevated
	TSH elevated
	T_3 elevated
	T_4 elevated

adenomas are the most common cause of secondary hyperthyroidism. The laboratory abnormalities in secondary hyperthyroidism are elevated levels of TSH, T_3 and T_4, but reduced levels of TRH.

Tertiary hyperthyroidism results from excessive secretion of TRH. The laboratory abnormalities in tertiary hyperthyroidism are elevated levels of TRH, TSH, and T_3 and T_4.

8. What are the causes of hypothyroidism?

Primary hypothyroidism is due to intrinsic thyroid gland failure. The most common causes are irradiation, surgery, and "burnt out" thyroiditis. Other causes include iodine deficiency or excess, amiodarone, lithium, and antithyroid medications. The laboratory abnormalities in primary hypothyroidism are elevated levels of TSH and low T_3 and T_4 levels.

Secondary hypothyroidism is due to inadequate levels of TSH with a normal thyroid gland. This can be caused by pituitary failure or pituitary surgery. The laboratory abnormalities in secondary hypothyroidism are low levels of T_3, T_4, and TSH but elevated levels of TRH.

Tertiary hypothyroidism is due to hypothalamic failure. The laboratory abnormalities in tertiary hypothyroidism are low levels of T_3, T_4, TSH, and TRH.

9. What are the preoperative considerations in a patient with thyroid disease?

The first, and most important, consideration is whether the patient is clinically euthyroid. Patients who are euthyroid or minimally hypothyroid are generally at no increased perioperative risk. However, patients who are clinically hyperthyroid may have dysrhythmias, hypertension, ischemia, high-output cardiac failure, and ultimately may develop thyroid storm. Conversely, patients who are clinically hypothyroid may have bradycardia, hypotension, low-output cardiac failure, and resistance to catecholamines.

Patients who are hyperthyroid must be treated preoperatively. For elective cases, this should include PTU or methimazole until the patient is euthyroid, which may take 6–8 weeks of therapy. The addition of β-blocking agents may also be necessary. For urgent or emergent cases, the patient should be treated with β-blocking agents.

Profoundly hypothyroid patients should receive intravenous T_4 before surgery. Patients should be observed carefully for dysrhythmias or angina.

Any patient with a goiter must be evaluated for airway compromise. Large goiters can cause distortion of the airway, making intubation difficult or impossible. Goiters also make emergency surgical access of the airway difficult if not impossible and therefore should not be considered a viable emergency back-up plan. Retrosternal goiters can cause collapse of the airway after induction of general anesthesia. Symptoms such as dysphagia, wheezing, stridor, and positional dyspnea are worrisome and necessitate further evaluation (see below). Physical examination should include the standard evaluation of the airway, as well as position of the trachea. Any plan for an awake fiberoptic intubation should be discussed with the patient preoperatively.

Patients who are euthyroid or hyperthyroid can safely receive preoperative anxiolysis. However, premedication in

Causes of Hypothyroidism and Their Laboratory Findings

Cause	Laboratory findings
Primary	
Irradiation	TSH elevated
Surgery	T_3 low
"Burnt out" thyroiditis	T_4 low
Iodine deficiency or excess	
Pharmacologic	
Amiodarone Lithium Anti-thyroid medications	
Secondary	
Pituitary failure	TSH low
Pituitary surgery	T_3 low
	T_4 low
	TRH elevated
Tertiary	
Hypothalamic failure	TRH low
	TSH low
	T_3 low
	T_4 low

patients who are hypothyroid should be avoided because they may have an exaggerated and life-threatening response to anxiolysis.

10. What are appropriate preoperative tests for a patient with thyroid disease?

Patients with thyroid disease should have recent evaluation of TSH and free T_4 levels. These should be nearly normal for elective surgery. Patients who have been on long-term thyroid-hormone replacement do not need recent hormone levels, unless there has been a change in symptoms.

Hypothyroidism can cause anemia and thrombocytopenia, as well as hyponatremia, hypoglycemia, and cholestasis. Thus, hypothyroid patients should have a complete blood count, platelet count, electrolytes, glucose, and liver function tests evaluated preoperatively.

An electrocardiogram should be done looking for the presence of atrial fibrillation, premature complexes, ischemia, or ventricular hypertrophy. Other cardiac testing should be considered for patients with cardiac symptoms.

All patients with a goiter or abnormal airway physical examination should have radiological evaluation of the trachea, either by radiography, CT, or MRI. Patients with large or retrosternal goiters should have a CT scan or MRI. These studies will help guide the choice of anesthesia (regional or general), intubation technique, and endotracheal tube size.

11. What are the intraoperative concerns with coexisting thyroid disease?

The first concern is airway management. The first decision to be made is whether to secure the airway before or after induction of anesthesia. This decision will be determined primarily by the results of the physical examination and radiological studies. There are many different modalities available for safely securing the abnormal airway. They include: awake or asleep fiberoptic intubation, awake intubation through a laryngeal mask airway (LMA), or inhalation induction followed by direct laryngoscopy. The uncompromised airway can be maintained with an endotracheal tube or an LMA. Endotracheal tubes should be reinforced or secured so that they cannot kink when warmed to body temperature. With an LMA, there is the risk of laryngospasm from surgical manipulation or nerve damage.

Thyroidectomy can be performed under bilateral superficial cervical plexus block and unilateral deep cervical plexus block. Bilateral deep cervical blocks should be avoided because of the risk of causing bilateral recurrent laryngeal nerve blockade. This technique requires a motivated patient, and a surgeon and anesthesiologist comfortable with the technique.

Patients who are clinically hyperthyroid presenting for emergency surgery will be oversensitive to β-adrenergic stimulation. They will have an exaggerated response to endogenous catecholamines released during the stress response, as well as to exogenous catecholamines administered for hypotension. Phenylephrine may be preferable, since it does not cause β-adrenergic stimulation. Hypothyroid patients, on the other hand, will be insensitive to catecholamines and will require larger doses than normal.

The minimal alveolar concentration (MAC) of inhalation agents does not change. However, these patients may require support or control of hemodynamic parameters when normal doses of anesthetics are administered. The volume of distribution and clearance of drugs may be affected by thyroid status.

12. What are the postoperative concerns?

The postoperative concerns after thyroid surgery are as follows:

- The possibility of thyroid storm occurring is still present.
- Injury to the recurrent laryngeal nerve during surgery causes vocal cord paralysis, and occurs transiently in 3–4% of thyroidectomies. Unilateral injury causes ineffective cough, hoarseness, and risk of aspiration. Bilateral injury causes airway obstruction. Injury to the nerve may be due to traction or transection, and should be suspected if the surgeon had difficulty identifying the nerves.
- Postoperative bleeding may result in rapidly expanding hematomas that can quickly obstruct the airway. Postanesthesia care unit (PACU) and ward staff should monitor the patient for airway compromise. Opening

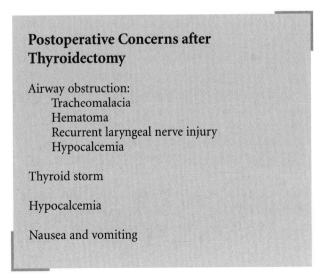

Postoperative Concerns after Thyroidectomy

Airway obstruction:
    Tracheomalacia
    Hematoma
    Recurrent laryngeal nerve injury
    Hypocalcemia

Thyroid storm

Hypocalcemia

Nausea and vomiting

the wound will usually temporarily relieve the airway obstruction. Ultimately, the patient's trachea should be reintubated and the patient returned to the operating room for evacuation of the hematoma and control of the bleeding. Edema from venous congestion may result in continued airway obstruction.

■ Large, long-standing goiters can cause tracheomalacia leading to postoperative airway obstruction. This complication more commonly occurs with retrosternal goiters. In cases of suspected tracheomalacia, the patient should demonstrate the ability to breathe around the endotracheal tube with the balloon deflated prior to extubation. Airway obstruction from tracheomalacia may require reintubation, tracheostomy, or stenting of the airway.

■ Postoperative hypocalcemia from parathyroid injury or inadvertent resection is common, and usually transient. Hypocalcemia may present in the PACU as airway obstruction. Calcium levels should be checked starting 2 hours postoperatively, with replacement as necessary.

■ There is an increased incidence of nausea and vomiting. There are multiple ways of reducing this risk, including use of propofol for the anesthetic, avoidance of nitrous oxide, and treatment with antiemetics.

SUGGESTED READINGS

Farling PA: Thyroid disease. Br J Anesth 85:15–28, 2000

Jameson JL, Weetman AP: Disorders of the thyroid gland. pp. 2060–2083. In Braunwald E, Fauci AS, et al. (eds): Harrison's Principles of Internal Medicine, 15th edition. McGraw-Hill, New York, 2001

Woeber KA: Thyrotoxicosis and the heart. N Engl J Med 327:94–98, 1992

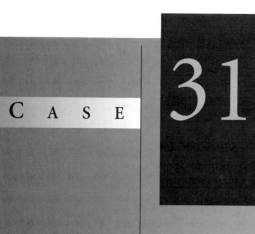

CASE 31 CALCIUM METABOLISM

Leon K. Specthrie, MD

A 68-year-old man presents for elective parathyroidectomy. The patient was diagnosed with parathyroid adenoma after a blood test in preparation for elective cataract surgery revealed hypercalcemia. Further blood tests demonstrated an elevated parathyroid hormone (PTH) level, and technetium-sestamibi scans showed hyperactivity in the right lower gland. The patient also has a history of well controlled hypertension.

QUESTIONS

1. What is the role of calcium in the body?
2. Where is calcium found in the body?
3. How is calcium regulated?
4. What are the symptoms of hypercalcemia? How is this treated?
5. What are the symptoms of hypocalcemia? How is this treated?
6. What are the causes of hyperparathyroidism?
7. What are the anesthetic considerations for parathyroid resection?
8. What are the postoperative concerns after parathyroid resection?

1. What is the role of calcium in the body?

Calcium, a divalent cation, is essential for the formation of bone, one of the largest organ systems in the body. Bone has important structural and protective functions in the body.

Intracellular calcium is essential for the interaction of actin and myosin causing muscle contraction. Intracellular calcium is also an important second messenger for many hormones and neurotransmitters.

2. Where is calcium found in the body?

Approximately 99% of the calcium in the body is found in the bones. The mineral phase of bone is composed of hydroxyapatite $(Ca_{10}(PO_4)_6(OH)_2)$ and other minerals. Hydroxyapatite is deposited in close association with an organic phase composed primarily of collagen. Osteoblasts create new bone and osteoclasts cause bone resorption.

The remainder of the calcium is found in extracellular fluid (1%) and intracellular fluid (0.1%). Half of the extracellular calcium is in the free ionized form. This is the important form for physiologic processes. About 40% of extracellular calcium is bound to albumin and globulins. Binding to albumin is decreased by acidosis and increased by alkalosis. Increases or decreases in serum protein will change total serum calcium without changing ionized calcium. For this reason, the most meaningful laboratory test for calcium is serum ionized calcium, which is widely available.

Intracellular free calcium concentrations are about 0.01% of extracellular concentrations. Calcium is actively transported out of the cell by ATP-dependent pumps. Muscle cells sequester calcium in the sarcoplasmic reticulum. This calcium is easily available during muscle contraction, but not present as free calcium during rest.

3. How is calcium regulated?

Total body calcium is determined by the relative balance of calcium absorption and calcium excretion. The average adult diet contains 600–800 mg per day, although calcium supplementation can raise this to 2,000 mg per day. Absorption of this calcium in the small intestine is variable, and is determined by vitamin D levels. Typical absorption is 40–50% of dietary intake. Calcium is excreted in the gastrointestinal tract and urine. Greater than 90% of calcium filtered by the glomerulus is reabsorbed by the nephron. Since the kidney cannot conserve calcium efficiently enough to compensate for low dietary intake or absorption problems, a negative calcium balance will result.

Calcium in the extracellular fluid is in constant equilibrium with bone. The relative balance of bone deposition or resorption is determined by parathyroid hormone (PTH) and vitamin D. Vitamin D can be obtained from the diet or synthesized in the liver and skin, with the help of sunlight. Vitamin D is metabolized to the inactive form, 25(OH)D, by the liver, which is then metabolized to the active form, $1,25(OH)_2D$, by the kidney. Production of $1,25(OH)_2D$ is enhanced by PTH, and possibly by hypocalcemia directly. $1,25(OH)_2D$ stimulates calcium and phosphate absorption in the small intestine and calcium resorption from bone. $1,25(OH)_2D$ also increases renal resorption of filtered calcium.

Hypocalcemia stimulates the parathyroid to secrete PTH. This peptide hormone causes resorption of calcium from bone, increased intestinal absorption of calcium, and increased resorption of filtered calcium in the kidney. PTH is involved in phosphate homeostasis, causing increased renal excretion. PTH excretion will increase in response to increased dietary phosphate because enhanced deposition of calcium and phosphate in bone leads to mild hypocalcemia. PTH also stimulates the production of $1,25(OH)_2D$.

Parathyroid-related protein (PTHrP) is functionally and structurally similar to PTH. This hormone is produced by numerous cell types, but little, if any, circulates in normal humans. Large tumors can produce enough PTHrP to cause significant blood levels and significant hypercalcemia.

Calcitonin is a peptide hormone that inhibits resorption of calcium from bone and in the kidney. Calcitonin is produced in the thyroid, and its production is stimulated by hypercalcemia. The role of calcitonin in normal physiology is minimal, and there is no adverse outcome when it is absent following total thyroidectomy. Calcitonin is useful as a treatment for severe hypercalcemia.

4. What are the symptoms of hypercalcemia? How is this treated?

Increases in free ionized calcium can cause gastrointestinal and neurologic symptoms. The normal level for total serum calcium is 9–10.5 mg/dL (2.2–2.6 mmol/L), and for ionized calcium is 4.5–5.6 mg/dL (1.1–1.4 mmol/L). These values vary slightly among laboratories. Gastrointestinal manifestations can be either excitatory (nausea and vomiting) or inhibitory (anorexia and

Hypercalcemia

Symptoms

Gastrointestinal
    Excitatory
        Nausea and vomiting
    Inhibitory
        Anorexia
        Constipation

Central nervous system
    Hypotonia
    Lethargy
    Coma

Calcium phosphate deposits in kidneys, blood
    vessels, and other organs

Treatment

Hydration

Furosemide

Bisphosphonate

Calcitonin

Hemodialysis/peritoneal dialysis

constipation). The nervous system is depressed with hypotonia, lethargy, and even coma.

Symptomatic hypercalcemia is more likely to be due to malignancy than is asymptomatic hypercalcemia. Malignancy can cause hypercalcemia via PTHrP or by invasion of bone by primary or metastatic tumors. Symptomatic hypercalcemia can also be due to acute vitamin D or oral calcium intoxication. Hypercalcemia is exacerbated by dehydration.

Long-standing hypercalcemia can cause calcium phosphate deposition in the kidneys, blood vessels, and other organs. This also happens in renal failure when patients have normal calcium concentrations but elevated phosphate concentrations.

Treatment of hypercalcemia is somewhat dependent on the cause. Mild hypercalcemia (<12 mg/dL) can be managed by hydration. More severe hypercalcemia can be treated acutely with escalating aggressiveness, depending on symptoms and calcium concentrations. First, patients can receive aggressive hydration and forced diuresis with furosemide. Potassium and magnesium are depleted during this treatment and may need to be replaced. Next, patients can receive a bisphosphonate, usually pamidronate. Finally, severe hypercalcemia can be treated with parenteral calcitonin. Hemodialysis or peritoneal dialysis is a useful treatment for severe hypercalcemia in patients with impaired renal function. After acute treatment, correctable causes of hypercalcemia can be accomplished surgically.

5. What are the symptoms of hypocalcemia? How is this treated?

Decreased free ionized calcium causes nervous system excitability. Symptoms include anxiety, muscle spasms, paresthesias, and seizures. Physical examination can demonstrate Chvostek's and Trousseau's signs. Chvostek's sign is contraction of the facial muscles in response to tapping over the facial nerve anterior to the ear. Trousseau's sign is elicited by occluding blood flow to the hand for 3 minutes with a blood pressure cuff. A positive sign is flexion spasm of the metacarpo-phalangeal joints. Muscle irritability can result in bronchospasm or even laryngospasm. The electrocardiogram shows prolongation of the QT interval.

Mild, asymptomatic hypocalcemia following parathyroidectomy can be treated with oral calcium supplementation. Symptomatic hypocalcemia can present after inadvertent injury to or removal of all the parathyroid glands in a patient. When symptomatic, hypocalcemia should be treated parenterally. Typically, a solution of calcium chloride 1 mg/mL in D5W is infused at 0.5–2 mg/kg/hr. Vitamin D supplementation should be started if a calcium chloride infusion does not improve symptoms or is needed for more than a few days.

6. What are the causes of hyperparathyroidism?

Primary hyperparathyroidism is most commonly due to hyperplasia of a single gland. This isolated hyperplasia is usually a benign adenoma. The inferior parathyroid glands are the most common sites for adenomas. Some adenomas present in and around the thyroid and thymus, and even behind the esophagus. Locating these adenomas during surgery can be difficult. Parathyroid carcinoma is a rare cause of hyperplasia. Familial forms of hyperparathyroidism tend to have multiple glands involved.

The multiple endocrine neoplasia (MEN) syndromes are the most common causes of hereditary hyperparathyroidism. MEN 1 consists of hyperparathyroidism, tumors of the pituitary, and tumors of the pancreas. MEN 2A consists of hyperparathyroidism, medullary carcinoma of the thyroid, and pheochromocytoma. The various disorders can present at different times, so the associated disorders should be considered in patients with familial hyperparathyroidism.

Chronic renal failure causes secondary hyperparathyroidism. Renal failure leads to chronically elevated phosphate levels. Increased deposition of calcium and

Hypocalcemia

Symptoms

Central nervous system
    Paresthesias
    Seizures
    Chvostek's sign
    Trousseau's sign

Respiratory
    Bronchospasm
    Laryngospasm

Cardiac
    Prolonged QT interval

Musculoskeletal
    Muscle spasm

Treatment

Oral calcium supplements

Calcium chloride infusion

Vitamin D

phosphate in bone, because of the increased phosphate concentrations, leads to hypocalcemia. The lack of $1,25(OH)_2D$, which is produced in normal kidneys and stimulates gastrointestinal absorption of calcium, exacerbates the hypocalcemia. This chronic hypocalcemia leads to chronic stimulation and hyperplasia of the parathyroid glands.

Long-standing secondary hyperparathyroidism can cause the parathyroid glands to become unresponsive to correction of hypocalcemia. This condition is referred to as tertiary hyperparathyroidism, and is treated surgically. Typically, the parathyroid glands are resected, and a portion of one is auto-transplanted into the forearm.

A rare cause of reversible hyperparathyroidism is treatment with lithium. There appears to be a high incidence of parathyroid adenomas with chronic lithium treatment. The mechanism for this is not clear.

7. What are the anesthetic considerations for parathyroid resection?

It is important to know the indication for the surgery. If the patient has secondary hyperparathyroidism from end-stage renal disease, it is important to consider all the implications of renal failure and its comorbidities. These patients are likely to have hypertension, diabetes mellitus, and coronary artery disease, as well as metabolic derangements from renal failure.

For patients presenting with primary hyperparathyroidism, it is important to know the calcium concentration and whether the patient is symptomatic. Hypercalcemia causing significant symptoms should be corrected preoperatively. Isolated parathyroid adenomas that have been localized preoperatively can be excised under general anesthesia, regional anesthesia with unilateral deep and superficial cervical blocks, or sedation and local anesthesia. The experience and comfort level of the surgeon and patient expectations play a large role in the choice of anesthetic plan. Surgery for all four glands or for poorly localized adenomas is more easily performed under general anesthesia. It is difficult to obtain adequate regional anesthesia bilaterally. Bilateral deep cervical plexus blocks can cause bilateral recurrent laryngeal nerve paralysis or bilateral phrenic nerve paralysis, and are relatively contraindicated. More surgeons are becoming comfortable with performing bilateral neck exploration under local anesthesia.

It is now commonplace to monitor PTH levels before and after adenoma resection. After successful resection, PTH levels should fall by half within 10 minutes. A large-bore intravenous catheter in an antecubital vein usually provides adequate blood flow to obtain specimens. Alternatively, it is sometimes necessary to place a catheter in a foot, or perform repeat venipuncture in a foot to obtain specimens. Rarely, an arterial line can be placed for the case, but the risk-benefit ratio must be carefully considered. The arms are usually tucked by the patient's side and are inaccessible during surgery.

8. What are the postoperative concerns after parathyroid resection?

Postoperative hypocalcemia can result from inadvertent removal of all parathyroid tissue. In this case, serum calcium will fall below 8 mg/dL. With an experienced surgeon this is a rare occurrence.

Transient mild hypocalcemia often results from chronic suppression of the remaining glands by chronic hypercalcemia. Oral calcium supplementation is usually adequate treatment for this. Symptomatic hypocalcemia should be treated with parenteral calcium. Prolonged hypocalcemia (more than several days) should be treated with calcitriol, a vitamin D analogue.

SUGGESTED READING

Braunwald E, Fauci AS, Kasper DL, Hauser SL, Long DL, Jameson JL: pp. 2205–2220. In Harrison's Principles of Internal Medicine, 15th edition. McGraw-Hill Professional, New York, 2001

Kulkarni RS, Braverman LE, Patwardhan NA: Bilateral cervical plexus block for thyroidectomy and parathyroidectomy in healthy and high risk patients. J Endocrinol Invest 19:714–718, 1996

Lo Gerfo P: Bilateral neck exploration for parathyroidectomy under local anesthesia: a viable technique for patients with coexisting thyroid disease with or without sestamibi scanning. Surgery 126:1011-1014, 1999

32

PERIOPERATIVE CORTICOSTEROID ADMINISTRATION

Andrew B. Leibowitz, MD

Adel Bassily-Marcus, MD

A 68-year-old man presents for a laparoscopic cholecystectomy. He has been taking prednisone 10 mg per day for the treatment of polymyalgia rheumatica. He has no other medical history.

QUESTIONS

1. Where and what kind of steroids are naturally produced?
2. What are the physiologic effects of glucocorticosteroids?
3. What steroids are available for administration and what are their equivalent doses?
4. How much cortisol is normally produced and what is Addison's disease?
5. What are Cushing syndrome and Cushing disease?
6. Does this patient require "stress" dose steroids?
7. How long after discontinuation of steroids should a patient be considered adrenally suppressed and treated accordingly?
8. What clinical scenarios frequently require steroid administration?
9. How is adrenal reserve evaluated?
10. If this patient develops septic shock from a bile leak in the postanesthesia care unit (PACU), should steroids be withheld or administered?

1. Where and what kind of steroids are naturally produced?

The adrenal cortex produces three different classes of steroids built from the basic cholesterol molecule. These three classes are glucocorticosteroids (cortisol), mineralocorticoids (aldosterone) and androgens (testosterone). The adrenal medulla produces catecholamines via an entirely different metabolic pathway starting with the amino acid tyrosine and under different neurohumoral control.

2. What are the physiologic effects of glucocorticosteroids?

Glucocorticosteroids are produced by the adrenal glands in response to stimulation by adrenocorticotropic hormone (ACTH). ACTH is secreted by the pituitary in response to corticotropin-releasing hormone (CRH), which is produced in the hypothalamus. Glucocorticosteroids primarily affect intermediary metabolism. Glucocorticosteroids diffuse through the cell membrane and bind to specific glucocorticosteroid receptors, creating a complex that migrates to the nucleus and alters gene transcription. Resulting physiologic effects include a rise in the blood glucose, mobilization of fatty acids, catabolism, and anti-inflammation.

3. What steroids are available for administration and what are their equivalent doses?

Dexamethasone (Decadron), methylprednisolone (Solumedrol), prednisone and hydrocortisone (intravenous

Relative Potencies of Steroid Preparations

Dexamethasone	1
Methylprednisolone	4
Prednisone	5
Hydrocortisone	20

Cushing Syndrome and Cushing Disease

Etiology
    Cushing syndrome
        Iatrogenic: exogenous steroid administration
        Non-iatrogenic: excessive ACTH secretion
    Cushing disease
        Excessive pituitary secretion of ACTH
Features
    Truncal obesity
    Hirsutism
    Weakness
    Hypertension
    Abdominal striae
    Edema
    Hyperglycemia

form is Solucortef, oral form is Cortef) are the four main steroids available for administration. Their relative potencies are 0.75, 4, 5, and 20, respectively. For example, a patient taking prednisone 5 mg orally per day who needs to be changed to an intravenous form of identical potency would receive hydrocortisone 20 mg intravenously.

4. How much cortisol is normally produced and what is Addison's disease?

Under normal conditions approximately 30 mg of cortisol is produced daily. During periods of extreme stress (e.g., thoracic aortic surgery or septic shock) up to 300 mg may be produced over the course of 24 hours.

Addison's disease results from chronic lack of endogenous cortisol (and usually aldosterone) production and results in fatigue, weakness, anorexia, increased skin pigmentation, hypotension, hypoglycemia, hyponatremia, and hyperkalemia. The majority of cases are idiopathic.

Addisonian "crisis" is an acute adrenocortical insufficiency resulting in these same findings but with a more severe presentation in which shock, coma, and death can occur. Acute adrenocortical insufficiency may occur in the face of an absolute or relative lack of glucocorticosteroids. Chronic exogenous steroid administration impairs the adrenal gland's ability to respond with increased production of glucocorticosteroids during periods of stress. In such instances, additional exogenous steroid administration will be necessary to prevent the above-mentioned sequelae.

5. What are Cushing syndrome and Cushing disease?

Cushing syndrome is caused by excessive cortisol levels. The most common etiology is iatrogenic secondary to excessive steroid administration. The most common non-iatrogenic cause is bilateral adrenal hyperplasia due to excessive pituitary or ectopic ACTH secretion. The term Cushing *disease* is reserved for patients with pituitary tumors causing excessive ACTH secretion.

The most notable features of Cushing syndrome are truncal obesity, hirsutism, weakness, hypertension, abdominal striae, edema, and hyperglycemia.

6. Does this patient require "stress" dose steroids?

Laparoscopic cholecystectomy without surgical complication, such as large blood loss, will usually not result in any significant increase in endogenous cortisol production. Therefore, the administration of full dose "stress" steroids (i.e., hydrocortisone 100 mg intravenously every 8 hours) is not indicated for this patient. However, most sources recommend a modest increase in steroid administration. For example, the patient may be instructed to take prednisone 10 or 15 mg orally on the day of surgery, and perhaps the day after, or the equivalent dose of another steroid.

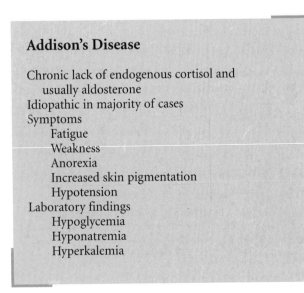

Addison's Disease

Chronic lack of endogenous cortisol and
    usually aldosterone
Idiopathic in majority of cases
Symptoms
    Fatigue
    Weakness
    Anorexia
    Increased skin pigmentation
    Hypotension
Laboratory findings
    Hypoglycemia
    Hyponatremia
    Hyperkalemia

7. How long after discontinuation of steroids should a patient be considered adrenally suppressed and treated accordingly?

The duration and dose of steroid therapy determine the duration and degree of suppression that results. Short courses of high doses of prednisone, such as may be administered to treat poison ivy (e.g., prednisone 50 mg per day for 5 days), have been shown to cause abnormal response to ACTH stimulation testing for up to 5 days. Recovery after prolonged exposure to oral steroids is highly variable, but may take as long as 1 year. Exposure to lower doses of steroids from inhalers and enemas results in an unknown degree of adrenal suppression. In the absence of ACTH testing, the underlying principles this author adheres to are as follows: (1) only the most major of surgical procedures require doses of hydrocortisone in the 200 mg per day range for 2 or more days; (2) 1–2 day courses of intermediate-dose steroids carry very little risk; (3) a common anti-nausea prophylactic dose of dexamethasone (e.g., 8 mg IV) alone will more than suffice to treat adrenal suppression in almost all commonly performed surgeries including hernia repair, cholecystectomy, lumpectomy, and hysterectomy.

8. What clinical scenarios frequently require steroid administration?

Steroids may be administered for a variety of therapeutic effects:

- Prevention or treatment of postoperative nausea and vomiting
- Reduction of swelling (e.g., traumatic intubation or laryngeal surgery)
- Prevention of transplant rejection
- Asthma
- Colitis
- Arthritis
- Septic shock
- Adult respiratory distress syndrome.

9. How is adrenal reserve evaluated?

The most commonly performed outpatient test for adrenal reserve is a urinary free cortisol collection over 24 hours. For hospitalized patients, the ACTH stimulation test is most commonly performed to determine the presence of adequate adrenal function. This screening test entails the measurement of a baseline plasma cortisol, followed by a measurement at 30 and 60 minutes after the intravenous administration of 250 µg of cosyntropin, an ACTH analog. During periods of stress, the baseline plasma cortisol level should exceed 20 µg/dL and all patients should have a rise in their plasma cortisol level of at least 7 µg/dL above their baseline.

10. If this patient develops septic shock from a bile leak in the postanesthesia care unit (PACU), should steroids be withheld or administered?

Administration of steroids for the treatment of septic shock has long been debated. Although it has been recognized that steroid administration could restore vascular responsiveness to catecholamine administration and allow the withdrawal of vasopressor therapy, clinical trials have generally revealed that greater potential harm than benefit occurred.

Recently Annane et al. (2002) performed a landmark multicenter, randomized, double-blind, and placebo-controlled trial to assess whether "low" doses of corticosteroids

---

Suggested Steroid Treatment in Septic Shock

Perform ACTH stimulation test

In patients requiring vasopressor therapy start:
  Hydrocortisone 50 mg intravenously every 6 hours
  Fludrocortisone 50 mg orally once daily (if enteral access and absorption present)

Stimulation test results
  Baseline cortisol level <20 mg/dL
              or   Continue therapy for 7 days
  Rise from baseline level <9 µg/dL

  Baseline cortisol level >20 µg/dL
              or   Discontinue therapy
  Rise from baseline level >9 µg/dL

improve survival from septic shock. In this investigation, patients in septic shock underwent a cosyntropin stimulation test. Patients were randomized to receive either hydrocortisone 50 mg by intravenous bolus every 6 hours and fludrocortisone 50 μg orally once daily or a placebo.

Of the 299 patients, 229 were found to be relatively adrenal-insufficient and classified as "nonresponders." A nonresponse to the cosyntropin stimulation test was defined as a rise in the serum cortisol level of 9 μg/dL or less. Patients who were nonresponders (i.e., adrenal-insufficient) had a statistically significant ($P = 0.04$) lowered mortality rate when administered steroids (53% vs. 63% at 28 days, and 58% vs. 70% at the end of the ICU stay in the steroid vs. placebo group). Patients who were responders (i.e., adrenal-sufficient) had a statistically insignificant increased mortality when administered steroids (61% vs. 53% at 28 days and 69% vs. 59% at the end of the ICU stay in the steroid vs. placebo group).

Based primarily on this investigation, the Society of Critical Care Medicine now recommends hydrocortisone administration in the treatment of vasopressor-resistant shock.

While final conclusive evidence is lacking, this author recommends performing an ACTH stimulation test followed by administration of hydrocortisone 50 mg intravenously every 6 hours to all patients requiring vasopressors in the management of presumed septic shock. After obtaining the results of the stimulation test (which usually takes 24–48 hours), steroids will be continued for 7 days in patients with a baseline plasma cortisol level of less than 20 μg/dL, or a rise from the baseline level of less than 9 mg/dL. Patients who do not meet these criteria will have their steroids discontinued.

SUGGESTED READINGS

Annane D, Sebille V, Charpentier C, et al.: Effect of treatment with low doses of hydrocortisone and fludrocortisone on mortality in patient with septic shock. JAMA 288:862–871, 2002

Axelrod L: Perioperative management of patients treated with glucocorticoids. Endocrinol Metab Clin North Am 32:367–383, 2003

Cooper MS, Stewart P: Corticosteroid insufficiency in acutely ill patients. N Engl J Med 348:727–734, 2003

Lamberts SWJ, Bruining HA, De Jong FH: Corticosteroid therapy in severe illness. N Engl J Med 337:1285–1292, 1997

Marik PE, Zaloga GP: Adrenal insufficiency in the critically ill: a new look at an old problem. Chest 122:1784–1796, 2002

Streck WF, Lockwood DH: Pituitary adrenal recovery following short-term suppression with corticosteroids. Am J Med 86:910–914, 1979

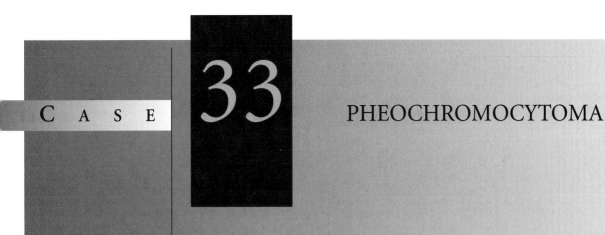

CASE 33

PHEOCHROMOCYTOMA

George V. Gabrielson, MD
Leon K. Specthrie, MD

A 67-year-old man with a presumptive diagnosis of a pheochromocytoma presents for elective adrenalectomy the following morning. His past medical history is unremarkable, except for symptoms leading to the establishment of his clinical diagnosis. Approximately 6 months before admission, the patient suffered from spontaneous episodes of headaches, sweating, and frequent palpitations. Because of these symptoms, he sought the advice of his internist, who ordered a series of tests that included determination of urinary catecholamines and metabolite concentrations. Results of these tests were elevated above normal values, and a subsequent computed tomography scan of the abdomen confirmed the presence of an adrenal mass. The internist started the patient on oral phenoxybenzamine therapy (10 mg by mouth, twice daily) in preparation for the surgical resection.

QUESTIONS

1. What is a pheochromocytoma?
2. Describe the clinical presentation of and diagnostic criteria for pheochromocytoma.
3. Pheochromocytoma is associated with what other syndromes?
4. What conditions may mimic pheochromocytoma?

5. How are patients with pheochromocytoma prepared for surgery?
6. Describe the intraoperative management goals.
7. Outline the anesthetic choices for pheochromocytoma.
8. What are the special postoperative problems associated with resection of a pheochromocytoma?
9. How is a previously unsuspected and undiagnosed pheochromocytoma managed following induction of anesthesia?

1. What is a pheochromocytoma?

Preganglionic sympathetic fibers synapse in the adrenal medulla. Under normal circumstances, this neuroendocrine tissue produces approximately 80% epinephrine and 20% norepinephrine, which function as hormones instead of neurotransmitters.

Most pheochromocytomas are adrenal medullary tumors, although a small percentage appear in the spleen, ovary, bladder, and right atrium. They usually arise from chromaffin cells, although 6% arise from other neuroendocrine tissue. These tumors usually secrete more norepinephrine than epinephrine, similar to the normal tissue. Infrequently, pheochromocytomas secrete predominantly epinephrine or dopamine. They may occur independently or as part of a multiple endocrine neoplastic (MEN) syndrome (see below).

2. Describe the clinical presentation of and diagnostic criteria for pheochromocytoma.

The classic presentation of pheochromocytoma is a triad of symptoms including headache, diaphoresis, and palpitations. This triad plus the presence of hypertension are almost pathognomonic. However, fewer than 20% of patients present with these symptoms. The remainder present with only one or two signs or symptoms and require vigilance to diagnose.

Hypertension, either sustained or paroxysmal, is the most common presenting sign (90%) with pheochromocytoma, although the tumor accounts for only 0.1–0.5% of all cases of hypertension. The most common symptom is headache, secondary to hypertension. Other symptoms attributable to severe hypertension are nausea, vomiting, and slow palpitations. Hypertension may be precipitated by abdominal palpation, postural alterations, exercise, drugs, surgery, or micturition in the case of bladder tumors. Tumors producing predominantly epinephrine or dopamine are more likely to cause palpitations, diaphoresis, and, rarely, panic attacks.

Chronic exposure to elevated levels of catecholamines predisposes to cardiomyopathy. Chronic norepinephrine stimulation leads to hypertrophic changes, and chronic epinephrine and dopamine stimulation leads to high-output failure. Rarely, the tumor will present with congestive heart failure, myocardial infarction, or cerebral hemorrhage.

Diagnostic confirmation requires laboratory studies. Norepinephrine, epinephrine, and dopamine can be measured directly in serum or urine. Measurement of these catecholamines is sensitive in patients with sustained hypertension, but may give false-negative results in patients with paroxysmal symptoms. Norepinephrine and epinephrine are metabolized by catechol-O-methyltransferase to normetanephrine and metanephrine, respectively. In turn, these are both metabolized to vanillylmandelic acid (VMA), which is excreted in the urine. Dopamine, which can also be measured directly, is metabolized to homovanillic acid (HVA), which is often confused with VMA. Urinary screening of these metabolites is very sensitive but not very specific because numerous stress-related conditions may lead to their elevation. Metabolism of catecholamines to free metanephrines occurs within the tumor cells, and is independent of catecholamine release. Thus, measurement of free serum metanephrines is reliable in almost all patients. Methyldopa or monoamine oxidase inhibitors interfere with urinary VMA determinations.

CT and magnetic resonance imaging (MRI) can detect even very small lesions (0.5 cm or less in diameter) and are particularly useful in locating adrenal lesions. Tumors are extra-adrenal in 10–15% of cases, and many of these are missed on CT or MRI. Additional tests to determine the presence and location of these small tumors include metaiodobenzylguanidine (mIBG) scintigraphy, and positron emission tomography (PET) using ^{11}C-hydroxyephedrine. These will highlight active neuroendocrine tissue. In complex diagnostic cases, differential venous sampling for catecholamines may also give clues to the tumor location.

Most pharmacologic tests for diagnosing pheochromocytoma are outmoded. Administration of histamine, tyramine, or glucagon risks hypertensive crises from stimulation of the tumor. One useful and safe pharmacologic challenge is the clonidine suppression test. Clonidine administration will produce a lowering of plasma catecholamine levels in hypertensive patients without a pheochromocytoma, but have no effect in patients with the tumor.

3. Pheochromocytoma is associated with what other syndromes?

This tumor arises from neural crest cells and is considered neuroendocrine in origin. Thus, diseases of other neuroendocrine tissues or organs are associated with a higher incidence of pheochromocytoma. MEN types II and III are syndromes that include pheochromocytomas. MEN II is a triad of medullary cancer of the thyroid, parathyroid adenoma, and pheochromocytoma. MEN III includes pheochromocytoma and medullary cancer of the thyroid in addition to mucocutaneous syndromes, multiple neuromas (von Recklinghausen's disease), marfanoid habitus, and hypertrophied corneal nerves. Pheochromocytomas are also seen in association with von Hippel-Lindau syndrome, which includes cerebral and retinal angiomatosis, pancreatic and renal cysts, and epididymal cystadenoma. When caring for patients with these associated conditions, one should maintain a high degree of suspicion for the presence of a pheochromocytoma.

4. What conditions may mimic pheochromocytoma?

In situations where the blood pressure is severely or acutely elevated, the differential diagnosis should include the possibility of pheochromocytoma. Other conditions that can cause this include severe essential hypertension, preeclampsia of pregnancy, thyrotoxicosis, intracranial hypertension, withdrawal of certain antihypertensive agents, or exogenous administration of vasopressor medications resulting from a drug-swap.

5. How are patients with pheochromocytoma prepared for surgery?

Mortality associated with pheochromocytoma resection has been reduced from 20%, in reports 20 years ago, to 0–1% in recent reports. There has been a similar reduction in reported major morbidity such as myocardial infarction and stroke. This dramatic reduction probably represents

Associated Syndromes

MEN II
    Pheochromocytoma
    Medullary thyroid cancer
    Parathyroid adenoma

MEN III
    Pheochromocytoma
    Medullary thyroid cancer
    Mucocutaneous syndromes
    Multiple neuromas (von Recklinghausen's
      disease)
    Marfanoid habitus
    Hypertrophied corneal nerves

von Hippel-Lindau syndrome
    Pheochromocytoma
    Cerebral and retinal angiomatosis
    Pancreatic and renal cysts
    Epididymal cystadenoma

some publication bias, but is largely due to gradual preoperative vasodilation and intravascular volume repletion. Chronic exposure to norepinephrine produces chronic vasoconstriction and hypovolemia. Rapid attempts to vasodilate and restore intravascular volume can produce complications and may serve little purpose. If the patient is not suffering from an acute hypertensive emergency, it is best to allow for a more gradual correction of the volume status.

Outpatient administration of phenoxybenzamine, an α-adrenergic blocking agent, has been the standard preoperative therapy for pheochromocytoma. The initial dose is approximately 20 mg/day, and this is titrated gradually to control blood pressure. Common side-effects include postural hypotension and nasal stuffiness. Therapy often requires a 2-week period.

Phenoxybenzamine has two characteristics that make it less than ideal. First, it is a nonselective α-blocker, so it prevents the α_2-mediated inhibition of norepinephrine and epinephrine release. Thus, most patients need simultaneous β-adrenergic blockade. Phenoxybenzamine is also a noncompetitive inhibitor that binds covalently. This causes more frequent and more resistant postoperative hypotension than other alternative therapies. Phenoxybenzamine should be withheld for at least 12 hours before surgery.

Prazosin and doxazosin, selective α_1-adrenergic blockers, may be substituted for phenoxybenzamine. These are competitive inhibitors with shorter half-lives, and cause less postoperative hypotension. Both these drugs can be continued until the morning of surgery. Patients treated with these agents usually do not require β-blockade, unless their tumor secretes epinephrine or dopamine.

Treatment with calcium-channel blockers has been advocated in several small published series and case

Preoperative Preparation

α-Adrenergic blockade
    Phenoxybenzamine
    Nonselective α-blocker
    Noncompetitive inhibitor covalently bonded
    Side-effects: postural hypotension, nasal
      stuffiness
    β-Blockade may be needed simultaneously
    Postoperative resistant hypotension
    Hold 12 hours before surgery

    Prazosin, doxasin
    Selective α_1-adrenergic blockers
    Competitive inhibitors, shorter half-lives
    β-Blockade not usually necessary
    Continue until the morning of surgery

Calcium channel blockers
    Control hypertension
    Vasodilation
    Less fluid resuscitation needed

Angiotensin-converting enzyme
    May cause more intraoperative hypotension
      than other treatments

β-Blockers
    Esmolol, labetalol
    Should not be initiated without α-blockade
      and fluid resuscitation
    May result in paroxysmal hypertension and
      ventricular failure

Immediate control of blood pressure
    Sodium nitroprusside, nitroglycerin,
      nicardipine, phentolamine
    Hypotension treated with intravascular volume
      replacement
    Tachycardia treated with β-blockers

reports. This treatment provides control of hypertension and vasodilation, but may necessitate less fluid replacement and cause less hypotension than treatment with phenoxybenzamine. With only small studies, there is no strong evidence to recommend this over α-blockade.

Angiotensin-converting enzyme inhibitors have also been used for preoperative blood pressure control and vasodilation. There is no apparent benefit to using these agents, and they may cause more intraoperative hypotension than other treatment options.

Immediate control of systemic blood pressure may be achieved for emergency cases through intravenous administration of vasodilators with a rapid onset and short duration of action. Drugs that fit this profile include sodium nitroprusside, nitroglycerin, nicardipine, and the pure α-blocker phentolamine. Postural hypotension is treated with intravascular volume repletion. A common side-effect of most of these medications is tachycardia. The relative risk that tachycardia imposes on these patients must be considered and potentially treated with intravenous β-blocking drugs.

Presently four β-blockers are available: esmolol, propranolol, metoprolol, and labetalol. These drugs differ widely in their characteristics and duration of action. Esmolol is β1-selective and has a very short duration of action. Propranolol is intermediate in duration but nonselective. While metoprolol is β1-selective, it is perhaps too long-lasting to be useful in this condition. Labetalol is nonselective in its β-blockade and has an additional beneficial effect of mild α-blockade. β-Blockade should never be initiated before at least partial α-blockade and intravascular resuscitation. β-Blockade with unopposed α-adrenergic stimulus can produce paroxysmal hypertension and acute left ventricular failure.

6. Describe the intraoperative management goals.

After adequate preoperative peripheral vasodilatation and replacement of intravascular volume, the primary intraoperative goal is to prevent and treat sympathetic activity. Manipulations such as establishment of invasive monitoring, induction of anesthesia, endotracheal intubation, positioning, and surgical stimulus increase sympathetic outflow. Invasive arterial pressure monitoring is important due to frequent and dramatic fluctuations in blood pressure. The requirement for other invasive monitoring is based on the patient's pre-existing medical condition. Placement of invasive monitors is accomplished under heavy sedation to minimize anxiety, which predisposes patients to sympathetic activity.

Combined epidural and general techniques provide partial protection from sympathetic outflow and are advocated by some, but they have drawbacks. Epidurals can complicate fluid management and judgment of anesthetic depth. Preoperative placement of epidural catheters can cause dramatic increases in sympathetic activity, even with sedation.

Most of the large published series of pheochromocytoma management are of open adrenal resections. Laparoscopic adrenalectomy has become the surgical standard of care. Benefits of laparoscopy are a shorter postoperative course and less postoperative pain compared with open procedures. However, recent studies show this minimally invasive technique is no more hemodynamically stable than open surgery. Pneumoperitoneum with carbon dioxide (CO_2) is a potent sympathetic stimulus, and causes an exaggerated response in patients with pheochromocytoma. Manipulation of the tumor in laparoscopy causes as much release of catecholamines from the tumor as in open surgery. Management of these stimuli is similar to the management in open procedures, with short-acting vasodilation and β-blockade.

Vancomycin and histamine releasers, such as curare, atracurium, and morphine, are best avoided. Episodes of hypotension often result in severe rebound hypertension from sympathetic compensation. Similarly, droperidol, an α-adrenergic blocker, must be used with caution. Succinylcholine fasciculations might cause catecholamine release from a pheochromocytoma through mechanical effects. Sympathomimetics, such as ephedrine, and vagolytics, such as atropine, also predispose to tachycardia and hypertension.

Tumor manipulation frequently results in catecholamine release causing hypertension and tachycardia. This reaction should be anticipated and treated. A short-acting agent such as phentolamine or sodium nitroprusside, with or without β-blockade, is a good choice.

Following ligation of the tumor's venous drainage, the emphasis switches from protecting against hypertension to treating hypotension. The patient is catecholamine-depleted because the contralateral adrenal has been chronically suppressed by the pheochromocytoma. The sudden absence of endogenous catecholamines and the general sympathetic depression caused by anesthesia result in passive vasodilatation with the potential for hypotension. Persistent chemical sympathectomy from regional techniques can exacerbate hypotensive episodes. Hypotension is treated with reduction of anesthetic depth, intravascular volume infusion, and peripheral vasoconstriction with norepinephrine or phenylephrine. Hypotension improves upon emergence from anesthesia, when sympathetic tone returns.

7. Outline the anesthetic choices for pheochromocytoma.

Because this disease is rare, few data are available from controlled studies as to the benefit of one anesthetic over another. From numerous case reports and retrospective reviews one can reach several conclusions. One is that there is little difference in the choice of anesthesia for this condition with respect to outcome or incidence of intraoperative complications. What matters far more is the previously discussed preoperative vasodilation and intravascular volume expansion. Epidural anesthesia has not been shown to be more effective than general anesthesia in reducing hemodynamic complications or the requirements for vasoactive medications.

All the potent inhalation agents available today have been used safely with this condition. Halothane appears to be the least acceptable, mostly because of its negative inotropic properties and potentiation of catecholamine-induced ventricular dysrhythmias. Both enflurane and isoflurane have been used extensively with little documented advantage of one agent over the other. The use of the newer inhalation agents, sevoflurane and desflurane, has been described in case reports.

Narcotic anesthesia may have some specific theoretical advantages over inhalation anesthesia, including few or no negative inotropic effects and reduced dysrhythmogenic potential. Droperidol releases catecholamines from the adrenal medulla and should be avoided. It is probably more important for the anesthesiologist to choose a technique that he or she is most comfortable with and that is suitable for resection of an intra-abdominal tumor than to try to achieve minor theoretical advantages from unfamiliar drugs.

The choice of neuromuscular blocking agent varies widely. Succinylcholine has been used safely with this condition, but fasciculations may cause a release of catecholamines from the tumor. Some nondepolarizing muscle relaxants, especially curare and atracurium, may cause the release of histamine, which in turn may cause a release of catecholamines and subsequent hypertension. These drugs should be avoided when possible. Pancuronium, with its vagolytic side-effects, may cause tachycardia, which may be confusing. Vecuronium, rocuronium, and cisatracurium are logical choices for muscle relaxation.

8. What are the special postoperative problems associated with resection of a pheochromocytoma?

The most common problem seen in the postoperative period is mild hypotension. Significant hypotension usually does not last beyond emergence from anesthesia. As discussed previously, hypotension is treated initially with fluid therapy and only occasionally requires an inotrope or vasopressor infusion. Hypertension in the post-tumor resection period suggests the presence of residual or additional tumor. In this case, α- and β-adrenergic blockade are continued. Sodium nitroprusside is added as required. Hypoglycemia may occur in the postoperative period and may be due to sudden withdrawal of catecholamines and possibly to the metabolic effects of β-blockers.

9. How is a previously unsuspected and undiagnosed pheochromocytoma managed following induction of anesthesia?

If severe acute hypertension occurs immediately after the administration of one of the so-called trigger drugs or with manipulation of a particular tumor or tissue, the anesthesiologist should maintain a strong suspicion of a pheochromocytoma. If severe sudden hypertension occurs before skin incision, the patient may be best served by canceling the operation and initiating immediate therapy. Later, the appropriate diagnostic tests may be pursued. When intraoperative hypertension occurs from a previously unsuspected pheochromocytoma, it must be treated as discussed previously, avoiding β-blockers as a primary mode of treatment. The patient's urine should be saved to help in later diagnosis of the disease.

Patients with undiagnosed pheochromocytoma may also present with profound hypotension after induction of anesthesia. This hypotension is due to chronic intravascular depletion and is treated with fluids. Catecholamines administered for treatment may confuse the issue, and should be minimized when there is a suspicion of pheochromocytoma.

SUGGESTED READINGS

Bittar DA: Innovar-induced hypertensive crises in patients with pheochromocytoma. Anesthesiology 50:366–369, 1979

Feldman JM: Diagnosis and management of pheochromocytoma. Hosp Pract 24:175–179,182,187–189, 1989

Loris JL, Hamoir EE, Hartstein GM, et al.: Hemodynamic changes and catecholamine release during laparoscopic adrenalectomy for pheochromocytoma. Anesth Analg 88:16–21, 1999

Prys-Roberts C: Phaeochromocytoma: recent progress in its management. Br J Anesth 85:44–57, 2000

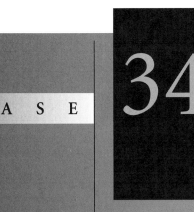

C A S E 34

FULL STOMACH

Laurence M. Hausman, MD

A 37-year-old, 65-kg woman with a small bowel obstruction presents to the operating room for an exploratory laparotomy, lysis of adhesions and possible bowel resection. Her past medical history is unremarkable. Her past surgical history is significant for a cholecystectomy 3 years ago under general anesthesia, and a cesarean section 1 year ago under spinal anesthesia. Both procedures were without complication. She has a nasogastric tube in place, which is draining approximately 25 cc/hr of bilious fluid. She was on no medications upon admission. Vital signs are a heart rate of 97 beats per minute, blood pressure of 130/65 mmHg and a respiratory rate of 12 breaths per minute. The hematocrit is 39%.

QUESTIONS

1. What are the mechanisms a conscious person has to prevent regurgitation and pulmonary aspiration?
2. What are the risk factors for regurgitation and pulmonary aspiration during general anesthesia?
3. When can aspiration occur during the perioperative period?
4. What are the problems associated with pulmonary aspiration?
5. If aspiration occurs, what are the usual course, treatment and prognosis?
6. How should the nasogastric tube (NGT) be managed during induction?

7. What pharmacologic interventions can be made to decrease the risk of aspiration?
8. What is the reason for applying cricoid pressure during a rapid sequence induction, and what are some of the problems associated with it?
9. What is the effect of commonly used pharmacologic agents during anesthesia on lower esophageal sphincter tone?
10. What would be an acceptable anesthetic plan for this patient?

1. What are the mechanisms a conscious patient has to prevent regurgitation and pulmonary aspiration?

The lower esophageal sphincter (LES) is the primary barrier to gastro-esophageal reflux. The LES is 2–5 cm long, and moves upward with inspiration and downward with expiration. Upon swallowing, the esophagus undergoes peristaltic contractions to allow the passage of food and the LES relaxes. This sphincter traverses the diaphragm and has a resting pressure greater than gastric pressure. The difference in these pressures (LES pressure minus gastric pressure) is known as "barrier pressure." In normal subjects, an increase in abdominal pressure will trigger an increase in LES pressure, thus maintaining barrier pressure. Reflux occurs when the barrier pressure decreases, either when the LES pressure decreases or the gastric pressure increases.

The angle at which the esophagus meets the stomach also protects against reflux. If the angle is oblique, high gastric pressures are required to cause reflux. If, however,

Mechanisms for Protection of Reflux and Aspiration in the Awake Patient

Lower esophageal sphincter tone

Gastro-esophageal angle

Diaphragmatic crura

Upper esophageal sphincter

Airway reflexes
Cough
Expiration reflex
Laryngospasm and apnea
Spasmodic panting

TABLE 34.1	Conditions Associated with Regurgitation and Pulmonary Aspiration

Obesity
Depressed level of consciousness
History of gastritis/ulcer
Bowel obstruction
Pregnancy – greater than 12 weeks gestation
Pain/stress
Emergency surgery
ASA IV-V
Esophageal disorders/previous esophageal surgery
Recent meal
Diabetes mellitus
Ileus
Trauma
Concurrent opioid administration
Symptomatic hiatal hernia
Male gender?

the angle is small (as often occurs in patients with morbid obesity or a gravid uterus), reflux may occur at lower gastric pressures.

The upper esophageal sphincter is another mechanism to protect against regurgitation. Virtually all commonly used general anesthetics including muscle relaxants cause relaxation of this sphincter.

Another protective mechanism is the diaphragmatic crura that tighten the lower esophagus to prevent reflux.

Finally, there are intrinsic airway reflexes used to protect the airway against aspiration in the event of regurgitation. These include coughing (a period of brief inspiration followed by a forceful expiration), the expiration reflex (expiration without inspiration), laryngospasm and apnea (with closure of both the false cords and the true cords) and spasmodic panting (rapid shallow breathing).

2. What are the risk factors for regurgitation and pulmonary aspiration under general anesthesia?

General anesthesia is associated with the loss of protective upper airway reflexes. Therefore, a patient who regurgitates under a general anesthetic is at risk for aspirating the regurgitant. Any condition associated with an increase in intragastric volume and intragastric pressure may result in regurgitation and pulmonary aspiration (Table 34.1)

3. When can aspiration occur during the perioperative period?

Aspiration can occur at any time during the perioperative period. Specifically it can occur before induction, during induction before laryngoscopy, during mask ventilation, during laryngoscopy, during extubation, or after tracheal extubation.

4. What are the problems associated with aspiration?

Aspiration during general anesthesia is very rare with estimates ranging from 1:4,000 to 1:9,000. However, when it does occur it is a serious problem. Aspiration of large gastric particles can completely obstruct the airway anywhere along the tracheo-bronchial tree making ventilation difficult or impossible. Furthermore, a chemical pneumonitis resulting from aspiration of gastric contents, known as Mendelson's syndrome, can occur. This syndrome may occur if the gastric aspirate has a pH <2.5 and a volume >0.4 ml/kg or 25 cc in the adult.

5. If aspiration occurs, what are the usual course, treatment and prognosis?

If aspiration occurs, treatment is symptomatic. The oral pharynx should be suctioned at the time of the aspiration. If the patient is supine, the head should be turned to the side to facilitate suctioning. The patient should also be placed in the Trendelenburg position to allow pooling of the regurgitant in the oropharynx, thereby lessening the volume aspirated. Irrigation of the airway is *not* advised since it may cause spreading of the aspirate and a more profound pulmonary destruction. Bronchoscopy may be needed to remove large particulate matter. Supplemental oxygen should be administered. Mechanical ventilation is

Signs of Clinically Significant Pulmonary Aspiration

Bronchospasm

Decreased SpO_2 >10% on room air

A-a gradient >300 mmHg

CXR – atelectasis or infiltrate

often necessary. β_2 inhalers may be helpful for treatment of bronchospasm. The routine use of steroids has *not* been shown to be beneficial. Antibiotics should only be started after evidence of infection by positive culture.

If a clinically significant aspiration has occurred, signs usually occur within 2 hours of the event. Signs include bronchospasm, a drop in oxygen saturation of greater than 10% from baseline on room air, an alveolar-arterial (A-a) gradient of >300 mmHg on 100% O_2, and a chest radiograph usually revealing atelectasis or an infiltrate (most commonly a right lower lobe infiltrate). Intrapulmonary damage can progress to interstitial and alveolar edema, with hyaline membrane formation and destruction of lung tissue. Adult respiratory distress syndrome (ARDS) often occurs in patients requiring more than 24 hours of mechanical ventilation. The prognosis in patients with pulmonary aspiration is usually good if there is good health preoperatively. A poor outcome has been associated with the presence of significant comorbid conditions.

6. How should the nasogastric tube (NGT) be managed during induction?

There are different thoughts regarding the management of the NGT during the induction of general anesthesia. The NGT should be suctioned prior to induction. There are those who, after this initial suctioning of the NGT, would remove it. This is based on the theory that there is a decrease in both lower and upper esophageal sphincter tone with an NGT in situ. In addition, it is felt that the NGT will interfere with esophageal compression from the cricoid pressure applied during a rapid sequence induction. These concerns have not been proven. Alternatively, some recommend leaving the NGT in place. This will allow for the continuous drainage of gastric fluid and air thus decreasing the increase in gastric pressure associated with induction. Still others suggest withdrawing the NGT to the mid-esophageal level (approximately

30 cm from the nares) to decrease esophageal pressure during induction and thereby decreasing the risk of esophageal rupture.

7. What pharmacologic interventions can be made to decrease the risk of aspiration?

Pharmacologic agents may be administered to decrease gastric volume (either by decreasing production or by increasing emptying), increase gastric pH, or increase LES tone.

- Metoclopramide, a derivative of procainamide, facilitates gastric emptying by causing gastric peristalsis and relaxation at the pylorus. Metoclopramide also increases LES tone. It should be avoided in cases of bowel obstruction. Because it is a dopaminergic antagonist, it should be avoided in patients with Parkinson's disease or depression. It can also cause extrapyramidal side-effects. The positive effects of this drug are inhibited by narcotics, which delay gastric emptying.
- Cimetidine or ranitidine are competitive H_2-blockers that will decrease basal gastric acid secretions that occur in response to gastrin and food, thereby increasing gastric pH. They should be administered 30–60 minutes prior to induction of general anesthesia.
- Sodium citrate is a *non*-particulate antacid that will increase gastric pH. A non-particulate formulation is important since aspiration of the particulate alkalis may also produce a chemical pneumonitis. One drawback of this antacid is that it must be taken orally, thereby increasing gastric volume. It should be administered within 30 minutes of the induction of general anesthesia.
- Omeprazole, rabeprazole, and lansoprazole are proton pump inhibitors that block H^+-K^+-adenosine triphosphatase activity at the secretory surface of the parietal cells in the stomach. These drugs decrease the volume and increase the pH of gastric secretions.
- Glycopyrrolate, an anticholinergic, will increase gastric pH by inhibiting vagally mediated gastric acid production. Atropine, however, is ineffective.

8. What is the reason for applying cricoid pressure during a rapid sequence induction, and what are some of the problems associated with it?

The cricoid cartilage is the only complete cartilaginous circular ring in the trachea. As a result, posterior/rostral pressure applied to it will occlude the upper esophagus against the cervical vertebrae in an effort to prevent regurgitation of gastric contents into the oropharynx. Interestingly, cricoid pressure has been shown to decrease LES tone and may actually promote reflux. However, if gastro-esophageal reflux should occur while cricoid pressure is being held, regurgitation into the pharynx should

Pharmacologic Agents for Aspiration Prophylaxis

Metoclopramide	Increases gastric emptying
H$_2$-blockers Cimetidine Ranitidine	Increase gastric pH
Sodium citrate	Increases gastric pH Increases gastric volume
Proton pump inhibitors Omeprazole Rabeprazole Lansoprazole	Increase gastric pH Decrease gastric volume
Glycopyrrolate	Increases gastric pH

TABLE 34.2   Effect on LES of Commonly Used Pharmacologic Agents

Increase LES and *increase* barrier pressure
  α-Adrenergic agonists
  Anti-emetics
  Cholinergics
  Edrophonium
  Histamines
  Metoclopramide
  Metoprolol
  Neostigmine
  Pancuronium
  Succinylcholine
Decrease LES and *decrease* barrier pressure
  Atropine
  β-Adrenergic agonists
  Dopamine
  Glycopyrrolate
  Inhalation agents
  Nitroglycerine
  Opioids
  Sodium nitroprusside
  Thiopental
No effect on LES
  Atracurium
  Cimetidine
  Propranolol
  Ranitidine
  Vecuronium

be prevented. In the case of a difficult intubation, cricoid pressure can make ventilation more difficult.

Cricoid pressure is poorly tolerated in the awake patient and can cause the patient to retch. This retching can increase intra-esophageal pressure and result in an esophageal rupture. In the starved supine patient the maximum intragastric pressure is 25 mmHg. Increasing gastric volume by 750 ml can increase the intragastric pressure to 35 mmHg. Regurgitation is associated with 40 mmHg of intragastric pressure and can be prevented by 30 newtons (N) of force on the cricoid. Older studies recommend 40 N of force. However, this much force is poorly tolerated, often distorts the laryngeal anatomy making intubation difficult, and may predispose the patient to an esophageal rupture. One solution is to provide 20 N of force to the awake patient. This relatively small amount of force will give some protection against regurgitation; however, if intra-esophageal pressure gets too high, regurgitation *will* occur but esophageal rupture *will not*. When the patient loses consciousness, the force on the cartilage should be increased to 30 N until the trachea is successfully intubated.

9. What is the effect of commonly used pharmacological agents during anesthesia on lower esophageal sphincter tone?

Table 34.2 lists the commonly used pharmacological agents and their effect on LES tone. Propofol will lower both esophageal and gastric pressure and, therefore, have no effect on barrier pressure.

10. What would be an acceptable anesthetic plan for this patient?

Choice of induction of general anesthesia in a patient with a full stomach is dependent upon several factors, among which is the patient's airway evaluation. The airway evaluation should always include a thorough history of the patient's prior intubations, making certain to elicit any history of difficult intubations. If the patient has an acceptable airway, pharmacologic prophylaxis should be administered and preoxygenation/denitrogenation is followed by a rapid sequence induction with cricoid pressure. At the time of induction, there should be an assistant present to provide the cricoid pressure. Suction should be immediately available in case of regurgitation. The induction agent selected should have a rapid predictable onset time. Commonly used agents are thiopental, propofol, etomidate and ketamine. The muscle relaxant used should also have a fast onset. Classically, the neuromuscular blocking agent used for rapid sequence inductions has been succinylcholine. If, however, succinylcholine is contraindicated for any reason, a fast-onset intermediate-acting neuromuscular blocking agent, such as rocuronium, can be used. When choosing these drugs, the dose must be increased. The disadvantage of using a nondepolarizing neuromuscular blocking agent is that its prolonged action may necessitate prolonged mask ventilation if intubation is unsuccessful.

If intubation is unsuccessful, help from an anesthesia colleague should be called for. Mask ventilation is initiated with cricoid pressure. The peak airway pressures should be kept <20 cm H_2O to limit ventilation of the stomach. Ventilation should be continued until the patient awakens. Further muscle relaxant should not be given. If mask ventilation is difficult, ventilation through an LMA is indicated. Intubation through a correctly seated LMA is possible. It is important to remember that both mask ventilation and LMA placement can be impeded by cricoid pressure.

If a difficult intubation is anticipated, either by history or physical examination, a rapid sequence induction is contraindicated. In this case, the most prudent approach would be to do an awake fiberoptic intubation. This poses some unique challenges in the patient with a full stomach. For an awake fiberoptic intubation to be successful, the patient's airway needs to be well topicalized with local anesthetic above and below the vocal cords. However, anesthetizing the entire airway, especially below the vocal cords, will cause a profound loss of all airway reflexes and may increase the risk of aspiration. There are those practitioners who believe that the awake, unsedated patient will know if they are about to vomit and can be encouraged to cough and turn their head to the side. These practitioners will proceed with topicalization of the entire airway. There are others who will only topicalize the airway above the vocal cords in an effort to preserve the tracheal reflexes in the event aspiration occurs. Therefore, topicalization of the airway *is* recommended for the patient with a full stomach, but the use of a transtracheal block is user dependent.

An inhalation induction by mask should not be done on a patient with a full stomach, except in specific circumstances such as a child with epiglottitis.

After the trachea has been intubated with a cuffed endotracheal tube, the anesthetic can be maintained in a number of ways including air/O_2, inhalation agent, opioid, and muscle relaxant. Although a cuffed tube will provide more protection than an uncuffed tube, aspiration may still occur around the cuff.

During extubation of the trachea, aspiration may also occur. It is thus imperative that the patient is able to protect their airway before the trachea is extubated. Therefore, the patient should be fully awake, responsive, and spontaneously breathing.

SUGGESTED READINGS

Cotton BR, Smith G: The lower oesophageal sphincter and anaesthesia. Br J Anaesth 56:37–46, 1984

Morgan M: Control of intragastric pH and volume. Br J Anaesth 56:47–55, 1984

Ng A, Smith G: Gastroesophageal reflux and aspiration of gastric contents in anesthetic practice. Anesth Analg 93:494–513, 2001

Nishina K, Mikawa K, Takao Y, Shiga M, Maekawa N, Obara H: A comparison of rabeprazole, lansoprazole, and ranitidine for improving preoperative gastric fluid property in adults undergoing elective surgery. Anesth Analg 90:717–721, 2000

Olsson GL, Hallen B, Hambraeus-Jonzon K: Aspiration during anaesthesia: a computer-aided study of 185, 358 anaesthetics. Acta Anaesthesiol Scand 30:84–92, 1986

Skinner HJ, Bedford NM, Girling KJ, Mahajan RP: Effect of cricoid pressure on gastro-oesophageal reflux in awake subjects. Anaesthesia 54:798–808, 1999

Vanner RG, Pryle BJ: Regurgitation and oesophageal rupture with cricoid pressure: a cadaver study. Anaesthesia 47:732–735, 1992

Warner MA, Warner ME, Weber JG: Clinical significance of pulmonary aspiration during the perioperative period. Anesthesiology 78:56–62, 1993

Dennis E. Feierman PhD, MD
George V. Gabrielson MD

A 65-year-old woman presented for open reduction internal fixation (ORIF) of a hip fracture, sustained during an accidental fall. Past medical history was significant for hepatitis C cirrhosis and heavy alcohol use. Cirrhosis developed after a blood transfusion received during gynecologic surgery approximately 15 years previously. She denied extrahepatic problems from liver disease such as variceal bleeding or encephalopathy. On physical examination, she weighed 55 kg and stood 152 cm tall. She was nonicteric and had minimal ascites. Selected laboratory examinations included a hematocrit of 34% after intravenous hydration, normal transaminase levels, and an albumin level of 3.2 g/dL. Her prothrombin time (PT) was 16 seconds over a control of 14 seconds, and platelet count was 90,000/mm^3.

QUESTIONS

1. Describe the basic hepatic functions that are of immediate concern to anesthesiologists.
2. Explain the liver's detoxifying and first-pass metabolic functions.
3. Describe common extrahepatic problems associated with chronic liver failure.
4. What should a preoperative evaluation of this patient include?
5. What effects do surgery and anesthesia have on normal liver function?
6. What are the concerns associated with viral hepatitis?
7. Describe acetaminophen- and halothane-associated hepatitis.
8. Is nitrous oxide, enflurane, or isoflurane hepatotoxic?
9. List the causes of postoperative hepatic dysfunction.
10. Are some anesthetic techniques free of hepatotoxic effects?
11. What coagulation problems are anticipated and how are they managed?
12. In the future, might liver transplantation become a viable option for this patient? What intraoperative anesthetic problems occur during liver transplantation?

1. Describe the basic hepatic functions that are of immediate concern to anesthesiologists.

Because of the myriad of liver functions that may be affected, no single laboratory test effectively measures the overall state of liver function. An understanding of hepatic functions and coexisting physiologic problems associated with liver failure will illuminate where the anesthetic concerns are and which preoperative test should be performed. In any given patient with hepatic disease, their ability to carry out normal hepatic functions will be characterized by the extent of liver failure. It is auspicious that the liver has an enormous reserve capacity. In experimental animal models, as well as in normal humans, the removal of greater than 80% of hepatic parenchyma is still compatible with normal liver function. Cirrhosis is characterized as scarring within the liver by fibrosis and the conversion of normal architecture into structurally abnormal modules throughout the liver. This abnormal architecture leads to obstruction of flow within the portal system and portal hypertension with all its clinical ramifications. The ultimate consequence of progressive liver diseases is hepatic failure and loss of liver function. Hepatic functions can be broken down into three main categories: endocrine, synthetic (anabolic), and metabolic (catabolic and detoxifying) functions.

Endocrine Functions

The liver has several endocrine functions and is a major target organ for glucose homeostasis. The liver produces somatomedin (insulin-like growth factor-1), a growth stimulator; thrombopoietin, which stimulates bone marrow to produce platelets; and angiotensinogen, which is closely involved in fluid and electrolyte balance.

Decreased production of angiotensinogen can have profound effects on the kidneys and fluid and electrolyte balance. Extravasation of fluid from the intravascular volume results in relative intravascular depletion. The kidney responds by producing increased amounts of renin. Two physiologic ramifications of increased renin production are constriction of the renal afferent arteries and fluid retention. Renin also converts angiotensinogen into angiotensin I. Angiotensin I diminishes renin production by the kidneys. Without production of angiotensinogen, the negative feedback that inhibits renin production is eliminated, and production of renin and its physiologic ramifications go unconstrained. This cycle can cause massive fluid retention, electrolyte abnormalities, and may play a role in the development of hepatorenal syndrome in end-stage liver disease (ESLD).

The liver plays a role in calcium homeostasis. It is responsible for the hydroxylation of vitamin D. Additionally, the liver is responsible for the homeostasis of other hormones. Thyroxine and triiodothyronine are deiodinated by the liver. Steroid hormones, such as testosterone, estradiol, glucocorticoids, and aldosterone, are first metabolized (inactivated) and conjugated in the liver and then excreted in the urine. In liver disease, normal estrogen and testosterone metabolism is prevented because of shunting to the systemic circulation, which results in gynecomastia.

Furthermore, the liver is a target organ for insulin and glucagon. These two hormones are involved in the metabolism and storage of carbohydrates. Glycogen is formed from glucose, under the influence of insulin, in a process called glycogenesis. Glycogen is broken down to glucose by glucagon in a process called glycogenolysis.

In this way, glucose becomes available for muscle and brain metabolism.

Anabolic Functions

The liver has numerous clinically important synthetic functions. It is involved in hemostasis by virtue of its anabolic functions. In addition to producing coagulation factors, the liver also synthesizes many anticoagulants, such as antithrombin III, α_1-antitrypsin, protein C and S, plasminogen, α_2-antiplasmin, and plasminogen activator inhibitor. Severe liver disease can lead to reduced synthesis of factors I (fibrinogen), II (prothrombin), V, VII, IX, X, XI, XII, XIII, prekallikrein, and high molecular weight kininogen. High molecular weight kininogen and factors II, VII, IX, and X are vitamin-K-dependent clotting factors. Vitamin K is a cofactor of an enzyme that catalyzes the γ-carboxylation of selected glutamyl residues in clotting factor precursors. When coagulopathies result from impaired hepatocellular function, exogenous vitamin K is unlikely to correct or improve the problem. Vitamin K-dependent clotting proteins have a substantially shorter serum half-life than albumin; therefore, coagulopathy can precede the development of other signs of liver failure, e.g., hypoalbuminemia. In cirrhosis, coagulopathy may be further aggravated by thrombocytopenia resulting from either decreased synthesis of thrombopoietin and/or from hypersplenism. Since the liver produces non-vitamin K-dependent clotting factors, severe liver disease may lead to decreased plasma concentrations of factor I (fibrinogen), V, XI, XII, and XIII. Initially, a damaged liver may actually produce increased amounts of fibrinogen; therefore, it is unusual for fibrinogen to be reduced significantly, unless there is an associated disseminated intravascular coagulation.

Several other clinically important proteins are made by the liver. They include acute phase reactants (C-reactive proteins, haptoglobin, ceruloplasmin, and transferrin), pseudocholinesterase, angiotensinogen (discussed above), α-acid glycoprotein, and albumin. The last two are the main drug-binding moieties. Derangements in albumin synthesis have several important clinical ramifications. It is the principal binding and transport protein for numerous substances, including some hormones, fatty acids, trace metals, bilirubin, and drugs. Many of the intravenous drugs employed by anesthesiologists are highly protein-bound. Low serum concentrations of plasma proteins, especially albumin, produce an increase in unbound drug concentrations and potentially exaggerate drug responses. This enhanced response may be seen with serum albumin concentrations of 2.5 g/dL or less. Additionally, decreased serum concentrations will lead to reduced oncotic pressure in the plasma, which may result in edema and ascites. When this is coupled with portal hypertension, there may be increased hepatic lymph production with extravasation into the peritoneal cavity. In a patient with ascites, the degree and ramifications of hypoalbuminemia may be accentuated by further loss of albumin in ascitic fluid.

Other important anabolic functions of the liver include production of saturated fatty acids, cholesterol, and bile salts, maintenance of glycogen storage (glucose storage), and production of ketones, i.e., β-hydroxybutyrate, which is the main energy source used by the brain during starvation. Decreased synthesis of bile salts can lead to malabsorption of fat and fat-soluble vitamins (vitamin K). Alterations in cholesterol production (and related substances) may lead to significant changes in the composition and morphology of erythrocytes. The presence of erythrocytes with spur and burr cell forms are usually an ominous sign of significantly advanced liver disease.

Abnormalities of glucose maintenance are common in cirrhosis. As stated above, carbohydrate metabolism and glucose production are important liver functions. Hypoglycemia, which is more commonly associated with acute fulminant hepatic failure, may occur with ESLD. Cirrhotic patients are at risk for perioperative hypoglycemia due to decreased hepatic glycogen stores (decreased capacity secondary to decreased liver mass or decreased intrinsic ability to synthesize glycogen), diminished response to glucagon, or compromised nutritional status. Additionally, these patients may have elevated serum lactate levels, reflecting the decreased capacity of the liver to utilize lactate for gluconeogenesis via the Cori cycle (Figure 35.1).

Catabolic Functions

The liver is responsible not only for elimination and metabolism of toxins and other xenobiotics absorbed by the gastrointestinal tract, but also for metabolism of drugs and alcohol.

The liver is the central organ responsible for biochemical intermediate metabolism. It shuffles many endogenous biological intermediate compounds into various pathways that lead to either the creation of new compounds or the complete metabolism of the intermediate ones. A perfect example of intermediate metabolism is the citrate pathway (Figure 35.2). Citrate is used as an anticoagulant in banked

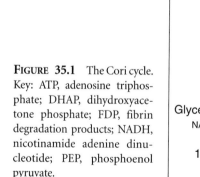

FIGURE 35.1 The Cori cycle. Key: ATP, adenosine triphosphate; DHAP, dihydroxyacetone phosphate; FDP, fibrin degradation products; NADH, nicotinamide adenine dinucleotide; PEP, phosphoenol pyruvate.

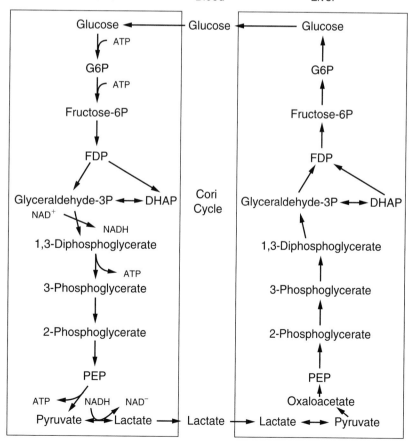

CITRATE INTERMEDIATE METABOLISM

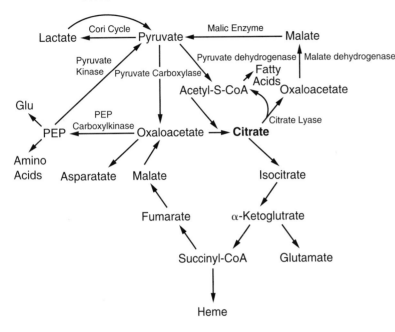

FIGURE 35.2   Citrate intermediate metabolism.

blood products. Citrate works as an anticoagulant via chelation of calcium, thereby blocking its availability for the coagulation cascade. Exogenously administered citrate, such as that from fresh frozen plasma or other blood products, is mainly metabolized by the liver. Citrate toxicity can occur when blood products are transfused at a rapid rate, or when the liver is unable to metabolize citrate appropriately. Toxicity results from chelation of ionized calcium by citrate. As citrate accumulates, ionized calcium levels decrease, resulting in a coagulopathy and myocardial depression leading to hypotension.

Carbohydrate and other biological intermediate metabolism is a vital function of the liver. The liver metabolizes glucose, fructose, lactate, citrate, acetate, and other biological intermediates. As function declines, the liver loses its ability to orchestrate intermediate metabolism. Frequently, cirrhotics may develop insulin resistance and consequently hyperglycemia and glucose intolerance. The hyperinsulinemia associated with ESLD suggests a decrease in the liver's intrinsic ability to handle a glucose load secondary to a decrease in hepatocellular function and/or mass. Lactic acid is produced peripherally but is metabolized in the liver. Elevated serum lactate levels may reflect the decreased capacity of the liver to utilize lactate and may result in metabolic acidosis (Figure 35.1).

The liver is responsible for amino acid degradation (and production of glucose), fatty acid metabolism (β-oxidation), and the production of ketones during prolonged fasting. The toxic byproduct of amino acid degradation is ammonia (NH_4^+). Disposal of ammonia via the production of urea is an important liver function.

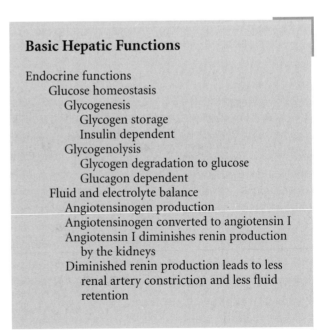

Basic Hepatic Functions

Endocrine functions
   Glucose homeostasis
      Glycogenesis
         Glycogen storage
         Insulin dependent
      Glycogenolysis
         Glycogen degradation to glucose
         Glucagon dependent
Fluid and electrolyte balance
   Angiotensinogen production
   Angiotensinogen converted to angiotensin I
   Angiotensin I diminishes renin production
     by the kidneys
   Diminished renin production leads to less
     renal artery constriction and less fluid
     retention

Continued

Basic Hepatic Functions—cont'd

Platelet production
    Thrombopoietin production
Calcium metabolism
    Hydroxylation of vitamin D
Thyroid homeostasis
    Thyroxine and triiodothyronine are
        deiodinated by the liver
Steroid hormone inactivation
    Testosterone
    Estradiol
    Glucocorticoids
    Aldosterone
Growth stimulation
    Somatomedin production
    Insulin-like growth factor-1

Synthetic (anabolic) functions
    Hemostasis
        Vitamin K-dependent factors synthesis
            II (prothrombin), VII, IX, and X
        Other factors synthesis
            I (fibrinogen), V, XI, XII, XIII
    Drug metabolism
        Pseudocholinesterase production
    Plasma protein production
        Albumin/α-acid glycoprotein
            Drug transport/binding
            Oncotic pressure changes
    Fatty acid metabolism
        β-Hydroxybutyrate production for brain
            metabolism during starvation
        Bile salt synthesis for vitamin K
            absorption

Metabolic (catabolic and detoxifying) functions
    Drug metabolism/detoxification
    Citrate metabolism
        Prevents calcium-mediated coagulopathies
        Prevents calcium-mediated myocardial
            depression
    Lactate detoxification
        Prevents lactic acidosis from muscle
            metabolism
    Ammonia detoxification
        Amino acids are degraded to ammonia
        Ammonia is transformed to urea

2. Explain the liver's detoxifying and first-pass, metabolic functions.

Other liver catabolic functions include the degradation of hemoglobin, production and elimination of bilirubin, clearance of fibrin split products and activated coagulation factors, and elimination of potential xenobiotics (alcohol/drugs) and toxins (e.g., endotoxin) absorbed from the gastrointestinal tract. While one of the main functions of the gastrointestinal tract is to absorb nutrients, it can also absorb toxins and other foreign material including drugs and other xenobiotics. Venous drainage from the gastrointestinal tract is channeled to the portal system which empties into the liver. With the exception of absorption that occurs in the mouth and in the distal part of the rectum, everything that is absorbed by the gastrointestinal tract must pass through the liver. The liver plays an active role in detoxifying foreign materials absorbed via the gastrointestinal tract. It is also responsible for first-pass metabolism of orally administered drugs. The bioavailability of a drug is the fraction of a given dose that reaches the general circulation. There are several factors than can influence bioavailability. One of the most important of these is first-pass metabolism. The cytochrome P450 (CYP) system found in the liver plays a significant role in first-pass metabolism and bioavailability of many drugs. However, when portal inflow into the liver is impeded, as seen in cirrhosis, collateral connections may constitute an important alternative route that bypasses the liver, thereby decreasing first-pass metabolism and increasing the bioavailability of drugs as well as increasing the risk of exposure to toxins.

CYPs are hemoprotein isoforms that are responsible for biotransformation of numerous endogenous and exogenous compounds. Isoforms that held the interest of many investigators are CYP2E1 and CYP3A. These isoforms are induced by ethanol. CYP2E1 is important in the metabolism of ethanol, toxins and potent inhaled anesthetics. In humans, the CYP3A family is the most abundant isoform and is involved in metabolizing numerous drugs, such as cyclosporine, midazolam, alfentanil, and lidocaine. Other drugs or substrates, such as phenobarbital and glucocorticoids, can also induce the CYP3A isoform. Since ethanol can induce CYP2E1 and CYP3A, its role in the metabolism, interaction, and toxicity of drugs that are regularly used by anesthesiologists and other physicians, and the impact of enzyme induction on these roles, are of immense interest. Management of patients with chronic and/or acute alcohol intake can be extremely challenging. Acute intoxication is analogous to partly anesthetizing a patient. However, the induction of CYP may cause drugs to be metabolized at an accelerated rate. A third consideration is that CYP induction may be offset by alcohol inhibiting drug metabolism by acting as a competitive substrate. Furthermore, the metabolic effects of CYP induction may be outweighed by alcohol-induced hepatic dysfunction. The great clinical importance of the interactions of drugs used in anesthesia (or any other area of medicine) with ethanol at the CYP level is further accentuated by the fact that 1 in 10–20 people consume ethanol on a daily basis.

The liver is a major site for the biotransformation of drugs and environmental toxins. Lipophilic compounds are transformed into hydrophilic compounds by a series of reactions. The ultimate goal of this process is excretion in either the bile or the urine. Phase 1 reactions, oxidation, reduction, dehalogenation, hydrolysis, etc., are mostly catalyzed by cytochrome P450. Products of phase I reactions can be inactive (transformation of fentanyl to norfentanyl) or active (transformation of diazepam to temazepam and oxazepam). Occasionally, phase I reactions will transform a compound into toxins (transformation of halothane to trifluoroacetyl (TFA) halide intermediate or of acetaminophen to N-acetyl-p-benzoquinone). Phase II biotransformations occur in the cytosol. They are conjugation reactions in which a covalent link between either the parent drug or metabolite (after a phase I transformation) and glucuronic acid, sulfate, glutathione, amino acids, or acetate is formed.

Pharmacokinetics can be altered by changes in absorption, first-pass metabolism, distribution, and elimination. In patients with liver disease, some or all of these kinetic mechanisms can be changed. In order to fully understand how liver disease affects pharmacokinetic parameters, one must understand the interactions of drug metabolism and how the liver extracts drugs from blood.

Drugs may be classified according to their liver extraction. The extraction ratio is defined as: $E = (C_a - C_v)/C_a$, where C_a is defined as the concentration in the hepatic artery and C_v is the concentration in the hepatic vein. High-extraction drugs usually have extraction ratios greater than 70%, whereas low-extraction drugs usually have extraction ratios that are less than 30%. Classification of drugs according to their extraction ratio is useful. Drugs with high extraction ratios are highly dependent on liver blood flow. Their clearance is independent of plasma protein binding and independent of liver metabolism. Induction or inhibition of P450 usually will not change clearance; however, extremely high inhibition will markedly decrease clearance of high (and low) extraction drugs by the liver. Scarring and abnormal architecture associated with cirrhosis leads to hepatic blood flow obstruction. Obstruction of portal flow produces shunting away from the liver. Portal blood accounts for approximately 70% of liver blood flow. Therefore, this will have a major effect on clearance of high-extraction drugs and first-pass metabolism. The clearance of low-extraction drugs is independent of liver blood flow. The amount of drug delivered to the liver under normal blood flow far exceeds the liver's intrinsic capacity to metabolize it. Low-extraction drugs are dependent on the intrinsic ability of the liver to metabolize the drug; therefore, induction or inhibition of cytochrome P450 usually will have a parallel change in clearance. Furthermore, low-extraction drugs are usually dependent on binding to plasma proteins. Drugs that are highly bound will have increased clearance in disease states that decreased the binding proteins and the fraction of bound drug, e.g., albumin. The liver is a major organ of the reticuloendothelial system (RES) and accounts for 85% of RES activity. The RES is a functional rather than an anatomic system that serves as an important bodily defense mechanism. In the liver, Kupffer cells, highly phagocytic macrophages that line the sinuses of the liver, take up large foreign particles and act as a first-line defense against bacteria absorbed from the gastrointestinal tract. Therefore, portal flow obstruction can lead to the shunting of toxins and bacteria absorbed by the gastrointestinal system directly into the systemic circulation.

3. Describe common extrahepatic problems associated with chronic liver failure.

A large number of extrahepatic problems are associated with ESLD, which may vary widely in severity and outcome.

Neurologic Problems

Changes in mental status are common but can be caused by a multitude of etiologies. Because there are pulmonary problems that are associated with ESLD, one should immediately rule out hypoxia or hypercardia as a cause for a change in mental status. Another life-threatening but easily correctable etiology is hypoglycemia. Hepatic encephalopathy is common but not necessarily terminal. It readily responds to neomycin and lactulose therapy. Cerebral edema, although rare, is often a preterminal event that is associated with acute fulminant liver failure and must be treated aggressively. Treatment consists of controlled mechanical hyperventilation and administration of osmotic diuretics. Encephalopathic patients are at increased risk for regurgitation and aspiration of gastric contents. The clinician should have a very low threshold for elective endotracheal intubation to protect the airway. Other causes of changes in mental status include acidosis, sepsis, and increased side-effects of drugs secondary to increased drug levels due to changes in pharmacokinetics. Additionally, one should always be on the lookout for ingestion of alcohol and/or drugs by the patient.

Pulmonary Problems

Numerous pulmonary problems can occur in patients with progressive liver disease. As mentioned previously, patients with mental status changes are at risk for aspiration. Chronic cirrhotics frequently hyperventilate due to accumulation of ammonia or acidosis. Nevertheless, PaO_2 values of 60–70 mmHg are common in these patients. The diaphragmatic compression by massive ascites accounts for many of the pulmonary problems encountered. This effectively reduces functional residual capacity (FRC) and predisposes to atelectasis and hypoxia. In addition, complex changes in the pulmonary arterial bed can occur. Two clinically important and distinct pulmonary syndromes occur: hepatopulmonary syndrome and portopulmonary hypertension.

Hepatopulmonary Syndrome   Arterial hypoxemia associate with ESLD can be multifactorial. However, severe hypoxemia is likely secondary to hepatopulmonary syndrome. Capillary dilatation causes a diffusion defect (a decrease in pulmonary diffusion capacity). Additionally, right-to-left intrapulmonary shunts may develop, leading to a noncorrectable arterial hypoxemia. The shunts may be either secondary to atelectasis, alveoli that are filled with fluid and/or exudate, or direct arteriovenous channels.

Portopulmonary Hypertension   Pulmonary hypertension is not uncommon in advance liver disease. This can be a result of possible cardiac manifestations of (alcohol) cirrhosis, the hyperdynamic circulation that results in high pulmonary flows, or vasoconstriction, medial hypertrophy and intimal fibrosis leading to potentially irreversible pulmonary hypertension. The latter, when associated with portal hypertension, is known as portopulmonary hypertension and is considered indistinguishable from primary pulmonary hypertension. It should be noted that severe arterial hypoxemia is usually not associated with portopulmonary hypertension.

Cardiac Problems

Cardiac disease may be difficult to diagnose in these patients because of the debilitating nature of the liver disease. Alcohol cirrhotics can develop a cardiomyopathy, which can lead to congestive heart failure. However, ESLD results in massive peripheral vasodilation with a reduced systemic vascular resistance (SVR). This effectively lowers left ventricular work and allows for cardiac disease to exist without immediate symptoms. A heightened suspicion for the presence of cardiac impairment is warranted.

Patients with ESLD usually have a hyperdynamic circulation that is characterized by a high cardiac output and low SVR. The primary sites for the reduction in SVR are the splanchnic circulation and arteriovenous shunts, which are coupled with a decrease in the viscosity of blood secondary to anemia and the vasodilating effects of glucagon, vasoactive intestinal peptides (VIP), substance P, and prostaglandins. The combination of vasodilation and the formation of new arteriovenous channels results in an increase in the intravenous compartment. Fluid retention eventually increases the plasma volume; however, the larger increase in the intravascular compartment with respect to the increase in plasma volume results in a relative intravascular depletion.

Renal Problems

A host of abnormalities in renal function, ranging from mild renal insufficiency and electrolyte imbalances to hepatorenal syndrome, are common. Hepatorenal syndrome usually occurs in the setting of severe liver disease without any obvious renal etiology. Cirrhosis can be associated with a decrease in the glomerular filtration rate (GFR) and renal blood flow (RBF) progressing to acute oliguria. Frequent problems resulting from aggressive treatment of ascites are prerenal azotemia and hyponatremia. Because these patients usually have relative intravascular depletion, treatment is directed at intravascular volume replacement. Aggressive administration of salt-containing solutions is unwarranted unless required to maintain intravascular volume. Rapid correction of hyponatremia is dangerous and may result in central pontine myelinolysis and significant neurologic injury.

The pathogenesis of hepatorenal syndrome is incompletely understood. There is strong evidence to support the theory that the relative intravascular volume depletion is a major determinant of the initial renal hypoperfusion. Hormonal mechanisms have also been implicated. The kidney responds to intravascular depletion by increasing renin production, which causes constriction of the renal afferent arteries and fluid retention. Furthermore, production of renin goes unconstrained due to the decrease in the negative feedback from angiotensin I. In fact, patients with cirrhosis and impaired renal functions manifest the most profound elevations of renin. The physiologic ramifications of this cycle are massive fluid retention, electrolyte abnormalities, and a possible role in the development of hepatorenal syndrome in ESLD.

Hematologic Problems

Other common extrahepatic problems in ESLD include a complex coagulopathy, which is in part due to decreased synthesis of clotting factors. Decreased production of platelets (decreased thrombopoietin), platelet sequestration by the spleen, and disseminated intravascular coagulation (DIC) adversely complicate coagulation problems.

Metabolic Problems

Metabolic acidosis (metabolic alkalosis can be seen early in the disease process), whether due to renal dysfunction or the liver's inability to handle lactic acid and compounds, is commonly seen in ESLD.

Extrahepatic Problems Associated With Liver Disease

Neurologic
  Hepatic encephalopathy
  Cerebral edema

Pulmonary
  Hypoxia
    Aspiration pneumonia
    Restrictive lung disease
      Reduced functional residual capacity as
        diaphragm is pushed cephalad
  Hepatopulmonary syndrome
    Capillary dilatation
    Pulmonary edema
    Pulmonary shunting
  Portopulmonary hypertension
    Pulmonary hypertension and portal
      hypertension

Cardiac
  Peripheral vasodilatation and reduced systemic
    vascular resistance
  High cardiac output

Renal
  Diuretic commonly used
  Chronic renal insufficiency
  Acute renal failure (hepatorenal
    syndrome)
  Electrolyte abnormalities

Coagulopathies
  Decreased production of clotting factors
  Decreased thrombopoietin leading to
    thrombocytopenia
  Platelet sequestration in spleen
  Disseminated intravascular coagulation

Metabolic acidosis
  Decreased capacity to degrade lactate
  Renal failure

4. What should a preoperative evaluation of this patient include?

Preoperative evaluation of patients with liver disease focuses on symptoms of liver dysfunction. Examples are easy bruising, bleeding problems, mental status changes, and dyspnea on exertion or at rest. Portal hypertension predisposes to upper gastrointestinal bleeding from esophageal varices. Additionally, portal flow obstruction can lead to the shunting of toxins and bacteria absorbed by the gastrointestinal system directly into the systemic circulation, putting these patients at increased risk for infection and sepsis.

In evaluating the patient with a history of liver disease, it is extremely important to note the degree of liver damage and remaining function. Although no specific single test can determine liver function, selected preoperative tests can give significant insight into the degree of liver function remaining.

Albumin is synthesized in the liver and has a long (20 days) half-life. Its serum levels are a result of balancing losses against production. Factors responsible for increased loss of albumin include massive ascites from various causes and renal disease. Decreased production can result from poor nutritional status and decreased hepatic synthesis. Thus, albumin levels may indicate the degree of hepatic dysfunction more in chronic liver disease than in fulminant hepatic failure.

A good laboratory indicator of liver function in both acute and chronic liver disease is the prothrombin time (PT). It is a measure of factors I, II, V, VII, and X. These factors are produced by the liver and require several intermediate steps, which is a reflection of the liver's synthetic function. Not only is the PT a good test of liver function, it is also a good prognosticator of outcome following surgery in patients with liver disease. It should be noted that vitamin K deficiency, disseminated intravascular coagulation, fibrinolysis, and coumadin administration all prolong PT independently of liver disease.

Transaminases are enzymes that help transfer amino groups from amino acids to ketoacids. In the setting of liver cell injury, transaminases leak into the plasma increasing blood levels. They serve as indicators of liver damage; however, they have significant limitations as determinants of liver function. In advanced chronic liver disease, transaminase levels may actually be normal or low. This is secondary to massive loss of liver parenchymal tissue. Although they have little prognostic value, transaminase levels are commonly followed throughout the perioperative course.

Just as risk of cardiac injury has been studied in noncardiac surgery, the risk of nonhepatic surgery in patients with significant liver disease has also been well studied. The Child's classification stratifies mortality risk of portosystemic shunting in patients with mild, moderate, or severe liver disease. Mortality ranged from 5% to 50%, depending on the severity of the disease. This classification has been modified, the Child-Turcotte-Pugh (CTP) score (Table 35.1), which now includes the PT and other variables. Patients with scores ≥7 are qualified to be listed for liver transplant, whereas those with a score ≥10 are considered to have significant liver disease.

TABLE 35.1	Child-Turcotte-Pugh Scoring System to Assess the Severity of Liver Disease		
	1 point	2 points	3 points
Encephalopathy	None	1–2	3–4
Ascites	Absent	Minimal (or controlled by diuretics)	*At least moderate despite diuretic treatment*
Bilirubin (mg/dL)	<2	2–3	>3
Albumin (g/dL)	>3.5	2.8–3.5	<2.8
Prothrombin time (seconds prolonged)	<4	4–6	>6
or international normalized ratio (INR)	<1.7	1.7–2.3	>2.3
For primary biliary cirrhosis, primary sclerosing cholangitis, or other cholestatic liver diseases:			
Bilirubin (mg/dL)[a]	<4	4–10	>10

Modified from the UNOS web site http://www.unos.org

[a]For cholestatic liver diseases, (e.g., primary biliary cirrhosis, primary sclerosing cholangitis) these values for bilirubin are to be substituted for the values above.

Other useful preoperative tests would include a hematocrit, platelet count, glucose, electrolyte profile, and a blood urea nitrogen (BUN) and creatinine. An electrocardiogram (ECG) is recommended because of the associated cardiac problems in these patients. A detailed physical examination of the airway, neck, heart, and lungs should be performed.

Recently, a new system was established to improve evaluation and allocation of donor livers for patients with ESLD: the *m*odel for *e*nd-stage *l*iver *d*isease (MELD). A MELD score is obtained based on objective and verifiable medical data that evaluates the patient's risk of dying while waiting for a liver transplant. This numerical scale is currently used for liver allocation. Further information can be obtained from the UNOS (www.unos.org/resources).

5. What effects do surgery and anesthesia have on normal liver function?

Anesthesia and surgery affect the liver independently. The liver benefits from a dual blood supply. Most of its perfusion comes from the portal vein, which has little autoregulatory ability. The hepatic artery, however, has significant autoregulatory properties. Changes in blood flow to the liver are of major significance and will be considered in detail. Venous return from the splanchnic organs is via the portal vein. The portal vein delivers about 70% of the total hepatic blood flow, whereas the hepatic artery delivers the remaining 30% of hepatic blood flow. Although the portal vein delivers approximately 70% of the total hepatic blood flow, it only provides 50% of the delivered oxygen since it is venous blood returning from the splanchnic organs. Hepatic arterial blood flow is autoregulated; furthermore, decreases in portal flow can be partially compensated by increases in hepatic arterial blood flow. This increase in arterial flow is an attempt to maintain hepatic oxygen delivery.

Splanchnic circulatory disturbances are induced by surgical interventions. During laparotomy, surgical manipulation and placement of pads in the abdomen reduce hepatic blood flow. Upper abdominal surgery may limit hepatic blood flow by as much as 40%. Other common perioperative factors that limit hepatic perfusion are intermittent positive pressure ventilation (IPPV), α-adrenergic agonists, and hypocapnia. Laparoscopy or surgery in the prone position impairs hepatic blood flow as well.

Anesthetics have multiple effects on the liver, which can be divided into two main categories: blood flow and cellular metabolism. Extensive animal studies have shown that volatile anesthetics can produce marked reductions in total hepatic blood flow. It appears that volatile anesthetic agents have a direct dilatory effect on splanchnic vasculature and thereby reduce portal blood flow. This reduction is further accentuated by decreased cardiac output secondary to potent inhaled anesthetic agents. For example, halothane when administered to dogs at 2 minimum alveolar concentration (MAC) produced a 53% reduction in total hepatic blood flow, while isoflurane at the same MAC produced only a 22% reduction in hepatic blood flow. Compensation by enhanced hepatic artery flow is only partial. It appears that isoflurane is more effective at preserving hepatic blood flow than halothane. In humans, volatile anesthetics produce dose-dependent reductions in systemic and portal blood pressure, as well as flow. However, there is little proof that halothane has a more detrimental effect than isoflurane on liver blood flow in humans. Spinal and epidural anesthesia will produce reductions in hepatic blood flow commensurate with the degree of sympathetic blockade and decrease in blood pressure. These changes can be prevented by intravenous ephedrine.

6. What are the concerns associated with viral hepatitis?

Hepatitis is an inflammatory process of the liver. The major causes of hepatitis in this country are viral, alcoholic, and drug-induced. Its natural history is highly variable and depends on numerous factors including age, coexisting liver disease, alcohol consumption, and obesity. The progression of viral hepatitis to cirrhosis and ultimately to ESLD has been a tremendous burden to society.

Anesthesiologists are commonly called on to care for these individuals either in advance consultation or as part of scheduled anesthetics. Two major concerns are associated with viral hepatitis. The first is the risk to the patient and the second is the risk to all health care personnel. Viral hepatitis is a significant source of occupational illness that frequently leads to a carrier state.

Hepatitis A is the most common hepatic viral infection, accounting for approximately 40% of all cases of hepatitis in the United States. It is usually transmitted by fecal-oral routes and is commonly acquired by consumption of contaminated seafood. Its incubation period is approximately 15–45 days and generally produces a mild illness. It is commonly subclinical and very rarely causes hepatic failure via massive liver necrosis. The disease is usually benign, acute, self-limited and, unlike hepatitis B, does not lead to chronicity or a carrier state. Recovery is usually complete at 1–2 months. Diagnosis may be aided by the detection of hepatitis A antigen (HAsAg) during the acute phase or of the immunoglobulin G (IgG) or M (IgM) antibodies later.

Hepatitis B causes much more morbidity and mortality, is variable in presentation, and requires a complex serologic diagnosis. Fortunately, its incidence is decreasing with improved detection and vaccination of individuals perceived to be at risk. In New York State, hepatitis B vaccination is mandatory for all children. The incubation period of hepatitis B ranges from 45 days to 6 months. Initially, the disease presents with nonspecific symptoms such as malaise, nausea, vomiting, anorexia, and headaches. Upper quadrant pain and hepatic enlargement may be present. The symptoms may subside or progress to an icteric phase characterized by jaundice, pruritus, hepatomegaly, or other gastrointestinal symptoms. This phase may develop into fulminant hepatic failure or a convalescent period. Full recovery from hepatitis B occurs in 90% of patients within 3 months. Approximately 10% of individuals remain in a carrier state, develop chronic hepatitis (either active or persistent), manifest cirrhosis, or present with hepatocellular carcinoma.

Hepatitis B persisting for more than 6 months following an attack of acute viral hepatitis is considered to have become chronic. Chronic persistent hepatitis differs from chronic active hepatitis in that it has an excellent prognosis for eventual recovery. Transaminase levels may fluctuate but eventually return to normal. Biopsy results show inflammation without fibrosis. On the other hand, chronic active hepatitis carries a poor prognosis, varies widely in presentation, and often leads to cirrhosis, hepatocellular carcinoma, and death.

The majority of non-A, non-B viral hepatitis is now known to be caused by hepatitis C. The clinical spectrum of hepatitis C spans the entire gamut from asymptomatic to acute fulminant disease. Compared with hepatitis B, the early hepatitis caused by the hepatitis C viruses is mild, but it has a much higher propensity (approximately 40%) for transition to chronicity. The most common presentation of hepatitis C is a mild increase in transaminase levels on routine blood screening.

7. Describe acetaminophen- and halothane-associated hepatitis.

Acetaminophen Toxicity

Radical and reactive intermediates have been implicated in the hepatotoxicity of ethanol, acetaminophen (APAP), and halogenated hydrocarbons. Both radicals and reactive intermediates may result in the interruption of cell function. Toxicity secondary to radical/reactive intermediates is complex and is probably the result of multiple intracellular interactions. One mechanism whereby a drug can become deleterious is via metabolic activation to a toxic metabolite. For example, APAP can cause liver damage. Glucuronidation and sulfation are the major pathways used by the liver to metabolize APAP. APAP is also metabolized by CYP to a reactive intermediate N-acetyl-p-benzoquinone imine (NAPQI) of which CYP1A2, 2E1 and 3A4 have the highest activity. Under normal conditions, e.g., an adult ingesting 650–1000 mg of APAP, only trace amounts of NAPQI are produced. However, under different conditions, e.g., a suicide attempt with ingestion of 6,500–10,000 mg (12–20 Extra Strength Tylenol®), or enhanced enzyme activity, e.g., chronic alcohol consumption, the production of NAPQI is greatly increased and hepatotoxicity can be produced even with a therapeutic dose. The effects of chronic ethanol consumption on APAP toxicity can be complex. In the presence of ethanol, APAP-mediated hepatotoxicity is actually decreased. Ethanol acts as a competitive inhibitor of CYP. The toxic intermediate, NAPQI, is usually neutralized by intracellular glutathione (GSH). Nonetheless, under these extreme conditions intracellular GSH is rapidly depleted and NAPQI can then react with other intracellular constituents to cause cell damage. NAPQI has been shown to initiate lipid peroxidation, to damage DNA, as well as to alter cell proteins. In the event that the patient's GSH is not replenished by treatment with N-acetylcysteine (a precursor of GSH), the end result can be severe liver necrosis that results in the need for liver transplantation, or even death. Accidental overdose and hepatotoxicity remain major clinical problems.

Halothane Toxicity

Halothane is a potent inhaled anesthetic that is in common clinical use worldwide. Its use has declined over recent years for several reasons. Other than the fact that less toxic agents are available today, it is also known that halothane can cause hepatotoxicity. Nonetheless, its use outside the United States is common and its toxicity remains a concern.

There are two main theories as to how halothane causes hepatotoxicity. The first suggests that halothane toxicity is related to CYP's ability to metabolize halothane via two pathways, an oxidative pathway and a reductive pathway. There are three major CYPs involved in the metabolism of potent inhaled anesthetics: CYP2E1, CYP3A4, and CYP2A6. It appears that halothane and other inhalational anesthetics are largely metabolized by the ethanol-inducible CYP, CYP2E1. CYP3A4, the most abundant isoform found in the liver (and responsible for the metabolism of many drugs), is one of the main isoforms responsible for the reductive metabolism of halothane in human microsomes. CYP2A6 can metabolize halothane via both the reductive and the oxidative pathway. Under normoxic conditions halothane is mostly metabolized via the oxidative pathway. Under conditions of low oxygen tension (e.g., decreased hepatic blood flow, hypoxemia), metabolism is via a reductive pathway that produces a halothane radical. This radical can either react with a number of intracellular molecules or abstract a hydrogen to form 2-chloro-1,1,1-trifluoroethane (CTE) or undergo further reduction to form 2-chloro-1,1-difluoroethane (CDE). This radical probably causes toxicity in the same way that acetaminophen causes toxicity. Under conditions of oxidative stress and/or hypoxia, ATP and NADPH stores may be limited, which can result in a decrease in intracellular GSH. The relationship of GSH to halothane toxicity is dependent on the model being studied. In cultured rat hepatocytes, GSH status is not associated with halothane toxicity. In the guinea pig model, depletion of GSH increased protein-adduct formation and potentiated halothane toxicity that could be diminished by replenishing the GSH. The combination of decreased intracellular GSH with cellular stress secondary to increased halothane radicals can lead to cellular dysfunction and/or cell death, which may ultimately lead to liver necrosis.

The second theory of halothane toxicity is the immune theory. Severe halothane hepatotoxicity usually occurs following a second exposure. Pohl and others (1988) have shown that exposure to halothane can lead to production of trifluoroacetyl chloride, a compound that is capable of reacting with several intracellular proteins and forming trifluoroacetyl (TFA) adducts. These adducts are expressed on the cell surface and are capable of inducing the production of antibodies to these altered cell proteins. The antibody-antigen complex is capable of initiating immune reactions that can result in cell death. Indeed, patients who exhibit halothane toxicity have TFA adducts expressed in their liver, as well as antibodies to these adducts in their serum.

The latter theory has been postulated for the rare, fulminant, and often fatal immune-mediated hepatotoxicity. The former theory addresses the common nonfatal hepatotoxicity secondary to locally produced reactive intermediates. Regardless of whether halothane is metabolized via a reductive or an oxidative pathway, the result is reactive intermediates that could disrupt cell function.

8. Is nitrous oxide, enflurane, or isoflurane hepatotoxic?

Nitrous oxide has largely escaped implications as being hepatotoxic. However, the incidence of hepatic injury following halothane exposure is 1:35,000 for primary exposure and increases to 1:3,700 for patients with repeated exposures. Hepatic injury following enflurane exposure has a strikingly lower incidence approaching 1:800,000. These rare cases of hepatic injury following enflurane administration can present with histologic patterns similar to hypoxic injury in laboratory studies. There have been reports of fatal hepatitis after exposure to enflurane where anti-TFA antibodies have been found in the patient's sera. Examples of possible cross-sensitization reactions between halothane and enflurane, isoflurane, or desflurane have been reported. Isoflurane presents an even lower incidence of posthepatic necrosis. The reason for this is probably related to its much lower level of metabolism.

9. List the causes of postoperative hepatic dysfunction.

Numerous etiologies of hepatic dysfunction occur postoperatively. It is important to establish the cause quickly and to initiate therapy as soon as possible. Three major concerns are bilirubin overload, hepatocellular injury, and cholestasis. A common cause of postoperative jaundice is a relative overproduction of bilirubin from hemoglobin. This commonly results from blood transfusion reactions, hematoma resorption, and hemolysis. Old and damaged stored erythrocytes will break down and release hemoglobin. The liver easily handles small increases in bilirubin; however, if there is significant pre-existing hepatic disease or large amounts of blood are transfused, significant increases in unconjugated and conjugated bilirubin may result even with mild liver impairment secondary to anesthesia. Similarly, hematoma resorption may also contribute to postoperative jaundice in a patient who has significantly bled into a limb, e.g., hip or femur fractures. Significant hemolysis from blood transfusion reactions can also result in jaundice. An increase in unconjugated bilirubin without increases in conjugated bilirubin suggests the presence of Gilbert syndrome, which is present in 7–10% of otherwise normal patients.

Persistent jaundice following surgery of the hepatobiliary tree is usually an indication of retained common bile duct stones. Trauma to the bile duct during surgery may result in spasm and/or stenosis. High-dose fentanyl can, on rare occasions, result in sphincter spasm.

The most common abnormalities found on liver function tests performed postoperatively suggest that parenchymal liver cell damage is not a dominant feature. The mild degree of liver dysfunction probably reflects a nonspecific perioperative change in hepatic blood flow. Transient hepatic oxygen deprivation is common and usually resolves without specific treatment. Some authorities believe that the minor transient alterations in liver function tests are in fact manifestations of mild hepatotoxicity of a potent inhaled agent. Indeed, following exposure to halogenate anesthetics, transient elevations in liver transaminase levels are common. There are many reports of minor alterations in liver function tests even when intravenous anesthetic techniques are used, and probably reflect the nonspecific perioperative changes in hepatic blood flow. It should be noted that a "shock liver" syndrome secondary to prolonged marked hypotension can occur.

In some patients postoperative liver dysfunction is the result of having pre-existing liver disease that only becomes evident after surgery. The manifestations of overt disease, which both the patient and the clinician may have been unaware of preoperatively, may be precipitated by the detrimental effects of decreased hepatic blood flow on liver function. Additionally, patients may be in a latent phase of an illness and postoperative liver dysfunction may be the result of the natural progression of the pre-existing liver disease.

10. Are some anesthetic techniques free of hepatotoxic effects?

The most important factors in preserving hepatic function are probably maintenance of hepatic blood flow and oxygenation.

When applicable and not contraindicated, spinal anesthetics have been suggested as alternatives to general anesthesia; however, even conduction anesthesia risks hepatic injury. Spinal anesthesia can reduce hepatic blood flow by as much as 30%. Although spinal anesthesia is not noted to cause massive hepatic necrosis, it may lead to transient elevations in liver transaminase levels. Careful delivery of anesthetic agents is as important as the actual choice of agents or technique. Except for halothane, halogenated anesthetics can be employed. Other factors affect hepatic blood flow, and are important to consider as well. Excessive intrathoracic pressures may impede venous return and decrease hepatic blood supply. IPPV with positive end expiratory pressure (PEEP) will similarly affect hepatic blood supply and should be avoided if possible. Hyperventilation and hypocapnia increase hepatic arterial resistance and reduce blood flow to the liver, whereas hypercapnia will increase blood flow. Severe hypoxemia also decreases hepatic artery blood flow.

Concomitantly administered nonanesthetic drugs may affect blood supply to liver, and these should be considered. β-Blockers reduce hepatic blood supply and are often used in treatment of portal hypertension. α-Adrenergic agonists also reduce blood flow through the hepatic artery. Cimetidine, an H_2-receptor blocker, not only inhibits hepatic clearance of other drugs, but also reduces hepatic blood flow. A reasonable anesthetic plan for this patient would include maintenance of near preanesthetic blood pressure (which must be considered with the risk of additional bleeding), the avoidance of hyperventilation and hypoxemia, and the avoidance of drugs that are associated with hepatotoxicity (e.g., halothane or acetaminophen).

11. What coagulation problems are anticipated and how are they managed?

ORIF of the hip has potential for significant blood loss, even in patients with normal liver function. Prolongation of the PT by even as little as 2 seconds over control is a significant elevation in this patient. Her elevated PT coupled with a decreased platelet count suggests the possibility of hemostatic problems. To avoid massive blood loss and potential associated morbidity, optimization of coagulation is required, and prior consultation with a hematologist, although not required, is reasonable.

This patient's prolonged PT is probably related to her liver disease and diminished liver function. Administration of vitamin K several hours before surgery may be partially effective, if at all. Her hemostatic defect may respond to transfusion of fresh frozen plasma. Fresh frozen plasma contains significant amounts of soluble coagulation factors. Fibrinogen deficiency may be corrected with cryoprecipitate, which contains fibrinogen, fibronectin, von Willebrand's factor and factor VIII. Factor VIII deficiencies are usually not a problem in liver disease unless the patient has hemophilia or is in DIC.

Patients with severe preoperative thrombocytopenia may benefit from prophylactic platelet transfusion. Typical thresholds for such prophylaxis are set at platelet counts between 50,000 and 80,000/mm³. If nonsurgical bleeding develops in the setting of massive transfusion, a dilutional thrombocytopenia can be expected to have developed and the appropriate laboratory test should be ordered to confirm the diagnosis. Patients with a dilutional thrombocytopenia can be expected to stop bleeding after an appropriate platelet transfusion.

Platelets, fresh frozen plasma, and cryoprecipitate carry the risk of disease transmission and must be used appropriately. Furthermore, fresh frozen plasma contains significant quantities of citrate and may cause citrate toxicity in patients with significant liver disease. Therefore, because of the associated risk inherent in the use of blood products, in this particular case there are those who might refrain from transfusing blood products until nonsurgical intraoperative bleeding occurs.

12. In the future, might liver transplantation become a viable option for this patient? what intraoperative anesthetic problems occur during liver transplantation?

Liver transplantation is viewed as a viable treatment option for patients with ESLD. Although this patient does not presently have ESLD, she may well do in a few years or even less. Liver transplantation is no longer experimental. With the advance of excellent immunosuppressive drugs, overall graft survival rates now exceed 80%. Life expectancy and quality are greatly improved in recipients of liver transplants.

Numerous anesthetic problems should be anticipated in conjunction with liver transplantation. The spectrum of patients presenting for transplantation is wide, ranging from the seemingly healthy to those with acute fulminant hepatic failure. The myriad and complex medical problems accompanying liver disease, as discussed above, require treatment prior to and during transplantation. However, once a liver becomes available, postponing surgery to correct medical conditions prolongs graft ischemic time and increases the risk of graft failure.

Transfusion requirements of this operation vary widely, and usually require additional personnel for the management of transfused blood products. The median number of packed red blood cell (PRBC) units transfused varies between 10 and 20 per transplant. The average value is higher because some patients had extremely large transfusion requirements (>150 units PRBC). Coagulation abnormalities seen during this operation are numerous and complex. Preoperatively, patients usually are deficient in both coagulation factors and platelets. Development of intraoperative dilutional coagulopathies exacerbates this problem. During the anhepatic phase, citrate toxicity is commonly seen and must be promptly treated. Additionally, fibrinolysis begins and peaks immediately on reperfusion of the donor graft. Severe hemodynamic changes usually occur on reperfusion and, if prolonged, are called the reperfusion syndrome. With prompt recognition and treatment, hematologic and hemodynamic changes are generally remediable.

SUGGESTED READINGS

Coalson DN: Chapter 22. In Collins VJ (ed): Physiologic and Pharmacologic Bases of Anesthesia. Williams and Wilkins, Philadelphia, 1996

Firestone L, et al.: Chapter 55. In Miller RD (ed): Anesthesia, 5th edition. Churchill Livingstone, Philadelphia, 2000

Hudson, RJ: Chapter 11. In Barash PG, Cullen BF, Stoelting RK (eds): Clinical Anesthesia, 4th edition. JB Lippincott, Philadelphia, 2001

Martin JL, et al.: Hepatotoxicity after desflurane anesthesia. Anesthesiology 83:1125, 1995

Maze M, Bass, N: Chapter 54. In Miller RD (ed): Anesthesia, 5th edition. Churchill Livingstone, Philadelphia, 2000

Neuberger J, Kenna JG: Halothane hepatitis: a model of immune mediated drug hepatotoxicity. Clin Sci 72:263, 1987

Pohl, LR, et al.: The immunologic and metabolic basis of drug hypersensitivities. Annu Rev Pharmacol Toxicol 28:367, 1988

Stoelting RK, Dierdorf SF: Chapter 18. In Anesthesia and Coexisting Disease, 4th edition. Churchill Livingstone, Philadelphia, 2002

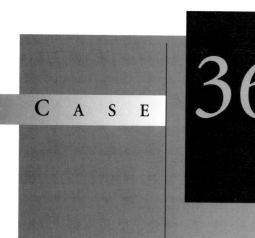

ABDOMINAL AORTIC
ANEURYSM

Ronald A. Kahn, MD

A 71-year-old man with a history of hypertension, stable angina, hypercholesterolemia, and smoking presents with a 6 cm infrarenal aortic aneurysm for conventional aortic repair.

QUESTIONS

1. What is the natural history of untreated abdominal aortic aneurysm (AAA)?
2. Outline the preoperative evaluation of the patient with an AAA.
3. Which anesthetic techniques are appropriate for AAA surgery?
4. Which monitoring devices are recommended for AAA surgery?
5. Explain the hemodynamic consequences of aortic cross-clamping.
6. Describe the options for postoperative analgesia.

1. What is the natural history of untreated abdominal aortic aneurysm (AAA)?

The natural history of all aneurysms is to expand in size. The tendency to rupture is primarily dependent on wall stress, which increases as the aneurysm enlarges, according to Laplace's law:

$$\text{Tension} = \text{Pressure} \times \text{Radius}/2 \times \text{Wall Thickness}$$

The average growth rate of aortic aneurysms is 0.4 cm per year. A follow-up study of high-risk patients reported an overall rupture rate of 3% and a surgical mortality (elective surgery for aneurysm size >6 cm or with symptoms) of 4.9%. Thirty-four percent of mortalities were due to causes unrelated to the aneurysm. The 5-year survival for untreated AAA >6 cm was less than 10%, while the 5-year survival for untreated AAA <6 cm was 50%. Elevated diastolic blood pressure, aneurysm anteroposterior diameter >5 cm, and obstructive pulmonary disease were independent predictors of rupture. Predicted 5-year rupture rates varied from 2% when these risk factors were absent to 100% when all three risk factors were present.

2. Outline the preoperative evaluation of the patient with an AAA.

Patients presenting for aortic surgery almost always have coexisting medical conditions that can significantly affect anesthetic management. These include diseases of the cardiovascular, pulmonary, renal, and central nervous systems. The goal of preoperative evaluation is to detect coexisting diseases, assess the risk of adverse outcomes, optimize the patient's medical status, and devise an anesthetic technique that minimizes complications. It is not always possible to obtain a complete preoperative evaluation when surgery is required on an urgent basis, thus preoperative optimization of medical problems is not always feasible.

It is imperative to evaluate the patient's myocardial reserves prior to aortic surgery. Risk factors for myocardial ischemia include previous myocardial infarction, angina, congestive heart failure, male gender, smoking, hypercholesterolemia, diabetes mellitus, and limited exercise tolerance. Patients at low risk for myocardial ischemia may proceed to surgery without further evaluation; however, this represents a very small group of patients. Additionally, those who have had a negative stress test within 2 years of surgery or who have had coronary artery bypass surgery within 5 years of surgery without postoperative symptoms most likely do not require further investigation for myocardial ischemia. While stress testing is probably most appropriate for patients with moderate risk, coronary angiography is recommended for patients at high risk for myocardial ischemia.

There are two components to stress testing: the "stressing" of the myocardium and the detection of myocardial ischemia or infarction. The "stressing" can be performed by either mechanical means (such as exercise via treadmill or hand-crank) or pharmacologic means. The pharmacologic stress may involve drugs such as dobutamine that increase myocardial oxygen demand or drugs that cause "myocardial steal" such as dipyridamole. Detection of myocardial ischemia may be performed by electrocardiogram (ECG), nuclear studies, or echocardiography. Ischemic myocardium is characterized by a lack of uptake of nuclear tracers with stressing and uptake of nuclear tracers with rest; this is known as a reversible defect. Fixed defects, i.e., no uptake during stressing or rest, is consistent with old infarction. Echocardiography reveals ischemic myocardium as significant changes in wall motion during stressing. In each of these studies it is important to determine whether there is myocardium at risk, i.e., myocardium that may become ischemic with stress, as opposed to myocardium that is infarcted. If patients have significant areas of myocardium at risk, further optimization (either pharmacologic or interventional) is warranted prior to surgery.

3. Which anesthetic techniques are appropriate for AAA surgery?

All antihypertensive and anti-anginal medications should be continued until the time of surgery. Preoperative sedation should be based on the patient's clinical condition and concurrent medical diseases. Some form of anxiolysis should be administered, as hypertension and tachycardia may increase the risk of aneurysm leakage or rupture, or induce myocardial ischemia in patients with concurrent coronary artery disease. Patients presenting for aortic surgery may be very unstable hemodynamically due to ongoing hemorrhage, myocardial ischemia, and/or congestive heart failure. Organ malperfusion is also a major problem. It is, therefore, recommended that patients who present for emergency aortic surgery are intensely monitored in order to control blood pressure and resuscitate appropriately.

In patients with aortic disease, the paramount goal is the maintenance of hemodynamic stability, while providing amnesia, analgesia, and immobility. As the aorta remains at risk of rupture or extension of the dissection, blood pressure must be strictly controlled. β-Adrenergic blockade and vasodilators are the mainstays for minimizing the driving force and the ejection velocity of blood, while maintaining adequate perfusion pressure. At the other end of the spectrum are patients who present in hypovolemic shock due to leaking or rupture of the aorta. In this situation, maintaining volume status, securing the airway, and immediate surgical control are the main goals.

All patients presenting for emergency aortic surgery are considered to have a full stomach, while elective cases must be considered individually. Avoidance of hemodynamic aberrations during induction and tracheal intubation is desirable. Any number of anesthetic agents can accomplish these goals and the choice is a personal decision that is dependent on the clinical situation. High-dose opioid techniques are still commonly employed for those patients in whom postoperative ventilatory support is anticipated; however, normothermic, hemodynamically stable patients may be considered for early extubation. Vasoactive medications, such as nitroprusside, nitroglycerin, and esmolol should be prepared preoperatively, including diluted amounts for bolus administration (Table 36.1).

4. Which monitoring devices are recommended for AAA surgery?

Standard monitors are placed for all patients presenting for aortic surgery. ECG with the ability to monitor limb and precordial leads (II and V_5 at the minimum) is desirable to detect myocardial ischemia and dysrhythmias. Foley catheterization is also prudent in order to assess volume status and to provide an early indication of renal malperfusion. Because of the increased incidence of myocardial ischemia, coagulopathy, and wound infection, patients should remain normothermic perioperatively.

Anesthesia for aortic surgery is frequently complicated by sudden blood pressure lability. Shifts in intravascular volume, effects of anesthetic agents, and/or surgical manipulations are the major causes. Sudden hemorrhage may induce severe hypovolemia at almost any time. Dramatic reductions in preload may be due to blood loss from intercostal artery back-bleeding, aortic disruptions, extensive anastomotic suture leaks, evaporative losses, and third-spaced fluids. Large-bore intravenous access is extremely important in aortic surgery. Aortic rupture may occur at any time and the ability to rapidly infuse intravenous fluids, blood, or blood products is necessary. One or two large-bore peripheral intravenous (IV) lines are recommended along with some form of central venous access. A rapid infusion system with a heat exchanger should be immediately available. Blood salvaging techniques for

TABLE 36.1	Basic Anesthetic Considerations for AAA Surgery

Preoperatively
  Continue antihypertensive medications (especially
    β-blockers and vasodilators)
  Continue anti-anginal medications
  Anxiolysis
  Large-bore intravenous access
Monitoring
  Standard monitors
  Foley catheter
  Arterial catheter
  Central venous catheter
  Pulmonary artery catheter
  Transesophageal echocardiography
Intraoperatively
  Maintain hemodynamic stability
  Vasoactive substances
    Nitroglycerin
    Nitroprusside
    Esmolol
    Phenylephrine
  Intravascular volume
    Crystalloids/colloids
    Blood and blood products
    Rapid infusion system with heat exchanger
    Blood salvage
  High-dose opioids if postoperative ventilation planned
  Normothermia, relatively small fluid shifts, and
    hemodynamic stability
   Consider early extubation

autotransfusion should be used. The easiest technique for blood salvaging is a centrifugal device, which scavenges and washes erythrocytes. The disadvantages of this technique are the delays related to filling the centrifugal bowl, processing the blood, as well as the loss of plasma volume, proteins, coagulation factors, and platelets. Normovolemic hemodilution may theoretically decrease the need for banked blood, but has been severely criticized.

This surgical population also includes many patients with occlusive coronary artery disease, in whom hemodynamic aberrations may induce myocardial ischemia by adversely affecting the myocardial oxygen supply and demand balance. The use of aggressive perioperative β blockade may decrease postoperative cardiac complications. A safe and reliable method of measuring acute changes in the blood pressure is required during aortic surgery. Intra-arterial monitoring accomplishes this goal by providing a continuous, beat-to-beat indication of the arterial pressure and waveform. Furthermore, an indwelling arterial catheter enables frequent sampling of arterial blood for laboratory analyses.

Central vein cannulation is routinely performed during aortic surgery. It allows for measurement of cardiac filling pressures (using a central venous catheter or a pulmonary artery catheter), provides a reliable route for drug delivery, and offers a site for rapid fluid administration. Ideally, central venous access can be accomplished with a large-bore cannula ("introducer") in the right internal jugular vein or left subclavian vein.

Central venous pressures (CVPs) do not give direct indications of left heart filling pressures, but they may estimate left-sided filling pressures in patients with good left ventricular function. CVP has been shown to correlate with left-sided filling pressures during a change in volume status in patients with coronary artery disease (CAD) and ejection fractions (EF) >0.4. Other studies have not shown a consistent relationship between the CVP and the pulmonary capillary wedge pressure (PCWP).

Pulmonary artery catheterization (PAC) should be strongly considered in patients with decreased ventricular function, pulmonary hypertension, severe valvular disease, or advanced systemic organ dysfunction. Monitoring right-sided pressures as the sole indication of volume status is probably not sufficient because right heart pressures do not reflect left heart preload. PACs may also be used to determine afterload, cardiac output by thermodilution, and oxygen delivery by measuring pulmonary artery oxygen saturation. Although PACs are used frequently in AAA surgery, no study has demonstrated better outcomes when they are employed.

Transesophageal echocardiography (TEE) is a very useful monitoring modality during aortic surgery. Ventricular dysfunction and regional wall motion abnormalities may be diagnosed. TEE produces images of the heart and great vessels, affording such information such as regional wall motion abnormalities, indirect measurements of stroke volume and EF, valvular abnormalities, and aortic and pericardial pathology. Ventricular function and intravascular volume status are probably the best indications for using TEE during these procedures. Personnel without proper training or credentials should exercise caution in using TEE in this modality.

5. Explain the hemodynamic consequences of aortic cross-clamping.

The most consistent hemodynamic response to acute aortic occlusion is an abrupt increase in afterload with a resultant increase in proximal aortic pressure. During supraceliac aortic occlusion, there is an increase in preload due to volume redistribution from veins distal to the site of aortic occlusion. The increases in afterload, preload, and possibly contractility resulting from aortic occlusion may exacerbate myocardial oxygen demand and possibly result in myocardial ischemia. Because of the expected increases in preload from aortic occlusion, the pre-occlusion preload should be maintained low. Venodilators such as nitroglycerin (NTG) may be titrated in order to further decrease preload and arterial dilators may be used to control increases in afterload. During aortic occlusion, attention should be directed toward maintaining preload, which may be complicated by continued blood loss.

Intraoperative hypotension may result from multiple causes. Hypovolemia, myocardial depression, and decreases in afterload should be considered. Reperfusion is associated with hypotension. Hypotension may be caused by central hypovolemia due to blood pooling in reperfused tissues, hypoxia-mediated vasodilation, and accumulation of vasoactive or myocardial-depressant metabolites, such as lactate. Treatment should be directed toward rapid correction of hypovolemia, acidosis, and hypocalcemia, as well as the judicious administration of vasoactive drugs. If there is difficulty obtaining hemodynamic stability, the aorta can be temporarily re-occluded while resuscitation continues (Table 36.2).

Renal insufficiency may occur as a result of abdominal aortic reconstruction. It is possible that pharmacologic agents may provide renal protection during repair. Although mannitol may result in greater diuresis on postoperative day 1 and has less subclinical glomerular and renal tubular damage, it most probably has no effect on postoperative blood urea levels, serum creatinine concentration, or creatinine clearance. There is little evidence of the effectiveness of furosemide as a renal protective agent.

Theoretically, the perioperative use of low doses of dopamine may confer renal protection in high-risk individuals. Low-dose dopamine (1–3 μg/kg/min) dilates

---

TABLE 36.2   Hypotension After Aortic Unclamping

Etiologies
  Hypovolemia
    Blood loss
    Evaporative losses
    Reperfusion syndrome
      Pooling in reperfused tissues
      Hypoxia-mediated vasodilators
      Myocardial depressant metabolites (lactic acid)
  Myocardial depression
  Decreased afterload
Therapy
  Volume infusion
  Vasoconstrictors
    Phenylephrine
  Inotropic support
  Reclamp aorta
  Treat acidosis

---

renal afferent arterioles and increases renal blood flow, independent of its cardiac effects. Dopamine infusion during aortic clamping results in a significant rise in urine sodium output, potassium output, creatinine clearance, and urine volume. The use of perioperative dopamine during aortic surgery is associated with increases in effective renal plasma flow and glomerular filtration rate as well as fractional excretion of sodium during the postoperative period; however, no studies have demonstrated a renal protective effect of low-dose dopamine. It is most likely that renal-dose dopamine administration during the perioperative period confers no advantage over the maintenance of euvolemia in most vascular patients during infrarenal AAA repair.

Visceral ischemia (which does not occur with infrarenal aortic clamping) may initiate fibrinolysis. Antifibrinolytic agents should be strongly considered if supraceliac occlusion is anticipated. Aminocaproic acid, tranexamic acid, and aprotinin are all effective in decreasing fibrinolytic activity.

6. Describe the options for postoperative analgesia.

Intravenous narcotic administration has the advantage of rapid uptake and attainment of therapeutic levels. However, this mode of administration is also associated with rapid declines in drug concentration during which patients may experience pain. Although using larger doses of narcotics may increase the duration of analgesia, higher doses may be associated with a greater number of adverse side-effects. To minimize these side-effects, small frequent doses of narcotic may be administered via a patient-controlled pump, i.e., patient controlled analgesia (PCA). This technique allows patients greater comfort control during their hospital course and may prevent overmedication. Although this technique is safe, respiratory depression may occur, so routine postoperative nursing care should include careful monitoring of respiratory status.

An attractive alternative to the use of intravenous narcotics is epidural administration of analgesics. Local anesthetics, narcotics, and other agents such as α_2-agonists have been described as effective in significantly decreasing the intensity of postoperative pain. Although this method can provide profound pain relief, it may be associated with significant side-effects. Local anesthetics may cause sympathetic blockade (with resultant decreases in preload and afterload that may result in hypotension and tachycardia), motor blockade, and local anesthetic toxicities. Epidural narcotics may cause pruritus, nausea, vomiting, urinary retention, or respiratory depression. These side-effects can usually be treated with conventional therapy (e.g., antihistamines or antiemetics) or specific narcotic antagonists. Epidural narcotics have the advantage of specificity of action, without the major hemodynamic changes and motor blockade that may be associated with local anesthetics.

Preoperative epidural catheter insertion for postoperative analgesia is probably safe when perioperative anticoagulation is anticipated. Epidural anesthesia may increase coronary blood flow, but there is contradictory evidence on the effect of epidural anesthesia on myocardial ischemia during noncardiac surgery. There have been multiple reports of attenuation in the stress response with peri- and postoperative epidural anesthesia and analgesia during vascular surgery. Supplemental epidural anesthesia may significantly attenuate catecholamine release during aortic occlusion and reperfusion. This reduction in the stress response by epidural anesthesia/analgesia may decrease postoperative hypercoagulability.

SUGGESTED READINGS

Bellomo R, Chapman M, Finfer S, Hickling K, Myburgh J: Low-dose dopamine in patients with early renal dysfunction: a placebo-controlled randomised trial. Australian and New Zealand Intensive Care Society (ANZICS) Clinical Trials Group. Lancet 356:2139, 2000

Bernstein EF, Chan EL: Abdominal aoric aneurysm in high risk patients: outcome of selective management based on size and expansion rate. Ann Surg 200:255, 1984

Bois S, Couture P, Boudreault D, et al.: Epidural analgesia and intravenous patient-controlled analgesia result in similar rates of postoperative myocardial ischemia after aortic surgery. Anesth Analg 85:1233, 1997

Eagle KA, Brundage BH, Chaitman BR, et al.: Guidelines for perioperative cardiovascular evaluation for noncardiac surgery: report of the American College of Cardiology/American Heart Association Task Force on Practice Guidelines (Committee on Perioperative Cardiovascular Evaluation for Noncardiac Surgery). J Am Coll Cardiol 27:910, 1996

Frank SM, Fleisher LA, Breslow MJ, et al.: Perioperative maintenance of normothermia reduces the incidence of morbid cardiac events: a randomized clinical trial. JAMA 277:1127, 1997

Gelman S: The pathophysiology of aortic cross-clamping and unclamping. Anesthesiology 82:1026, 1995

Mangano DT, Layug EL, Wallace A, Tateo I: Effect of atenolol on mortality and cardiovascular morbidity after noncardiac surgery. Multicenter Study of Perioperative Ischemia Research Group. N Engl J Med 335:1713, 1996

Practice guidelines for perioperative transesophageal echocardiography: a report by the American Society of Anesthesiologists and the Society of Cardiovascular Anesthesiologists Task Force on Transesophageal Echocardiography. Anesthesiology 84:986, 1996

Practice guidelines for pulmonary artery catheterization: a report by the American Society of Anesthesiologists Task Force on Pulmonary Artery Catheterization. Anesthesiology 78:380, 1993

37

ENDOVASCULAR AORTIC STENT PLACEMENT

Ronald A. Kahn, MD

An 83-year-old man presents for therapy of a 7 cm descending thoracic aortic aneurysm. He has a history of coronary artery disease, congestive heart failure, chronic obstructive pulmonary disease, hypertension, and previous abdominal aortic aneurysm repair. The descending aortic aneurysm begins 5 cm distal to the left subclavian artery and extends for 30 cm. Because of the patient's concurrent medical conditions, an endovascular repair is planned, with several self-expanding endografts. He tolerates the procedure without incident. In the postanesthesia care unit, the patient becomes febrile, mildly hypotensive, and develops oozing at the surgical sites.

QUESTIONS

1. Explain the concept of endovascular aortic repair.
2. What are the recognized perioperative surgical complications associated with endovascular repairs?
3. What are the outcomes following thoracic endovascular aortic repair?
4. What anesthetic techniques are used for endovascular graft insertions?
5. What problems are anticipated during proximal graft deployment?
6. Explain the special role of transesophageal echocardiography in endovascular stent placement.

7. Is the incidence of spinal cord ischemia different after endovascular thoracic aortic repairs compared with open repairs?
8. What is the "post-implantation syndrome"?

1. Explain the concept of endovascular aortic repair.

Endovascular aortic repair is a new alternative to conventional surgical repair of aortic pathology. Endovascular grafts are less invasive compared with conventional arterial reconstruction. They are inserted through small incisions from remote arterial access sites. This technique obviates the need for aortic occlusion, decreases blood loss, avoids significant fluid shifts that occur with visceral manipulation, thus lowering the risk of significant hemodynamic changes perioperatively, and prevents respiratory impairment from abdominal incisions.

Because of the uncertainty of long-term outcome, younger patients with minimal or no medical comorbidities may be better candidates for open repair because of its established track record. Patients with severe medical comorbidities may be better candidates for endovascular reconstruction. Not all patients with aortic pathology have suitable anatomy for endovascular repair. In order for an endovascular repair to be successful, the device must form a tight seal between the graft and the native artery. The proximal neck (i.e., proximal "landing zone") must be at least 15 mm in length and the aneurysm neck diameter should be no larger than the largest endograft available. Similarly, the distal attachment site must be non-aneurysmal and of sufficient length to accommodate the graft. No important aortic side branches, such as an accessory renal artery or inferior mesenteric artery, can be present in the aortic segment that is to be excluded. In practice, excessive aneurysm neck tortuosity, severe calcification, aneurysmal necks greater than 26–27 mm in diameter and less than 10–15 mm in length may be relative contraindications for endovascular repair. Finally there must be at least one large, straight iliac artery that can accommodate passage (i.e., act as a conduit) of the endograft delivery system.

2. What are the recognized perioperative surgical complications associated with endovascular repairs?

Although endovascular aortic repair is less invasive than open repair, it is nonetheless associated with significant perioperative complications. Prior to insertion of the endovascular device, the operator may be unable to pass the sheath or delivery device through the arteries because of iliac or aortic anatomy and/or pathology. Alternatively, the possibility of iatrogenic arterial rupture always exists with intra-arterial manipulations, which may necessitate emergent resuscitation and immediate conversion to an open procedure, thus increasing the morbidity and mortality associated with the repair.

Injury to the aorta and end organs may occur with guidewire insertion and device manipulation via either embolization or obstruction. Distal embolization of aortic material to the bowel, lower extremities, or other organs is not uncommon. Although the endovascular device may

---

Surgical Complications of Endovascular Stent Placement

Arterial rupture

Guidewire induced complications
    Injury to aorta and end organs
    Cerebral injury
    Aortic valve injury
    Pericardial tamponade

Cerebral injury secondary to retrograde thromboembolism, large volumes of contrast, vigorous flushing

Renal injury
    Graft migration
    Renal artery dissection
    Occlusion of renal arteries
    Contrast

---

obstruct hypogastric artery flow, complications have not been reported. It is possible that either retrograde thromboembolism as a result of graft manipulation, large volumes of contrast injection, vigorous flushing, or the passage of guidewires through a diseased aortic arch may result in cerebral injury. Furthermore, inadvertent guidewire placement into the heart has occurred with injury to the aortic valve or pericardial tamponade.

Renal injury, either segmental or total, may occur as a complication of endovascular aortic repair. Graft migration, renal artery dissection, and improper placement of the proximal portion of the endovascular device can occlude the renal arteries. This may lead to renal insufficiency and the possibility of further procedures to correct the problem. A significant amount of contrast is used during these procedures to define aortic anatomy, providing another possible mechanism for renal injury.

3. What are the outcomes following thoracic endovascular aortic repair?

Endovascular repair may be a viable option for repair of thoracic aortic pathology. Dake et al. (1994) reported 6 month, 1 year, and 2 year survival rates of 86%, 81%, and 73% respectively after endovascular thoracic aortic aneurysm repair. The predictors of death were: patients who were not surgical candidates, the use of cardiopulmonary bypass (which was used in patients who underwent combined ascending aortic and arch surgery with endovascular thoracic aortic aneurysm repair), patients with large aneurysms or large aneurysm neck diameters, and older age. The major complications of the procedure were early death (9%), neurologic (10%), and pulmonary (12%). The 9% endovascular mortality was not much different from the reported 11% mortality incidence of open repair. However, it should be noted that 16% of the endovascular patients were operated on an emergency basis and 60% of these patients were not candidates for open repair. In this context, a 9% mortality rate is not unreasonable. It was suggested that the high incidence of stroke might be caused by catheter or sheath manipulations in the aortic arch and ascending aorta, excessive anticoagulation, or possibly surgical manipulation of the carotid or subclavian arteries.

4. What anesthetic techniques are used for endovascular graft insertions?

Different anesthetic techniques have been described for aortic stent-graft placement including local anesthesia, regional anesthesia, and general anesthesia. Since the early procedures often required long surgical times, general anesthesia was usually administered to improve patient compliance. Increasing surgical experience and more sophisticated devices allowed for regional anesthetics (including epidural, spinal, and continuous spinal anesthetics) as well as local anesthetics supplemented by sedation. Choice of anesthetic technique is dependent on the planned surgical intervention and the patient's comorbid conditions. Surgery for arterial stents that require percutaneous placement of catheters through limited incisions may be tolerated with local anesthesia and sedation. The need for extensive inguinal exploration and dissection or for the construction of a femoral artery to femoral arterial conduit may favor either regional or general anesthesia. If surgical dissection is extended into the retroperitoneum, a higher level of regional anesthesia or general anesthesia will be necessary to provide adequate anesthesia. Many of these procedures may take a long time to perform. If the patient is undergoing local anesthesia or regional anesthesia, adequate intravenous sedation is necessary because of agitation secondary to restlessness and pain from lying in one position for a prolonged period of time.

5. What problems are anticipated during proximal graft deployment?

Hemodynamic stability to preserve organ function is the primary goal for aortic endovascular stent placement. Various comorbid conditions make this particularly important. Special attention must be directed towards evaluating the function and reserves of cardiac, pulmonary, neurologic, and renal systems. Fluid requirements are potentially large because significant amounts of blood can be lost, often concealed, during these procedures. In addition, emergent conversion to open repair secondary to aortic rupture is always possible.

Distal migration of the endograft during proximal deployment may not include the aneurysm sac, causing endoleakage. Older endovascular stent-grafts employed large balloon angioplasty catheters to expand and secure the proximal stent attachment system of the endovascular graft to the underlying normal vessel wall. These balloons have a large cross-sectional area, predisposing them to distal aortic migration as forward aortic blood flow pushes in downstream. Device malposition secondary to inadvertent migration may result in either occlusion of major arterial branches or incomplete aneurysm exclusion. Induced hypotension during device deployment has been successfully used by some centers to assist in proximal endovascular stent-graft placement and may reduce the magnitude of migration. However, significant endovascular stent-graft movement may nonetheless occur because of continued aortic blood flow. The risk of malposition may be decreased by induced hypotension using short-acting vasodilators, ventricular quiescence (achieved by either pharmacologic induction of sinoatrial and atrioventricular nodal inhibition with high-dose adenosine), or induced ventricular fibrillation. Most likely, no interventions are necessary for self-expanding devices placed in the infrarenal aorta.

6. Explain the special role of transesophageal echocardiography in endovascular stent placement.

With the rapid evolution of ultrasound technology and the advent of transesophageal echocardiography (TEE), perioperative dynamic views of the cardiovascular system are now obtainable that have previously been unavailable by conventional transthoracic ultrasonography. Because the esophagus is in close approximation to the aorta, TEE has become an excellent tool for diagnosing pathology of the distal aortic arch, the descending thoracic aorta, and the proximal abdominal aorta. TEE can provide instantaneous views of the aorta and location of the guidewires and endografts prior to deployment in relation to the normal and diseased thoracic aorta. While the long-axis view may aid in placement of the angiography catheter and delivery device, these devices may not be visualized unless they are in the precise plane of the ultrasonic beam or if there is significant artifact. To overcome these pitfalls, higher frequencies and intermittent use of the transverse imaging plane can help identify where the tip of the catheter and delivery system lie within the aorta.

TEE appears to have distinct advantages over perioperative angiography. TEE provides exact vessel and lesion sizing and localization, which is difficult to obtain during single-plane angiography. In contrast to angiography, both endograft leakage (using Doppler color flow imaging) and iatrogenic dissections may be diagnosed by TEE. It can also be used to estimate endograft sizing and evaluate the endograft location. Large intercostal arteries have been imaged, thus avoiding inadvertent obstruction by the aortic stent-graft; however, consistent visualization of intercostal arteries is not possible in all patients. After stent-graft placement, exclusion of flow from the aorta into the aneurysm can be easily confirmed using color Doppler flow imaging in most patients. Finally, since most of these patients have severe concomitant cardiac disease, perioperative TEE allows dynamic assessment of cardiac function.

7. Is the incidence of spinal cord ischemia different after endovascular thoracic aortic repairs compared to open repairs?

The reported incidence of postoperative neurologic injuries after endovascular thoracic aortic reconstruction is similar to that of open thoracic aortic repair. With descending aortic reconstruction, intercostal arteries that supply the anterior spinal cord may be sacrificed, resulting in spinal cord injury. Probable risk factors for paraplegia include the length of the thoracic endograft placed and a history of previous abdominal aortic aneurysm repair.

Anecdotal evidence exists for the reversal of spinal cord symptoms by cerebrospinal fluid (CSF) drainage after endovascular thoracic aortic repair. In our practice, patients who are judged to be at high risk for postoperative

Post-implantation Syndrome

Characteristics
    Fever
    Elevated C-reactive protein
    Leukocytosis
    Absence of infectious agent

Duration: 2–10 days postoperatively

Treatment: Nonsteroidal anti-inflammatory drugs

Exaggerated response:
    Distributive shock
    Respiratory failure
    Disseminated intravascular coagulopathy

paraplegia (based upon endograft length and history of abdominal aortic aneurysm repair) receive perioperative induced hypertension, CSF drainage, and steroid and mannitol administration.

8. What is the "post-implantation syndrome"?

The post-implantation syndrome is commonly observed after endovascular aortic repair. It is characterized by fever, elevated C-reactive protein levels, and leukocytosis in the absence of an infectious agent. It is usually mild and self-limited, lasting from 2 to 10 days postoperatively and responds to nonsteroidal anti-inflammatory drugs. Occasionally an exaggerated response may result in life-threatening distributive shock, respiratory failure, and disseminated intravascular coagulopathy. It is hypothesized that endovascular aortic aneurysm repair induces a significant inflammatory response resulting in endothelial cell activation from intra-aneurysmal device manipulation. Although rare, the post-implantation syndrome may present as a consumptive coagulopathy. Endovascular exclusion of a large aortic aneurysm may result in significant thrombus in the excluded aneurysm sac, which may initiate fibrinolysis. Repeated instrumentation of the aorta, which may occur with difficult placement of an endograft, may result in endothelial damage resulting in stimulation of a procoagulant response.

SUGGESTED READINGS

Dake MD, Miller DC, Semba CP, et al.: Transluminal placement of endovascular stent-grafts for the treatment of descending thoracic aortic aneurysms. N Engl J Med 331:1729, 1994

Greenberg R: Clinical decision making and operative approaches to thoracic aortic aneurysms. Surg Clin North Am 78:805, 1998

Greenberg R, Resch T, Nyman U, et al.: Endovascular repair of descending thoracic aortic aneurysms: an early experience with intermediate-term follow-up. J Vasc Surg 31:147, 2000

Kahn RA, Moskowitz DM: Endovascular aortic repair. J Cardiothorac Vasc Anesth 16:218, 2002

Moskowitz DM, Kahn RA, Konstadt SN, et al.: Intraoperative transesophageal echocardiography as an adjunct to fluoroscopy during endovascular thoracic aortic repair. Eur J Vasc Endovasc Surg 17:22, 1999

Tiesenhausen K, Amann W, Koch G, et al.: Cerebrospinal fluid drainage to reverse paraplegia after endovascular thoracic aortic aneurysm repair. J Endovasc Ther 7:132, 2000

38

TRANSURETHRAL RESECTION OF THE PROSTATE

Laurence M. Hausman, MD

A 74-year-old man is scheduled to undergo a transurethral resection of the prostate (TURP) for benign prostatic hypertrophy. He has a history of coronary artery disease with stable angina and hypertension. Current medications include metoprolol 5 mg twice a day and amlodipine 10 mg once a day. The physical examination is unremarkable. Heart rate is 74 beats per minute, blood pressure is 160/75 mmHg, and the respiratory rate is 12 breaths per minute. He is 177.5 cm tall and weighs 72 kg.

QUESTIONS

1. Describe the TURP syndrome and its treatment.
2. What other complications can occur during a TURP?
3. What types of irrigating fluids have been used for a TURP?
4. What are the toxicities associated with glycine?
5. What are the anesthetic options for a patient undergoing a TURP?
6. If a regional anesthetic is selected, what level of anesthesia is required?
7. One hour and 15 minutes into the procedure, the patient's serum Na^+ level is 102 mEq/L. How would one correct the Na^+ level to 135 mEq/L?

1. Describe the TURP syndrome and its treatment.

The TURP syndrome is a collection of signs and symptoms that occur when excessive amounts of irrigating fluids are absorbed through the opened prostatic venous sinusoids. This absorption of fluids may result in water intoxication, hyponatremia, and hypo-osmolality.

The decrease in sodium levels during a TURP ranges from 3.65 to 10 mEq/L. Several mechanisms for this have been postulated. Hyponatremia may be due either to simple dilution of the blood by the irrigating solution or to diffusion of sodium into the irrigating solution at either the surgical site, or into the periprostatic and/or retroperitoneal spaces. The degree of hyponatremia is related to the rate of absorption of the irrigating fluid and not to the absolute amount absorbed.

The effects on the central nervous system include headache, restlessness, agitation, confusion, seizures, and eventually coma. These findings are thought to be caused by cerebral edema, with a concomitant increase in intracerebral pressure. As the neurologic condition worsens, the patient may develop decerebrate posturing, clonus and a positive Babinski sign. Ocular examination often reveals bilateral dilated and sluggishly reactive pupils as well as papilledema. Electroencephalogram (EEG) often shows low-voltage activity. If coma occurs, it usually resolves within hours to days, but can be permanent. The incidence of neurologic injury is more closely related to the rate of sodium decrease rather than the degree of hyponatremia.

Central Nervous System Effects of TURP Syndrome

Headache

Restlessness

Agitation

Confusion

Seizures

Coma

Decerebrate posturing

Clonus

Babinski sign

Sluggishly reacting pupils

Papilledema

Cardiovascular Effects of TURP Syndrome

Na^+ <120 mEq/L
    Hypotension
    Pulmonary edema
    Congestive heart failure

Na^+ <115 mEq/L
    Widened QRS complex
    Ventricular ectopy
    T-wave inversion

Na^+ <100 mEq/L
    Respiratory arrest
    Cardiac arrest

Hyponatremia and fluid overload have deleterious consequences on the heart. The initial cardiovascular effects of fluid overload include hypertension and bradycardia. However, serum sodium (Na^+) levels of 120 mEq/L are associated with a negative inotropic effect on the heart causing hypotension, pulmonary edema, and congestive heart failure (CHF). Serum Na^+ levels of less than 115 mEq/L are associated with electrocardiogram (ECG) changes, such as a widened QRS complex, ventricular ectopy, and T-wave inversion. When serum Na^+ falls below 100 mEq/L, respiratory and cardiac arrest may occur.

If the patient develops signs and symptoms of the TURP syndrome, the surgical procedure should be concluded as soon as possible. Treatment should then be directed at raising the serum Na^+ level and correcting the volume overload by fluid restriction and the administration of a loop diuretic, such as furosemide. In severe cases of hyponatremia, administration of a hypertonic saline solution (3–5% sodium chloride) may be necessary. Rapid correction of hyponatremia has been associated with cerebral edema and central pontine myelinolysis. All other treatment is dictated by the patient's symptomatology. Supplemental oxygen should be considered and the patient may even require tracheal intubation and mechanical ventilation.

2. What other complications can occur during a TURP?

Approximately 7% of all patients undergoing a TURP suffer a major complication. The 30-day mortality rate has been estimated to be 0.1–0.8%. This is a marked improvement over earlier studies that showed a mortality rate of approximately 2.5% during the 1960s. Patients undergoing a TURP are often advanced in age, and have coexisting cardiopulmonary disorders making them more likely to experience complications. Since many patients are on chronic diuretics, they are often dehydrated with electrolyte abnormalities preoperatively.

Other complications associated with this procedure are as follows:

Bladder Perforation

Bladder perforation occurs in approximately 1% of all TURP procedures. It may be caused by overdistention of the bladder with irrigating fluid, or as a result of surgical instrumentation. An early sign of bladder perforation is a decrease in return of irrigating fluid from the bladder. The abdomen will become distended and often rigid. If the procedure is being performed under a regional anesthetic, the patient may complain of pain and/or experience nausea and vomiting. Hypotension followed by hypertension is common.

Most perforations are extraperitoneal and benign in nature. This type of perforation causes pain in the periumbilical region. However, pain in the upper abdomen or referred pain to the shoulder may be a sign of an intraperitoneal perforation, a potentially fatal complication. Diagnosis should quickly be confirmed by cysto-urethrography and treated with a suprapubic cystostomy.

Bleeding

The prostate is a highly vascular organ. Since a large amount of irrigation is used, it is difficult to determine the actual blood loss. Intraoperative blood loss corresponds to the size of the gland as well as to the resection time. It has been estimated that the blood loss is approximately 2–5 ml/min of resection time and 20–50 ml/g of prostate tissue. Blood loss is linearly related to prostate size up to 35 grams, at which point blood loss tends to exceed the linear correlation. Patients with resection times of greater than 90 minutes or a prostate size of more than 60 grams have been found to have a significant increase in morbidity associated with bleeding.

Coagulopathy

Subclinical coagulopathy occurs in approximately 6% of patients undergoing a TURP, while clinical coagulopathy occurs approximately 1% of the time. This condition seems to correlate with the mass of the resected prostatic tissue. It is more likely to occur if the resected tissue is greater than 35 grams. Coagulopathy may be due to a dilution of coagulation factors and platelets.

Primary fibrinolysis has also been implicated as a cause of coagulopathy. Plasminogen activator, which is responsible for converting plasminogen into plasmin, is released during these procedures. The treatment of choice for primary fibrinolysis is ε-aminocaproic acid.

Secondary fibrinolysis may occur as a result of disseminated intravascular coagulopathy (DIC). DIC is caused by the systemic absorption of prostate tissue, which is rich in thromboplastin. Proof of this theory lies in the fact that these patients often have a low level of plasminogen activator, platelets, and fibrinogen – common findings in DIC. If DIC is suspected, the treatment is symptomatic. Fluid and blood products are administered as needed. Heparin administration may be beneficial.

Transient Bacteremia and Septicemia

The prostate, rich in bacteria, may cause a postoperative bacteremia via the prostatic venous sinusoids. An indwelling urinary catheter will enhance the risk. Approximately 6–7% of patients will go on to develop sepsis. Treatment consists of antibiotics and supportive care.

Toxicity of Irrigating Fluids

The major toxicity of the irrigation fluids used today is secondary to massive absorption causing fluid overload, hyponatremia, and hypo-osmolality. The incidence of hypo-osmolality and its associated neurologic sequelae has decreased since the use of nonelectrolyte iso-osmotic irrigating fluids. However, fluid overload and hyponatremia still remain a problem. As much as 8 liters of irrigating fluid may be absorbed during a TURP, causing an average weight gain of about 2 kg. Twenty to thirty percent of this fluid is absorbed directly into the vascular space. The remainder is absorbed into the periprostatic and the peritoneal space (interstitial space). Several factors contribute to the rate of absorption of irrigating fluid by the patient. These include the prostate size, integrity of the prostatic capsule, and the height of the irrigating fluid container. Greater amounts of irrigating fluid are absorbed when the prostate is large because of its richer blood supply, and if the prostate capsule is violated.

There are maneuvers that may be carried out to limit the amount of irrigating fluid absorbed. The first is to restrict the height of the fluid container above the surgical field. This will decrease the hydrostatic pressure driving the fluid into the sinuses. When the height of the bag is greater than 60 cm, absorption is greatly enhanced. The second is to limit the length of the resection time to less than 150 minutes, as some investigators have found that 10–30 cc of irrigation fluid is absorbed per minute of resection time.

Sorbitol and mannitol, both sugar alcohols, have been associated with the development of lactic acidosis and hyperglycemia. Specific effects of glycine will be discussed later.

Hypothermia

Patients may develop hypothermia under either general or neuraxial anesthesia. This can be exacerbated by using irrigating fluids at room temperature. Using warmed

---

Complications of TURP

Bladder perforation
    Extraperitoneal or intraperitoneal

Bleeding
    Related to size of the gland and resection time

Coagulopathy
    Dilution of coagulation factors
    Primary fibrinolysis
    Disseminated intravascular coagulopathy

Transient bacteremia and septicemia

Toxicity of irrigating fluids
    Hypervolemia
    Hyponatremia

Hypothermia

irrigating fluid can decrease heat loss and shivering. It is a theoretical concern that warming the irrigating fluids would cause vasodilation, thereby increasing blood loss. However, this has not been shown to be a clinical concern. In fact, since hypothermia may cause shivering, which increases venous pressure, there may be an increased blood loss if the irrigating fluids are not warmed.

3. What types of irrigating fluids have been used for a TURP?

The ideal irrigating fluid would be isotonic, electrically inert, nontoxic and transparent. Unfortunately, this type of solution does not exist. Originally, distilled water was used. However, absorption of distilled water caused hyponatremia and hemolysis of red blood cells. This severe complication led to the use of iso-osmotic solutions such as saline or lactated Ringer solution. However, since these solutions are highly ionized, they caused dispersion of the high-frequency current from the resectoscope. The present generation of irrigating fluids is electrically inert as well as isotonic. These solutions include glycine and Cytal (the most commonly used) as well as glucose, mannitol, urea, and sorbitol.

4. What are the toxicities associated with glycine?

Intravascular absorption of 1.5% glycine solution has been implicated as a possible cause for many of the neurologic manifestations associated with a TURP, including transient blindness. Glycine, a nonessential amino acid, readily crosses the blood–brain barrier. It has a distribution similar to γ-aminobutyric acid, a naturally occurring inhibitory neurotransmitter. Transient blindness may be a result of the inhibitory effect of glycine on the central nervous system or via its direct inhibitory effect on the retina. The effect of glycine on the retina appears to be unrelated to its plasma concentration.

Glycine is metabolized to ammonia, which may lead to hyperammonemia in some patients. The mechanism by which hyperammonemia develops is unclear. One mechanism postulated is that ammonia is converted to urea in the liver via the ornithine cycle, in a reaction requiring arginine. This mechanism of action is supported by the fact that patients with an arginine deficiency have been found to be more likely to develop hyperammonemia. Common signs and symptoms of ammonia toxicity include nausea and vomiting. As the ammonia level rises above 500 μmol/L coma may occur. Coma typically resolves when the ammonia level decreases to below 150 μmol/L.

The cardiovascular effects of glycine are myocardial depression and nonspecific ECG changes, such as T-wave depression.

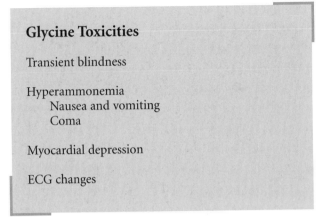

Glycine Toxicities

Transient blindness

Hyperammonemia
    Nausea and vomiting
    Coma

Myocardial depression

ECG changes

5. What are the anesthetic options for a patient undergoing a TURP?

Regional anesthesia has long been considered the anesthetic of choice for this procedure. The clear advantage of this technique is the ability to monitor for the early signs of hyponatremia such as irritability and headache. If these occur, a serum Na^+ level should be checked and hyponatremia, if confirmed, should be treated expeditiously. It is important to remember that the development of combativeness intraoperatively should not be assumed to be inadequate anesthesia. Deepening the anesthetic level with sedation could have a catastrophic effect.

As discussed earlier, another potentially fatal complication of a TURP is bladder perforation. If a T_{10} level of sensory blockade is achieved, the patient would still be able to complain of abdominal or shoulder pain. This complaint would alert the anesthesiologist and the surgeon to the probability of a bladder perforation, and would allow for prompt diagnosis and treatment.

As with other pelvic procedures, regional anesthesia has been shown to decrease blood loss and the incidence of deep vein thrombosis. The decrease in blood loss is most likely secondary to the decrease in blood pressure as well as the decrease in both central and peripheral venous pressure associated with neuraxial anesthesia. A number of different reasons have been postulated for the decreased incidence of deep vein thromboses. One reason may be the increase in peripheral blood flow resulting from the sympathetic blockade. Other reasons include an increase in prothrombin time, a measure of the extrinsic pathway of coagulation, and a decrease in platelet count.

Another clear advantage of regional anesthesia is postoperative pain control. Good postoperative pain control will also allow the patient to avoid the sympathetic response to pain, such as tachycardia and hypertension, which could increase the likelihood of myocardial ischemia in susceptible patients.

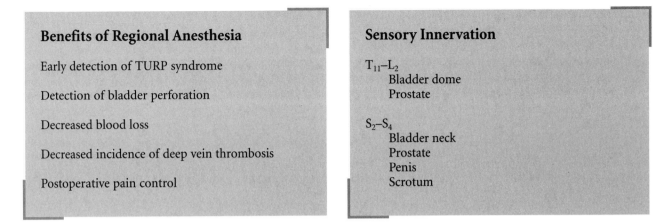

Benefits of Regional Anesthesia

Early detection of TURP syndrome

Detection of bladder perforation

Decreased blood loss

Decreased incidence of deep vein thrombosis

Postoperative pain control

Sensory Innervation

T_{11}–L_2
   Bladder dome
   Prostate

S_2–S_4
   Bladder neck
   Prostate
   Penis
   Scrotum

The presence of comorbid condition(s) in the patient may necessitate a general anesthetic. It must be appreciated that the early neurologic signs and symptoms associated with hyponatremia, hypo-osmolality or bladder perforation will no longer be available to the anesthesiologist. When a general anesthetic is chosen, a smooth emergence is desirable. If the patient awakens coughing and "bucking" on the endotracheal tube, venous pressure will increase and bleeding may develop.

6. If a regional anesthetic is selected, what level of anesthesia is required?

The level of anesthesia required is dependent on the anatomy and sensory innervation of the involved structures. The structures that need to be blocked are the bladder, prostate, penis, and urethra. The dome of the bladder receives its sensory innervation via T_{11}–L_2, while the neck of the bladder is via S_2–S_4. The prostate receives its sensory innervation via T_{11}–L_2 and S_2–S_4. Finally, a sensory block of the penis and scrotum will require blocking S_2–S_4.

Based upon this anatomy, a block to the level of T_{10} is usually sufficient for a TURP. If a lower level is attained, the stretch of the bladder from the irrigating fluids will not be well tolerated. Since a block at the level of S_4 is also required, a spinal is preferred over an epidural anesthetic, since there is often an incomplete block of the sacral nerve roots.

7. One hour and 15 minutes into the procedure, the patient's serum Na^+ level is 102 mEq/L. How would one correct the Na^+ level to 135 mEq/L?

The sodium deficit must first be calculated using the following equation:

$$Na^+_{deficit} \; mEq = total\; body\; water\; (TBW) \times (Na^+_{desired} - Na^+_{observed})$$

TBW comprises 60% of lean body weight in the average male and 50% of lean body weight in the average female. In this example, the patient's sodium deficit is:

$$1,425.6\; mEq = (72\; kg \times 0.6) \times (135 - 102)$$

Hypertonic saline (3% NaCl) contains 513 mEq/L of Na^+. Therefore, the volume of hypertonic saline required to replace a Na^+ deficit of 1,425.6 mEq is 2.78 liters. The maximum safe rate of rise in a patient's serum sodium is 0.5 mEq/L/hr. In this case, the serum Na^+ should be corrected over 66 hours. Therefore, the hypertonic saline should run at a rate of 1,425.6/66 = 21.6 cc/hr.

In situations of significant hyponatremia associated with seizures and/or progressive neurologic deterioration, it may be necessary to correct the Na^+ deficit more rapidly (up to 3 mEq/L/hr). This rapid correction should not exceed 2 hours and should be stopped if the neurologic symptoms resolve sooner.

SUGGESTED READINGS

Allen TD: Body temperature changes during prostatic resection as related to the temperature of the irrigating solution. J Urol 110:433–435, 1973

Gehring H, Nahm W, Baerwald PF, Schneeweiss A, Roth-Isigkeit A, Schmucker P: Irrigation fluid absorption during transurethral resection of the prostate: spinal vs. general anaesthesia. Acta Anaesthesiol Scand 43:458–463, 1999

Hahn RG: Relations between irrigation absorption rate and hyponatremia during transurethral resection of the prostate. Acta Anaesthesiol Scand 32:53–60, 1988

Hahn RG, Essen P: ECG and cardiac enzymes after glycine absorption in transurethral prostatic resection. Acta Anaesthesiol Scand 38:550–556, 1994

Heathcote PS, Dyer PM: The effect of warm irrigation on blood loss during transurethral prostatectomy under spinal anesthesia. Br J Urol 58:669–671, 1986

Henderson DJ, Middleton RG: Coma from hyponatremia following transurethral resection of the prostate. Urology 15:267–271, 1980

Hurlbert BJ, Wingard DW: Water intoxication after 15 minutes of transurethral resection of the prostate. Anesthesiology 50:355–356, 1979

Kirollos MM, Campbell N: Factors influencing blood loss in transurethral resection of the prostate (TURP): auditing TURP. Br J Urol 80:111–115, 1997

Madsen PO, Naber KG: The importance of pressure in the prostatic fossa and absorption of irrigation fluid during transurethral resection of the prostate. J Urol 109:446–452, 1973

Malhotra V: Transurethral resection of the prostate. Anesthesiol Clin North Am 18:883–897, 2000

Ovassapian A, Joshi CW, Brumer EA: Visual disturbances: an unusual symptom of transurethral prostatic resection reaction. Anesthesiology 57:332–334, 1982

Radziwill AJ, Vuadens P, Borruat FX, Bogousslavsky J: Visual disturbances and transurethral resection of the prostate: the TURP syndrome. Eur Neurol 38:7–9, 1997

Rhymer JC, Bell TJ, Perry KC, Ward JP: Hyponatremia following transurethral resection of the prostate. Br J Urol 57:450–452, 1985

Roesch RP, Stoelting RK, Lingeman JE, et al.: Ammonia toxicity resulting from glycine absorption during a transurethral resection of the prostate. Anesthesiology 58:577–579, 1983

Smyth R, Cheng D, Asokumar B, Chung F: Coagulopathies in patients after transurethral resection of the prostate: spinal versus general anesthesia. Anesth Analg 81:680–685, 1995

Sterns RH, Riggs JE, Schochet SS Jr.: Osmotic demyelination syndrome following correction of hyponatremia. N Engl J Med 314:1534–1542, 1986

Still AJ, Modell JA: Acute water intoxication during transurethral resection of the prostate using glycine solution for irrigation. Anesthesiology 38:98–99, 1973

Toyoaki U, Ohori M, Soh S, Sato T, Masatsugu I, Ao T, Koshiba K: Factors influencing morbidity in patients undergoing transurethral resection of the prostate. Urology 53:98–105, 1999

Trepanier CA, Lessard MR, Brochu J, Turcotte G: Another feature of TURP syndrome: hyperglycemia and lactic acidosis caused by massive absorption of sorbitol. Br J Anesth 87:316–319, 2001

MORBID OBESITY

Allan P. Reed, MD

A 28-year-old woman weighing 300 pounds (136 kg) and standing 5 feet 5 inches (165 cm) presents for bariatric surgery. She has a history of diabetes mellitus, hypertension, and obstructive sleep apnea.

QUESTIONS

1. How is morbid obesity (MO) defined?
2. Name the diseases associated with MO.
3. Describe the pathophysiology of obstructive sleep apnea.
4. How is obstructive sleep apnea diagnosed?
5. Outline the effect of MO on functional residual capacity.
6. Is MO an indication for awake intubation?
7. What special equipment does the anesthesiologist require to anesthetize patients for bariatric surgery?
8. Describe an anesthetic plan for bariatric surgery.

1. How is morbid obesity (MO) defined?

Morbid obesity is defined in terms of body mass index (BMI). BMI is calculated by establishing a ratio between the patient's weight and height as follows:

Body mass index (BMI) = weight in kg/height in m^2

This patient's BMI is calculated as:

$$BMI = 136 \text{ kg}/(1.65 \text{ m})^2 = 50$$

BMI values are classified as follows:

- BMI of 18.5–24.9 = normal
- BMI of 25.0–29.9 = overweight
- BMI of 30.0–34.9 = class I obesity
- BMI of 35.0–39.9 = class II obesity
- BMI of 40.0 or greater = class III obesity.

BMI values of 40 or greater are indications for bariatric surgery. Those with significant comorbidities become acceptable candidates for bariatric surgery at a BMI value of 35.

2. Name the diseases associated with MO.

MO typically affects multiple organ systems. The respiratory system frequently develops upper and lower airway problems. Upper airway issues include various degrees of upper airway obstruction and obstructive sleep apnea. Lower airway problems manifest as restrictive lung disease, atelectasis, and obesity hypoventilation syndrome. One or more of these problems can result in hypoxemia. Frequently, this occurs during sleep. Hypoxic episodes lead to sympathetic discharge and arousal. When this cycle recurs several times during the night, restful sleep becomes interrupted and patients suffer from daytime somnolence,

TABLE 39.1	Comorbidities Associated with Morbid Obesity
Respiratory system	Restrictive lung disease
	Obstructive sleep apnea
	Obesity hypoventilation syndrome
Cardiovascular system	Systemic and/or pulmonary hypertension
	Ischemic heart disease
	Pulmonary embolus
	Congestive heart failure
Central nervous system	Cerebrovascular accidents
Endocrine system	Diabetes mellitus
Gastrointestinal system	Hiatus hernia
Musculocutaneous system	Osteoarthritis
Malignancies	Breast
	Prostate
	Uterus
	Colon and rectum

irritability, impaired cognition, and reduced concentration. They are accident-prone and frequently suffer trauma, which brings them to the operating room.

Cardiovascular diseases such as hypertension, coronary artery disease, dysrhythmias, pulmonary artery hypertension, right ventricular hypertrophy, right ventricular failure, left ventricular hypertrophy, left ventricular failure, and pulmonary emboli occur frequently. Hypoxemia exacerbates many of the cardiovascular problems. Cerebrovascular accidents, diabetes mellitus, and hiatus hernia occur frequently. Surgery is frequently required for arthritis of weight-bearing joints or malignancies. MO patients have a high incidence of malignancies originating in the breasts, prostate, uterus, cervix, colon, and rectum (Table 39.1).

3. Describe the pathophysiology of obstructive sleep apnea.

Under normal circumstances breaths are initiated by contraction of the diaphragm and intercostal muscles, thereby increasing the thoracic size. Negative pleural pressure results and is transmitted from the lower airways to the pharynx. The pharynx consists of mucosa and soft tissues that lack bony attachments, allowing them to move readily. Negative pressure in the pharynx draws these tissues into its lumen, as if the pharynx were imploding. If unopposed, upper airway obstruction would result. Compensation for such soft tissue movement is accomplished by constricting the upper airway dilator muscles,

which maintain upper airway patency. Upper airway dilator muscles include the tensor palatini, which brings the soft palate off the nasopharyngeal wall, the genioglosssus, which advances the tongue off the oropharyngeal wall, and the hyoid muscles, which move the epiglottis off the laryngopharyngeal wall. During sleep, MO patients lose control of their upper airway dilator muscles and upper airway obstruction results.

4. How is obstructive sleep apnea diagnosed?

The first clinical indicator of obstructive sleep apnea, loud snoring, is frequently reported by the patient's sleeping partner. Definitive diagnosis is obtained by sleep studies, which look for apnea and hypopnea. Apnea is the total cessation of gas flow through the airway, despite attempts to breathe. Hypopnea is reduction of gas flow through the airway while breathing. Diagnostic criteria generally include five or more episodes of apnea lasting 10 seconds or more, associated with a 4% decrease in oxygen saturation by pulse oximetry (SpO_2). Other criteria include 15 or more episodes of hypopnea attaining at least a 50% decrease in flow lasting 10 seconds or longer, and associated with a 4% decrease in SpO_2.

Although most patients with obstructive sleep apnea are morbidly obese, many lean patients suffer from this problem. It tends to occur in middle-aged and elder adults. Obstructive sleep apnea may be exacerbated by sedatives, hypnotics, alcohol, or muscle relaxants. Young patients with craniofacial abnormalities sometimes manifest obstructive sleep apnea, also.

5. Outline the effect of MO on functional residual capacity.

MO reduces functional residual capacity (FRC). During the course of normal tidal ventilation, the lung inflates and deflates. During exhalation of a normal tidal volume the lung deflates partially, but much of it remains inflated. The amount of gas remaining in the lung after expiration of a normal tidal volume is the FRC. Normally, the FRC maintains lung inflation above the closing volume. Closing volume is that lung volume at which terminal air units collapse. Reduced FRC associated with MO allows the lungs to deflate and reach closing volume during exhalation. The result is alveolar collapse, ventilation/perfusion mismatching, and hypoxemia.

FRC is further reduced in the supine position and by paralysis. Consequently, MO patients are at increased risk for hypoxemia during anesthesia and surgery.

6. Is MO an indication for awake intubation?

Neither absolute body weight nor absolute BMI are independent indicators for awake intubation. The vast majority of MO patients undergo rapid sequence induction with cricoid pressure. Obesity is a recognized predictor of difficult mask ventilation, so another supraglottic airway device may be needed to provide oxygenation if intubation fails. Typically, laryngeal mask airways (LMAs) are used for this purpose, but any one of a number of alternatives is a reasonable choice. The ProSeal LMA offers certain advantages over other devices. It could divert regurgitated gastric contents away from the larynx and provides the potential for passing a gastric tube into the stomach. LMAs and other supraglottic airway devices remain relatively contraindicated for elective use in MO patients, but are acceptable choices for emergency use.

The need for awake intubation is determined by the airway examination. When traditional predictors of difficult intubation exist, awake intubation may be a good alternative. Occasionally, a patient's neck may be so fat that thyromental distance, hyomental distance, and sternomental distance cannot be assessed. In such cases, this author prefers flexible fiberoptic intubation with the patient awake and spontaneously breathing.

7. What special equipment does the anesthesiologist require to anesthetize patients for bariatric surgery?

Most operating room tables are rated for 250 pounds (115 kg). Placing patients whose weight exceeds this limit on a standard table risks collapse and harm to the patient. Specially designed operating room tables that support heavier patients are recommended. The operating room table should also be equipped with a motor to change table positions. Traditional hand cranks do not offer enough mechanical advantage to adjust table positions and frequently break under heavier loads.

Ramps are recommended to achieve optimal sniffing position. These ramps are created by placing folded blankets under the patient's shoulders, neck, and occiput. The idea is to bring the patient's chin to a higher point than the chest. Without ramps, a MO patient lying supine will often be positioned with the chin in close proximity to the chest, creating two problems. First, the mouth opening is reduced, thereby limiting space in the mouth for a laryngoscope blade and tracheal tube. Also, the assistant's hand providing cricoid pressure takes up space needed to open the mouth and exacerbates the problem. Second, as the laryngoscope is placed in the mouth and directed over the chin, it contacts the chest. In other words, the chest occupies space needed to position the laryngoscope and becomes an obstruction to laryngoscope placement. Ramps allow the chest to fall below the space needed to place a laryngoscope, thereby avoiding this problem.

Previously, large blood pressure cuffs were recommended for all MO patients. These often gave inconsistent measurements necessitating intra-arterial blood pressure monitoring. Additionally, MO patients frequently have conical-shaped arms that prevent proper positioning of the blood pressure cuff. When deflated, the cuff tends to slip distally, covering the elbow and forearm. More recently, normal-sized blood pressure cuffs have been used on the forearm for MO patients. This technique generally gives consistent readings that are closely matched to those of indwelling arterial catheters.

A wide range of airway equipment is required. Among the numerous supraglottic airway devices that exist, several should be available. Although medium facemasks fit most patients, some MO patients will require large facemasks. It is best to have several sizes of oral airways. Available models include single hard plastic molded types, traditional Guedel types, and adjustable Chou airways. LMAs and esophageal-tracheal Combitubes are the more traditional fallback supraglottic devices. Newer devices include pharyngeal airways, EZ tubes, Cobras, laryngotracheal tubes (LTs), and many more. Although tracheostomy sets come within the surgeon's purview, they should be readily available also. Numerous laryngoscope blades and sizes may be applicable to MO patients, but in this author's experience almost everyone can be intubated with a Macintosh 3 or Miller 2 blade. Additional possibilities include a Bullard laryngoscope, Wu Scope, Glidescope, and flexible fiberoptic laryngoscope. Stylets help guide tracheal tubes into the larynx. Although semirigid models are the most commonly used in the United States, specially designed malleable stylets that extend beyond the tracheal tube tip are helpful. They include the 'Reusch' stylet and gummed elastic bougie.

Neuromuscular blockade monitors guide administration of muscle relaxants and help determine extubation criteria at the end of surgery. Anesthesia machines equipped with air are important to avoid using nitrous oxide, which distends the bowel. One hundred percent oxygen predisposes to oxygen toxicity, which is avoided by diluting oxygen in air. Continuous infusion pumps are optional, depending on the anesthetic technique planned. Orogastric tubes are needed to decompress the stomach prior to insertion of trochars and to evacuate the stomach prior to surgical manipulation. Warming blankets help prevent heat loss to the environment during laparotomy and to cold gases that are insufflated into the peritoneum during laparoscopy.

Following surgery, patients who are unable to move themselves to the next bed need to be transported to it. Several people working together can lift the patient, but using an inflatable air mattress makes the job much easier. The bed to which they are moved must be extra large and rated for the patient's weight. The bed's back should be capable of rising, allowing for the sitting or semi-Fowler's position. For the postanesthesia care unit, large chairs rated for the patient's weight are also desirable.

8. Describe an anesthetic plan for bariatric surgery.

Patient preparation begins well before entering the operating room. Preoperative functional status of the upper airway, lower airway, and cardiovascular system help predict perioperative outcome and should be assessed. Although controversial, some form of aspiration prophylaxis is commonly administered. Often this is simply a non-particulate antacid by mouth, just prior to entering the operating room. Most patients walk into the operating room and lie down on the operating room table. Intravenous access is frequently difficult, but rarely requires central venous cannulation. Large blood pressure cuffs are useful for many patients, but for others large cuffs slide distally and become unreliable. In such cases, normal-sized cuffs are placed on the forearm. Infrequently, intra-arterial cannulation is required for blood pressure measurements. Standard electrocardiogram electrodes and pulse oximeter probes generally work well on MO patients.

Preoxygenation is achieved employing an anesthesia facemask with an airtight seal. Three vital capacity breaths or 3 minutes of tidal breathing is rarely sufficient. Effective preoxygenation requires varying amounts of time, depending on several factors. A clinically useful endpoint for preoxygenation is an expired oxygen concentration of 90% or above.

Although some might argue it is unnecessary, anesthesia is generally begun with a rapid sequence induction, utilizing cricoid pressure. Any one of multiple induction agents can be administered. Determining induction doses based on total body weight may result in overdosing, while selecting induction doses predicated on ideal body weight can result in underdosing. For most agents, dosing is predicated on lean body mass. As a rule of thumb, lean body mass frequently approximates 100 kg in men and 80 kg in women. Actual doses of induction agents are modified based on myocardial reserves. Succinylcholine is an excellent choice for laryngoscopy, although nondepolarizing neuromuscular blockers can be used as well. A Macintosh 3 blade or a Miller 2 blade provides adequate laryngoscopic views in most patients and is a good way to start out. Tracheal tubes of various sizes are prepared with one or more stylets.

Just about any anesthetic agent or adjuvant can be used for bariatric patients. Since the goal is to have them awake and extubated at the end of surgery, short-acting agents are preferable. The duration of action of midazolam and its active metabolite often extends into the emergence phase, thereby delaying awakening, and in combination with opioids depresses respiration. For these reasons, midazolam seems to be counterproductive as an anesthetic adjuvant during bariatric surgery. Muscle relaxants are necessary for laparotomy and helpful for laparoscopy. Opioids are useful as anesthetic adjuvants and required for postoperative analgesia. Even laparoscopy patients suffer from significant abdominal wall soreness and benefit from analgesia. Air is used instead of nitrous oxide to avoid bowel distention. Potent inhalation agents are generally used.

MO patients are prone to soft tissue infections, necessitating antibiotic prophylaxis. Two grams of cephalosporin or equivalent is commonly administered intravenously prior to incision. The stomach is decompressed before inserting trochars to help prevent gastric damage by these sharp instruments. Additionally, the evacuated stomach takes up less space in the abdomen, thereby providing improved surgical vision and facilitates manipulations of the organ. Forced-air warming blankets help prevent heat loss during laparotomy and laparoscopy.

For lean patients, intraoperative tidal volumes are generally based on weight. To do so for MO patients results in excessive tidal volumes and very high inspiratory pressures. In fact, selection of tidal volume should be predicated on patient height. As a general rule of thumb, short patients do well with tidal volumes approximating 500 ml and tall patients do well with tidal volumes approximating 700 ml. Although these starting points are adequate for many MO patients, they should be adjusted depending upon the individual's requirements. Selecting a tidal volume must account for oxygenation, ventilation, and inspiratory pressures. Some authors advocate larger tidal volumes as prophylaxis against intraoperative decreases in FRC, that often result in hypoxemia. This was challenged by Sprung et al. (2003), who showed that large tidal volumes did not improve oxygenation during laparoscopy. An alternative to large tidal volumes is the use of positive end expiratory pressure (PEEP). PEEP can improve oxygenation, but tends to increase inspiratory pressures, predisposing to pneumothorax, and decreases venous return to the heart, resulting in decreased blood pressures.

Emergence and extubation are critically important. At the completion of surgery, bariatric patients still suffer from the same preoperative problems with which they started, plus others. Residual anesthetic agents depress respiratory drive and diminish upper airway dilator muscle efficiency. Lingering muscle weakness impairs coughing and deep breathing, as well as interfering with upper airway dilator muscle function. Abdominal wall pain from laparotomy or abdominal wall soreness from laparoscopy predispose to splinting and all its associated problems. Consequently, MO patients are at risk for hypoxemia in the postoperative period. To prevent this problem, those who do not meet extubation criteria remain intubated and ventilated postoperatively. Those who satisfy extubation criteria are extubated and given supplemental oxygen to breathe by nasal cannula or facemask. They are nursed in the upright position to help restore FRC and ventilation/perfusion matching.

SUGGESTED READINGS

Benumof JL: Obstructive sleep apnea in the adult obese patient: implications for airway management. J Clin Anesth 13:144, 2001

Brodsky JB, Lemmens HJM, Brock-Utne JG, Vierra M, Saidman LJ: Morbid obesity and tracheal intubation. Anesth Analg 94:732, 2002

Donati F: Tracheal intubation: unconsciousness, analgesia and muscle relaxation. Can J Anesth 50:99, 2003

National Institutes of Health; National Heart, Lung, and Blood Institute: Clinical guidelines on the identification, evaluation, and treatment of overweight and obesity in adults: the evidence report. www.nhlbi.hih.gov/guidelines/obesity/ob_gdlns.pdf

Sprung J, Whalley DG, Falcone T, Wilks W, Navratil JE, Bourke DL: The effects of tidal volume and respiratory rate on oxygenation and respiratory muscle mechanics during laparoscopy in morbidly obese patients. Anesth Analg 97:268, 2003

40

LAPAROSCOPY

Ilene K. Michaels, MD

A 32-year-old woman 157 cm tall, weighing 80 kg presents for a diagnostic laparoscopy because of a history of right-sided abdominal pain. A gynecologic and general surgeon will be performing the operation.

QUESTIONS

1. What procedures are amenable to the laparoscopic technique?
2. How is laparoscopy initiated?
3. Why is carbon dioxide (CO_2) the gas used for insufflation?
4. What are the cardiovascular changes associated with laparoscopic surgery?
5. What are the regional circulatory changes that occur during laparoscopy?
6. What are the pulmonary effects associated with laparoscopic surgery?
7. What are the benefits of laparoscopic surgery?
8. What are the complications of laparoscopic surgery?
9. What anesthetic techniques can be used for laparoscopic surgery?
10. What is the controversy regarding the use of nitrous oxide?
11. What is the etiology and treatment of post-laparoscopy pain?

1. What procedures are amenable to the laparoscopic technique?

Since the late 1980s, less invasive surgical methods have taken the place of traditional "open" operations, significantly reducing the risks of morbidity and mortality. These new procedures are being performed on patients of all ages. They do not come without a price, however; altered changes in cardiovascular and pulmonary dynamics are inherent in the laparoscopic approach and the benefits must be weighed against the risks. Awareness of the physiologic changes that occur during laparoscopy will enable us to further improve the outcomes of these operations.

The following is a list of the most commonly performed laparoscopic surgical procedures:

Intra-abdominal:

- Cholecystectomy
- Vagotomy
- Appendectomy
- Colectomy
- Inguinal hernia repair
- Adrenalectomy
- Nephrectomy
- Prostatectomy
- Pancreatectomy
- Bariatric surgery
- Nissen fundoplication

- Para-esophageal hernia repair
- Splenectomy
- Liver resection
- Cystectomy with ileal conduit

Gynecologic

- Ectopic pregnancy
- Ovarian cystectomy
- Reversal of ovarian torsion
- Salpingo-oophorectomy
- Hysterectomy
- Myomectomy
- Sacrocolpopexy
- Lymphadenectomy, staging
- Ablation of endometriosis

2. How is laparoscopy initiated?

The most frequent surgical complications are associated with the creation of the initial pneumoperitoneum. Being familiar with the surgical technique enables one to better anticipate these untoward events.

Carbon dioxide (CO_2) is insufflated through a Veress needle, which is blindly inserted just beneath the umbilicus into the peritoneal cavity. Confirmation of intraperitoneal placement of the Veress needle may be done in several ways. Firstly, the "pop" of piercing fascia and peritoneum may be appreciated. This is the most "unscientific" of the approaches, yet probably the most common method used. Secondly, a drop of water may be left on the hub of the Veress needle. As the peritoneum is entered, the negative pressure that exists within the cavity will "suck in" the drop. This is said to be the safest of the methods described. Lastly, after insertion of the Veress needle, on initial insufflation, the intraperitoneal pressures should not be greater than 8–9 mmHg. Once insufflation begins, percussion of air in the abdomen is a promising sign. An abrupt, very high increase in abdominal pressure with the onset of gas flow may signify extraperitoneal insufflation. A "Hassan" mini-laparotomy technique has been advocated for pneumoperitoneum creation to avoid the injuries associated with the blind Veress needle insertion. An electronic variable-flow insufflator terminates flow when a preset intra-abdominal pressure of 12–15 mmHg has been reached. A cannula, or trocar, is then inserted in place of the needle. A video laparoscope is inserted through the cannula, and the operative field is visualized via the camera and monitoring systems.

3. Why is carbon dioxide (CO_2) the gas used for insufflation?

Many gases have been utilized to create the pneumoperitoneum to facilitate the exposure necessary for surgical laparoscopy. These gases include helium, argon, nitrous oxide (N_2O), and CO_2. Each gas has problems associated with its use. Nitrous oxide supports combustion. Helium and argon are insoluble and are more likely to be associated with adverse events following embolic phenomena. CO_2 provides the safest profile. It is safe during electrocautery and laser surgery and can easily be eliminated through the lungs. Additionally, CO_2 is rapidly absorbed into the bloodstream. Its absorption is greater during extraperitoneal insufflation (laparoscopic inguinal hernia repair) compared with intraperitoneal insufflation. Extraperitoneal insufflation occurs when gas accumulates accidentally in the subcutaneous tissues or in the potential space between the fascia and the peritoneum, as is the goal for inguinal hernia repair. This absorption proves beneficial if moderate hypercapnia is maintained because the resulting cardiovascular stimulation helps to offset some of the hemodynamic burden imposed by the pneumoperitoneum. However, intraoperative hypercapnia is not completely benign. In patients with poor reserve (i.e., ischemic heart disease), whose arterial CO_2 ($PaCO_2$) levels approach 55–65 mmHg, there is a significant increase in systolic blood pressure, heart rate, and cardiac output. Hypercarbia causes sympathetic nervous system stimulation as manifest by a 2- to 3-fold increase in plasma catecholamine concentrations. When the $PaCO_2$ is >65 mmHg, cardiodepressive effects predominate with possible cardiovascular collapse or fatal dysrhythmias. Hypercapnia also causes pulmonary vasoconstriction that may worsen right ventricular ischemia or pulmonary hypertension. Patients with increased intracranial pressure may also be adversely affected by increases in $PaCO_2$.

End-tidal CO_2 ($ETCO_2$) provides an estimation of $PaCO_2$ levels. In relatively healthy individuals, the $PaCO_2$–$ETCO_2$ gradient approximates 3–5 mmHg, and is not affected during short laparoscopic procedures. However, in patients with severe cardiopulmonary disease or in prolonged operations, the $PaCO_2$–$ETCO_2$ gradient increases in an unpredictable manner and the usual $PaCO_2$–$ETCO_2$ relationship may be lost.

Not all increases in $PaCO_2$ result from increased absorption. Absorption is responsible for the increases in $PaCO_2$ that occur initially, until a plateau level is reached 15–30 minutes after the onset of gas insufflation. Any significant increases thereafter require a search for the cause. The differential diagnosis of hypercarbia is:

- Absorption of CO_2
- Hypoventilation
- Increased dead space
- CO_2 embolism
- Pneumothorax, pneumomediastinum, pneumopericardium
- Subcutaneous emphysema
- Exhausted CO_2 absorber
- Unidirectional valve dysfunction
- Malignant hyperthermia

4. **What are the cardiovascular changes associated with laparoscopic surgery?**

Although laparoscopic surgery is tolerated well by most, it may produce adverse consequences in those with limited cardiac reserve. The hemodynamic changes occurring during laparoscopy result from the combined effects of:

- Pneumoperitoneum
- Systemic absorption of CO_2
- Patient positioning

Mechanical Effects of the Pneumoperitoneum

Cardiovascular changes are proportional to the intra-abdominal pressure (IAP) attained. Peritoneal insufflation to IAPs >10 mmHg induces significant alterations in hemodynamics. As IAP increases, the cardiovascular changes associated with the pneumoperitoneum are biphasic in nature. Cardiac output decreases to 50% of preoperative levels 5 minutes after the onset of CO_2 insufflation and then gradually increases back toward baseline 10 minutes after the onset of insufflation.

Increased IAP causes compression of the abdominal arterial and venous vessels. Aortic compression contributes to an increase in systemic vascular resistance (SVR), which may result in a decrease in cardiac output. A second cause of increased SVR is compression of the splanchnic circulation, in both the venous and arterial systems. The effect of an increase in SVR on cardiac output is dependent upon the patient's volume status. A modest fall is seen in normovolemic patients, with a more pronounced fall in hypovolemic patients. Neurohumoral factors, such as circulating catecholamines, renin/angiotensin, and vasopressin, may also influence the cardiovascular response to the pneumoperitoneum.

Venous compression causes a decrease in venous return, and a consequent decrease in preload. Paradoxically, central venous pressure (CVP) and pulmonary capillary occlusion pressure (PCOP) rise during insufflation. This increase is secondary to a cephalad shift of the diaphragm due to increased intra-abdominal contents and pressure. This translates into increased intrathoracic pressures. Consequently, pressures obtained by transvenous catheters may not be reflective of true volume status. Increasing the circulating volume prior to establishment of the pneumoperitoneum may attenuate the decreases in venous return and cardiac output.

Dysrhythmias, more commonly bradycardias or asystole, occur most often during early insufflation. This may be the result of sudden stretching of the peritoneum with an abrupt increase in vagal tone. If treatment is necessary, vagolytic drug therapy and decreasing the IAP are often helpful.

The induction of the pneumoperitoneum has the least consequences if done with the patient in the level, supine position.

Effects of the Absorption of CO_2

The absorption of CO_2 has effects at various sites in the body, often with opposing results. The direct effects are initially inhibitory causing decreases in heart rate, contractility, and SVR. Counteracting these effects is the stimulation of the sympathetic nervous system, causing increases in heart rate, contractility, and SVR. If acidosis should develop, the parasympathetic effect may be enhanced.

Tachycardias and premature ventricular contractions resulting from CO_2 are usually benign, yet in the presence of severe hypercapnia, may be fatal. This hypercapnia may potentiate the vagal stimulation associated with peritoneal insufflation and can produce bradydysrhythmias or asystolic arrest.

The Hemodynamic Effects of Patient Positioning

The site of surgery determines the patient's position during laparoscopic surgery. The Trendelenburg position is used for pelvic and inframesocolic procedures (e.g., ovarian cystectomy or appendectomy); the reverse Trendelenburg position is used for supramesocolic operations (e.g., cholecystectomy). These positions may contribute to the hemodynamic changes associated with laparoscopic procedures.

The cardiovascular effects of the Trendelenburg position are multifactorial. The changes associated with this position are related to the degree of head-down tilt, patient's age, intravascular volume status, associated cardiac disease, ventilation techniques and anesthetic drugs. In the healthy patient, the Trendelenburg position favors venous return and improves cardiac output. If intact baroreceptor responses are maintained, compensatory responses are activated, and there is a decrease in heart rate and vasodilation. With all reflexes intact, the overall effect of the Trendelenburg position is insignificant. However, in patients with coronary artery disease, the increase in central blood volume is associated with a deleterious increase in myocardial oxygen demand as the ventricular volume is increased.

The reverse Trendelenburg position results in a decrease in venous return that is reflected as a decrease in mean arterial pressure and cardiac output. In healthy patients, the reduction in cardiac output is insignificant. In those with pre-existing cardiac disease, these changes may not be benign. The already diminished cardiac output may be lessened further, reducing already compromised end-organ perfusion.

The lateral tilt has minimal hemodynamic effects. It may occasionally counteract the adverse effects of the reverse Trendelenburg position. Extreme right lateral positioning may obstruct the vena cava, decreasing venous return.

In summary, the alterations in cardiovascular function are dependent on the patient's status (intravascular volume, pre-existing disease, neurohumoral factors) and surgical factors (IAP, patient position, CO_2 absorption, ventilation strategy, nature and duration of the procedure).

5. What are the regional circulatory changes that occur during laparoscopy?

Cerebral

Laparoscopy causes an increase in intracranial pressure (ICP). Firstly, the absorption of CO_2 and the resultant hypercarbia cause an increase in cerebral blood flow and consequently ICP. Secondly, the pneumoperitoneum increases ICP, with or without an increase in $PaCO_2$. The increase in IAP determines the extent of increase in ICP. High IAP compresses the inferior vena cava causing an increase in lumbar spinal pressure, which decreases drainage of cerebrospinal fluid from the lumbar plexus. In turn, there is decreased cerebrospinal fluid drainage and increased ICP. This increase is unresponsive to hyperventilation, yet ICP is higher when ventilation is inadequate. High IAP also causes a cephalad shift of the diaphragm, increasing intrathoracic pressure, also increasing ICP.

Hepatoportal

There is controversy in the literature regarding the effects of increased IAP on splanchnic perfusion. Some believe that the CO_2 pneumoperitoneum causes vasodilating effects that counteract the effects of increased IAP on perfusion. Others believe that there is a decrease in splanchnic flow that results both from mechanical compression of the mesenteric vasculature and from humoral factors, i.e., antidiuretic hormone causing superior mesenteric artery constriction.

Renal

There is a decrease in renal blood flow when IAP >15 mmHg. There is a decline in glomerular filtration rate (GFR), urine output, creatinine clearance, sodium excretion, and the potential for volume overload in the face of excessive fluid administration. Patients with pre-existing renal dysfunction should have optimization of their hemodynamics during pneumoperitoneum and the use of nephrotoxic drugs should be avoided.

Lower limb

The development of pneumoperitoneum causes a decrease in femoral venous flow increasing the risk of deep vein thrombosis. This is especially problematic if the patient is placed in the reverse Trendelenburg position because of blood pooling in the lower extremities. Intermittent sequential compression stockings should be used.

6. What are the pulmonary effects associated with laparoscopic surgery?

Many components of laparoscopic surgery adversely affect pulmonary function. The increased IAP and volume produced by the pneumoperitoneum elevate the diaphragm, decreasing lung capacities (especially functional residual capacity (FRC)), increasing pulmonary airway pressures, and decreasing pulmonary compliance. The healthy individual may remain unaffected by these conditions; however, the obese or those with pre-existing pulmonary disease may exhibit compromised pulmonary function. The increases in airway pressures are most problematic in those with bullous lung disease. At pressures >40 cm H_2O, these patients are at risk for bleb rupture and pneumothorax. To adjust for these increases one must either decrease the tidal volume, inspiratory flow rate, or liters per minute of fresh gas flow, or ask the surgeons to decrease the IAP.

The Trendelenburg position predisposes to worsening pulmonary compliance and V̇/Q̇ mismatch. The pneumoperitoneum and shift of the abdominal contents cephalad both increase atelectasis and increase the risk of right mainstem endobronchial intubation. The latter occurs as a result of cephalad movement of the carina. Conversely, the reverse Trendelenburg position is beneficial for lung mechanics.

Desaturation is not infrequent during laparoscopy. The differential diagnosis of hypoxemia is as follows:

- Pre-existing conditions: morbid obesity, chronic obstructive pulmonary disease
- Hypoventilation: positioning, pneumoperitoneum, endotracheal tube obstruction, inadequate ventilation
- Intrapulmonary shunting: decreased FRC, endobronchial intubation, pneumothorax
- Decreased cardiac output: hemorrhage, dysrhythmias, myocardial depression
- Technical equipment failure: circuit disconnect, delivery of hypoxic gas mixture

Laparoscopic surgery can reduce postoperative pulmonary complications by avoiding the restrictive pattern of breathing that usually follows open upper abdominal surgery. Atelectasis is more common and more severe in patients who undergo open surgery. Not only are the spirometric measures of lung function preserved, but also global respiratory strength is greater 24 and 48 hours after laparoscopic surgery than after open cholecystectomy. The use of epidural anesthesia to supplement general anesthesia does not improve lung function after the open operation.

7. What are the benefits of laparoscopic surgery?

The benefits of laparoscopic surgery are:

- Decreased postoperative respiratory dysfunction
- Decreased postoperative pain
- Decreased analgesic use and sequelae: lethargy, nausea, vomiting and constipation
- Decreased postoperative ileus and adhesions resulting from less bowel exposure and manipulation
- Earlier ambulation
- Shorter hospital stays
- More rapid return to normal activities
- Reduced metabolic response, e.g., ↓hyperglycemia
- Possibly preserved immune response and nitrogen balance

8. What are the complications of laparoscopic surgery?

The complications associated with laparoscopic surgery are:

- Overall mortality rate 0.1–1.0 per 1,000 cases
- Postoperative nausea and vomiting (40–75% of patients)
- Shoulder pain
- Bowel perforation 0.06–0.4% with a mortality rate of 5%
- Bladder/ureter injuries 2 per 10,000 cases
- Vascular injuries
- Gynecologic injuries 0.64%
- Gastrointestinal, urologic injuries 0.03–0.06%
- Significant hemorrhage in 2–9 per 1,000 cases, often delayed
- Nerve injuries from improper positioning: peroneal/femoral neuropathies, meralgia paresthetica
- Subcutaneous emphysema from extraperitoneal insufflation
- Pneumothorax, pneumomediastinum
- Venous gas embolism
- Volume overload from excessive fluid administration, decreased insensible losses and decreased urine production
- ↑ICP
- Deep vein thrombosis
- Increased risk of regurgitation from ↑IAP along with the Trendelenburg position

Subcutaneous Emphysema

Subcutaneous emphysema (SQE) is a known complication of laparoscopic surgery. It may occur as a result of accidental extraperitoneal insufflation or may be considered unavoidable in certain laparoscopic procedures that require intentional extraperitoneal insufflation, such as inguinal hernia repair. SQE is identified by the development of crepitus over the abdominal wall, excessive changes in airway pressures, or by increasing $ETCO_2$ concentrations over time.

When SQE does occur, the area for diffusion of CO_2 increases and this may lead to hypercarbia and respiratory acidosis.

In most cases, no specific intervention is necessary other than the discontinuation of N_2O, if it is being used. SQE resolves soon after deflation of the abdomen. However, as there exists a "continuum of fascial planes," SQE could potentially extend from the abdomen to the thorax and neck, resulting in pneumothorax or pneumomediastinum. If SQE is suspected, a chest radiograph should be obtained for confirmation. Although the treatment may not change, having the diagnosis is important for future management of untoward events, for example, cardiovascular collapse. The presence of SQE does not necessarily contraindicate extubation, yet it should be emphasized that it may predispose to laryngeal swelling, difficult spontaneous respirations, and difficult reintubation. It is recommended that controlled mechanical ventilation be maintained until hypercarbia is corrected to avoid the increase in work of breathing, especially in compromised patients.

Pneumothorax

Pneumothorax is a rare yet potentially life-threatening complication of laparoscopic surgery with increasing incidence over recent years as a result of an increasing number of procedures involving dissections at the esophageal junction (e.g., Nissen fundoplication). Pneumothorax occurs when gas traverses into the thorax, either through a tear in the visceral peritoneum, disruption of the parietal pleura during dissection around the esophagus, or through a congenital defect in the diaphragm. Pneumothorax may be asymptomatic or may be associated with hypotension or cardiac arrest resulting from the impairment of cardiac filling and limitation of lung excursion. When CO_2 pneumothorax occurs without pulmonary trauma, spontaneous resolution may occur within 30–60 minutes after abdominal deflation. If the pneumothorax is large or symptomatic, thoracocentesis should be performed without delay. N_2O, if used, should be discontinued and the IAP should be reduced. Ventilation should be adjusted to correct hypoxemia, applying positive end-expiratory pressure (PEEP) if necessary. If the pneumothorax results from trauma to the lung itself, PEEP should be avoided.

Venous Gas Embolism

A rare, yet potentially fatal complication of laparoscopy is that of venous gas embolism (VGE). The estimated incidence is 0.002–0.08%. When it occurs, it brings with it the potential for significant hemodynamic compromise. VGE develops most commonly during the first few minutes after the development of the pneumoperitoneum. This occurs more frequently in patients who have had prior abdominal surgery.

Gas bubbles enter the venous system via vessel tears in the abdominal wall or peritoneum and enter the heart and pulmonary circulation. When clinically significant, the right ventricular outflow tract is obstructed, producing a constellation of signs and symptoms: a "mill-wheel murmur," sudden hypotension, decrease in cardiac output, tachycardia or other dysrhythmias, pulmonary edema, hypoxemia, increased airway pressures, and jugular venous distention and facial plethora/cyanosis from inflow obstruction to the right heart. The $ETCO_2$ response is biphasic. Firstly, an initial increase in $ETCO_2$ occurs secondary to the pulmonary excretion of CO_2. Then, a decrease in $ETCO_2$ occurs because of a decrease in cardiac output and an increase in physiologic dead space. When this occurs, the N_2O should be discontinued (if being used), and the patient should be placed in the left lateral decubitus position, with steep head-down tilt to prevent entry of the bubbles into the pulmonary arterial circulation. The patient should be hyperventilated to eliminate CO_2. If a central venous catheter is in place, it should be aspirated in an attempt to remove gas emboli. Hyperbaric oxygen, cardiopulmonary bypass, and external cardiac massage are all measures that may be necessary in extreme situations.

9. What anesthetic techniques can be used for laparoscopic surgery?

General, regional, and local anesthesia have all been used successfully and safely for laparoscopy.

General Anesthesia

General anesthesia with endotracheal intubation and controlled ventilation is one of the more commonly used techniques. Here, the airway is protected and $ETCO_2$ can be controlled to levels approximating 35 mmHg. IAP and airway pressures should be monitored. IAP should be kept below 20 mmHg, ideally between 12 and 15 mmHg. Increases in IAP should be avoided by ensuring an adequately deep plane of anesthesia. The need for muscle relaxation is controversial. Peak inspiratory pressures >40 cm H_2O predispose to barotrauma and should be reported to the surgeon if they occur. This is of particular importance in those with pre-existing bullous disease or in those with a history of barotrauma. The management of increased peak airway pressures may involve decreasing intra-abdominal pressure, lessening the Trendelenburg positioning, and decreasing tidal volumes and inspiratory flow rates.

The laryngeal mask airway (LMA) is an alternative to endotracheal intubation. This device does not protect the airway from aspiration of gastric contents. Controlled ventilation and monitoring of $ETCO_2$ are possible. As peak airway pressures are frequently greater than 20 cmH_2O during these operations, there is no guarantee that the airway seal provided by the LMA will be preserved. Consequently, its use is strongly cautioned. If employed, it should be reserved for thin individuals without intrinsic increased risks for aspiration. In emergency situations, however, an airway maintained with an LMA is better than no airway at all.

Regional Anesthesia

Gynecologic laparoscopic procedures can be performed under spinal or epidural anesthesia. The advantage of regional anesthesia is the reduced need for sedatives and narcotics when compared with local anesthesia with supplemental sedation. However, shoulder tip pain and discomfort secondary to abdominal distention are incompletely alleviated under epidural anesthesia. A sensory block from T_4 to L_5 is needed and may also be uncomfortable. The hemodynamic effects of the pneumoperitoneum under epidural anesthesia have not been studied. It is necessary to have a cooperative and motivated patient, a skilled laparoscopist, and minimal IAPs and Trendelenburg positioning for this method to be successful. Patients considered a "full stomach" are not the best candidates for this technique. The increases in intra-abdominal and intragastric pressures along with the frequently used Trendelenburg positioning and the need for significant intravenous sedation all increase the risks of regurgitation and potential aspiration when the airway is unprotected.

Monitored Anesthesia Care

Local anesthesia with sedation offers several advantages compared with general anesthesia: quicker recovery, decreased incidence of postoperative nausea and vomiting, and fewer hemodynamic changes. The sequelae of general anesthesia, such as sore throat, muscle pain, and airway trauma, may also be avoided.

Success with local anesthesia also requires a relaxed, cooperative and motivated patient, a supportive operating room staff, and a skilled surgeon. Any laparoscopic procedure that requires multiple puncture sites, considerable organ manipulation, steep tilt, or extensive pneumoperitoneum should not be managed with this method. Diagnostic laparoscopy and sterilization procedures are two operations that may be performed under this technique.

10. What is the controversy regarding the use of nitrous oxide?

NO_2 is commonly used to provide amnesia, enhance analgesia, and to reduce the requirements of other inhaled or intravenous agents. When utilized during laparoscopic surgery, operative conditions have the potential to become suboptimal. Air-containing spaces (e.g., bowel loops) contain approximately 78% nitrogen and 21% oxygen. Because N_2O is 37 times more soluble in blood than is nitrogen, N_2O diffuses into these spaces faster than nitrogen leaves, resulting in intestinal distention, potentially impairing surgical access. This becomes of special consideration during the longer, mid/upper abdominal laparoscopic procedures (lysis of adhesions, colon resection). Many gynecologic surgeons have little difficulty performing lower pelvic surgery with N_2O as a component of the anesthetic.

11. What is the etiology and treatment of post-laparoscopy pain?

A major advantage of laparoscopic surgery compared with open procedures is the reduction in postoperative pain. However, pain is still a problem. The etiology of the pain is multifactorial and amenable to maneuvers that may decrease its incidence.

Pneumoperitoneum Factors

With insufflation, there is distention of the abdomen with a resultant phrenic nerve neuropraxia. A 20% stretch of the nerve results in occlusion of the endoneural vessels and consequent nerve ischemia. The greater the time the nerve has to adapt to the stretch, the less likely nerve injury will occur. The use of reduced insufflation rates and sub-diaphragmatically administered local anesthetics may aid in the reduction of pain.

The phrenic nerves may be damaged by the acid milieu created by the dissolution of CO_2 used for insufflation. Potential neural injury may be minimized by shorter exposure to the implicated gases.

If the insufflating gas is not evacuated adequately, the intra-abdominal acidosis and consequent irritation may persist for a prolonged period of time causing damage. Residual gas may also result in loss of peritoneal surface tension and support to the abdominal viscera, also contributing to postoperative pain. The greatest reduction in postoperative pain is seen when warmed, humidified gases are used.

Operative Factors

Local anesthesia administered into the incision sites before the wounds are created is believed by some, but not all, to be associated with significant reduction in postoperative pain. More commonly the wounds are injected with local anesthetic just prior to closure. Only small amounts of anesthetic are necessary for the small wounds associated with laparoscopic procedures and minimal side-effects are therefore expected. The use of local anesthetic infiltration is therefore recommended.

Anesthetic Factors

Nonsteroidal anti-inflammatory medications administered after the induction of anesthesia have useful opioid sparing and anti-inflammatory effects. Ibuprofen is a reasonable alternative to fentanyl in the reduction of both postoperative pain and nausea after outpatient procedures.

SUGGESTED READINGS

Cunningham AJ: Anesthetic implications of laparoscopic surgery. Yale J Biol Med 71:551–578, 1998

Efron DT, Bender JS: Laparoscopic surgery in older adults. J Am Geriatr Soc 49:658–663, 2001

Joris JL: Anesthesia for laparoscopic surgery. pp. 2003–2023. In Miller RD (ed): Anesthesia, 5th edition. Churchill Livingstone, Philadelphia, 2000

Joshi GP: Complications of laparoscopy. Anesthesiol Clin North Am 19:89–105, 2001

Mouton WG, Bessell JR, Otten KT, Maddern GJ: Pain after laparoscopy. Surg Endosc 13:445–448, 1999

O'Malley C, Cunningham AJ: Physiologic changes during laparoscopy. Anesthesiol Clin North Am 19: 1–19, 2001

Smith I: Anesthesia for laparoscopy with emphasis on outpatient laparoscopy. Anesthesiol Clin North Am 19:21–41, 2001

Wolf JS Jr: Pathophysiologic effects of prolonged laparoscopic operation. Semin Surg Oncol 12:86–95, 1996

CASE 41

CARCINOID SYNDROME

Barbara Alper, MD

A 38-year-old woman presents with flushing, diarrhea, and abdominal pain. Her past medical history is pertinent for ectopic pregnancy and hypothyroidism. Colonoscopy reveals a mass in the ileocolic region and increased levels of 5-hydroxyindoleacetic acid (5-HIAA) are found in the urine. A presumptive diagnosis of carcinoid syndrome is made and the patient admitted for laparotomy.

QUESTIONS

1. What are carcinoid tumors?
2. What is carcinoid syndrome?
3. In what locations do carcinoid tumors occur?
4. What are the major anesthetic concerns in patients with carcinoid syndrome?
5. What is the mechanism of action of somatostatin?
6. What precautions are prudent for anesthetizing patients with carcinoid syndrome?
7. How is chemoembolization used to treat metastatic carcinoid syndrome?

1. What are carcinoid tumors?

Carcinoid is a slow-growing tumor arising from enterochromaffin cells identified by silver staining of cytoplasmic granules within the cells. These cells release vasoactive substances, which have amine precursors. The substances include serotonin, prostaglandin, histamine, and kallikreinins. Histologically, carcinoid tumors that arise from the ileum demonstrate dense nests of cells with uniform size and nuclear appearance. Histochemically, they typically exhibit an argentaffin reaction in which the cells convert silver salts to a metallic silver color. A positive argentaffin reaction is not required for diagnosis. Tumors arising from the embryonic foregut usually contain few argentaffin cells.

Bronchogenic carcinoid can range from having typical carcinoid features to being indistinguishable from oat cell carcinoma of the lung. Tumors arising from the ileum or jejunum produce more common manifestations of carcinoid syndrome, such as cutaneous flushing, intestinal hypermobility, and hypotension caused by serotonin release. Tumors arising from the stomach usually tend to produce histamine, causing hypotension and less commonly wheezing. Carcinoid syndrome was originally thought to be due to serotonin and histamine only. These agents predominate in the syndrome; however, more recently other hormone and vasoactive polypeptides have been identified. The mediators include prostaglandins, bradykinins, tachykinins, adrenocorticotropic hormones, and vasoactive intestinal peptide (VIP). Serotonin is produced from tryptophan by a hydroxylation and decarboxylation reaction. It is broken down ultimately to 5-HIAA by the enzymes monoamine oxidase and alcohol dehydrogenase (Figure 41.1). The measurement of 5-HIAA in the urine is used to monitor the disease process clinically.

Histamine release is seen more commonly with foregut carcinoid tumors and is thought to cause bronchospasm associated with flushing. Serotonin causes vasodilation and vasoconstriction; therefore, both hypotension and hypertension can be seen. Serotonin has no effect on cardiac function itself at normal levels; however, at elevated levels it can cause positive chronotropic and inotropic responses. Other effects due to high serotonin levels are increased gut motility, and secretion of sodium chloride (NaCl), potassium (K^+), and water by the small intestine. Hyperglycemia can also occur from elevated adrenergic levels as well. Patients may exhibit prolonged effects from anesthesia with excessive postoperative drowsiness. Bradykinins can cause severe hypotension secondary to extreme vasomotor relaxation or vasodilation. Flushing can occur due to enhanced nitric oxide synthesis. Bronchospasm can follow, especially in patients with cardiac disease or asthmatics.

2. What is carcinoid syndrome?

Tumors of the small intestine, principally the ileum, which have metastasized to the liver, produce the syndrome. Carcinoid tumors in the liver present direct access of vasoactive substances to the circulation. The hormones secreted by primary gastrointestinal carcinoid tumors reach the liver by way of the portal vein where they are usually inactivated. Once metastases to the liver have occurred, hormones secreted by hepatic involvement have direct access to the systemic circulation, thus producing the signs and symptoms of the carcinoid syndrome. Serotonin, which is the most common substance producing carcinoid syndrome, can cause changes in the skin, gastrointestinal tract, respiratory tract, and heart. The most frequent clinical feature is cutaneous flushing. The typical flush is erythematous and involves the head and neck. The color may change from red to violet. Prolonged flushing may be associated with lacrimation and periorbital edema. This is the phenomenon known as the vasomotor paroxysmal syndrome.

Many patients with carcinoid tumors do not exhibit generalized symptoms of the syndrome. Only about 8% of patients with carcinoid tumors actually display the carcinoid syndrome itself. Seventy-five percent of these patients have cutaneous flushing, 67% have intestinal hypermotility leading to dehydration and metabolic acidosis. Forty-one percent have cardiac involvement, usually on the right side of the heart, most commonly the tricuspid or pulmonic valves. This is thought to be due to chronic serotonin stimulation of the endocardium. Tricuspid insufficiency is more common than pulmonic stenosis. The left-sided heart valves are usually spared, possibly due to pulmonary parenchymal cells, which inactivate vasoactive substances. Only 18% of patients with carcinoid syndrome present with wheezing. This is seen more frequently with gastric tumors. Some patients with carcinoid tumors may present with iron deficiency anemia from gastrointestinal bleeding

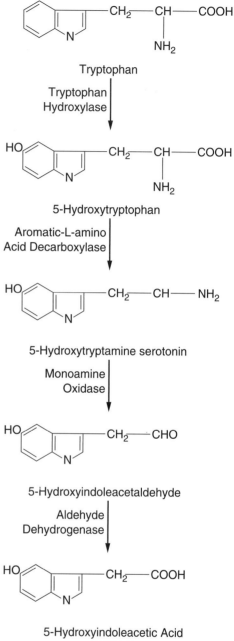

FIGURE 41.1   The metabolic pathway of serotonin.

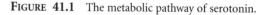

or vitamin B_{12} and folic acid deficiencies. Clotting disorders can also occur caused by malabsorption of the fat-soluble vitamins. In rare cases, pellagra can occur from niacin deficiency.

3. In what locations do carcinoid tumors occur?

Tumors most commonly arise from the embryonic midgut, i.e., small intestine – ileum, jejunum, with the highest incidence occurring in the appendix. Occasionally, these tumors arise from the foregut, i.e., the stomach, pancreas, thyroid, bronchus and from ovarian or testicular teratomas. Bronchogenic carcinoid is indistinguishable from undifferentiated small cell carcinoma of the lung. Pathologically, gastric tumors tend to produce histamine rather than serotonin-derived products, which are more common in tumors of the small intestine. Small cell tumors and bronchogenic carcinoid of the lung are associated with the syndrome of inappropriate antidiuretic hormone (SIADH). These patients commonly present with euvolemic hyponatremia. Treatment requires vasopressin, an antidiuretic hormone (ADH) inhibitor, secreted from the posterior pituitary gland. Chronic hyponatremia is common in these patients. Hyponatremia is particularly problematic for patients undergoing transurethral resection of the prostate (TURP). During TURP, absorption of glycine through the prostatic vascular bed can exacerbate the hyponatremia. Severe or acute hyponatremia can present with confusion and seizures.

The small intestine, particularly the ileum, is by far the most common site for carcinoid tumors of any clinical significance. These tumors tend to be small and tend to metastasize after reaching 2 cm in size. They have a strong tendency toward multicentricity, invading the mesentery and producing intermittent bowel obstruction, which is a common clinical presentation. As metastatic disease progresses, mesenteric lymph nodes become involved, and finally the liver. Bone is the next most frequent metastatic site. The more unusual metastatic locations include the breast, orbit of the eye, and the myocardium. Extrahepatic metastases occur in the bone where they tend to be osteoblastic rather than osteolytic. Tumors can also spread to the adrenal glands, ovaries, spleen, pancreas, and the lung.

Clinical Manifestations of Carcinoid Syndrome

Cutaneous flushing

Hypotension

Intestinal hypermotility
    Diarrhea
    Dehydration
    Metabolic acidosis

Cardiac involvement
    Tricuspid insufficiency
    Pulmonic stenosis
    Supraventricular tachycardia

Wheezing

Hyperglycemia

Iron deficiency anemia – gastrointestinal bleeding

Bowel obstruction

Vitamin B_{12} and folic acid deficiencies

Clotting disorders – malabsorption of fat-soluble vitamins

Pellagra – niacin deficiency

4. What are the major anesthetic concerns in patients with carcinoid syndrome?

Although carcinoid tumors are relatively rare, patients with this disease frequently have concurrent medical problems. Thirty percent have carcinoid heart disease. The cause is unclear. Right-sided fibrous plaque deposited on the tricuspid valve and right ventricular walls is the most common finding. Tricuspid regurgitation is the most common valvulopathy associated with carcinoid tumors. If the pulmonary valve is involved, stenosis rather than regurgitation is more prevalent. Carcinoid plaques are rarely found on the left side of the heart, but do occur.

Anesthetic concerns include right-sided heart failure and pulmonary hypertension. It is important to avoid increases in pulmonary vascular resistance to prevent hypoxemia. High-dose nitrous oxide may predispose to pulmonary hypertension. Patients with significant tricuspid regurgitation should be kept well hydrated and tachycardia should be avoided. These patients are more susceptible to supraventricular dysrhythmias as well. Endocarditis prophylaxis should be undertaken with a penicillin or variant, and under some circumstances an aminoglycoside. Treatment of hypotension with catecholamines may produce worse physiologic problems. Catecholamines stimulate secretion of substances from carcinoid tumors. Among these substances are mediators that produce hypotension and other components of the carcinoid syndrome. Consequently treatment of hypotension with catecholamines can produce a paradoxical exacerbation of hypotension.

Gastric carcinoid generally releases histamine, thus bronchospasm can occur, which does not respond well to β-agonists or aminophylline. It is prudent to avoid drugs which release histamine such as d-tubocurarine, atracurium, mivacurium, and morphine. H_1-blockers, H_2-blockers, and

Major Anesthetic Concerns in Patients With Carcinoid Syndrome

Hypotension
  Prevention
    Octreotide
    Prehydration
    Avoid catecholamines
  Treatment
    Volume infusion
    Phenylephrine
    Octreotide
    Angiotensin
    Avoid catecholamines

Bronchospasm
  Prevention
    Octreotide
    Avoid histamine-releasing drugs
      d-tubocurarine
      atracurium
      mivacurium
      morphine
    H_1-blockers, H_2-blockers, and steroids are
      unreliable
  Treatment
    Does not respond well to β-agonists or amino-
      phylline
    Octreotide

Hypertension
  Prevention
    Octreotide
  Treatment
    Octreotide
    Nitroglycerin
    Sodium nitroprusside

steroids have been used prophylactically to avoid severe reactions, but are unreliable. Succinylcholine should also be used with caution, as abdominal wall fasciculations can increase intra-abdominal pressure, thus squeezing the tumor causing further hormone release. Pretreatment with a nondepolarizing neuromuscular blocker can decrease fasciculations. If hypotension occurs intraoperatively it is important to give volume and avoid the use of catecholamines or β-agonists. The use of angiotensin in a dose of 1.5 mg/kg may improve hypotension. Prehydration is of great benefit in these patients as a generalized fluid deficit occurs due to secondary hormone release from the tumor. Invasive monitoring to assess cardiovascular status

is helpful in some patients with cardiac disease, due either to carcinoid or intrinsic myocardial disease itself. Acute intraoperative hypertension is often associated with bronchospasm, which is probably due to serotonin release. If hypertension occurs acutely, the use of vasodilating agents, such as nitroglycerin or sodium nitroprusside, is recommended.

5. What is the mechanism of action of somatostatin?

Octreotide is a synthetic analog of somatostatin, which is a natural growth inhibitor that also competitively inhibits release of several hormones. It decreases serotonin levels and relieves the symptoms of carcinoid syndrome. Somatostatin has been shown to suppress diarrhea associated with VIP tumors. It has a transient half-life; therefore, intravenous infusions are required for treatment of acute crises. For preoperative prophylaxis, octreotide 50–150 µg every 8 hours subcutaneously is recommended. If patients are on long-term therapy, the dose can be adjusted accordingly. Side-effects include ascending cholangitis or cholelithiasis because somatostatin inhibits gallbladder contractions. Other side-effects include nausea, vomiting, pain, diarrhea, and bradycardia. This occurs more commonly with larger doses. Symptoms are variable in different patients. Steatorrhea is occasionally observed, but this is generally mild and not associated with significant nutritional impairment. Somatostatin suppresses the response of leutinizing hormone (LH) to gonadotropic releasing hormone (GnRH). It decreases splanchnic blood flow and inhibits the release of serotonin, gastrin, VIP, and pancreatic polypeptide. VIP-omas tend to cause watery diarrhea rather than steatorrhea, which is common with metastatic carcinoid tumors. Octreotide reduces growth hormone levels in patients with acromegaly as well.

6. What precautions are prudent for anesthetizing patients with carcinoid syndrome?

The severity of the symptoms does not predict difficulties encountered during the anesthetic or complications that may follow. Patients with minor signs and symptoms may have significant intraoperative problems. 5-HIAA levels provide an indicator of the disease progression; however, they do not predict the physiologic response to tumor manipulation during surgery.

The anesthetic technique should minimize mediator release in response to the stress of induction, tracheal intubation, and emergence. It is prudent to premedicate patients with octreotide. If succinylcholine is used, a defasciculating dose of a nondepolarizer should be administered to prevent the increase in intra-abdominal pressure that can lead to squeezing of the tumor thereby releasing additional vasoactive polypeptide. Administration of topical local anesthetics or intravenous lidocaine helps prevent cate-cholamine responses to intubation and extubation. Cardiovascular instability, especially hypotension, is common, so that invasive monitoring such as arterial lines, central venous pressure monitoring, or pulmonary artery catheters may be necessary. Anesthetic maintenance should be performed with a nitrous oxide–narcotic technique to maintain hemodynamic stability.

7. How is chemoembolization used to treat metastatic carcinoid syndrome?

Selective hepatic artery chemoembolization has been used in patients with liver metastases from carcinoid syndrome for years. It provides palliation of symptoms from hormone-releasing tumors. Embolization-induced tumor ischemia improves the quality of life. The most promising chemotherapeutic agents to date include cisplatinum and doxorubicin. However, 5-fluorouracil (5-FU), mitomycin C, and adriamycin have been used in combination as well.

A recent study by Douglas et al. (1998) treated 15 patients with intra-arterial chemotherapy. Patients received 5 days of intra-arterial 5-FU 1 g/m^2 followed by adriamycin 60 mg/m^2, cisplatinum 100 mg, mitomycin C 30 mg, and polyvinyl alcohol (Invalim) 200–710 μm. Patients were given octreotide 150–2000 μg subcutaneously every 8 hours before, during, and after the procedure. Symptoms improved in 8 of 12 patients with diarrhea, in 9 of 12 patients with abdominal pain, in 7 of 12 patients with cutaneous flushing, and in 4 of 7 patients with malaise. Biochemical markers were followed up at 3 months. Improvement occurred in 60% for 5-HIAA levels, 75% for chromogranin A, and 50% for neuron nonspecific enolase titers. Follow-up was at 16 months with 13 deaths occurring from 1 week to 71 months after treatment. As for survival, chemoembolization with chemotherapy improved short-term quality of life and not long-term survival in patients with advanced hepatic carcinoid disease.

SUGGESTED READINGS

Douglas JG, Anthony LB, Blair TK, et al.: Hepatic artery chemoembolization for the management of patients with advanced metastatic carcinoid tumors. Am J Surg 5:408, 1998

Gerstle JT, Kauffman GL Jr., Koltum WA: The incidence, management and outcome of patients with gastrointestinal carcinoids and second primary malignances. J Am Coll Surg 180:427, 1995

Ruszniewski P, Malka D: Hepatic artery chemoembolization in the management of advanced digestive endocrine tumors. Digestion 62 [Suppl 1]:79, 2000

Vaughan DJ, Brunner MD: Anesthesia for patients with carcinoid syndrome. Int Anesthesiol. Clin 35:129, 1997

Venook AP: Embolization and chemoembolization therapy for neuroendocrine tumors. Curr Opin Oncol 11:38, 1999

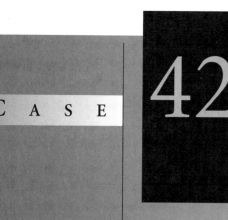

KIDNEY TRANSPLANTATION

Barbara Alper, MD

A 58-year-old obese man with non-insulin-dependent diabetes, hypertension, coronary artery disease, and end-stage renal disease presents for cadaveric kidney transplantation. His last hemodialysis was 2 days prior to admission.

QUESTIONS

1. How does diabetes affect renal transplantation?
2. Why is timing of hemodialysis important for renal transplantation?
3. Discuss the treatment of hyperkalemia and its associated metabolic problems.
4. What are the major anesthetic concerns for renal transplantation?
5. What are the implications of long ischemic times during renal transplantation?

1. How does diabetes affect renal transplantation?

Patients with Type I diabetes mellitus (juvenile or insulin-dependent) and end-stage renal disease (ESRD) are good renal transplantation candidates. Patients with Type II diabetes mellitus (adult onset or non-insulin-dependent) were not considered good candidates for renal transplantation until recently. In the past, less than 15% of these patients received renal allografts. Type II diabetes mellitus is associated with a higher incidence of vasculopathies, especially involving the renal arteries, which complicate graft anastomoses. With improved anesthetic and surgical techniques, graft survival rates for Type II diabetics with ESRD have improved dramatically. Non-insulin-requiring diabetes tends to occur in older patients as compared with Type I diabetes. Consequently, Type II diabetics frequently present with concomitant medical problems.

Previously, left ventricular dysfunction was also a contraindication to renal transplantation. However, uremic cardiomyopathy has been proven to be reversible with successful renal allografts.

2. Why is timing of hemodialysis important for renal transplantation?

By its very nature, cadaveric transplantation is more urgent than living donor transplantation. There is less preoperative time for preparation and planning with cadaveric versus living related donor transplantation. The potential for hyperkalemia is an important consideration. Morbidity and mortality is improved by hemodialysis within 24 hours of surgery. If potassium (K^+) levels are 6 mEq/L or greater, or if electrocardiogram (ECG) abnormalities exist, such as peaked T waves or cardiac dysrhythmias, it is prudent to perform dialysis prior to transplantation.

Intravascular volume overload is another important problem addressed by dialysis. Preoperative intravascular volume overload predisposes to congestive heart failure, which decreases cardiac output to the new kidney and complicates further volume loading used to prevent ischemia of the transplanted organ. An average of 3–5 liters of crystalloid is required before renal artery and vein anastomoses. Associated uremic pericarditis further complicates fluid management and is another indication for preoperative dialysis.

3. Discuss the treatment of hyperkalemia and its associated metabolic problems.

Patients with chronic renal failure experience an extraordinarily wide range of serum K^+ levels ranging from 2.5 to 6.0 mEq/L. Acute hyperkalemia suppresses electrical conduction and can ultimately cause cardiac arrest. Associated ECG changes include prolonged PR intervals, widened QRS complexes, and peaked T waves before ventricular fibrillation actually occurs. Fatal dysrhythmias may occur without these gradual changes.

Extracellular acidosis results in an increased concentration of hydrogen ion (H^+), which moves into the cell along its concentration gradient. To preserve electrical neutrality, K^+ moves out of the cell. In this way, extracellular acidosis promotes extracellular hyperkalemia. In acute metabolic acidosis, serum K^+ increases approximately 0.5–0.8 mEq/L for every drop in pH of 0.1 units. Normally the ratio of intracellular to extracellular K^+ concentration is approximately 40:1 or 160:4 mEq/L in vivo. This is maintained by an energy-dependent Na^+–K^+-ATPase pump at the cell membrane, which brings K^+ intracellularly against its concentration gradient.

In chronic renal failure patients, aggressive treatment of hyperkalemia is appropriate. The treatment for acute hyperkalemia consists of the intravenous administration of insulin 5–10 units with 25 mL of 50% dextrose, sodium bicarbonate 44.6 mEq/L, and calcium chloride 500 mg. Insulin promotes transmembrane cellular transport of K^+ intracellularly, thus reducing serum levels of K^+. Calcium chloride is given to reduce the arrhythmogenic potential.

4. What are the major anesthetic concerns for renal transplantation?

Anesthetic management for patients receiving kidney transplantation is similar to that for patients with chronic renal failure. Many patients have diabetes mellitus, so there is a need to monitor blood glucose concentrations in the perioperative period. Preoperative hemodialysis optimizes uremic coagulopathies due to platelet dysfunction, improves acid–base imbalance, reduces intravascular volume, and corrects serum K^+ levels. Both general and regional anesthesia have been used successfully during renal transplantation.

When general anesthesia is chosen certain anesthetic considerations come into play. A useful approach is the administration of volatile inhalation agents combined with nitrous oxide and short-acting opioids. Patients with diabetic gastroparesis require aspiration prophylaxis and rapid sequence induction with cricoid pressure. Pretreatment with a nonparticulate antacid, such as bicitrate, and a prokinetic, such as metoclopramide, to increase lower esophageal tone and increase gastrointestinal motility are recommended. These drugs will increase gastric pH and decrease gastric volume. If serum K^+ levels are equal to or greater than 5.5 mEq/L, succinylcholine may be contraindicated. K^+ levels can increase by as much as 0.5–1.0 mEq/L after a single dose of succinylcholine, predisposing to hemodynamically significant acute hyperkalemia and its complications. Choice of muscle relaxant pivots on the unpredictable nature of renal function after renal transplantation. Intermediate-acting muscle relaxants degraded by Hoffman elimination, such as cisatracurium or atracurium, are more predictable than a renally excreted nondepolarizing neuromuscular blocker, such as pancuronium. Rocuronium and vecuronium are acceptable choices also.

Regardless of the muscle relaxant selected, doses should be carefully titrated. Patients should be closely observed for

---

Hyperkalemia

Dangerous as levels approach 7 mEq/L
Cardiac effects
    Bradycardia
    Ventricular fibrillation
    Cardiac arrest

ECG manifestations
    Peaked T waves
    Prolonged PR interval
    Loss of P waves
    Diminished R waves
    QRS widening
    Prolonged QT
    P-QRS-T complex approaches sine wave

Treatment
    Antagonize K^+
        Calcium chloride: 0.5–1 g IV
    Shift K^+ intracellularly
        Hyperventilation
        Sodium bicarbonate 44.6 mEq
        Regular insulin 5–10 units and 25 mL of
            50% dextrose
    Remove
        Dialysis
        Sodium polystyrene sulfonate (Kayexalate)
            20–50 g with sorbital

Major Anesthetic Concerns for Renal Transplantation

Preoperative preparation
  Electrolyte abnormalities
    Sodium (Na^+)<131 mEq/L or >150 mEq/L
    Potassium (K^+)<2.5 mEq/L or >5.9 mEq/L
    Predispose to dysrhythmias and depress cardiac
      output
  Dialysis
    Correct electrolyte abnormalities
    Treat acidosis
    Reverse intravascular fluid overload
  Treat hyperglycemia
  Anemia is chronic and well tolerated
  Treat coagulopathies

Anesthetic considerations
  Intravenous access
    Avoid extremities with fistulas and shunts
      if possible
  Intravenous fluids
    Avoid K^+-containing solutions
    Postoperative dialysis may be required
  Gastroparesis
    Aspiration prophylaxis
  Hyperkalemia
    K^+ levels greater than 5.5 mEq/L may
      contraindicate succinylcholine
  Coagulopathy
    May contraindicate regional anesthesia
  Benzodiazepines
    Highly protein bound
    Active metabolites undergo renal elimination
    Administer in small doses
  Meperidine
    Active metabolite normeperidine renally
      excreted
    Accumulation of normeperidine leads to
      seizures
  Muscle relaxants
    Succinylcholine
      May increase K^+ level by 1 mEq/L
    Recommended
      Atracurium and cisatracurium – Hoffman
        elimination
      Mivacurium – hydrolysis by plasma
        cholinesterases
      Rocuronium – primarily hepatic excretion
      Vecuronium – primarily biliary and hepatic
        excretion

Not recommended
  d-tubocurarine
  Pancuronium
Volatile agents
  Recommended
    Isoflurane and desflurane
  Contraindicated
    Enflurane and sevoflurane – metabolized to
      free fluoride ion
Induction agents
  Propofol, etomidate, and barbiturates are
    highly protein bound
  Hypoalbuminemic patients require smaller
    doses than usual
Opioids
  Morphine and meperidine may have enhanced
    effects in hypoalbuminemic patients
  Fentanyl and remifentanil pharmacokinetics
    essentially unchanged
Cholinesterase inhibitors
  Duration of action prolonged
Vasoactive agents
  Norepinephrine, epinephrine, phenylephrine,
    ephedrine
    Constrict kidney vessels
    Reduce renal blood flow
  Dopamine
    0.5–3 µg/kg/min
    Dilates renal arterioles
    Improves renal blood flow
  Sodium nitroprusside
    Contains cyanide which is metabolized to
      thiocyanate
    Thiocyanate is excreted by the kidneys
    Thiocyanate is neurotoxic
Fluid load prior to vascular anastomoses
Just after artery and vein anastomoses
  Diuretics
    Mannitol and furosemide
  Steroids
    Methylprednisolone
  Dopamine (rarely needed)
Wisconsin solution
  Can produce hypersensitivity reactions in
    recipients

early postoperative skeletal muscle weakness. The duration of anticholinesterase drugs used to antagonize nondepolarizing neuromuscular blockers is prolonged.

K+-containing intravenous fluids should be used with caution, if at all. Anephric patients require approximately 8 mL/kg per day of fluid to replace insensible water losses, which can be accomplished with hyponatremic solutions, such as dextrose in water. For other intraoperative fluid requirements, normal saline may be preferable to lactated Ringer's solution when hyperkalemia is a concern. Tissue oxygen delivery is improved with adequate volume replacement. Central venous pressure (CVP) monitoring is sometimes used to optimize fluid management. Poor cardiac reserves may indicate the need for pulmonary artery monitoring. Diuretics are administered to improve urine outflow in the newly transplanted kidney. Mannitol, an osmotic diuretic, is used frequently. A loop diuretic, such as furosemide or ethacrynic acid, may be added to mannitol. Unlike loop diuretics, mannitol does not depend on renal tubular concentrating ability to produce a diuresis.

Regional anesthesia has been used successfully during renal transplantation. It frequently avoids the need for tracheal intubation and the associated hemodynamic changes. However, there are disadvantages to regional anesthesia. Sympathetic blockade secondary to regional anesthesia predisposes to hypotension, especially at times of intravascular volume fluxes. It may be necessary to administer more fluid to optimize blood pressure. Consequently, when sympathetic tone returns and the vascular space shrinks in size, pulmonary edema may occur. Epidural and spinal techniques are contraindicated in the presence of uremic coagulopathy secondary to platelet dysfunction. It may be necessary to supplement regional anesthetics with intravenous agents, which depress respiration and thus increase the possibility of respiratory support.

5. What are the implications of long ischemic times during renal transplantation?

Cardiac arrest can occur after renal artery and vein anastomoses. It usually happens subsequent to releasing the vascular clamp and is most likely due to acute hyperkalemia. K+-containing solutions used to preserve the kidney during cold ischemic time may be washed out to the general circulation. If the external iliac artery was clamped, additional K+ can be released into the circulation after unclamping from an ischemic limb. The result is hypotension and metabolic acidosis from an acute washout of vasodilating substances. Although cold ischemic time can extend up to 48 hours, 30 hours is a better predictor of successful transplantation.

Warm ischemic time refers to the time from cold ischemic time to the revascularization of the kidney in vivo. This includes the renal artery and vein anastomoses but not that of the ureter. It is important to limit warm ischemic time to less than 45 minutes. Longer warm ischemic times are associated with poorer outcomes. Blood pressure control is also imperative. Cardiac output must be maintained to provide adequate perfusion of the newly transplanted kidney. The use of vasoconstrictors is discouraged during kidney transplantation; however, it is sometimes necessary to maintain adequate blood pressures.

SUGGESTED READINGS

Monk TG, Weldon BC: The renal system and anesthesia for urologic surgery. pp. 1005–1017. In Barash PG, Cullen BF, Stoelting RK (eds): Clinical Anesthesia, 4th edition. Lippincott, Williams & Wilkins, Philadelphia, 2001

Prough DS: Physiologic acid–base and electrolyte changes in acute and chronic renal failure patients. Anesthesiol Clin North Am 8:809–834, 2000

Singh AJ, Brenner BM: Transplantation and the treatment of renal failure. pp. 1562–1567. In Braunwald E (ed): Harrison's Principles of Internal Medicine, 15th edition. McGraw-Hill, New York, 2001

Sladen RN: Oliguria in the ICU: systemic approach to diagnosis and treatment. Anesthesiol Clin North Am 18:739–752, 2000

Sprung J, Kapural L, Bourke DL, O'Hara JF Jr.: Anesthesia for kidney transplant surgery. Anesthesiol Clin North Am 18:919–951, 2000

Stoelting RK, Dierdorf SF: Renal disease. pp. 371–372. In Stoelting RK, Dierdorf SF (eds): Anesthesia and Co-existing Disease, 4th edition. Churchill Livingstone, Philadelphia, 2002

43

OPEN-EYE INJURY AND INTRAOCULAR PRESSURE

Andrew Herlich, MD

A 25-year-old carpenter sustained a ruptured globe while working. He had recently eaten lunch. No other injuries were incurred. He smoked two packs of cigarettes per day.

QUESTIONS

1. What is the mechanism by which intraocular pressure (IOP) is normally maintained?
2. What pathologic conditions constitute a true ocular emergency versus a relative urgency?
3. What neuromuscular blocking agents are appropriate for the patient who is at risk for loss of intraocular contents? How does one minimize the deleterious side-effects of these agents in the presence of a ruptured globe?
4. What nonanesthetic agents might the ophthalmologist use to maximize surgical outcome?

1. What is the mechanism by which intraocular pressure (IOP) is normally maintained?

IOP contributes to the refracting properties of the eye. Significant intraocular hypotension or hypertension may lead to blurred vision or refractive discrepancies. The normal range of IOP is 10–22 mmHg. IOP is much higher than tissue pressure, which is 2–3 mmHg, and intracranial pressure, which is 7–8 mmHg. Pressures greater than 25 mmHg are considered abnormal. There are diurnal variations of modest proportion, 2–3 mmHg. IOP is highest in the morning secondary to the dilatation of pupils during sleep, carbon dioxide (CO_2) retention, the recumbent position, immobility of the eye, and pressure of the eyelid. Each systole can increase the pressure by another 1–2 mmHg, while inspiration can lower IOP by 5 mmHg.

IOP is normally maintained by several factors. One factor is external pressure exerted by periorbital structures, such as the extraocular muscles, venous congestion of the orbital veins, closure of the eyelid, or contraction of the orbicularis ocularis muscle. A second factor is scleral rigidity. The sclera is normally distensible, but as IOP rises it becomes rigid, thereby exacerbating intraocular hypertension. A third factor is the volume of intraocular fluid, such as blood, aqueous humor, and the semisolid structures, which include the lens, the vitreous, and intraocular tumors.

Alterations in fluid contents are crucial to IOP. Intraocular blood is mainly present in the choroid plexus, and the state of dilatation or contracture of these vessels will determine the blood volume in the eye. Although IOP is maintained at a relatively uniform level regardless of the degree of hypertension, an acute rise in arterial blood pressure may increase IOP. Over time, if arterial hypertension is chronic, IOP will normalize after adaptation of the choroidal vessels.

TABLE 43.1	Clinically Important Factors That Increase Intraocular Pressure	
Factor	**Mechanism**	**Etiology**
External pressure	Extraocular muscle and Orbicularis ocularis contraction Venous congestion Blepharospasm	Succinylcholine (without defasciculation), Etomidate, ketamine Coughing, vomiting Trendelenburg position
Internal constituents	Systemic hypertension Aqueous humor volume Mydriasis	Light anesthesia, hypoxia, hypercarbia, essential hypertension, ephedrine, phenylephrine, atropine, pancuronium, distended urinary bladder
Physiologic factors	Elevated $PaCO_2$ Trendelenburg position Metabolic alkalosis Respiratory acidosis	Sedatives, hypnotics, narcotics

Impaired venous drainage increases IOP. Coughing or straining will raise IOP by elevating venous pressure (Table 43.1). A mild cough can raise IOP by 34–40 mmHg. Similarly, retching, coughing, or vomiting during induction of anesthesia may cause a rise in IOP which persists for many minutes. This may be particularly true in patients with a history of smoking.

Another important intraocular constituent is aqueous humor, two-thirds of which is formed in the posterior chamber, and one-third of which is produced in the anterior chamber. It is secreted from epithelial cells of the ciliary process. After formation in the posterior segment, aqueous humor circulates through the pupil into the anterior chamber, which is subsequently drained at the angle of the eye and at the spaces of Fontana. The spaces of Fontana are channels in the trabecular mesh. Impaired drainage through this trabecular mesh results in glaucoma. Aqueous humor continues to pass into Schlemm's canal and the ophthalmic, cavernous, and jugular veins.

Aqueous humor is similar in composition to plasma, without its proteins. Aqueous humor secretion is an energy-requiring process mediated through a sodium pump mechanism. Its production requires both cytochrome oxidase and carbonic anhydrase. Changes in solute concentration of plasma can affect the formation of aqueous humor and, consequently, the IOP. Thus, mannitol or glycerol is used for lowering IOP. Acetazolamide may also lower IOP. Each of the aforementioned agents has metabolic consequences.

Pupillary dilatation narrows the trabecular mesh and spaces of Fontana, predisposing the patient to glaucoma. Agents causing pupillary constriction (miosis)

improve aqueous drainage, whereas agents producing pupillary dilatation (mydriasis) impair aqueous drainage.

2. What pathologic conditions constitute a true ocular emergency versus a relative urgency?

True ocular emergencies requiring immediate treatment are thermal or chemical corneal burns and central retinal artery occlusion. Copious fluid washing will treat the former, while simple needle aspiration of the globe will decrease the IOP, relieving arterial obstruction in the latter.

Ruptured globes are a relative urgency. Delaying surgery for several hours may be satisfactory in some cases. The waiting period depends upon the patient's vision at the time of initial evaluation. The patient must be kept calm to prevent coughing, straining, nausea, or vomiting, all of which will predispose to greater extrusion of intraocular contents. If the patient has had a recent meal, delaying surgery for several hours may be of overall benefit to the patient without compromising the surgical outcome. This will allow for gastric emptying and aspiration prophylaxis before induction of general anesthesia.

A thorough preoperative evaluation before induction of general anesthesia is prudent. Special radiographic studies, such as computed tomography (CT), ocular ultrasound, and angiography might be needed to delineate additional injuries of the orbit and craniofacial complex. Proceeding without these studies may be ill-advised and life-threatening in certain circumstances. In some cases, surgical procedures allow both the ophthalmologist and craniofacial surgeon to proceed in concert. In other instances, the ophthalmologist may need to defer to surgeons treating more life-threatening injuries.

3. What neuromuscular blocking agents are appropriate for the patient who is at risk for loss of intraocular contents? How does one minimize the deleterious side-effects of these agents in the presence of a ruptured globe?

Selection of a neuromuscular blocking agent for the patient at increased risk for both aspiration of abdominal contents and extrusion of ocular contents has long been controversial. For many years, succinylcholine, which is recognized to increase IOP by causing tonic contractions of extraocular muscles, was thought to be contraindicated, and the use of nondepolarizing agents was recommended. The dilemma occurred at a time when only relatively long acting agents, such as pancuronium, d-tubocurarine, and dimethylcurarine were available. Over the last 15 years, with the introduction of the intermediate-acting agents, suitable substitutes have become available. Caveats to the use of these agents under the circumstances of this case suggest that very large doses (4 times the ED_{95}) of these drugs must be used to effect good intubating conditions. Consequently, there may be a prolonged duration of neuromuscular blockade. Using larger intubating doses of rocuronium offers intubating times and conditions similar to succinylcholine but prolongs the duration of action to similar times as vecuronium. Using similar doses of mivacurium has a shorter duration of action than rocuronium but mivacurium has a longer onset time that may be crucial to securing the airway. In general, the issue of succinylcholine and the open globe is no longer controversial. Clinicians may rest assured that there are no contraindications to its use. Two separate studies by Libonati et al. (1985) and Donlon (1986) demonstrated that succinylcholine offers ideal intubating conditions with minimal risk. This is true provided that defasciculation with a nondepolarizing neuromuscular blocker and administration of lidocaine and fentanyl were accomplished before intubation.

The ideal neuromuscular blocking agent will be one that offers rapid onset, short duration, and absence of fasciculations. Prolonged or difficult laryngoscopy will have a more deleterious effect on raising IOP and subsequent extrusion of intraocular contents than the choice of neuromuscular blocking agent itself. It is important to remember during preoxygenation that suboptimal placement of the facemask can result in pressure on the globe, predisposing to extrusion of intraocular contents.

In this particular patient with a smoking history, airway reactivity increases the risk of coughing during patient management. The use of intravenous lidocaine and fentanyl will aid in cough suppression. Equally important is the timing of laryngoscopy and endotracheal intubation, which requires use of a neuromuscular blockade monitor. Although laryngotracheal topical anesthesia may reduce airway reactivity, it is probably ill advised. The act of spraying the larynx and trachea with local anesthesia in the awake state may cause retching or coughing. Abolition of laryngotracheal reflexes increases the risk of gastric content aspiration before endotracheal intubation and after extubation in both the awake and anesthetized patient.

Intravenous induction agents, such as propofol, thiopental, and methohexital, reduce IOP. Narcotics, sedatives, and major tranquilizers also lower IOP, as long as ventilation is controlled because increases in $PaCO_2$ will raise IOP.

Ketamine may cause nystagmus and blepharospasm, resulting in suboptimal surgical conditions. Etomidate, which reduces IOP, may cause myoclonus, which may ultimately result in an increase in IOP. Additionally, both ketamine and etomidate have been associated with higher rates of postoperative nausea and vomiting, which also detract from their usefulness in the case of the ruptured globe.

As previously stated, any form of respiratory acidosis will increase IOP, and respiratory alkalosis will decrease IOP. Normal ranges of $PaCO_2$ will have little effect on IOP. Interestingly, metabolic acidosis actually reduces IOP, whereas metabolic alkalosis will increase IOP.

Hypoxemia and hyperthermia will lead to increased IOP. Hypothermia will reduce IOP.

4. What non-anesthetic agents might the ophthalmologist use to maximize surgical outcome?

Intravenous agents, such as mannitol, dextran, urea, as well as oral glycerol, will increase plasma osmotic pressure, decrease aqueous humor formation, and reduce IOP

TABLE 43.2	Factors That Lower Intraocular Pressure

Osmotic agents
  Mannitol
  Dextran
  Urea
  Glycerol
Carbonic anhydrase inhibitors
  Acetazolamide
Miotics
  Narcotics
Laryngeal reflex suppression
  Narcotics
  Lidocaine
  Barbiturates
  Propofol
Acid–base balance
  Respiratory alkalosis
  Metabolic acidosis
Hypothermia

(Table 43.2). Intravenous acetazolamide will also lower IOP. Acetazolamide inhibits carbonic anhydrase and therefore interferes with the sodium pump responsible for aqueous humor formation.

SUGGESTED READINGS

Aboul-Eish E: Physiology of the eye pertinent to anesthesia. Int Ophthalmol Clin 13:1–20, 1973

Donlon JV: Succinylcholine and open eye injury. Part II. Anesthesiology 64:254, 1986

Edmondson L, Lindsay SL, Lanigan LP, et al.: Intra-ocular pressure changes during rapid sequence induction of anaesthesia. A comparison between thiopentone and suxamethonium and thiopentone and atracurium. Anaesthesia 43:1005–1010, 1988

Kilickan L, Baykara N, Gurkan Y, et al.: The effect on intraocular pressure of endotracheal intubation or laryngeal mask use during TIVA without the use of muscle relaxants. Acta Anaesthesiol Scand 43:343–346, 1999

Libonati MM, Leahy JJ, Ellison N: Use of succinylcholine in open eye surgery. Anesthesiology 62:637–640, 1985

McGoldrick K: Anatomy and physiology of the eye. In McGoldrick K (ed): Anesthesia for Ophthalmologic and Otolaryngological Surgery. WB Saunders, Philadelphia, 1992

McGoldrick K: Anesthetics and intraocular pressure: management of penetrating eye injuries. In McGoldrick K (ed): Anesthesia for Ophthalmologic and Otolaryngology Surgery. WB Saunders, Philadelphia, 1992

Schultz P, Ibsen M, Østergaard D, Skovgaard LT: Onset and duration of action of rocuronium—from tracheal intubation, through intense block to complete recovery. Acta Anaesthesiol Scand 45:612–617, 2001

Vachon CA, Warner DO, Bacon DR: Succinylcholine and the open globe: tracing the teaching. Anesthesiology 99:220, 2003

44

RETINAL DETACHMENT

Andrew Herlich, MD

A 33-year-old woman with severe myopia presents for scleral buckle repair of a spontaneous retinal detachment. Her medical, surgical, and anesthesia history are otherwise unremarkable.

QUESTIONS

1. What are the advantages and disadvantages of general anesthesia for scleral buckle repair?
2. Describe the oculocardiac reflex and its treatment.
3. What are the potential complications of retrobulbar anesthesia? Are there any other ophthalmic blocks that are satisfactory with less morbidity?
4. What types of retinal detachments are amenable to elective repair?
5. Briefly describe the series of events that occur during retinal detachment surgery.
6. Reattachment of the retina occasionally requires intraocular gas. What are the different types of gases that can be used, and what are the anesthetic implications of their use?

1. What are the advantages and disadvantages of general anesthesia for scleral buckle repair?

There are a number of disadvantages of scleral buckle repair under regional anesthesia. In patients undergoing repeat procedures, surgical time may exceed 2 hours, predisposing the patient to muscle and ligament strain of the back while lying on the hard operating room table. Giant retinal tears require changing position from supine to prone which can be anxiety-provoking for some individuals. Severe traction required to approach the posterior retina can provoke the oculocardiac reflex and/or pain. A thin sclera in the operated eye or blindness in the other eye makes the consequences of unintentional globe perforation during retrobulbar block unacceptable in many cases. For all of these reasons, general anesthesia may be preferred.

Although offering freedom from many of regional anesthesia's disadvantages, general anesthesia is associated with several of its own problems. Postoperative pain, nausea, retching, bucking, and coughing are all recognized consequences of general anesthesia that predispose individuals to increased intraocular pressure.

2. Describe the oculocardiac reflex and its treatment.

The afferent pathway of the oculocardiac reflex begins with the long and short ciliary nerves, which transmit impulses to the ciliary ganglion followed by the Gasserian ganglion. The Gasserian ganglion sends impulses along the first division, ophthalmic division, of the fifth cranial nerve (trigeminal nerve) to the main sensory nucleus of the fifth cranial nerve in the floor of the fourth ventricle. The efferent pathway begins in the nucleus ambiguus, the motor nucleus of the vagal nerve, and transmits impulses to the vagal cardiac depressor nerves. Maneuvers that are most likely to evoke the oculocardiac reflex are tension on the extraocular muscles or pressure on the cornea. Retrobulbar block may both treat and evoke the oculocardiac reflex. This reflex manifests clinically as bradycardia with ventricular escape beats, nodal rhythm, or asystole. Treatment of these dysrhythmias is best initiated by requesting the surgeon to refrain from the maneuver that precipitated the reflex, such as traction on a muscle or severe scleral depression during indirect ophthalmoscopy to examine the retina. Although the reflex will eventually fatigue, life-threatening bradycardic dysrhythmias can be prevented with small doses of intravenous atropine or glycopyrrolate. Prophylactic intramuscular atropine or glycopyrrolate have generally not been successful in the prevention of the reflex when compared with intravenous dosing. The oculocardiac reflex may be more likely to occur under general anesthesia in the face of hypoxemia and hypercarbia.

Predisposing factors include hypoxemia, hypercarbia, deep anesthesia, and light anesthesia. Persistent, nonfatiguing episodes may respond to retrobulbar anesthesia.

3. What are the potential complications of retrobulbar anesthesia? Are there any other blocks that are satisfactory with less morbidity?

The onset time of retrobulbar blockade is 5–10 minutes. Retrobulbar blockade has a low failure rate of less than 1% in skilled hands. However, retrobulbar anesthesia is associated with a number of complications. The recognized complications of retrobulbar blockade are:

- Central retinal artery occlusion
- Retrobulbar hemorrhage
- Subdural or subarachnoid injection
- Seizures
- Intraneuronal injection
- Globe puncture
- Oculocardiac reflex

Peribulbar block is a good alternative to retrobulbar block and is associated with fewer complications. To perform a retrobulbar blockade, local anesthetic is injected into the eye's muscle cone. Peribulbar blockade is performed by injecting local anesthetic around the eye.

The failure rate of peribulbar block is as high as 10%, and the onset time is 10–12 minutes, which is slower than that of retrobulbar block. An alternative to the retrobulbar and peribulbar block is the more recently popularized sub-Tenon block. The sub-Tenon block is performed somewhat similarly to a retrobulbar block. In the sub-Tenon block a blunt-tipped cannula is inserted between the fused conjunctiva and anterior Tenon capsule. It is advanced to midway between the insertion of the medial and inferior rectus muscles into a thin channel to the posterior sub-Tenon space. Success rates are reported as high as 98.8%.

4. What types of retinal detachments are amenable to elective repair?

Peripheral retinal detachments and macular detachments exceeding 24 hours can be treated electively. Recent or impending macular detachment requires urgent attention.

5. Briefly describe the series of events that occur during retinal detachment surgery.

After re-examination with indirect ophthalmoscopy, while the patient is anesthetized, cryothermy or diathermy is used to allow the retina to oppose pigment epithelium. Retinal tears are covered with a scleral buckle, which is sutured into place. A small incision perforating the scleral-choroidal region drains accumulated subretinal fluid, allowing the retina to oppose the scleral buckle and close the tear.

6. Reattachment of the retina requires intraocular gas. What are the different types of gases that can be used, and what are the anesthetic implications of their use?

The surgeon may use intraocular air, sulfurhexafluoride (SF_6), octafluorocyclobutane (C_4F_8), or perfluoropropane (C_3F_8). Since these gases are mixed with air in concentrations that normally do not expand, they will expand in volume with the coincident use of nitrous oxide (N_2O). If the procedure is performed under general anesthesia, N_2O should be discontinued at least 10–15 minutes prior to intraocular gas injection. In the case of C_3F_8 and SF_6, N_2O is contraindicated for at least 30 days to prevent subsequent increases in intraocular pressure. Intraocular gases are resorbed very slowly. Occasionally, intraocular silicone is injected, which does not resorb.

Postoperatively, intraocular gas may be directed to a particular portion of the retina by adjusting the patient's position. Prone, lateral decubitus, and sitting are commonly prescribed positions. Such departures from standard postanesthetic nursing care mandate an awake, cooperative patient.

Regional anesthesia techniques are most compatible with these postoperative requirements.

Nausea and vomiting are not only frequent sequelae of anesthesia but may also indicate increased intraocular pressure secondary to overinflation with intraocular gas. Nausea and vomiting often follow scleral buckling without gas injection and may be reduced by administration of perioperative ketorolac to diminish traction and inflammatory-related pain.

SUGGESTED READINGS

Aboul-Eish E: Physiology of the eye pertinent to anesthesia. Int Ophthalmol Clin 13:1–20, 1973

Feitl ME, Krupin T: Retrobulbar anesthesia. Ophthalmol Clin North Am 3:83, 1990

Guise PA: Sub-Tenon anesthesia: a prospective study of 6,000 blocks. Anesthesiology 98:964–968, 2003

McGoldrick KG, Mardirossian J: New technology: understanding ophthalmic procedures and their anesthetic implications. p. 266. In McGoldrick KG (ed): Anesthesia for Ophthalmic and Otolaryngologic Surgery. WB Saunders, Philadelphia, 1992

Seaberg RR, Freeman WR, Goldbaum MH, et al.: Permanent postoperative vision loss associated with expansion of intraocular gas in the presence of a nitrous oxide-containing anesthetic. Anesthesiology 97:1309–1310, 2002

Vote BJ, Hart RH, Worsley DR, et al.: Visual loss after use of nitrous oxide gas with general anesthetic in patients with intraocular gas still persistent up to 30 days after vitrectomy. Anesthesiology 97:1305–1308, 2002

45

TYMPANOMASTOIDECTOMY

Andrew Herlich, MD

A 52-year-old anxious man presents for revision of a previous tympanomastoidectomy on an ambulatory basis. The patient is otherwise in good general health. He has undergone several previous procedures with general anesthesia. Each previous procedure has resulted in postoperative nausea and vomiting.

QUESTIONS

1. Is the anxious patient a good candidate for surgery under monitored anesthesia care (MAC)?
2. What general anesthetic techniques are most likely to minimize postoperative nausea and vomiting (PONV)?
3. Are regional anesthetics less likely to result in PONV in this patient?
4. Why is control of blood loss important during middle ear surgery?
5. Are long-acting neuromuscular blocking agents contraindicated in middle ear surgery?
6. Describe the conduction of general and regional anesthesia for middle ear surgery.

1. Is the anxious patient a good candidate for surgery under monitored anesthesia care (MAC)?

This particular patient is quite anxious and is anticipating postoperative nausea and vomiting (PONV). His baseline agitation may prevent a quiescent state during microsurgery. Oversedation could easily precipitate hypoxia and hypercarbia, resulting in loss of patient cooperation. Intravenous narcotics might exacerbate nausea and vomiting.

Intraoperative and postoperative nausea, vomiting, and dizziness are recognized complications of middle ear surgery. Prophylactic administration of antiemetics may be helpful in addition to benzodiazepine sedatives. 5-Hydroxytryptamine (5HT) blockers, such as ondansetron, granisetron, or dolasetron, may prove to be useful; however, insufficient data exist to warrant their prophylactic use in middle ear surgery. 5HT blockers when combined with dexamethasone have an excellent record of preventing PONV in the general population. Low-dose propofol infusion during the procedure, as part of the sedative technique, may also help to keep the patient calm and reduce the risk of PONV.

2. What general anesthetic techniques are most likely to minimize postopertive nausea and vomiting?

Clearly, the patient at high risk for PONV should receive an anesthetic designed to minimize this problem. Many of these patients are ambulatory and may have higher gastric volumes and lower gastric pHs as a result of prolonged fasting. This may be obviated by permitting clear fluids until 2–3 hours prior to surgery. Atropine or glycopyrrolate has been shown on occasion to reduce PONV by preventing increased vagal tone. Prophylactic use of atropine or glycopyrrolate, however, may reduce the gastroesophageal barrier pressure.

Avoiding mask ventilation in the patient with an uncomplicated airway may reduce the risk of insufflating large volumes of anesthetic gas into the stomach before intubation of the trachea. Immediately after securing the airway, orogastric tube decompression will reduce gastric distention. The orogastric tube may be left in situ for passive drainage intraoperatively. Capping or clamping a sump defeats its intended purpose of continuous passive drainage. Constant suction may result in gastric mucosal injury.

Avoidance of nitrous oxide (N_2O) may be warranted to help minimize nausea and vomiting. Due to its insolubility, nitrous oxide tends to diffuse into closed air spaces, thereby increasing gaseous volume and/or pressure. Diffusion into the gastric bubble may exacerbate gastric distention predisposing the patient to PONV. Passage into the middle ear, especially in combination with Eustachian tube dysfunction, can cause dislodgement of the tympanic graft. After graft placement, sudden discontinuation of N_2O causes massive negative inner ear pressure. Graft implosion may occur resulting in PONV and pain.

The use of propofol as an induction agent and possibly a maintenance agent may reduce the risk of PONV. Anxiolytics, such as midazolam, may successfully treat the anxiety of nausea and vomiting.

Total intravenous anesthesia that includes propofol and remifentanil infusions as opposed to balanced anesthesia with a volatile agent produces significantly less PONV.

Many medications and maneuvers have been used to control PONV after surgery. A slow, deliberate transfer from the operating room to the postanesthesia recovery unit (PACU) with care turning corners will help prevent emesis. Administration of supplemental oxygen may also reduce the incidence of PONV. Assuming there are no surgical misadventures such as an endolymphatic sac disruption or cerebrospinal fluid leak, the anesthesiologist should consider combination therapy for treatment. Use of dexamethasone prophylactically as a single dose may be quite helpful. Rescue of symptoms in the PACU may include inexpensive medications such as dimenhydramine or diphenhydramine. The use of transdermal scopolamine may be quite useful as well, assuming the patient does not have glaucoma or bladder outlet obstruction.

3. Are regional anesthetics less likely to result in PONV in this patient?

Despite the elimination of general anesthesia, the risk of PONV is only somewhat less likely due to many reasons. Firstly, this patient is quite anxious; anxiety probably has a major role in nausea and vomiting. Additionally, caloric effects of injection of local anesthesia close to the vestibular system may stimulate the vestibular organ. Surgical suction may also induce caloric effects since passage of air may also lower temperature in the middle ear. Consequently, the vestibular system may be stimulated.

Manipulation of the ossicles results in vertigo in those patients who undergo ossiculoplasty and, as a result, PONV.

Finally, diffusion of local anesthesia through the round window membrane also contributes to PONV. Different local anesthetics diffuse at different rates and there may be different degrees of PONV depending upon the local anesthetic involved.

4. Why is control of blood loss important during middle ear surgery?

Unlike many other types of surgery, the anticipated amount of blood lost during middle ear surgery is usually of little hemodynamic consequence. Nevertheless, even small amounts of hemorrhage impair the surgeon's visualization through a dissecting microscope. Blood loss may be controlled by several methods. One popular technique is the injection of a vasoconstrictor, such as epinephrine 1:200,000, at the surgical site. Postural changes, such as a 10°–15° moderate head-up tilt may be beneficial. Patients who are free from major organ system impairment tolerate deliberate hypotension best. Pre-existing cardiovascular, central nervous system, renal, or pulmonary diseases are relative contraindications to induced hypotension. Combining deliberate hypotension and head-up tilt is a popular technique. However, these maneuvers may increase the risk of venous air embolism because central venous pressure is reduced and the operative field is elevated above the level of the heart. Induced hypotension in the presence of hypovolemia results in poor organ perfusion and organ hypoxia. Potent inhalation agents, sodium nitroprusside, nitroglycerin, α-adrenergic blockers, or β-adrenergic blockers have been employed for induced hypotension.

Complications of deliberate hypotension include impaired vital organ function, central nervous system thrombosis, renal vessel thrombosis, dizziness, and prolonged emergence. Properly selected patients who are at low risk for these complications, and the use of deliberate hypotension, contribute to an improved surgical outcome.

5. Are long-acting neuromuscular blockers contraindicated in middle ear surgery?

Although readily identifiable in a normal ear, the facial nerve may be difficult to locate in a diseased ear. External electrical stimulation of the facial nerve trunk and its muscular innervation may be required. Concurrent use of a long-acting neuromuscular blocker interferes with this test and is, therefore, contraindicated. Deep potent inhalation anesthesia is generally selected for middle ear surgery. Pre-existing facial nerve palsy eliminates such considerations and allows for the use of muscle relaxants. Debilitated patients may not tolerate the myocardial depressant effects of deep inhalational anesthesia, necessitating the employment of neuromuscular blockade. Under such circumstances, maintenance of 1 or 2 twitch responses to train-of-four stimulation should allow for facial muscle contraction during facial nerve stimulation. Before the use of neuromuscular blockers, the risks and benefits should be discussed with the surgeon and the patient.

6. Describe the conduction of general and regional anesthesia for middle ear surgery.

The epinephrine given for control of bleeding is generally combined with local anesthetics, which minimizes surgical stimulation from the operative site. Use of laryngotracheal anesthesia may eliminate endotracheal-tube-induced pain and coughing. The simultaneous employment of these two techniques markedly reduces inhalation agent requirements. Mild to moderate hypotension frequently ensues. Attempts at decreasing the inspired partial pressure of volatile anesthetic agent may be met with patient motion or bucking. The surgical result could be disastrous. Consequently, deep anesthesia must be maintained and the blood pressure supported with occasional small doses of ephedrine or phenylephrine. If hypotension persists, a low-dose infusion of phenylephrine may be helpful.

At the termination of surgery, emergence from anesthesia should ideally be free from coughing and straining in order that the tympanic membrane graft remains in place. Intravenous or intratracheal lidocaine may be used to help prevent these complications if the patient is not at increased risk for aspiration of gastric contents.

Regional anesthesia for radical tympanomastoidectomy and other similar procedures may be accomplished with lidocaine 1% with epinephrine 1:200,000 (5 μg/cc). To block the branches of the trigeminal nerve and the cervical plexus that innervate the auricle, multiple skin wheals connected by subcutaneous infiltration are made around the mastoid process. The total volume of local anesthesia is 5–8 mL. The superior two-thirds of the anterior surface of the auricle may be anesthetized by infiltrating local anesthesia over the posterior aspect of the zygoma and connecting the skin wheal with subcutaneous infiltration along the anterior border of the auricle to its inferior border. The auriculotemporal nerve supplies the anterior portion of the auditory canal and can be infiltrated with 2 mL at the osseous-cartilaginous region. The floor of the external auditory canal and the inferior portion of the tympanic membrane are supplied by the vagus nerve.

Two milliliters of local anesthetic is infiltrated in the inferior portion of the canal.

The remainder of the tympanic membrane may be anesthetized by direct application of 4% lidocaine spray or 4% cocaine. Occasionally, extensive radical mastoid surgery may require an incision that is more posterior. Consequently, the lesser occipital and greater occipital nerves may need to be blocked. Subcutaneous infiltration from the mastoid process to the greater occipital protuberance along the superior nuchal line will create adequate anesthesia. Five to eight milliliters of a local anesthetic will successfully accomplish this block.

SUGGESTED READINGS

Gonzalez RM, Bjerke RJ, Drobycki T, et al.: Prevention of endotracheal tube-induced coughing during emergence from general anesthesia. Anesth Analg 79:792–795, 1994

Henzi I, Walder B, Tramèr MR: Dexamethasone for the prevention of postoperative nausea and vomiting: a quantitative systematic review. Anesth Analg 90:186–194, 2000

Jellish WS, Leonetti JP, Avramov A, et al.: Remifentanil-based anesthesia versus a propofol technique for otologic surgical procedures. Otolaryngol Head Neck Surg 122:222–227, 2000

McGoldrick KG, Miller JG: Anesthesia for otologic surgery. p. 130. In McGoldrick KG (ed): Anesthesia for Ophthalmic and Otolaryngologic Surgery. WB Saunders, Philadelphia, 1992

Mukherjee K, Seavell C, Rawling E, et al.: A comparison of total intravenous with balanced anaesthesia for middle ear surgery: effects on postoperative nausea and vomiting, pain, and conditions of surgery. Anaesthesia 58:176–180, 2003

Munson ES: Transfer of nitrous oxide into body air cavities. Br J Anaesth 46:202–209, 1974

Tramèr MR: A rational approach to the control of postoperative nausea and vomiting: evidence from systematic reviews. Part 1. Efficacy and harm of antiemetic interventions, and methodological issues. Acta Anaesthesiol Scand 45:4–13, 2001

Tramèr MR: A rational approach to the control of postoperative nausea and vomiting: evidence from systematic reviews. Part 2. Recommendations for prevention and treatment, and research agenda. Acta Anaesthesiol Scand 45:14–19, 2001

Watcha MF, White PF: Postoperative nausea and vomiting: Its etiology, treatment, and prevention. Anesthesiology 77:162–184, 1992

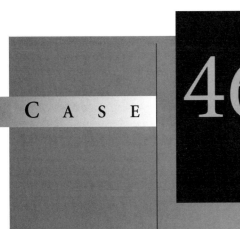

Allan P. Reed, MD

A 35-year-old woman presents for laparoscopic lysis of adhesions. Her first laparotomy occurred 10 years prior to this admission. At that time, the process of tracheal intubation consumed 1 hour. She awakened with a very sore throat, but does not know the details of the intubation. The old records are unavailable.

QUESTIONS

1. What are the predictors of difficult mask ventilation?
2. Discuss the risk factors for difficult intubation.
3. Are the risk factors for difficult intubation reliable predictors of difficult intubation?
4. How is the anticipated difficult intubation approached?
5. Describe the management options for a patient who, after induction of anesthesia, unexpectedly cannot be intubated with a Macintosh blade. This patient has a good mask airway.
6. Following induction of anesthesia, ventilation by facemask and intubation are impossible. What maneuvers may help?
7. How is successful tracheal intubation verified?
8. Following a difficult intubation, how is postoperative extubation managed?

1. What are the predictors of difficult mask ventilation?

One of the most important predictors of the difficult airway is a history of difficult airway. The opposite is not necessarily true. A history of problem-free airway management is suggestive of future ease, but not a guarantee. Many factors that contribute to difficulty are progressive. Examples of such problems include rheumatoid arthritis and obesity. An airway history should be elicited from all patients. Review of prior anesthesia records is frequently helpful. They may describe previously encountered problems, failed therapies, and successful solutions.

Difficult facemask ventilation occurs when a practitioner cannot provide sufficient gas exchange due to inadequate mask seal, large volume leaks, or excessive resistance to the ingress or egress of gas. This occurs with an incidence of 0.08–5%. The wide range is probably due to conflicting definitions of difficult mask airway. Risk factors for difficult mask ventilation include full beard, massive jaw, edentulousness, skin sensitivity (burns, epidermolysis bullosa, fresh skin grafts), facial dressings, obesity, age greater than 55 years, and a history of snoring. Other criteria that suggest the possibility of difficult facemask ventilation include large tongue, heavy jaw muscles, history of obstructive sleep apnea, poor atlanto-occipital extension, some types of pharyngeal pathology, facial burns, and facial deformities. Multiple types of pharyngeal problems can produce difficult facemask ventilation. They include

Predictors of Difficult Facemask Ventilation

Obesity
Beard
Edentulousness
History of snoring
History of obstructive sleep apnea
Skin sensitivity (burns, epidermolysis bullosa, fresh skin grafts)
Massive jaw
Heavy jaw muscles
Age greater than 55 years
Large tongue
Poor atlanto-occipital extension
Pharyngeal pathology
    Lingual tonsil hypertrophy
    Lingual tonsil abscess
    Lingual thyroid
    Thyroglossal duct cyst
Facial abnormalities
    Facial dressings
    Facial burns
    Facial deformities

lingual tonsil hypertrophy, lingual tonsillar abscess, lingual thyroid, and thyroglossal duct cyst. Many of these cannot be diagnosed by classical airway examination techniques. The presence of any one factor is suggestive of difficult mask ventilation. The more factors present at the same time, the greater the likelihood of difficulty. Increased mandibulo-hyoid distance has been associated with obstructive sleep apnea, the pathophysiology of which may be related to difficult mask ventilation.

Traditional facemask airway management is generally safe and effective. In the unusual instances when it is not, tracheal intubation remains the fallback option. Although this scheme works well in most cases, approximately 15% of difficult intubations are also difficult mask airways.

2. Discuss the risk factors for difficult intubation.

Sniffing Position

The presence or absence of airway pathology does not influence the definition of difficult tracheal intubation. It occurs when multiple attempts at intubation are required. Traditional laryngoscopy is performed in order to visualize the laryngeal opening. The laryngoscopist is positioned outside the airway, above the patient's head. To see through the airway, light must travel from the glottic opening to the laryngoscopist's eye. This technique requires an uninterrupted linear path between the larynx and laryngoscopist because light generally travels in a straight line. Most manipulations performed attempt to satisfy this criterion.

The airway contains three visual axes. They are the long axes of the mouth, oropharynx, and larynx. In the neutral position, these axes form acute and obtuse angles with one another. Light cannot bend around these angles under normal circumstances. In order to bring all three axes into better alignment, Magill suggested "Sniffing the morning air position." True sniffing position requires both cervical flexion and atlanto-occipital extension. Cervical flexion approximates the pharyngeal and laryngeal axes. Atlanto-occipital extension brings the oral axis into better alignment with the other two. Normal atlanto-occipital extension measures 35°. With optimal alignment of the airway's visual axes, it becomes possible to look through the airway into the laryngeal opening. Reduced atlanto-occipital gap or prominent C1 spinous processes impairs laryngoscopy if vigorous attempts at extension are performed because the larynx is forced anteriorly causing the trachea to bow.

Inability to assume the sniffing position is a predictor of difficult intubation. Examples of problems that prevent sniffing position include cervical vertebral arthritis, cervical ankylosing spondylitis, unstable cervical fractures, protruding cervical discs, atlanto-axial subluxation, cervical fusions, cervical collars, and halo frames. Morbidly obese patients sometimes have posterior neck fat pads that prevent atlanto-occipital extension.

The ability to achieve the sniffing position is easily tested: simply have the patient flex the lower cervical vertebrae and extend at the atlanto-occipital joint. Pain, tingling, numbness, or inability to achieve these maneuvers predicts difficult intubation.

The benefits of the sniffing position have been dogma for over 70 years. More recently, Adnet et al. (2001) and Chou and Wu (2001) have independently questioned its utility.

Mouth Opening

Mouth opening is important because it determines the available space for placing and manipulating the laryngoscope and tracheal tube. A small mouth opening may not accommodate either one. Mouth opening also facilitates visualization of the uppermost part of the airway. Mouth opening relies on the temporomandibular joint (TMJ), which works in two ways. It has both a hinge-like movement and a gliding motion. The gliding motion is known as translation. Its hinge-like movement allows the mandible to pivot on the maxilla. The more the mandible swings away from the maxilla, the bigger the mouth opening. The adequacy of mouth opening is assessed by measuring the inter-incisor distance. An inter-incisor distance of 3 cm provides sufficient space for intubation, in the absence of other complicating factors. This corresponds approximately to the width of 2 finger breadths. The 2 finger breadth test is performed by placing the examiner's 2nd and 3rd digits between the patient's central incisors. If they fit, there should be adequate room to perform laryngoscopy. If they do not fit, then laryngoscopy may be difficult. Factors that interfere with mouth opening include masseter muscle spasm, TMJ dysfunction, and various integumentary ailments, such as burn scar contractures and progressive systemic sclerosis. Masseter muscle spasm may be relieved by induction of anesthesia and administration of muscle relaxants. TMJ mechanical problems remain unaltered by medications. Some patients demonstrate adequate mouth opening when awake, but not after anesthetic induction. The problem can oftentimes be relieved by pulling the mandible forward. A mouth opening that was sufficient for a previous anesthetic may not be after temporal neurosurgical procedures.

Dentition

Instrumentation of the airway places teeth at risk for damage. Multiple problems result from dental injury. Teeth may be dislodged or broken. Such teeth cannot be used for chewing, may be painful, and will be costly to repair. Beyond these issues, broken teeth can fall into the trachea, migrate to the lung, and predispose to abscesses. Poor dentition is at risk for damage as the mouth is opened and as the laryngoscope blade is introduced. Teeth that can be extracted easily with digital pressure should probably be removed. During laryngoscopy in the presence of poor dentition, extra efforts are made to avoid placing pressure on the maxillary incisors. In doing so, the laryngoscope is manipulated into a less than ideal position resulting in poor visualization of the glottis.

Prominent maxillary incisors complicate laryngoscopy in another way. They protrude into the mouth and block the line of sight to the larynx. In order to overcome this problem, laryngoscopists must adjust their line of sight. To accomplish this, the laryngoscopist's eye is brought to a new position that is higher than the original one. The laryngoscopist then looks tangentially over the protruding maxillary incisor. This creates two new points in the adjusted line of sight and, thus, a new straight line of sight. The new line of sight brings the laryngoscopist's view to a more posterior laryngopharyngeal position. This results in a view that is posterior to the larynx. Consequently, the larynx is not visualized and a difficult laryngoscopy is produced. In much the same way, edentulous patients tend to be easy intubations, because the laryngoscopist can adjust the line of sight to a more advantageous angle.

Tongue

The tongue occupies space in the mouth and oropharynx. The base of the tongue resides close to the glottic aperture.

During traditional direct laryngoscopy, the base of the tongue falls posteriorly obstructing the line of sight into the glottis. Visualizing the larynx requires displacing the base of the tongue anteriorly, so that the line of sight to the glottis is restored. The tongue is frequently displaced with a hand-held rigid laryngoscope, to which Macintosh and Miller blades are the most commonly attached. Laryngoscopes push the tongue anteriorly and, in so doing, move it from a posterior obstructing position to a new anterior non-obstructing position within the mandibular space. The mandibular space is that area between the two rami of the mandible. Even with the tongue maximally displaced into the mandibular space, visualization of the larynx is sometimes inadequate.

Usually, a normal-size tongue fits easily into a normal-size mandibular space, whereas a large tongue would fit poorly. After filling the space, a large tongue still occupies some of the oropharyngeal airway causing obstruction. For this reason, a large tongue (macroglossia) is a predictor of a difficult intubation. Similarly, a normal-size tongue fits poorly into a small mandibular space. It too occupies some of the oropharyngeal airway, thereby obstructing the line of sight. Consequently, a small mandible (micrognathia) is a predictor of a difficult intubation. In essence, a tongue that is large compared with the size of the mouth, oropharynx, and mandible takes up excessive space in the oropharynx and interferes with visualization.

The base of the tongue resides so close to the larynx that inability to adequately displace it anteriorly creates another problem. As the base of the tongue hangs down over the larynx, the glottis is hidden from view. The glottic aperture is then anatomically anterior to the base of the tongue, hence the term "anterior larynx." Under such circumstances the larynx is anterior to the base of the tongue and cannot be seen because the tongue hides it. Glottic and supraglottic masses that force the base of the tongue posteriorly can create difficult intubations as well. Some of the masses that may be encountered include lingual tonsils, epiglottic cysts, and thyroglossal duct cysts.

After filling the mandibular space with the tongue, additional pressure on the laryngoscope blade lifts the mandible anteriorly. In this setting, mandibular displacement is dependent upon the TMJ. In addition to its hinge-like motion, the TMJ also works in a gliding (translational) movement. It is the gliding motion that allows the mandible to slide anteriorly across the maxilla. If the joint does not translate, the mandible cannot be displaced anteriorly and the tongue cannot be moved out of the line of sight.

Recognizing the implications of tongue size to successful laryngoscopy, Mallampati et al. in 1985 and Samsoon and Young in 1987 devised classification systems to predict difficult laryngoscopy, utilizing this concept. A difficult laryngoscopy occurs when it is not possible to visualize any portion of the vocal cords. Mallampati and Samsoon reasoned that a large tongue could be identified upon visual inspection of the open mouth. Both classification systems relate the size of tongue to the oropharyngeal structures identified. A normal-size tongue allows for visualization of certain oropharyngeal structures. As the tongue size increases, some structures become hidden from view. Consequently, both investigators proposed systems that reason backwards from this premise.

Application of the Mallampati and/or Samsoon classification system(s) is easy and painless. The patient is seated in the neutral position. The mouth is opened as wide as it can and the tongue is protruded as far as possible. Phonation is discouraged because it raises the soft palate and allows for visualization of additional structures. The observer looks for specified anatomic landmarks. They are the fauces, pillars, uvula, and soft palate. The Mallampati classification system utilizes three groups and the Samsoon classification system employs four groups (Figure 46.1). Both systems suggest that as the tongue size increases, fewer structures are visualized and laryngoscopy becomes more difficult. Mallampati scores tend to be higher in pregnant versus nonpregnant patients.

Just as the size of tongue can be estimated, so too can the size of the mandible. This is accomplished by asking the patient to extend their head at the atlanto-occipital joint and identifying the mandibular mentum and thyroid cartilage. The Adam's apple (thyroid notch) is the most superficial structure in the neck and serves as a good landmark for the thyroid cartilage. The vocal cords lie just caudad to the thyroid notch. The distance between the thyroid cartilage and mentum (thyromental distance) is measured in one of three ways. The measurement can be made with a set of spacers, a small pocket ruler, or with the observer's fingers. The normal thyromental distance is 6.5 cm. A thyromental distance of greater than 6 cm is predictive of an easy intubation. A thyromental distance of 6 cm or less is suggestive of a difficult intubation. Oftentimes, rulers are not present at

the bedside. In the absence of a ruler, practitioners can judge the thyromental distance with their fingers. By knowing the width of one's middle three fingers, which frequently approximates 6 cm, the thyromental distance can be compared with the fingers' span. In this way, clinically relevant approximations can be taken into account when examining patients for the purpose of predicting difficult intubation. The usefulness of predicting difficult intubation based on thyromental distance has been challenged. Data extracted from Rocke et al.'s 1992 paper and El-Ganzouri's 1996 paper show that thyromental distance (receding mandible) offers a 7% or less probability of predicting difficult intubation. Chou in 1993 and Brodsky in 2002 describe patients whose thyromental distances were well in excess of 6.5 cm and who were difficult intubations.

Similar measurements and predictions have been made utilizing the hyoid bone and mandible, as well as the sternum and mentum. Chou and Wu (2001) suggest that a long mandibulohyoid distance predicts a large hypopharyngeal tongue, which hides the glottis during laryngoscopy and thereby produces a difficult intubation. They reason that the tongue is hinged to the hyoid bone, so that a long hyomandibular length represents a caudad-lying tongue. With the base of the tongue positioned farther inferiorly, it occupies more space in the oropharyngeal airway. Consequently, it obstructs the laryngoscopist's line of sight. The hyoid bone is more difficult to feel than the thyroid cartilage and is oftentimes impossible to locate. The sternum and mentum are generally easy to find, but the sternomental distance has not been substantiated as a good predictor of difficult intubation by other investigators.

The ability to translate the TMJ is easily assessed prior to induction. The patient is asked to place the mandibular incisors (bottom teeth) in front of the maxillary incisors (upper teeth). Inability to perform this simple task is usually from one of two sources. First, the TMJ may not glide, thereby

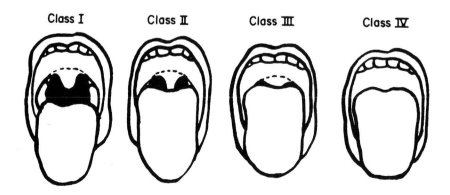

FIGURE 46.1 Samsoon classification of pharyngeal structures. (From Samsoon GLT, Young JRB: Difficult tracheal intubation: a retrospective study. Anaesthesia 42:487, 1987.)

predicting a difficult intubation. Second, some patients find it difficult to coordinate the maneuver, in which case there is no implication for a difficult intubation.

The upper lip bite test was proposed as a modification of the TMJ displacement test. The upper lip bite test is performed by asking the patient to move the mandibular incisors as high on the upper lip as possible. The maneuver is similar to biting the lip. Contact of the teeth above or on the vermilion border is thought to predict adequate laryngoscopic views. Inability to contact the vermilion border is thought to predict poor laryngoscopic views. Both the TMJ translation test and the upper lip bite test assess TMJ glide, which is an important consideration during laryngoscopy. Table 46.1 summarizes a quick, easy, bedside scheme for predicting difficult intubation.

3. Are the risk factors for difficult intubation reliable predictors of difficult intubation?

Although it makes intuitive sense to perform, and is consistent with best medical practices, airway evaluation frequently falls short of its intended goal. Numerous rating systems based on recognized prediction criteria have been investigated. Most suffer from recurrent problems.

The first problem is nomenclature. A standardized definition of the "difficult airway" did not exist until 1993. At that time it was explained as a situation in which a conventionally trained anesthesiologist experienced difficulty with mask ventilation, difficulty with tracheal intubation, or both. For years, individual investigators needed to establish their own definition of "difficult intubation" each time studies were conducted. Consequently, the endpoints of their work were not necessarily comparable to other investigations in the field, making comparative analysis of studies impossible. In 1993, the American Society of Anesthesiologists' (ASA) Committee on Practice Guidelines for Management of the Difficult Airway offered a generally acceptable definition. Ten years later the definition was altered slightly. In 2003, "difficult tracheal intubation" referred to any intubation that required multiple attempts. This is a good clinical definition but lacks the precision required for scientific investigation. For example, some practitioners may perform a single laryngoscopy and, based upon the view obtained, elect to forego further attempts at laryngoscopy. Such cases may be handled with a supraglottic airway device, regional anesthesia, or other techniques. This situation does not meet the definition of difficult intubation, when in fact it would have if one more attempt at intubation was performed. Thus, the ASA's definition serves as a good clinical understanding of difficult intubation, but lacks the rigid, encompassing concerns required for scientific investigation. "Failed intubation" is an easier term to understand. A failed intubation exists when laryngoscopists give up and admit that traditional intubation will not be successful. The endpoint is clear and occurs with an incidence of 1:280 in obstetric patients and 1:2,230 in the general operating room population.

The second problem is identifying features that predict difficult intubation. This is frequently accomplished by attempting to recognize characteristics found in patients who have proven to be difficult intubations. The problem with such an approach is the lack of information about the same characteristics in patients who are easy intubations. As Turkan points out, we do not even know the normal values for many prediction criteria. A better method is to

---

TABLE 46.1   Predictors of Difficult Intubation

Criteria	Factors that Suggest Difficult Intubation
History	History of difficult intubation
Length of upper incisors	Relatively long
Inter-incisor distance	Less than two finger breadths or less than 3 cm
Overbite	Maxillary incisors override mandibular incisors
TMJ translation	Inability to extend mandibular incisors anterior to maxillary incisors
Mandibular space	Small, indurated, encroached upon by mass
Cervical vertebral range of motion	Cannot touch chin to chest or cannot extend neck
Thyromental distance	Less than 3 finger breadths (less than 6 cm)
Mallampati/Samsoon classification	Mallampati III/Samsoon IV: relatively large tongue, uvula not visible
Neck	Short, thick

Adapted from American Society of Anesthesiologists Task Force on Difficult Airway Management: Practice guidelines for management of the difficult airway. Anesthesiology 98:1269–1277, 2003.

apply multivariate analysis to patient populations in a prospective manner. In that way, a single factor can be compared for difficult and easy intubations. Various rating systems attempt to combine multiple predictors into a formula. To date, none are satisfactory.

The third problem is validating the tests, once they are promulgated. Validation tests performed on the same patient population used to identify them are misleading. This is like counting the number of envelopes in a particular mail box, predicting that all mailboxes contain that number of envelopes, and then validating the prediction by re-counting the envelopes in that same mailbox. Validation must be performed by counting the envelopes in multiple different mailboxes. In the same way, validation of difficult intubation predictors must be performed in multiple different patient populations. The experimental patient sample cannot be used to validate experimental results. Different sample populations are needed for that.

The fourth problem is the experimental methods. Individual practitioners differ and clinical practice has shown that a particular patient who is difficult to intubate in the hands of one laryngoscopist may be successfully intubated by another laryngoscopist. In this way, experimental designs utilizing more than one laryngoscopist introduce a source of variation, which detracts from attempts to control experimental conditions. Relying on a single laryngoscopist obviates this problem, but limits the number of patients that can be enrolled into a single study. Another source of experimental error is observer variation. Observations performed by different experimenters are subject to variations and introduce another source of erroneous data. The best way to prevent this problem is for all observations to be performed by a single experimenter. This too may limit the number of patients enrolled in a single study.

Statistical tests for assessing the usefulness of criteria include sensitivity and positive predictive value. Sensitivity is the ratio of correctly identified difficult intubation patients to all the difficult intubation patients within the entire patient population. For example, take a patient population in which 5 are difficult to intubate. If a particular predictor of difficult intubation correctly identifies all 5 patients, then its sensitivity is 100%. If the test correctly identifies only 2 of the 5 patients, then its sensitivity is 2/5 or 40%. Positive predictive value is the probability that difficult intubation patients identified by the test are in fact difficult to intubate. If the test predicts that 5 patients will be difficult to intubate and all 5 of those patients are difficult to intubate then its positive predictive value is 100%. If the test predicts that 10 patients will be difficult to intubate but only 5 of them are difficult to intubate, then its predictive value is 5/10 or 50%. Unfortunately, statistical tests such as sensitivity and positive predictive value applied to classic prediction criteria have yielded disappointing results.

In 1984, Cormack and Lehane described a grading system for comparing laryngoscopic views as follows:

- Grade I: the entire glottic opening
- Grade II: the posterior laryngeal aperture but not the anterior portion
- Grade III: the epiglottis but not any part of the larynx
- Grade IV: the soft palate but not the epiglottis

Early evidence indicated good correlation between Mallampati/Samsoon classes and laryngoscopic grades. In other words, as the Mallampati/Samsoon classes increased in number, the prediction was that corresponding laryngoscopic grades would also increase in number, for any given patient. This concept formed the basis for using Mallampati/Samsoon classes to predict difficult intubation. In 1992, Rocke et al. disproved that relationship. Rocke and colleagues investigated several classic predictors of difficult intubation and demonstrated that none of the ones they studied were reliable predictors of difficult intubation (Figure 46.2). Classic prediction criteria essentially deal with surface anatomy. They screen for some factors that are associated with difficult intubation, but fail to address others. Some potential problems are hidden from surface anatomy examinations. Subglottic, glottic, and supraglottic abnormalities, such as tracheal stenosis, lingual tonsil hypertrophy, or epiglottic prolapse into the glottic opening, cannot be diagnosed by standard physical examinations for predicting difficult intubation. Pathophysiologic factors such as mobile TMJ discs or disc fragments can produce severely limited mouth opening following induction of anesthesia, when none existed before. Precise measurements of atlanto-axial motion sometimes fail to predict difficult intubation. These factors and others may be unrecognized by standard tests but complicate intubation, nonetheless. At the time of this writing, *no single factor reliably predicts difficult intubation. The likelihood of a difficult intubation increases when multiple predictors are present in a patient at the same time.*

4. How is the anticipated difficult intubation approached?

Anticipated difficult intubations with proven or suspected difficult mask ventilation are best approached with the patient awake and spontaneously breathing. Proper preparation of the airway before instrumentation is critical. Preparation begins approximately 1 hour before arrival in the operating room. At that time, antisialagogues are administered as premedication. Their use is intended to desiccate the mucosa before administration of topical local anesthetics. An intervening layer of secretions acts as a physical barrier preventing contact between local anesthetic and mucosa. Without direct contact of the two, inadequate airway anesthesia results and predisposes the patient to coughing, gagging, and withdrawal. Furthermore, copious

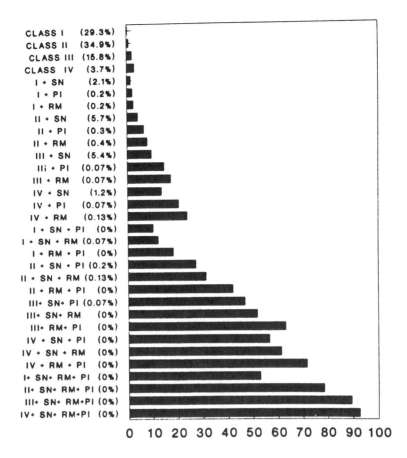

FIGURE 46.2 The probability of experiencing a difficult intubation for combinations of risk factors and their observed incidence (percentages). Abbreviations: SN, short neck; PI, protruding maxillary incisors; RM, receding mandible. (From Rocke DA, Murray WB, Rout CC, Gouws E: Relative risk analysis of factors associated with difficult intubation in obstetric anesthesia. Anesthesiology 77:67, 1992.)

secretions impair the view through flexible fiberoptic laryngoscopes. Depending on the degree of pre-existing airway compromise, preoperative sedation may be contraindicated.

After adequate antisialagogue effect, airway anesthesia is most easily achieved by nebulizing 4 mL of 4% lidocaine. Another equally effective option is to atomize the same solution. Superior laryngeal nerve blocks and transtracheal nerve blocks are sometimes required.

If the nasal approach is planned, the risk of epistaxis can be minimized with topical application of 0.5% phenylephrine, 4% cocaine, or 0.05% oxymetazoline (Afrin). In the absence of local nasal pathology, flexible fiberoptic nasal tracheal intubation is generally less difficult than the oral route.

After achieving satisfactory airway anesthesia, most intubation techniques progress well to successful completion. Blind techniques, retraction blades, or fiberscopes are commonly employed.

Friable tumors, abscesses, and impending obstructive airway tumors often require awake tracheostomy.

5. Describe the management options for a patient who, after induction of anesthesia, unexpectedly cannot be intubated with a Macintosh blade. This patient has a good mask airway.

Having induced general anesthesia in a patient and then discovered a difficult intubation, it is imperative to maintain oxygenation and ventilation. This is generally accomplished with a facemask and 100% oxygen. Successful oxygenation during controlled ventilation and desaturation during intubation attempts are monitored with pulse oximetry. During traditional laryngoscopy, external posterior and/or lateral displacement of the larynx may bring it into view. Improved sniffing position may be helpful.

A multitude of retraction blades exist and vary in length and shape. They are used to displace the base of the tongue and epiglottis anterior to the line of vision. The most familiar types are the Macintosh and Miller blades. Difficulty with the Macintosh blade often arises when its tip fails to elevate the hyoid bone, which indirectly raises the epiglottis. Often, a straight blade elevates a floppy epiglottis when curved blades fail to do so. Difficulty with the straight blade frequently comes from impacting on teeth. The Siker blade was developed to view the "anterior larynx" but is extremely difficult to use because the laryngoscopist must learn to work with a mirror image. The Bellscope, a bent straight blade, offers the advantages of the Macintosh and Miller blades, as well as improved anterior vision by employing angulation and a prism, rather than a mirror. The Bullard and Wu laryngoscopes incorporate a fiberoptic viewing system and a broad retraction blade. Consequently, sniffing position is not as important when using these laryngoscopes. They may be of greatest potential benefit for those whose head must remain flat on the bed, such as the patient with cervical spine fractures. A working channel is provided for suctioning, administration of local anesthetics, or insufflation of oxygen. Both the Bullard and Wu laryngoscopes require a mouth opening sufficiently wide to accommodate the broad retraction blade and endotracheal tube. Blood and secretions in the airway tend to impair the view through fiberoptic systems. Upper airway edema or adipose tissue may sometimes encroach on the view of traditional retraction laryngoscopes, which are open on the right side. A two-piece tubular laryngoscope such as the Wu scope can overcome this problem.

Various stylets may be used. The hollow stylet, gummed elastic bougie, or similar devices should be available in all anesthetizing locations. High-technology variations, such as illuminating stylets, work well in the average adult but are associated with false-positives and false-negatives in the very thin and obese. Illuminating stylets function on the principle of transillumination. As the light bulb enters the trachea, transilluminated light remains bright and circumscribed. If the stylet enters the esophagus, the light becomes more diffuse. Factors impairing its usefulness include anterior cervical scars, obesity, neck tumors, blood, or secretions. Macintosh first described this technique in 1957. Over the ensuing five decades, it has not gained popularity.

If a flexible fiberoptic laryngoscopy is not planned, then blind spontaneously breathing nasal tracheal intubation is an alternative offering a good chance of success. Vasoconstriction of the nasal mucosa, selection of a small nasal tracheal tube (6 mm), and generous lubrication of the tube's distal portion are highly recommended. If flexible fiberoptic intubation is planned, then the risk of epistaxis may dissuade one from the nasal approach. Epistaxis might seriously impair mask ventilation and visualization by all means of laryngoscopy.

Retrograde guided techniques are highly successful but have not gained popularity. The cricothyroid membrane is pierced by a 16-gauge needle at a 30° angle pointing cephalad. Confirmation of proper placement is achieved by aspirating air into a syringe. The needle remains in situ, and a thin wire is passed through the needle until it exits the mouth or nose. The wire is clamped outside the neck to anchor its distal end. The endotracheal tube is advanced over the guidewire and into the trachea. Several predictable problems occur with this technique. After the wire is threaded retrograde through the airway, it may not exit the mouth or nose. Laryngoscopy and retrieval with a clamp may be necessary. Advancement of the endotracheal tube along the wire may be blocked by the arytenoids. To overcome this problem, the endotracheal tube is retracted 1–2 cm and rotated 90° counterclockwise. Progression beyond the vocal cords and into the trachea may be prevented by the guidewire as it exits the neck and tethers the endotracheal tube at a distance of 1–2 cm into the trachea.

Alternatively, the portion of the guidewire that exits the mouth or nose can be threaded through the working channel of a flexible fiberoptic laryngoscope. The scope is then advanced over the wire, under direct vision, through the vocal cords. In this way passage through the vocal cords and into the trachea is confirmed visually. Once positioned properly in the trachea, the endotracheal tube can be advanced over the fiberscope, and its proper location above the carina confirmed.

Compared with various retraction blades and stylets, flexible fiberoptic laryngoscopy has established a long and impressive success record with difficult intubations. Flexible fiberoptic laryngoscopy is applicable to the anesthetized and awake patient. In the anesthetized patient, it can be performed with interrupted controlled ventilation by facemask, such as with traditional rigid laryngoscopy. Alternatively, it can be accomplished using simultaneous controlled ventilation via anesthesia facemasks equipped with a self-sealing diaphragm.

Flexible fiberoptic intubation in the paralyzed patient is generally more difficult than in the spontaneously breathing patient because the anterior pharyngeal wall tends to collapse onto the posterior pharyngeal wall, thereby obstructing the view. Also, the larynx assumes a more anterior position, hindering its identification. Copious blood and/or secretions seriously impair vision through a flexible fiberoptic laryngoscope (FFL). FFLs contain suction channels, but unlike suction channels in the pulmonologist's bronchoscope, the FFL's channel is an inefficient one. Consequently, blood and secretions are aspirated better with a standard large-bore suction device, such as the one normally used for traditional rigid laryngoscopy. Passing oxygen through the FFL's working channel tends to push blood and secretions out of the way, prevents fogging, and enhances the patient's effective FiO_2. The sniffing position allows for further posterior displacement of the epiglottis, which could also obstruct the view. Consequently, cervical extension with the head flat on the bed is preferable for flexible fiberoptic laryngoscopy.

Alternatives to Endotracheal Intubation Under General Anesthesia

Continue anesthesia by facemask or other
    supraglottic devices
Regional anesthesia
Awake spontaneously breathing intubation (usually
    flexible fiberoptic intubation)
Tracheostomy
Cricothyroidotomy

Various aids to FFL insertion exist. Care must be taken to seat oral airways exactly in the midline to prevent lateral displacement of the fiberscope, which adds to the difficulty of intubation. In cases for which it is especially important to do so, none of the presently available oral intubation airways adequately elevate the base of the tongue. Insertion of the nasal tracheal tube before the fiberoptic scope risks epistaxis before passage of the insertion tube. Furthermore, placing nasal tracheal tubes too far eliminates adequate space for manipulating the scope between the nasal tracheal tube and larynx. Difficulty threading endotracheal tubes into the larynx may arise if the endotracheal tube's tip abuts the right arytenoid. To overcome this obstacle, the endotracheal tube should be retracted 1–2 cm and rotated 90° counterclockwise. This maneuver brings the tip anteriorly, away from the right arytenoid.

After exhausting one's personal repertoire of techniques, simply repeating methods that have already failed seems to have little chance of success. Additional instrumentation will lead to laryngeal and pharyngeal edema predisposing the patient to airway obstruction. The remaining options include continuing anesthesia by facemask; performing regional anesthesia; for urgent cases, awakening the patient and intubating with spontaneous breathing that day; awakening the patient and intubating with spontaneous respirations several days later to allow for resorption of airway edema; performing tracheostomy; and performing cricothyroidotomy. Initial tracheostomy is indicated for laryngeal fractures and for abscesses impinging on the airway.

The ASA's Difficult Airway Algorithm serves as a useful guideline (Figure 46.3).

6. Following induction of anesthesia, ventilation by facemask and intubation are impossible. What maneuvers may help?

Inability to both intubate and ventilate is a rare occurrence with a potentially tragic outcome. Several treatment options exist. A variety of oral and cricoid puncture methods have been described to assist with such situations.

Of the oral techniques, world-wide experience is greatest with two: the esophageal-tracheal combitube (ETC) and the laryngeal mask airway (LMA). The ETC is a device intended for blind insertion into the airway. It is potentially useful for ventilation and oxygenation whether located in the esophagus or trachea (Figure 46.4). The ETC is a double-lumen tube with an outside diameter of 13 mm. One lumen is open at both ends, like an endotracheal tube. The other lumen is open at the proximal end and occluded at the distal end. The ETC contains two inflatable cuffs. The proximal cuff is large and when situated properly is located in the pharynx, between the base of the tongue and soft palate. Inflation of this balloon seals the mouth and nose. A smaller, distal cuff seals the trachea or esophagus, depending upon its location. The lumen with the distal occlusion is perforated in a segment between the two cuffs.

If the ETC is placed in the esophagus, oxygen is administered through the closed-end lumen, which allows gas to escape from perforations in the pharyngeal portion (Figure 46.4A). Oxygen then enters the larynx and is prevented from entering the stomach by the distal balloon. The proximal balloon prevents gas escaping from the mouth or nose. If the ETC is placed into the trachea, oxygen is administered into the lumen open at both ends, which functions like a standard endotracheal tube (Figure 46.4B). The ETC, when placed in the esophagus, allows suctioning of gastric contents through the open-ended side, thereby helping to reduce the risk of aspiration pneumonitis. In the esophageal position, pulmonary toilet is impossible through the ETC.

Ventilation through the ETC has been adequate during anesthesia, intensive care, cardiopulmonary resuscitation, and mechanical ventilation. It has been used successfully to oxygenate and ventilate patients whose trachea could not be intubated and whose lungs could not be ventilated by facemask. At the time of this writing, it is available in two adult sizes.

Another device that is inserted blindly through the mouth is the LMA (Figure 46.5). The LMA is a 12-mm inner diameter tube attached to a mask. The mask has an inflatable balloon around its periphery. With the balloon deflated, the mask is advanced into the mouth and through the airway until obstruction to passage is encountered. At this point, the mask should be positioned cephalad to the esophagus and surrounding the larynx. The balloon is inflated in an attempt to create an airtight chamber around the larynx. The 12-mm tube now exits from the mouth and is connected to an anesthesia breathing circuit.

The LMA is available in adult and pediatric sizes. It works well in 90–98% of cases. This 2–10% failure rate is far greater than the incidence of inability to ventilate and intubate. Nevertheless, it has been successfully used for airway management in elective surgery, as well as in cases of predicted and unanticipated difficult intubation. The LMA

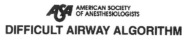

DIFFICULT AIRWAY ALGORITHM

1. Assess the likelihood and clinical impact of basic management problems:
   - A. Difficult Ventilation
   - B. Difficult Intubation
   - C. Difficulty with Patient Cooperation or Consent
   - D. Difficult Tracheostomy

2. Actively pursue opportunities to deliver supplemental oxygen throughout the process of difficult airway management

3. Consider the relative merits and feasibility of basic management choices:

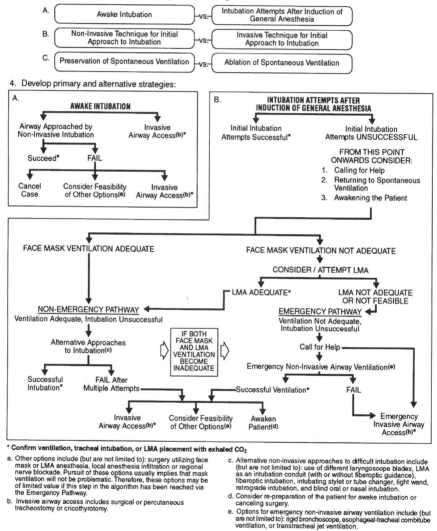

4. Develop primary and alternative strategies:

* Confirm ventilation, tracheal intubation, or LMA placement with exhaled CO_2

a. Other options include (but are not limited to): surgery utilizing face mask or LMA anesthesia, local anesthesia infiltration or regional nerve blockade. Pursuit of these options usually implies that mask ventilation will not be problematic. Therefore, these options may be of limited value if this step in the algorithm has been reached via the Emergency Pathway.

b. Invasive airway access includes surgical or percutaneous tracheostomy or cricothyrotomy.

c. Alternative non-invasive approaches to difficult intubation include (but are not limited to): use of different laryngoscope blades, LMA as an intubation conduit (with or without fiberoptic guidance), fiberoptic intubation, intubating stylet or tube changer, light wand, retrograde intubation, and blind oral or nasal intubation.

d. Consider re-preparation of the patient for awake intubation or canceling surgery.

e. Options for emergency non-invasive airway ventilation include (but are not limited to): rigid bronchoscope, esophageal-tracheal combitube ventilation, or transtracheal jet ventilation.

FIGURE 46.3 American Society of Anesthesiologists' Difficult Airway Algorithm. This is intended as a practice guideline for difficult airway management. LMA, laryngeal mask airway. (From American Society of Anesthesiologists Task Force on Difficult Airway Management: Practice guidelines for management of the difficult airway. Anesthesiology 98:1269–1277, 2003.)

has been used to assist blind intubation and FFL-guided intubation in patients whose larynxes could not be visualized by traditional rigid laryngoscopy.

If the LMA's inflatable balloon is not positioned properly, a large gas leak occurs around the mask, impairing ventilation. This leak is exacerbated by high inflation pressures. Malposition of the balloon increases the risk of gastric content aspiration into the lungs. Obstruction to gas flow may occur if the tongue or epiglottis is pushed back over the larynx as the mask is inserted. Difficulty in positioning the LMA occurred 18% of the time, and failure to properly position occurred 3% of the time. It will predictably offer little in cases of airway stenosis and gross anatomic distortion. LMAs are available in several varieties. The classic LMA is shown in Figure 46.5. A disposable model also exists. Advantages of disposable models include reduced cost for each one, as well as elimination of cross-contamination from inadequately cleaned and sterilized, reusable types. An intubating LMA was designed to facilitate tracheal tube passage through the glottis. Although it works well to maintain upper airway patency, ideal alignment with the trachea can be problematic. Deviations from ideal positioning hamper tracheal tube passage. The ProSeal LMA comes equipped with a distal port. The port is positioned just cephalad to the esophagus and allows egress of gastric contents that might collect in the pharynx.

A tube connected to the port provides access to the opening. With proper alignment, a gastric tube can be inserted through the ProSeal LMA and into the stomach for elimination of gastric contents.

Alternative supraglottic devices include COBRAs, pharyngeal airways, E-Z Tubes, Chou Airways, and others.

Of the more invasive techniques, cricothyroid puncture and transtracheal ventilation are well described. Successful use of transtracheal ventilation relies on preparation before the critical incident occurs. Equipment must be assembled and readily available to patients requiring its use. Devices are best stored in all anesthetizing locations and anywhere intubation might reasonably be anticipated.

Basic equipment consists of a 14-gauge over-the-needle catheter with luer lock adapter, non-compressible oxygen tubing, standard 15-mm connector, and a source of pressurized oxygen (Figure 46.6). Such systems deliver gas at very high pressures and tend to disconnect at portions that are not securely fastened.

With the patient in the supine position, the head is extended to expose the anterior neck. The thyroid cartilage is palpated and the finger run inferiorly until a depression (the cricothyroid membrane) is felt. Another dense substance (cricoid cartilage) is appreciated just caudad to the depression. A 14-gauge needle is placed through the skin perpendicular to all planes, and advanced until the cricothyroid

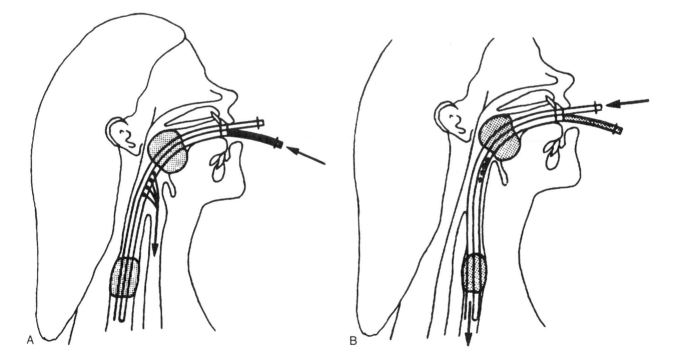

FIGURE 46.4 Esophageal-tracheal combitube. (A) The esophageal position. (B) The tracheal position. (From Eichinger S, et al.: Airway management in a case of neck impalement. Br J Anaesth 68:534, 1992.)

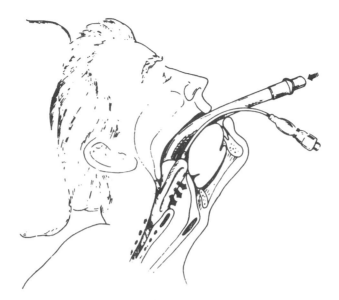

FIGURE 46.5 Laryngeal mask airway positioned posterior to the larynx. (From Cork R, Monk JE: Management of a suspected and re-suspected difficult laryngoscopy with the laryngeal mask airway. J Clin Anesth 4:231, 1992.)

membrane is punctured. Proper positioning within the trachea is confirmed by freely aspirating air through the needle. The needle is then removed, leaving the catheter positioned in the lumen of the trachea. The device is attached to the intravenous catheter and 100% oxygen administered under positive pressure. This is most conveniently accomplished by attaching the 15-mm connector to the anesthesia machine's common gas outlet and controlling the flow of oxygen with the oxygen flush valve. Not all anesthesia machines function well in this circumstance.

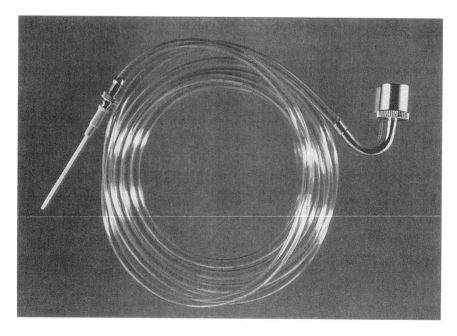

FIGURE 46.6 Cricothyroid puncture ventilation equipment (transtracheal ventilation).

Ventilation systems utilizing pressure step-down valves interposed between high-pressure oxygen sources, such as wall oxygen or oxygen tanks, can be attached to the same cricothyroid puncture catheter. The higher the pressure generated, the more likely the catheter will become dislodged, so a designated holder must be assigned to keep it in place.

If intubation and ventilation are impaired by tissues encroaching on the airway, then rigid bronchoscopy may provide for immediate life-saving ventilation and oxygenation.

7. How is successful tracheal intubation verified?

The most reliable method of confirming successful tracheal intubation is by direct laryngoscopy with a traditional rigid laryngoscope and visualizing the tracheal tube between the vocal cords. External posterior displacement of the larynx may improve the view. Alternatively, a FFL can be advanced through the endotracheal tube and tracheal rings and carina identified. Two other methods of confirmation, expired carbon dioxide detection and esophageal indicator bulb inflation, are slightly less reliable. Expired carbon dioxide detection can be quantitative or qualitative. These methods frequently provide digital readouts, wave forms, or colorimetric indicators. Alternatively, the esophageal indicator bulb attached to an indwelling tracheal tube will expand rapidly if the tube is located in the trachea. When positioned in the esophagus, it will generally fail to inflate or expand slowly. Tertiary methods of verifying tracheal tube placement are less reliable than those mentioned above and are listed in Table 46.2.

8. Following a difficult intubation, how is postoperative extubation managed?

Extubation requires an estimate of postoperative airway edema. Repeated instrumentation during intubation and surgical manipulation, independently and additively contribute to tongue base and laryngeal swelling. Airway edema may culminate in respiratory obstruction.

Patients at risk for edema are best managed with prolonged tracheal intubation or tracheostomy. Once edema has resolved, a trial of extubation or decannulation can be considered.

Before extubating the potentially edematous airway, the endotracheal tube cuff is deflated and gas escaping around the tube is sought. Absence of an audible gas leak may be an indicator of upper airway swelling. If a leak is detected and if the risk of reintubation is high, then the tracheal tube can be removed over a FFL. This technique allows for the administration of oxygen through the working channel while observing for airway collapse. In the event of respiratory difficulty, airway patency can be re-established by advancing the endotracheal tube over the FFL, which is still positioned in the trachea. A jet stylet or endotracheal tube

TABLE 46.2	Methods to Verify Correct Tracheal Tube Placement

Most reliable
  Direct visualization of tracheal tube between the vocal cords
  Observation of carina via a flexible fiberoptic laryngoscope passed through the tracheal tube
Very reliable
  Expired carbon dioxide detection by colorimetry or capnography
  Esophageal detector device
Reliable
  Auscultation of breath sounds
  Observation of chest expansion and contraction during inspiration and exhalation
  Epigastric auscultation and observation for gastric distention during respiration
  Tactile confirmation by assistant as tube is passed
  Respiratory bag inflation and deflation during spontaneous respiration
  Respiratory bag compliance and spontaneous refilling
  Exhaled gas via the tracheal tube during chest compression
  Condensation and evaporation of water during respirations
  Tracheal tube cuff palpation at the suprasternal notch
  Endobronchial intubation
  Pulse oximetry
  Chest radiograph

exchanger may be used in a similar fashion. Jet stylets and tube exchangers share several potential complications. Both reside between the vocal cords and can produce laryngospasm, which predisposes to two problems. First, jet ventilation in the presence of upper airway obstruction results in breath-stacking because there is no egress for gas from the lungs. Intrapulmonary pressures increase, thereby risking pneumothorax. Second, spontaneous respiratory efforts against a closed glottis can produce negative pressure pulmonary edema. This is usually amenable to relief of the obstruction, supplemental oxygen, diuretics, and morphine. Both jet stylets and tube exchangers, if extended beyond the tracheal tube, can produce other problems. The posterior tracheal wall is membranous and is easily punctured leading to pneumomediastinum and mediastinitis. Stimulation of the carina produces hypertension, tachycardia, vigorous coughing, and retching. Even with these devices in place, the tracheal tube may not advance through the glottis. It can get caught on the base of the tongue, laryngeal cartilages, and vocal cords.

SUGGESTED READINGS

Adnet F, Borron SW, Dumas JL, Lapostolle F, Cupa M, Lapandry C: Study of the "sniffing position" by magnetic resonance imaging. Anesthesiology 94:83, 2001

American Society of Anesthesiologists Task Force on Difficult Airway Management: Practice guidelines for management of the difficult airway. Anesthesiology 98:1269, 2003

Benumof L: Management of the difficult adult airway with special emphasis on awake tracheal intubation. Anesthesiology 75:1082, 1991

Brodsky JB, Lemmens HJ, Brock-Utne JG, Vierra M, Saidman LJ. Morbid obesity and tracheal intubation. Anesth Analg 96:732, 2002

Buckland RW, Pedley J: Lingual thyroid: a threat to the airway. Anaesthesia 55:1103, 2000

Chou HC, Wu TL: Mandibulohyoid distance in difficult laryngoscopy. Br J Anaesth 71:368, 1993

Chou HC, Wu TL: Rethinking the three axes alignment theory for direct laryngoscopy. Acta Anaesthesiol Scand 45:261, 2001

El-Ganzouri AR, McCarthy RJ, Tuman KJ, Tanck EN, Ivankovich AD: Preoperative airway assessment: predictive value of a multivariate risk index. Anesth Analg 82:1197, 1996

Khan ZH, Kashfi A, Ebrahimkhani E: A comparison of the upper lip bite test (a simple new technique) with modified Mallampati classification in predicting difficulty in endotracheal intubation: a prospective blinded study. Anesth Analg 96:595, 2003

Langeron O, Masso E, Huraux C, Guggiari M, Bianchi A, Coriat P, Riou B: Prediction of difficult mask ventilation. Anesthesiology 92:1229, 2000

Macintosch R, Richards HR: Illuminated introducer for endotracheal tubes. Anesthesia 12:223, 1957

Mallampati SR, Gugino LD, Desai SP, et al.: A clinical sign to predict difficult tracheal intubation: a prospective study. Can Anaesth Soc J 32:429, 1985

Reed AP, Han D: Preparation of the patient for awake fiberoptic intubation. Anesthesiol Clin North Am 9:69, 1991

Rocke DA, Murray WB, Rout CC, Gouws E: Relative risk analysis of factors associated with difficult intubation in obstetric anesthesia. Anesthesiology 77:67, 1992

Samsoon GLT, Young JRB: Difficult tracheal intubation: a retrospective study. Anaesthesia 42:487, 1987

ADENOTONSILLECTOMY

Andrew Herlich, MD

A 5-year-old boy presents to the emergency room with hematemesis. He has undergone an ambulatory adenotonsillectomy 7 days previously. After evaluation, he is scheduled to return to the operating room for control of post-adenotonsillectomy hemorrhage. He is anxious and ill-appearing. Physical examination reveals a heart rate of 120 beats per minute, blood pressure of 85/65 mmHg, and a respiratory rate of 32 breaths per minute.

QUESTIONS

1. What are the indications and contraindications for adenotonsillectomy?
2. Describe the essential elements of preoperative evaluation for adenotonsillectomy.
3. How is the patient premedicated for adenotonsillectomy?
4. What anesthetic alternatives are available for patients undergoing adenotonsillectomy?
5. What are the common postanesthetic care unit problems anticipated following adenotonsillectomy?
6. Which patients are suitable candidates for ambulatory adenotonsillectomy?
7. Describe the anesthetic management of a patient presenting with post-tonsillectomy hemorrhage.

1. What are the indications and contraindications for adenotonsillectomy?

Tonsillar and adenoidal tissues are actually a part of the lymphatic system known as Waldeyer's ring. At one time, adenotonsillectomy was the single most frequently performed surgical procedure. With the advent of antibiotics and more conservative thinking, its numbers have diminished. The most common indications for adenotonsillectomy today are adenotonsillar hyperplasia in conjunction with obstructive sleep apnea, suspicion of malignant disease, hemorrhagic tonsillitis, abnormal maxillofacial growth, and failure to thrive. Indications for tonsillectomy *without* adenoidectomy include recurrent/chronic tonsillitis, peritonsillar abscess, and streptococcal carriage. Indications for adenoidectomy *without* tonsillectomy include adenoiditis, recurrent or chronic rhinosinusitis and otitis media. Relative indications for adenotonsillectomy include chronic halitosis, speech impairment, dysphagia, and upper airway obstruction with relative adenotonsillar hyperplasia.

Significant contraindications to adenotonsillectomy are systemic infection, uncorrected coagulopathy, occult or frank cleft palate, and uncontrolled systemic diseases such as diabetes mellitus. Coagulopathies can be corrected preoperatively once the diagnosis is known. In the case of occult or frank clefts, tonsillar and adenoidal tissue may contribute to intelligible speech by filling the velopharyngeal space. Once they are removed, velopharyngeal incompetence occurs, resulting in less intelligible, hypernasal speech. A clue to the occult cleft is a bifid uvula.

In the event that adenoidectomy is necessary in the patient with a cleft, partial adenoidectomy to the level of Passavant's ridge is performed. Passavant's ridge is the hypertrophied portion of the posterior pharyngeal wall that is approximated by the soft palate (velum) during speech and deglutition.

Historically, severe adenotonsillar hypertrophy sometimes resulted in airway obstruction and led to alveolar hypoventilation syndrome, culminating in hypoxia and hypercarbia. Secondary pulmonary artery hypertension and right ventricular hypertrophy led to cor pulmonale. This sequence of events is rare today.

Patients with Down syndrome (trisomy 21) have narrow oral and nasal airways, predisposing to obstruction whenever tonsils and adenoids enlarge. These patients are at higher risk for cor pulmonale as a result of adenotonsillar hypertrophy.

Patients with abnormal facies related to trisomy 21 (Down syndrome), mandibulofacial dysostosis (Treacher-Collins syndrome), acrocephaly-syndactyly (Apert syndrome), dwarfism, or craniofacial dysostosis (Crouzon syndrome) possess abnormally small maxillary and mandibular relationships. In these patients, even normal-sized tonsillar and adenoidal tissue may be sufficient to cause airway obstruction. In these cases, adenotonsillectomy may be indicated even in the absence of adenotonsillar hypertrophy.

2. Describe the essential elements of preoperative evaluation for adenotonsillectomy.

Preoperative evaluation of the patient presenting for adenotonsillectomy focuses on airway obstruction. Air movement through the nasal cavity indicates that adenoidal tissue is not obstructing the nasopharynx. A history of dysphagia, sleep apnea, daytime somnolence, or snoring may predict difficult mask ventilation and/or difficult laryngoscopy and intubation.

Preoperative examination of the oral pharynx may reveal enlarged tonsillar tissues encroaching on the airway and predisposing to obstruction during induction. Jugular venous distention, pretibial edema, hepatojugular reflux, and the signs of right-sided congestive heart failure must be searched for to determine the possible need for preoperative digoxin and diuretics. Uncorrected congestive heart failure markedly increases the morbidity and mortality of any surgical procedure including adenotonsillectomy.

Hemorrhage is a major source of concern in the perioperative period. A coagulation history is essential for all patients, although the necessity for international normalized ratio (INR), prothrombin time (PT), and activated partial thromboplastin time (aPTT) is controversial without clinical correlation. Salicylate ingestion, which impairs platelet function, is a probable basis for postponement of an elective adenotonsillectomy. Other nonsteroidal compounds such as ibuprofen or parenteral ketorolac have been proven to be a significant risk for perioperative hemorrhage. However, early data suggest that the COX-2 inhibitors may not be a significant risk for perioperative hemorrhage and may be quite useful as a non-opiate perioperative analgesic.

The potential for dental trauma requires inspection of the oropharynx. Dentition should be carefully observed for ill-fitting removable prostheses, fixed dental prostheses such as crowns or bridges, and orthodontic appliances. Most importantly, the oropharynx should be inspected for grossly carious and loose teeth. Adenotonsillectomy is a common procedure in childhood when the primary teeth are exfoliating, risking accidental avulsion. Dental trauma may be the result of oropharyngeal airway placement, laryngoscopy, or the mouth gag used to maintain adequate surgical exposure.

3. How is the patient premedicated for adenotonsillectomy?

The goals of premedication are anxiolysis, analgesia, and drying of secretions.

Preanesthetic Evaluation Specific to the Patient for Tonsillectomy and Adenotonsillectomy

Upper airway obstruction
  Patent nasal airway
  Dysphagia
  Sleep apnea
  Restless sleeping positions
  Snoring
  Tonsils encroaching on the airway

Congestive heart failure
  Jugular venous distention
  Pretibial edema
  Hepatojugular reflux

Cor pulmonale
  Right ventricular hypertrophy

Bleeding diathesis

Loose teeth

Antisialogogues are valuable for patients undergoing adenotonsillectomy. A dry airway assists assessment and manipulation by both anesthesiologist and surgeon. Patients with obstructive sleep apnea should be carefully premedicated. Oral midazolam, a common premedicant used in pediatrics, may significantly compromise airway dynamics in the child with obstructive sleep apnea.

4. What anesthetic alternatives are available for patients undergoing adenotonsillectomy?

The anesthetic alternatives for adenotonsillectomy are varied. Induction of anesthesia may proceed following the application of a blood pressure cuff, precordial stethoscope, pulse oximeter, electrocardiogram, and temperature probe. The primary concern is airway patency, necessitating early initiation of capnography. Establishment of intravenous access is ideally accomplished before induction of anesthesia, but if not, this becomes a top priority after induction. Sometimes, uncooperative children and adults require inhalation induction without the benefit of prehydration or rapid-acting medications. Anticipated difficult mask airways and difficult intubations suggest the need for awake intubation under topical anesthesia. An inhalation induction with assisted ventilation represents an alternative approach. As anesthetic depth increases, pharyngeal muscles and soft tissues become lax, resulting in exacerbated airway obstruction. Oral or nasal airway placement carries the potential for worsening obstruction if sufficient anesthetic depth has not yet been achieved. A popular maintenance anesthetic in children includes sevoflurane, nitrous oxide, oxygen, and muscle relaxant. Propofol hastens the early return of airway reflexes, lucidity, and cooperation. Substituting rofecoxib, a selective COX-2 inhibitor, for opiates can minimize postoperative respiratory depression. Rofecoxib does not alter central respiratory drive and does not have significant antiplatelet effects. Its current major drawback may be cost.

Although 4% lidocaine spray to the larynx as well as lidocaine injection into the tonsillar bed helps to reduce afferent sensory input from the surgical field, they are potentially detrimental. Reduced airway sensation predisposes to aspiration pneumonia.

Over the years, recurrent problems with intraoperative endotracheal obstruction have popularized the use of preformed tubes, which adapt well to many mouth gags and minimize interference with surgical manipulations. Although the endotracheal tubes are unlikely to be kinked at the level of the mandibular incisors, potential still exists for endotracheal tube compression by the tongue blade in the hypopharynx. The increased risk for endotracheal tube dislodgement, kinking, and compression predisposes patients to hypoxia and hypercarbia, underscoring the importance of capnography and pulse oximetry. Precor-dial stethoscopes may detect a mainstem endobronchial intubation.

Ventricular dysrhythmias are a recognized complication of adenotonsillectomy. Their appearance frequently signals inappropriate depth of anesthesia, hypoxia, hypercarbia, or absorption of dysrhythmogenic drugs. Deepening the anesthetic readily treats light levels of anesthesia. Surgeons may administer epinephrine into the operative field. The resulting dysrhythmias are usually short-lived and generally require no treatment.

Swallowed blood frequently culminates in nausea and vomiting. To help minimize this problem, an orogastric tube is placed and the stomach contents aspirated before emergence. An awake extubation is preferable to protect against aspiration, but deep extubation is sometimes chosen. Deep extubation helps prevent violent coughing, profound straining, and bronchospasm during emergence. After deep extubation, the patient is placed in the lateral decubitus position, the table is moved to a slight head-down position, the head is turned to the side, and the upper hand is situated under the patient's chin. Administering intravenous lidocaine, which may also slightly impair emergence, can reduce the risk of laryngospasm. Humidified oxygen is administered in the postanesthesia care unit.

5. What are the common postanesthesia care unit problems anticipated following adenotonsillectomy?

Postanesthesia care unit problems specific to adenotonsillectomy are hemorrhage and airway obstruction. Oozing or frank hemorrhage into the airway may occur. Blood from adenotonsillar beds is usually swallowed. Consequently, blood loss is not measurable, and significant hemorrhage may remain undiagnosed. Tachycardia, diaphoresis, orthostatic hypotension, pallor, and hematemesis may be the presenting signs of postoperative hemorrhage. Often only small amounts of blood are seen on bed sheets.

Airway obstruction may result from many etiologies. During emergence from anesthesia, lax oropharyngeal tissues can prolapse into the airway, creating obstruction. Surgical edema and hematomas exacerbate the process.

Many drug regimens have been advocated to reduce postoperative nausea and vomiting. Dexamethasone and ondansetron have an excellent track record if given prophylactically for this specific type of surgery.

6. Which patients are suitable candidates for ambulatory adenotonsillectomy?

Although adenotonsillectomy has been performed on an ambulatory basis for many years, most are now performed on an ambulatory basis due to economic pressures. Appropriate reluctance exists to performing ambulatory adenotonsillectomy on patients less than 3 years of age. This group appears to be at increased risk for airway obstruction, hemorrhage and, most importantly, hypovolemia.

Hypovolemia often results from inadequate oral consumption. Regardless of age, children with coexisting medical conditions may be poor candidates for outpatient adenotonsillectomy. Conditions associated with narrow airways place patients at increased risk for obstruction postoperatively. Examples of these syndromes were mentioned in question 1. They include Treacher-Collins syndrome, Crouzon syndrome, Apert syndrome, Down syndrome, and mucopolysaccharidoses. Even normal amounts of pharyngeal lymphoid may obstruct the airway of patients with these problems. Subsequent postoperative edema may lead to severe obstruction. Observation in the intensive care unit may be warranted for patients with complicated medical problems, syndromes, and those who are unable to understand instructions.

For most patients undergoing ambulatory adenotonsillectomy, 4–8 hours of postanesthesia care unit observation are recommended before discharge from the hospital or ambulatory surgical facility.

7. Describe the anesthetic management of a patient presenting with post-tonsillectomy hemorrhage.

The majority of post-adenotonsillectomy hemorrhage occurs with a biphasic pattern. The most common bleeding falls within the first 8 hours after surgery. The next significant risk period is 7–10 days postoperatively when the eschar falls away from the surgical site. Post-adenotonsillectomy hemorrhage usually results from significant emesis, retching, or straining secondary to swallowed blood or pain. Adequate treatment of emesis and pain will reduce the risk of such hemorrhage. Coagulation studies may be warranted at this time.

Preparation for anesthetic induction begins with intravascular volume replacement. Although a blood transfusion may be required, crystalloid administration generally suffices. Nevertheless, compatible blood should be available. Essential monitoring consists of pulse oximetry, precordial stethoscope, noninvasive blood pressure cuff, electrocardiogram, and capnography. Formerly, uncooperative children received inhalation induction in the lateral decubitus position. The current recommendation for preoperative volume replacement virtually eliminates the need for an inhalation induction, which may increase the risk of hypotension, laryngospasm, and aspiration pneumonitis. Etomidate or ketamine should be selected for those who remain hypovolemic.

Rapid sequence induction with cricoid pressure and a cuffed endotracheal tube help reduce the risk of aspiration. Evacuation of stomach contents reduces postoperative nausea and vomiting. Narcotic-based maintenance anesthesia may facilitate awake extubation, while limiting coughing and retching on the endotracheal tube. "Stormy" emergences predispose patients to re-bleeding from the surgical site.

SUGGESTED READINGS

American Academy of Pediatrics, Section on Pediatric Pulmonology, Subcommittee on Obstructive Sleep Apnea: Clinical practice guideline: diagnosis and management of childhood obstructive sleep apnea syndrome. Pediatrics 109:704–712, 2002

Darrow DH, Siemens C: Indications for tonsillectomy and adenoidectomy. Laryngoscope 112:6–10, 2002

Gan TJ, Meyer T, Apfel CC, et al.: Consensus guidelines for managing postoperative nausea and vomiting. Anesth Analg 97:62–71, 2003

Joshi W, Connelly NR, Reuben SS, et al.: An evaluation of the safety and efficacy of administering rofecoxib for postoperative pain management. Anesth Analg 97:35–38, 2003

Lalakea LM, Marquez-Biggs I, Messner AH: Safety of pediatric short-stay tonsillectomy. Arch Otolaryngol Head Neck Surg 125:749–752, 1999

Marret E, Flahault A, Samama CM, et al.: Effects of postoperative, nonsteroidal antiinflammatory drugs on bleeding risk after tonsillectomy: meta-analysis of randomized, controlled trials. Anesthesiology 98:1497–1502, 2003

Møiniche S, Rømsing J, Dahl JB, et al.: Nonsteroidal antiinflammatory drugs and the risk of operative site bleeding after tonsillectomy: a quantitative systematic review. Anesth Analg 96:68–77, 2003

Rusy LM, Hoffman GH, Weisman SJ: Electroacupuncture prophylaxis of postoperative nausea and vomiting following pediatric tonsillectomy with or without adenoidectomy. Anesthesiology 96:300–305, 2002

Strauss SG, Lynn AM, Bratton SL, et al.: Ventilatory response to CO_2 in children with obstructive sleep apnea from adenotonsillar hypertrophy. Anesth Analg 89:328–332, 1999

Wilson K, Lakheeram I, Morielli A, et al.: Can assessment for obstructive sleep apnea help predict postadenotonsillectomy respiratory complications? Anesthesiology 96:313–322, 2002

Andrew Herlich, MD

A 40-year-old opera singer presents with vocal cord nodules. A laser laryngoscopy is planned. She has no other illnesses. Surgical history is significant for removal of impacted third molars under general anesthesia at age 16 years without difficulty.

QUESTIONS

1. What is a laser?
2. Describe the most common types of lasers used in medical practice.
3. Which lasers are used in laryngeal and tracheo-bronchial surgery?
4. What are the indications for laser laryngoscopy?
5. What are the hazards of laser laryngoscopy to patients, operating room personnel, and anesthesia equipment?
6. What anesthetic techniques are appropriate for patients undergoing laser laryngoscopy?
7. What maneuvers are instituted to treat an airway fire? Is the risk of fire any less likely with electrocautery?

1. What is a laser?

The word laser is an acronym, which stands for light amplification by stimulated emission of radiation. A laser differs from natural light in three ways:

- Lasers emit intense parallel beams of single-frequency radiation (light). Natural light disperses widely as it travels.

- Laser light is essentially monochromatic. Natural light contains a wide spectrum of wavelengths.
- Laser light is coherent and its photons oscillate synchronously. In natural light the photons oscillate randomly.

A laser system is composed of four different parts:

- The first part is the laser medium, which may be a gas, liquid, or solid. In solid medium lasers, ionic impurities known as *dopants* are used to generate the laser light. An example of a laser with a dopant is the neodymium-yttrium-aluminum-garnet (Nd-YAG) laser. The dopant determines the wavelength of the emitted radiation.
- The second portion is the optical cavity wherein the laser medium is confined. One of the mirrors in the optical cavity allows the laser beam to escape the cavity instead of being reflected by the other mirrors.
- The third portion of the laser system is a pumping source, which supplies electrical discharge or high-energy photons from a xenon flash lamp.
- The fourth portion is a light guide, which directs the laser beam to the site of surgery.

2. Describe the most common types of lasers used in medical practice.

Several types of lasers are used in medical practice. The carbon dioxide (CO_2) laser is most commonly employed for laryngoscopy. It has a long-wavelength light that is totally absorbed by cell water in the first few cell layers traversed. CO_2 lasers result in accurate explosive vaporization with minimal peripheral damage. Since the CO_2 laser beam is invisible it needs a marker, which is composed of a helium-neon aiming beam.

Near-infrared laser light from the Nd-YAG laser is used for coagulation of hemorrhagic lesions, such as necrotic respiratory tumors and gastrointestinal tract varices. It creates more thermocoagulation and less vaporization.

Shorter-wavelength lasers of the ruby or argon types are absorbed primarily by pigmented structures such as hemoglobin or darkly pigmented cells.

3. Which lasers are used in laryngeal and tracheo-bronchial surgery?

CO_2, Nd-YAG, argon, and potassium tetanal phosphate (KTP) lasers have all been used for airway surgery. Although CO_2 lasers offer the best precision, they cannot be focused through fiberoptic bronchoscopes. Argon, Nd-YAG, and KTP lasers can be delivered through fiberoptic devices and are selected for this purpose.

4. What are the indications for laser laryngoscopy?

Laser laryngoscopy is applicable for benign and malignant lesions. Specific indications for its use include cysts, laryngoceles, recurrent respiratory papillomatosis, subglottic hemangioma, benign cysts in the laryngoceles, vocal process granulomas, contact ulcers, and lymphangiomas. Malignant neoplasms, such as vocal cord cancer, and other obstructive airway lesions are also amenable to laser treatment. Conditions amenable to laser therapy include laryngomalacia, vocal cord paralysis, congenital and acquired anterior glottic webs, subglottic and glottic stenosis, as well as large laryngeal tumor debulking.

Speech applications of laser techniques include excision of vocal cord nodules and polyps, polypoid corditis, and dysphonia plicaventricularis.

5. What are the hazards of laser laryngoscopy to patients, operating room personnel, and anesthesia equipment?

Administrative organizations have taken steps to minimize laser-related problems. The US Food and Drug Administration (FDA), the American National Standards Institute (ANSI), as well as the National Fire Protection Association (NFPA) have developed rigorous safeguards to help protect patients and operating room personnel from laser-device-related injuries. The Occupational Health and Safety Administration (OSHA) has been empowered to protect operating room personnel from laser injury. Most health care facilities prohibit the use of lasers by uncredentialed practitioners.

One of the most dramatic and unique hazards of laser laryngoscopy is airway fire. Ideally, anesthetic techniques should minimize the risk of anesthetic gas combustion while providing adequate patient oxygenation. Frequently, these goals are conflicting and difficult to achieve because patients with the greatest need for laser laryngeal surgery often present with compromised vital organ function. To further complicate matters, these procedures are usually performed on an ambulatory basis.

Other laser hazards include unintentional perforation of adjacent structures, embolic phenomena (usually occurring during gynecologic surgery), inappropriate energy transfer, and atmospheric contamination. Perforation of an adjacent structure may occur as an esophageal perforation during posterior laryngeal laser surgery. Inappropriate energy transfer harms the patient or operating room personnel. Examples include ignition of an endotracheal tube or surgical drapes. Avoiding such hazards mandates depression of the laser foot pedal control only after aiming the target light beam.

Atmospheric contamination may be the single most common complication of laser surgery. Tissues vaporized by laser light emit a plume of smoke containing pyrogens and other materials, such as viral particles. These particles are released into the atmosphere and distributed to exposed skin of the patient and operating room personnel. Therefore, total body covering during laser procedures may be indicated. Operating room personnel should wear specially designed facemasks that are resistant to the laser plume's particulate matter, in an effort to reduce the risk of dissemination into the tracheobronchial tree.

Applying an aqueous-based lubricant, taping the eyes closed, and covering with moist gauze or metallic eye shields may avoid ocular damage to the patient. The patient's face, head, and neck should be surrounded with wet surgical towels to reduce the risk of ignition. Special wrap-around goggles designed for each laser frequency are available to protect the eyes of operating room personnel. Clear wrap-around goggles block far-wavelength light associated with CO_2 lasers. Specific color-tinted goggles protect against near-wavelength lasers, such as the Nd-YAG and argon lasers.

Lasers also jeopardize anesthesia equipment. Errant beams have ignited endotracheal tubes. Polyvinyl chloride (PVC) tubes burn most easily and consequently are least desirable for laser surgery. Red rubber and silicon endotracheal tubes are not as highly combustible as PVC types. Although metal tubes present the least combustion hazard, they do not eliminate the risk entirely, since their cuffs may still ignite. Covering the cuff with saline-soaked gauze and inflating it with saline instead of air reduces the potential for airway fire. Saline-soaked gauze can also be used to protect nonoperative airway sites. Wrapping the anesthesia breathing circuit in aluminum foil protects it from errant laser beams. The aluminum foil wrapping should also include the CO_2 sampling tubing, which is no less combustible than the anesthesia circuit. Similarly, nonmetallic

Complications of Laser Surgery

Airway fire

Perforation of adjacent structures

Embolism

Inappropriate energy transfer

Atmospheric contamination

endotracheal tubes may be surrounded with metallic tape. At the time of writing, only the Mericel® laser guard wrap is FDA-approved among all commercially available metallic wraps. Copper tape protects against CO_2, argon, and the KTP-Nd-YAG laser, but not the YAG laser alone. Metallic wraps increase the endotracheal tube's external diameter in some cases. A small number of laser-shielded endotracheal tubes are offered for sale. One such tube consists of aluminum powder in a silicon base. These tubes contain silicone cuffs which, if ruptured, can propel silica into the distal trachea.

6. What anesthetic techniques are appropriate for patients undergoing laser laryngoscopy?

The caveat to anesthesia for laser laryngoscopy is to supply a gas mixture with the lowest potential for combustion. Nitrous oxide (N_2O) is as combustible as oxygen. Preferable mixtures include air–oxygen, or helium–oxygen. Compared with nitrogen, helium possesses a higher thermal conductivity, predisposing to delayed ignition of the endotracheal tube by several seconds. Theoretically, helium's lower density will allow for less turbulent flow and lower resistance to flow through smaller endotracheal tubes. The ANSI recommends against using volatile anesthetics during laser airway surgery because they decompose into potentially toxic compounds when exposed to airway fires. Positive pressure ventilation can be provided without an endotracheal tube by employing a Sanders Venturi system. Ideally, the lowest inspired oxygen concentration required to safely oxygenate the patient should be used. Total intravenous anesthesia with propofol, remifentanil, or alfentanil might be preferred in most cases.

An immobile surgical field is necessary to ensure precise laser therapy. Even the slightest motion of the vocal cords may result in improper laser therapy. Despite its controversies, a succinylcholine infusion with precise train-of-four monitoring may deliver the intense neuromuscular blockade needed for this precise surgery.

7. What maneuvers are instituted to treat an airway fire? Is the risk of fire any less likely with electrocautery?

The first person to recognize an airway fire will probably be the surgeon. The surgeon must notify the anesthesiologists immediately, who should *cease ventilation and discontinue oxygen administration* to eliminate the source of combustion. In some circumstances, it may be necessary to disconnect the breathing circuit from the anesthesia machine. The flaming material must be removed from the airway and placed in a bucket of water, which should always be available for this purpose. Designated CO_2 fire extinguishers are also recommended. Immediately after removal of the tube, ventilate the patient with 100% oxygen by face mask and continue the anesthetic. Debris removal and airway examination are performed with a rigid bronchoscope. An airway burn requires reintubation to protect against potential airway obstruction from edema. On occasion, tracheostomy, bronchopulmonary lavage, or fiberoptic tracheobronchoscopy may be indicated. If the injury is severe, prolonged intubation and mechanical ventilation may be necessary, along with a course of high-dose steroids and antibiotics when cultures are positive. The long-term sequelae of burns may take weeks to manifest.

Electrocautery fire is no less risky than laser fire. Electrocautery fire may even be more common.

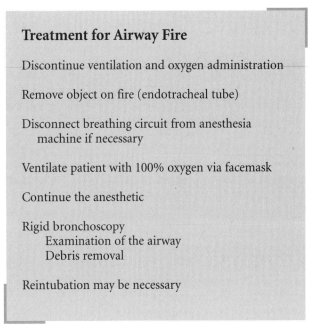

Treatment for Airway Fire

Discontinue ventilation and oxygen administration

Remove object on fire (endotracheal tube)

Disconnect breathing circuit from anesthesia machine if necessary

Ventilate patient with 100% oxygen via facemask

Continue the anesthetic

Rigid bronchoscopy
    Examination of the airway
    Debris removal

Reintubation may be necessary

SUGGESTED READINGS

Abramson AL, DiLorenzo TP, Steinberg BM: Is papillomavirus detectable in the plume of laser-treated laryngeal papilloma? Arch Otol Head Neck Surg 116:604–607, 1990

Dorsch JA, Dorsch SE: Understanding Anesthesia Equipment, 4th edition, pp 600–604. Williams and Wilkins, Philadelphia, 1998

Handa KK, Bhalla AP, Arora A: Fire during the use of Nd-YAG laser. Int J Pediatr Otolaryngol 60:239–242, 2001

Health Devices: Fire 21:3, 1992

Ilgner J, Falter F, Westhofen M: Long-term follow-up after laser-induced endotracheal fire. J Laryngol Otol 116:213–215, 2002

Mattucci KF, Militana CJ: The prevention of fire during oropharyngeal electrosurgery. ENT-Ear, Nose, and Throat J 82:107–109, 2003

Puura AI, Rorarius MG, Manninen P, et al.: The costs of intense neuromuscular block for anesthesia during endolaryngeal procedures due to waiting time. Anesth Analg 88:1335–1339, 1999

Schramm VL Jr, Mattox DE, Stool SE: Acute management of laser-ignited intratracheal explosion. Laryngoscope 91:1417–1426, 1981

Smith TL, Smith JM: Electrosurgery in otolaryngology–head and neck surgery: principles, advances, and complications. Laryngoscope 111:769–780, 2001

Carolyn F. Whitsett, MD

A red cell transfusion is initiated on a 72-year-old woman admitted for acute myocardial infarction with a hemoglobin of 7.0 g/dL. Approximately 30 minutes after the transfusion is started the patient becomes agitated and has a shaking chill. The blood pressure drops from 102/86 to 60/40 mmHg and the pulse increases from 86 to 120 beats per minute. The temperature increases from a pre-transfusion value of 37.5°C to 39.6°C. Urine collected in the Foley catheter is reddish in color, but urine in the collection bag is straw-colored. The transfusion is immediately discontinued and a transfusion investigation requested. The nurse discontinuing the blood notes that the crossmatch tag indicates the product was found compatible using a computer crossmatch.

QUESTIONS

1. How are standards for transfusion practice developed?
2. What steps should be taken when a transfusion reaction occurs?
3. How does the laboratory determine which direction the investigation should take?
4. How many different types of crossmatches are there and how does the laboratory decide which should be performed?

5. What are the immediate and delayed adverse effects of blood transfusion?

1. How are standards for transfusion practice developed?

US federal and state regulations require that blood products be prescribed and administered under medical direction. Standards require that each institution develop a protocol for administration of blood and blood components. Transfusion protocols in individual institutions are usually developed jointly by the nursing service and the blood bank/transfusion service and adopted by the institution for use by all medical personnel. Protocols include specific instructions for transfusing all components including the use of infusion devices, filters, blood warmers, and other ancillary equipment. They specify mechanisms for patient and product identification prior to infusion, instructions for patient monitoring during and at the end of the transfusion, and instructions on specific actions that are required if a transfusion reaction occurs. In general, patient records are required to contain the donor unit or pool identification number of the product, the product name, the date and time of transfusion, the amount transfused, the identification of the transfusionist, pre- and post-transfusion vital signs, and a description of any transfusion reaction that occurred.

2. What steps should be taken when a transfusion reaction occurs?

Whenever a reaction is suspected:

- The transfusion should be immediately discontinued.
- Intravenous access should be maintained.
- The patient information on the blood product label should be compared with the information on the patient wristband.
- The blood bank/transfusion service should be notified and a transfusion investigation should be requested.
- An entry documenting the reaction should be made in the medical progress notes.

The transfusion protocol for each institution generally specifies the type of samples needed for the preliminary investigation. In general, a post-transfusion blood sample (one tube with anticoagulants and one without) and a post-transfusion urine sample are requested. Depending on the type of reaction, other samples may be requested.

The laboratory should be provided with a full and accurate description of the reaction. This includes the patient's pre-transfusion status including: diagnosis, indication for transfusion, previous history of transfusion and transfusion reactions, pre-transfusion vital signs, and any changes in signs and symptoms that developed during the transfusion. It is helpful to know how long after the transfusion was initiated the symptoms developed and how much of the product was transfused. In addition, the response of the symptoms to discontinuation of the transfusion and medications given to treat the reaction, as well as the patient's current clinical condition, should be provided. Most transfusion investigation forms are designed to capture this information. The blood bank physician uses the clinical information, the type of product transfused, and the results of the preliminary laboratory investigation to develop a differential diagnosis that guides the laboratory investigation.

3. How does the laboratory determine which direction the investigation should take?

Each laboratory has standard operating procedures that define the extent of the preliminary laboratory investigation. The first step in any investigation is a clerical check. This check involves comparing identifying information on the transfusion request, blood product label, compatibility label, pre- and post-transfusion blood samples, and blood bank product release record. The purpose of the clerical check is to determine whether the product implicated in the investigation was transfused to the individual for whom it was intended.

The next step is a hemolysis check. The color of plasma/serum from pre- and post-transfusion samples is compared for hemolysis and direct antiglobulin testing is performed on the pre- and post-transfusion samples.

The ABO and Rh type are also repeated on the pre- and post-transfusion samples when the product implicated in the reaction is a red cell product. This testing is not routinely performed for non-red-cell products, such as plasma or platelets, unless there is evidence of red cell destruction. If there is evidence of a hemolytic reaction, the type and screen and compatibility tests are completed on the pre- and post-transfusion samples.

In summary, the preliminary laboratory investigation determines whether the implicated product was transfused to the appropriate patient and classifies the reaction as hemolytic or non-hemolytic. Additional testing is based on the patient's signs and symptoms, the differential diagnosis that this information suggests, and the specific product involved in the investigation.

4. How many different types of crossmatches are there and how does the laboratory decide which should be performed?

There are basically three types of crossmatch (compatibility) tests: the computer crossmatch, the immediate spin crossmatch, and the antiglobulin crossmatch. The antiglobulin crossmatch may use any one of several different enhancing media and may be performed in solution, on a solid phase support, or in a gel medium.

Standards require that every sample used for compatibility testing be tested for ABO group, Rh type, and unexpected antibodies to red cell antigens. A specific type of test is not recommended, but standards require that the test methods demonstrate clinically significant antibodies, and include incubation at 37°C preceding an antiglobulin test using unpooled reagent red cells. If red cell antibodies are detected, the method used for crossmatching must demonstrate ABO incompatibility, must detect clinically significant antibodies, and must include an antiglobulin test. If no clinically significant antibodies are detected, and there is no prior history of immunization to red cell antigens or of transfusion reactions, then at a minimum, the crossmatch technique must demonstrate ABO compatibility. The immediate spin crossmatch involves mixing donor red cells with patient serum followed by centrifugation, and examination of the suspension for red cell agglutination. This technique detects ABO incompatibility but does not detect incompatibility for other clinically significant blood groups. However, a computer system instead of the immediate spin crossmatch may be used to detect ABO incompatibility provided the following conditions have been met:

- The computer system must have been validated on-site to ensure that only ABO-compatible red cell products have been selected for transfusion.

- Two determinations of the recipient's ABO group are made, either by testing the same sample twice or by testing of two current samples.
- The system contains complete blood group information and unique identifiers for the product and the recipient.
- A method exists to verify correct entry of data.
- The system contains logic to alert users to discrepancies in the donor product testing record, and ABO incompatibility between donor and recipient. If no clinically significant antibodies are detected, but there is a past history of immunization to red cell antigens, or a history of transfusion reactions, an antiglobulin crossmatch must be performed.

5. What are the immediate and delayed adverse effects of blood transfusion?

Immediate Reactions

Immediate transfusion reactions are those that occur during or within 24 hours after transfusion whereas delayed reactions occur several days to years after the transfusion. The immediate adverse effects of blood transfusion are summarized in Table 49.1.

Acute Hemolytic Reaction Acute hemolytic transfusion reactions are the most frequent cause of fatal transfusion reactions reported to the FDA. These reactions result from either failure to detect blood group incompatibility or inadvertent transfusion of a blood product to the wrong patient. The risk of death from acute hemolytic reactions has been estimated to be 1:587,000–1:630,000 using data reported to the FDA. Data from the French Haemovigilance system reported approximately 1 death per 2 million units transfused. Most acute hemolytic reactions are caused by transfusion errors. Data from the United Kingdom Serious Hazards of Transfusion (SHOT) initiative indicated that 52% of events investigated involved incorrect transfusion of blood or blood component. An analysis of transfusion errors in New York State that resulted in transfusion of a blood product to other than the intended recipient indicated that erroneous transfusion occurred in 1 of 19,000 red cell units transfused. The frequency of fatal reactions was 1:1,800,000. Approximately half the errors occurred at the bedside and involved administration to the wrong recipient (38%) or phlebotomy errors (13%). Blood bank errors, including testing the wrong sample, transcription errors, and issuing the wrong unit, accounted for 29% of errors. Fifteen percent of events involved multiple errors.

The severity of the reaction is in general related to the amount of blood transfused. Mortality appears to be directly related to the volume of incompatible cells transfused. A review of 41 cases of hemolytic transfusion reactions causing renal failure demonstrated 25% mortality when 500–1,000 mL of blood was transfused and 44% mortality when more than 1000 mL was transfused. However, it is important to remember that fatalities have occurred when as little as 30 mL was transfused. Transfusion guidelines recommend that patients be monitored carefully during the first 15–30 minutes of a transfusion, so that there will be prompt recognition of a serious reaction.

It is important that clinicians recognize that blood group incompatibility, while common, is not the only possible cause of what appears to be a hemolytic transfusion reaction. The patient may have an intercurrent illness causing in vivo destruction of red cells. Autoimmune hemolytic anemias, congenital hemolytic anemias, drug-induced hemolysis, microangiopathic hemolytic anemias, and infections such as malaria or babesiosis where red cells are parasitized or clostridial infections where toxins hemolyze red cells, are among the disorders that may mimic an acute hemolytic transfusion reaction. Ventricular assist devices, membrane oxygenators, and artificial heart valves may also cause hemolysis. Factors that could cause non-immune hemolysis may also need to be considered. Improper storage of blood (very low temperatures at which blood freezes) or malfunction of a blood warmer may cause thermal destruction of red cells before transfusion. Infusing blood under pressure or through a small-gauge needle may also cause hemolysis. Finally, incompatible intravenous solutions will cause hemolysis if administered with blood.

Allergic and Anaphylactic Reactions Mild allergic reactions manifested primarily by urticaria are common following blood transfusion, occurring in approximately 1–3% of transfusions. Severe allergic reactions associated with hypotension, respiratory distress, and other cardiac and gastrointestinal symptoms of anaphylaxis are estimated to occur in 1:20,000 to 1:47,000 transfusions. In the French Haemovigilance system approximately 31% of reported events were allergic in nature. In most allergic reactions, patients appear to have preformed antibodies to a component of donor plasma, usually a plasma protein. In severe reactions, the patient may be IgA-deficient and have anti-IgA antibodies. On occasion the patient will have IgA but will lack one of the isotypic or allotypic determinants of the IgA class. Other patients have antibodies to other immunoglobulin classes or to proteins such as haptoglobin. Passive transfer of allergens or passive transfer of IgE antibodies in the donor product should also be considered. Although allergic reactions are generally thought to be IgE-mediated and histamine release from mast cells is the primary mediator, IgE antibody is not always demonstrable. Complement-derived anaphylatoxins such as C3a and C5a generated by immune complexes or other secondary mediators such as cytokines are responsible for anaphylactoid symptoms.

TABLE 49.1	Immediate Transfusion Reactions			
Type of Reaction	**Mechanism**	**Manifestations**	**Most Common Cause**	**Initial Management**
Acute hemolytic reactions	Immune reaction; pre-formed antibody in recipient causes destruction of donor cells; antibodies often bind complement; rarely, infusion of incompatible plasma	Fever, chills, rigor, dyspnea, nausea, flank, chest, or back pain, hypotension, tachycardia, bleeding, hemoglobinuria, diathesis, oliguria, renal failure	Transfusion of ABO-incompatible unit because of error in patient identification, sample/product labeling, or laboratory testing	Stop transfusion Maintain blood pressure with fluids, and vasopressor if needed Use mannitol, diuretics and fluid to maintain urine output Treat DIC with fresh frozen plasma, platelets and cryoprecipitate if there is active hemorrhage
Allergic (mild or moderate)	Recipient is allergic to substance in donor plasma	Hives, wheezing, swelling, generalized erythema and itching, hypotension	Transfusion of blood component containing plasma; reaction more common and severe with platelets and plasma than red blood cells	Stop transfusion Administer antihistamine (e.g., diphenhydramine) Epinephrine and steroids may be needed for moderately severe reaction
Anaphylactic	Recipient has pre-formed antibody to donor IgA or other plasma component such as haptoglobin or IgG; passive transfer of IgE antibodies from donor to recipient	Hypotension, bronchospasm, laryngeal and pulmonary edema, generalized erythema with or without hives	IgA-deficient recipient with anti-IgA antibodies	Stop transfusion and administer oxygen Maintain airway with endotracheal intubation Treat hypotension with volume expansion Administer epinephrine in dosage appropriate for symptoms
Circulatory overload	Volume of product or rate of administration excessive for patient's cardiovascular system	Tachycardia, cough, cyanosis, dyspnea, pulmonary edema, hypotension, hypertension	Rapid administration of blood product or intercurrent cardiac or pulmonary problems	Stop transfusion Maintain sitting position Administer oxygen Administer parenteral diuretic Add inotropic drugs if indicated
Febrile non-hemolytic	Recipient has antibodies to white blood cells that react with donor passenger leukocytes; cytokines	Chills, fever	Recipient is multi-transfused or immunized to white cell antigens by pregnancy or transplantation; more common with platelet transfusions	Stop transfusion Administer antipyretics

Hypotensive reaction related to bradykinin/cytokines	Generation of bradykinin in donor products by filtration; bradykinin is not degraded either because patient is taking angiotensin-converting enzyme inhibitor or had cardiopulmonary bypass	Hypotension, erythema, angioedema	Use of leukoreduction filter immediately prior to transfusion for patients on angiotensin-converting enzyme inhibitor	Stop transfusion Resuscitate as in anaphylactoid reaction Use pre-storage leukoreduced products (RBC, platelets) or wash product
Hypothermia	Infusion of large volume of blood/blood product in a short period of time	Chills, decrease in temperature, arrhythmia, metabolic acidosis	Rapid infusion of a large volume of blood	Use of in-line warmer
Metabolic disorders: citrate intoxication	Citrate complexes calcium leading to hypocalcemia	Numbness and tingling of extremities and around the mouth, muscle tremors, abdominal pain, nausea and vomiting, dysrhythmia, prolonged QT intervals, cardiac arrest	Massive transfusion; therapeutic plasma exchange	Decrease rate of transfusion Administer calcium
Metabolic disorders: hyperkalemia	Red cell potassium leaks into extracellular fluid during storage	Muscle weakness, bradycardia, dysrhythmia, ventricular dysrhythmia	Massive transfusion; decreased renal function	Use bicarbonate, dextrose and insulin to drive potassium intracellularly Consider washing RBCs if time permits
Sepsis	Bacterial contamination of blood products	Rigors, fever, tachycardia, hypotension, dyspnea, anxiety, back pain, nausea, malaise	Platelet products; fatal reaction caused by gram-negative organisms	Stop transfusion Maintain blood pressure Administer broad-spectrum antibiotics Consider treatment with activated Protein C
Transfusion-related acute lung injury (TRALI)	Immune-mediated, donor product contains antibodies to recipient granulocytes or HLA antigens	Acute respiratory distress with severe hypoxemia and bilateral pulmonary edema	Transfusion of plasma containing product such as platelets	Intensive respiratory support with supplemental oxygen including mechanical ventilation if needed Fluids for volume

DIC, disseminated intravascular coagulation; RBC, red blood cells.

Mild allergic reactions are usually treated with an oral or parenteral (intravenous or intramuscular) antihistamine (diphenhydramine 25–50 mg). If a patient has a documented history of recurrent allergic reactions, prophylactic administration of an antihistamine is indicated. The mild allergic reaction may be the only reaction where there is general agreement that the transfusion could be interrupted, an antihistamine given, and the transfusion restarted when symptoms subside. Severe allergic or anaphylactoid transfusion reactions should be treated as any other type of anaphylaxis is treated (i.e., epinephrine, volume expansion, oxygen supplementation and other respiratory support, etc.). Any patient having an anaphylactoid reaction should be tested for antibodies to IgA. Patients who have IgA antibodies must receive plasma and platelets from IgA-deficient donors. These products are usually available only from large regional blood centers. Red blood cells washed with 2 liters of normal saline will be satisfactory for transfusion. IgA-deficient patients who may need plasma derivatives pose a special problem because the standard labeling on these products does not indicate whether there may be trace amounts of IgA present. As little as 1 mg of IgA may trigger an allergic reaction. Clinicians should speak with the manufacturer's representative to determine whether a particular product and lot number is safe.

Circulatory Overload   Circulatory overload is a frequent complication of transfusion therapy. It usually occurs in elderly patients with renal insufficiency, diminished cardiac reserve, or severe anemia. Circulatory overload is often included in acute pulmonary problems in many reports and accurate data on the incidence are not available. However, a report from the Mayo Clinic suggested that it occurred in 1/3,168 patients receiving red cell transfusions. The early symptoms of volume overload are nonspecific and include an increase in blood pressure, headache, development of a new cough, and a sensation of pressure in the chest. The development of any of these signs and symptoms in a patient receiving transfusion therapy should be an indication to slow the infusion and monitor the patient more often. As cardiac decompensation progresses, dyspnea, orthopnea, tachycardia, cyanosis, and frank pulmonary edema may develop.

When the patient's signs and symptoms suggest circulatory overload, the transfusion should be stopped and the patient placed in a sitting position. Oxygen supplementation should be provided and diuretics given to reduce the intravascular volume. If diuretics are ineffective, consideration should be given to phlebotomy.

Febrile Non-hemolytic Reactions   The definition of a febrile non-hemolytic reaction is an increase in temperature of ≥1°C following transfusion that cannot be explained by the patient's clinical condition. This increase in temperature is usually accompanied by chills and rigors and sometimes headache, nausea, and vomiting. In most patients, fever develops during the transfusion. Usually the increase in temperature is ≤2°C. When the temperature increase is ≥2°C, bacterial contamination of the blood product and the development of an intercurrent infection must be considered. Some patients have chills, rigor, and feel cold but do not develop fever. The diagnosis of a febrile non-hemolytic reaction can be established only by excluding other types of transfusion reactions accompanied by fever. In a community hospital population, approximately 0.5–1.0% of red cell transfusions are associated with febrile non-hemolytic reactions. In chronically transfused patients, the frequency is much higher.

Recipient antibodies directed against antigens on donor leukocytes are generally considered to be the cause of febrile non-hemolytic reactions. Initially it was believed that endogenous pyrogens (interleukin-1β, interleukin-6, and tumor necrosis factor) from donor leukocytes caused the febrile reaction. Recently, it has been suggested that complement activation following the interaction of recipient antibodies with donor leukocytes causes activation of recipient monocytes. These activated monocytes are thought to release proinflammatory cytokines causing the reaction. Finally, since the widespread use of leukoreduction filters to eliminate these reactions, it appears that cytokines produced by donor leukocytes prior to leukoreduction may also cause febrile non-hemolytic reactions.

In the general population, only 15% of patients having a febrile reaction to a red cell product are likely to have a recurrent febrile reaction with the next transfusion. Therefore, many transfusion services do not recommend premedication or leukoreduction for the average patient until a second febrile reaction occurs. Febrile reactions are more common following platelet transfusions than red cell transfusions and are more common with older products than relatively fresh products. If reactions are mild, they can often be prevented by premedication with an antipyretic. If reactions are severe or if premedication does not prevent the reaction, leukoreduced products are indicated. In some multitransfused patients, it may be necessary to provide pre-storage leukoreduced products. Pre-storage leukoreduction will not remove all biologically active mediators because some of these are derived from platelets. Removal of most of the plasma from platelet products just prior to transfusion helps reduce reactions in patients not responding to pre-storage leukoreduction strategies.

Other Hypotensive Reactions   Hypotension not uncommonly accompanies severe immune reactions in which antibodies in the recipient react with donor cells or vice versa and transfusions where bacterial contamination of a blood product has been documented. In addition to these circumstances, hypotension has been described following the administration of leukoreduced products (both platelets and red cells), following the administration of plasma-containing products to patients taking angiotensin-converting enzyme (ACE) inhibitors and following the administration of plasma protein fraction to patients undergoing cardiopulmonary bypass. These reactions appear to be related to the generation of bradykinin under circumstances where enzymes important in bradykinin inactivation are either inhibited or a tissue containing these enzymes has been excluded from the circulation (cardiopulmonary bypass). Contact of plasma with negatively charged blood filters leads to contact activation of the intrinsic coagulation system and bradykinin generation. There are at least five metallopeptidases responsible for the inactivation and metabolism of bradykinin. ACE is responsible for the hydrolysis of 60% of bradykinin in normal subjects and inactivation by aminopeptidase P (APP) is a second major metabolic pathway. Clinical reports have documented unexplained hypotensive reactions in patients on ACE inhibitors receiving platelet products leukoreduced at the bedside and in patients undergoing therapeutic plasma exchange. In vitro studies have documented an increase in bradykinin levels following filtration of platelet concentrates. The generated bradykinin was rapidly degraded and was undetectable after 1 hour of storage.

Treatment of a hypotensive reaction in a patient on ACE inhibitors should include immediate discontinuation of the product and appropriate resuscitation. If additional red cells are needed, washing is advised. If platelets are needed, the product should be pre-storage leukoreduced or filtered an hour prior to administration. Reduction of the residual plasma on the platelet product may also be helpful.

Transfusion-Transmitted Bacterial Infection Sepsis related to bacterial contamination of blood products is the second most common cause of fatal transfusion reactions reported to the FDA. In the United States between 1976 and 1999, 10% of transfusion-related deaths were caused by bacterial contamination. It is estimated that 0.2% of whole blood collections are contaminated. Bacterial contamination of platelets is more common than contamination of red blood cells but prevalence estimates vary widely. Estimates for red cells vary from 0.002% to 1.0% and for platelets from 0.04% to 10%. Some studies have suggested that contamination of pooled platelet concentrates is more frequent than contamination of single donor platelets. The organisms contaminating blood products are usually from donor skin flora (i.e., *Staphylococcus* species, *Propionibacterium acnes*). However, asymptomatic donor bacteremia (*Yersinia enterocolitica*) and contamination of products from environmental sources (*Pseudomonas* species) may also lead to bacterial contamination of blood components.

The most common symptoms and signs associated with bacterial contamination of blood products are chills, fever, tachycardia, shock or hypotension, shortness of breath, back pain, and nausea and/or vomiting. Occasional patients may have an increase in blood pressure. Although these symptoms often develop immediately or within the first hour after transfusion is initiated, some patients may not develop symptoms or signs for several hours.

Two national studies of bacterial contamination of blood products performed in France and the United States provide the most current data on this complication of transfusion. In the United States from 1998 to 2000, suspected cases of bacterial contamination of blood products were reported to the Centers for Disease Control (CDC) by blood collection facilities and transfusion services associated with the American Red Cross, the American Association of Blood Banks, and the Department of Defense. This study was given the acronym BaCon (Assessment of the Frequency of Bacterial Contamination Associated with Transfusion Reaction). In France, there is a national mandatory reporting system for adverse reactions to transfusion. From November 1996–1998, all adverse reactions suspected to be related to bacterial contamination were investigated as part of the French BACTHEM Study.

The case definition for BaCon included the presence of one or more of the following signs or symptoms developing within 4 hours of transfusion: fever ≥39°C or a change of ≥2°C from the pre-transfusion value; rigors; tachycardia ≥120 beats per minute, or a change of ≥40 beats per minute from the pre-transfusion value; a rise or drop of ≥30 mmHg in systolic blood pressure. Of 56 reported cases, 34 were confirmed with the same organism being cultured from the recipient and the component. There were 9 deaths. The rate of transfusion-transmitted bacteremia (in events per million units distributed) was 9.98 for single donor platelets, 10.64 for pooled platelets, and 0.21 for red cells. The rate of fatal reactions was 1.94 for pooled platelets, 2.22 for single donor platelets, and 0.13 for red blood cells. Fatal transfusion reactions were more likely to be associated with contamination with gram-negative organisms.

Results from BACTHEM were similar. Of 158 suspected cases, 41 were confirmed. Twenty-five were associated with red blood cells and 16 with platelet products. This led to an estimated incidence rate per million components issued of 5.8 for red blood cells, 31.8 for apheresis platelets, and 71.8 for pooled platelet concentrate. Fatal reactions were uniformly associated with gram-negative organisms.

In comparing results from current studies and earlier published reports, the organisms identified as contaminants have changed over time. In earlier studies, *Yersinia enterocolitica* and *Pseudomonas* species were the predominant organisms isolated from red cells. In the BaCon study *Serratia* species accounted for most of the cases of red blood cell contamination and *Acinetobacter* was the second most frequent species cultured from blood components in the BACTHEM study. Currently, manufacturers are focusing on the development of systems to detect bacterial contamination in blood products and the development of nucleic acid binding compounds that will prevent the proliferation of bacteria accidentally introduced into units at the time of phlebotomy.

Transfusion-Related Acute Lung Injury   Transfusion-related acute lung injury (TRALI) is one of the most serious, underdiagnosed complications of transfusion. Typically, acute respiratory distress develops within 1–2 hours of starting a transfusion of a blood component that contains plasma, but some patients have developed symptoms as late as 6 hours after transfusion. Patients have severe hypoxemia and pulmonary edema. Hypotension and fever may also occur. The SHOT study from the UK reported that 11 of 169 (7%) reports involved acute lung injury. Data from the Mayo Clinic suggest that the incidence of TRALI may be 1:5,000 with plasma-containing transfusions. In Canada, data from Quebec reported 3 cases of TRALI in a population receiving 190,000 red cells and 3,000 units of plasma. At a hospital in Ontario, one case of TRALI was observed annually and 12,000 red cell units were transfused.

In most investigations, donor plasma has contained antibodies either to granulocytes or to HLA antigens (both class I and class II). In a small percentage of cases, the recipient serum has contained such antibodies (prior to transfusion). However, antibodies have not been identified in all cases, and it has been hypothesized that lipid products from neutrophils may cause TRALI. A case of TRALI following the administration of intravenous immune globulin was recently reported. Treatment for TRALI depends on the severity of the reaction. Supplemental oxygen and respiratory support including mechanical ventilation may be required. Hypotension is corrected and corticosteroids are usually given.

When a blood product is implicated in TRALI, a donor serum sample is obtained and tested for antibodies to leukocytes. Most such donors are multiparous women. When antibodies are identified, donors are usually no longer allowed to donate. If they have an unusual blood type, the red cells are collected and either frozen or washed, processes that eliminate residual plasma.

Delayed Reactions

Delayed adverse reactions to blood transfusion may be immunologic, related to transmission of a viral or parasitic disease, or caused by iron overload secondary to transfusion. Immunologic adverse effects include delayed hemolytic transfusion reaction (DHTR), immunization to red cell, platelet, leukocyte or plasma antigens, auto-immune phenomena triggered by alloimmunization, and graft-versus-host disease.

Delayed Hemolytic Transfusion Reactions   Delayed hemolytic transfusion reactions usually result from failure to detect existing antibody because the antibody concentration has dropped below the detection level for the method used in antibody screening and crossmatching tests. The transfusion stimulates antibody production causing an accelerated destruction of transfused cells. Common presenting signs and symptoms include unexplained fever, a decrease in hemoglobin unexplained by clinical events, and an increase in bilirubin several days to weeks after transfusion. When a patient blood sample is examined, a positive direct antiglobulin test is present and often antibody can be eluted from the transfused cells. Antibody may also be detectable in patient serum at this time. Delayed reactions are usually mild and may go unrecognized. Clinically detectable hemolysis is reported to vary from 1:5,000 to 1:10,000 transfusions. Some delayed reactions are serious, causing disseminated intravascular coagulation, renal failure, and death. In the first 2 years of the SHOT study, 51 of 366 (14%) reports concerned delayed hemolytic transfusion reactions; and in two cases death was attributed to the transfusion reaction.

Alloimmunization   Alloimmunization to antigens on red cells is estimated to occur in 1–1.6% per donor unit provided that D-negative units are given to D-negative recipients. However, immunization may become a serious problem when a patient requires chronic transfusion and the red cell phenotypes of the blood donors vary from that of the recipient population. For example, most patients with sickle cell disease are African-American and in most communities in the United States the majority of blood donors are Caucasian. Some specialists in the treatment of sickle cell disease have recommended prospective matching of clinically important blood groups for patients on chronic transfusion protocols to prevent immunization and lower the risk of delayed transfusion reactions. Immunization to HLA antigens through routine blood transfusion may also pose problems for patients. Red blood cells and platelet products contain a large number of white blood cells that normally express HLA antigens. Patients having many transfusions with unmodified red cell or platelet products may become immunized to antigens of the HLA system. Immunization to HLA antigens will make a patient with thrombocytopenia refractory to random donor platelet transfusions and may make finding a compatible solid organ donor impossible for a patient needing a heart, kidney, or small bowel transplant. The prophylactic use of leukoreduced red cell and platelet products may be indicated for these patient populations.

Immunization to platelet-specific antigens may also occur following transfusion. In addition to refractoriness to platelet transfusions this type of immunization may lead in rare instances to the disorder post-transfusion purpura. In post-transfusion purpura patients develop severe thrombocytopenia 5–10 days following transfusion. Patients are usually women who have been previously pregnant or transfused. Although several platelet-specific antigen systems have been reported to cause this disorder, in most cases patients lack a platelet-specific antigen HPA-1a (Pl^{A1}), and have made an anti-HPA-1a. HPA-1a is a high-frequency platelet-specific antigen with only 2% of the population being HPA-1a-negative. Through mechanisms that are not well understood the anti-HPA-1a destroys the transfused HPA-1a-positive transfused platelets and the patient's own HPA-1a-negative platelets. Post-transfusion purpura is usually self-limited with spontaneous recovery within 3 weeks. Occasional patients with severe symptomatic thrombocytopenia require treatment. High-dose intravenous immune globulin (IVIG) is the treatment of choice. Random platelets are generally HPA-1a-positive and will not increase the platelet count. Antigen-negative platelets may be helpful when given with IVIG.

Graft-Versus-Host Disease Transfusion-associated graft versus-host disease (TA-GVHD) is a rare but usually fatal complication of transfusion in which viable lymphocytes in donor blood products transfused to an immunologically compromised patient engraft. These foreign lymphocytes recognize the HLA antigens of the transfusion recipient as foreign and generate a characteristic immune response characterized by rash, fever, liver function abnormalities, diarrhea, and marrow dysfunction. Symptoms usually develop 8–10 days after transfusion. TA-GVHD was originally described in immunocompromised individuals. It was described in newborns having exchange transfusion, patients with congenital forms of immune deficiency, and patients immunosuppressed by intense chemotherapy. Subsequently, it was reported in immunologically normal individuals transfused with blood from an individual who was either HLA-identical or homozygous for a shared HLA haplotype. The risk of such matched transfusions in unrelated populations varies.

Treatment of TA-GVHD is rarely effective, with 90% of patients dying from the disorder. Transfusion guidelines are focused on prevention through blood product irradiation. Irradiation of blood products requires a specific physician order. However, most blood bank/transfusion services have developed guidelines for blood product irradiation. Transfusions to premature infants, neonates, individuals with congenital immune deficiency, recipients of hematopoietic stem cell transplants, patients receiving intense immunosuppressive chemotherapy (for leukemia, Hodgkin's disease, and other lymphomas), and directed blood product donations from family members are generally irradiated routinely. Physicians should be informed about irradiation guidelines at the institutions where they practice. Products for some patients may automatically be irradiated based on admitting diagnosis but other cases may require a specific order. It is always best to specifically order irradiated blood, rather than to depend on a standard operating procedure. This practice minimizes the opportunity for error.

Iron Overload Transfusion hemosiderosis is common when patients with hematologic disorders require chronic transfusion. Typically these are patients with hemoglobinopathies such as thalassemia or sickle cell disease. However, patients with myelodysplastic syndromes are also at risk for this disorder. Chronically transfused patients should have ferritin levels monitored and should be treated with iron-chelating agents such as desferoxamine when needed.

Transfusion-Transmitted Viral and Parasitic Infection Currently blood donations for allogeneic use have been tested by FDA-licensed tests and found negative for antibodies to human immunodeficiency virus (anti-HIV), hepatitis C virus (anti-HCV), human T-cell lymphotrophic virus (anti-HTLVI/II) and hepatitis B core antigen (anti-HBc), as well as HIV-antigen (HIV-1-Ag, also called p24 antigen) and hepatitis B surface antigen (HbsAg). Beginning in March 1999, nucleic acid amplification testing (NAT) for HIV and HCV has been performed on most of the blood collected in the United States under an investigational new drug application (IND) approved by the FDA. Traditional tests are performed on individual samples, but NAT testing is performed on pooled samples. Two manufacturers have developed test systems using NAT. Gen-Probe (San Diego, CA) developed a multiplex system that tests for HCV and HIV at the same time. Roche Molecular Systems (RMS, Pleasanton, CA) developed independent NAT tests for HIV and HCV. Since the implementation of NAT under FDA IND one case of HIV transmitted by blood transfusion has been reported in the United States. Although the new tests are very sensitive, the window period for HIV remains at 10–11 days. NAT testing is not yet legally mandated, but will be as soon as sufficient licensed kits are available to screen the entire US blood supply. In the meantime, the FDA is requiring that all allogeneic units be NAT-tested unless there is an extremely urgent situation such as the 9/11 terrorist attacks. At the present time, NAT testing for HBV on pooled samples does not appear to be superior to serologic tests for HbsAg. It is unclear when NAT testing for HBV will be introduced.

The Gen-Probe test for HIV and HCV was licensed in February 2002. Licensure of the RMS test is imminent. Table 49.2, derived primarily from the American Red Cross experience, provides data on the window period reduction with NAT using pooled testing for transfusion-transmitted viruses. For HIV the residual risk with NAT decreased from 1:1,300,000 to 1:1,900,000 per million red cells transfused. For HCV, the window period could become 10–12 days. Although the estimated reduction in the window period for HCV (time from infection to seropositivity) is calculated to be 32.5–40 days, there is a very high level of viremia in HCV infection, with virus becoming detectable 10–12 days after exposure. Thus NAT may reduce the HCV window period to 10–12 days. If these estimates are correct, the residual risk could be as low as 1:1,600,000.

TABLE 49.2	Viral Window Period and Estimated Residual Risk

Virus	Window (days) RBC transfused		Residual Risk	
	Pre-NAT	Post-NAT	Pre-NAT	Post-NAT
HIV	16	11–12	1:1,300,00	1:1,900,000
HCV	70	10–30	1:230,000	1:1,600,000[b]
HBV	45	(39)[a]	1:180,000	1:210,000
HTLV	–	–	–	1.6:1,000,000

NAT performed with minipools of 16–24 donor samples.
[a]Data from European Studies.
[b]Assumes a 10 day window period in repeat donors.

Blood is not routinely screened for cytomegalovirus (CMV) or parvovirus B19 even though these infections can be transmitted by transfusion. However, the standard of care is to provide CMV-seronegative blood for individuals who are CMV-seronegative and are either immunodeficient (infants, congenital or acquired immunodeficiency) or are candidates for hematopoietic stem cell transplantation or solid organ transplantation where the tissue donor is also CMV-seronegative. Blood centers screen part of their inventory for CMV to provide CMV-seronegative blood for these special patients. Most adult blood donors are CMV-seropositive. The prevalence of seropositivity for CMV varies in different geographic areas of the United States. Most of these donors have latent infections but there is not currently a test available to distinguish between donors who are infectious and those who are not. In the absence of CMV-seronegative blood, leukoreduced blood components are considered an appropriate alternative.

Other infections such as malaria, babesiosis, and trypanosomiasis may be transmitted by transfusion. There is no specific testing for malaria in the United States, and exclusion of infected donors is through the medical history. For other potential infections, local blood centers often add specific questions related to local infectious risks.

NAT for HIV and HCV was licensed in the United States in 2003. Investigative NAT testing for West Nile virus, which can be transmitted by transfusion and transplantation, is currently being conducted under FDA-IND in the United States. Systems for detecting bacterial contamination of platelets are now licensed.

SUGGESTED READINGS

American Association of Blood Banks: Standards for Blood Bank and Transfusion Services, 21st edition. American Association of Blood Banks, Bethesda, MD, 2002

American Association of Blood Banks: Technical Manual, 13th edition. pp. 557–634. American Association of Blood Banks, Bethesda, MD, 1999

Blood Bank Association of New York State, Inc.: Quarterly 35:15–21, 2001. Blood Bank Association of New York State, Albany, NY, 2001

Busch MP, Kleinman SH: Nucleic acid amplification testing of blood donors for transfusion-transmitted infectious diseases. Transfusion 40:143–159, 2000

Callum JL, Kaplan HS, Merkley LL, et al.: Reporting of near-miss events for transfusion medicine: improving transfusion safety. Transfusion 41:1204–1211, 2001

Cyr M, Eastlund T, Blais Jr C, et al.: Bradykinin metabolism and hypotensive transfusion reaction. Transfusion 41:136–156, 2001

Engelfriet CP, Reesink HW: International forum: transfusion-related acute lung injury (TRALI). Vox Sanguinis 81:269–283, 2001

Kuehnert MJ, Roth VR, Haley NR, et al.: Transfusion-transmitted bacterial infection in the United States, 1998 through 2000. Transfusion 41:1493–1499, 2001

Linden JV, Wagner K, Voytovich AE, et al.: Transfusion errors in New York State: an analysis of 10 years' experience. Transfusion 40:1207–1213, 2000

Noel L, Debeir J, Cosson A: The French Haemovigilance System. Vox Sanguinis 74 [Suppl. 2]:441–445, 1998

Perez P, Salmi RL, Follea G, et al.: Determinants of transfusion-associated bacterial contamination: results of the French BACTHEM case–control study. Transfusion 41:862–872, 2001

Williamson LM, Lowe S, Love EM, et al.: Serious hazards of transfusion (SHOT) initiative: analysis of the first two annual reports. Br Med J 319:16–19, 1999

50

INTRAOPERATIVE COAGULOPATHIES

Carolyn F. Whitsett, MD

A 72-year-old man is admitted with lower gastrointestinal bleeding. Endoscopy reveals a large ulcerated sessile polyp in the sigmoid colon. Routine preoperative laboratory studies were as follows: hemoglobin 11.5 g/dL, platelets 320 × 10^9/L, plasma prothrombin time (PT) 12 seconds (normal range 11–15 seconds), and activated partial thromboplastin time (aPTT) 58 seconds (normal range 32–46 seconds).

QUESTIONS

1. What should be included in the preoperative evaluation?
2. If the screening PT or aPTT is prolonged, which other coagulation tests should be ordered?
3. What are the most common intraoperative coagulopathies?
4. Which blood products are used to treat intraoperative coagulopathies?

1. What should be included in the preoperative evaluation?

The goal of the preoperative evaluation is to identify pre-existing conditions that could cause excessive bleeding or thrombosis in the perioperative period. Table 50.1 lists items that should be included. The complete medical history (personal and family), list of recent medications, physical examination results, and preoperative laboratory studies should be reviewed on every patient. In obtaining a medical history one must specifically inquire about over-the-counter medications, vitamins, other nutritional supplements, and homeopathic or natural remedies. Many patients do not consider these to be medications and forget to mention them. However, many of these natural remedies such as ginkgo biloba, garlic, ginseng, feverfew, and vitamin E inhibit platelet function and may cause bleeding if not discontinued prior to surgery.

The physical examination and blood chemistry profiles may identify other medical problems that could lead to surgical bleeding. Examination of the skin and mucous membranes may provide evidence of a hemorrhagic predisposition (vascular purpura, hereditary hemorrhagic telangiectasia), or collagen vascular disease. Splenomegaly, if present, may be associated with hereditary spherocytosis, myeloproliferative disorders, lymphoma, chronic leukemias, or liver disease with portal hypertension. Renal or liver abnormalities identified in the chemistry profile may suggest a need for specialized coagulation tests.

In the absence of a personal or family history of a bleeding disorder, coagulation tests are usually confined to a complete blood count, PT, and aPTT. Any abnormalities identified in the screening tests must be investigated and evaluated in terms of the operative procedure that is planned. Preoperative correction is advisable. If that is not possible, plans for intraoperative treatment and management must be developed. If there is a personal history of excessive bleeding, additional studies may be indicated even if screening tests are normal. The most common inherited abnormality of

TABLE 50.1	Preoperative Hemostasis Evaluation	
Patient history	Autoimmune and collagen vascular disease Blood disease Cardiac disease Epistaxis, recurrent or severe excessive bleeding after minor trauma Gastrointestinal disorders Liver disease Renal disease	Reproductive disorders Recurrent abortion Menorrhagia Postpartum hemorrhage Fetal death in utero, stillbirths Surgery Excessive bleeding Delayed wound healing Stroke Thrombosis Transfusion-types of products, reaction
Family history	Hemorrhagic disorders Thrombophilia Heart attacks Stroke	
Medications	Antiplatelet drugs Aspirin, clopidogrel, abciximab, COX-2 inhibitors, other nonsteroidal anti-inflammatory drugs Anticoagulants Heparin, coumadin, low-molecular-weight heparin Cardiac medications Homeopathic remedies Nutritional supplements Oral contraceptives	
Physical examination	Acral cyanosis or blisters Arthritic deformities Hepatosplenomegaly Malar rash Purpura/petechiae Telangiectasia Pulses Peripheral edema	
Laboratory tests	Complete blood count Prothrombin time Activated partial thromboplastin time Chemistry tests to evaluate liver and renal function Bleeding time Platelet function assays Mixing studies Factor assay Evaluation for thrombophilia	

coagulation is von Willebrand disease (vWD), with a prevalence of 1% in the general population. Approximately 1:1,000 individuals have clinically significant disease. In the most common form of the disease, the aPTT may be normal and assays for factor VIIIc, von Willebrand antigen, and ristocetin cofactor activity may be necessary to establish the diagnosis.

Medications known to inhibit platelet function should be discontinued in time to insure normal platelet function at the time of surgery. Patients should be advised about over-the-counter medications to avoid in the period immediately before surgery. If patients are on coumadin, vitamin K should be administered. If anticoagulation must continue until surgery, coumadin reversal and substitution of low-molecular-weight heparin, or regular heparin, may be advisable.

Finally, consultation with a hematologist to plan the management of patients with significant alterations in hemostasis or a predisposition to thrombosis is advisable.

2. If the screening PT or aPTT are prolonged, which other laboratory tests should be ordered?

When a prolonged PT or aPTT is encountered in the preoperative evaluation, the primary concern is to determine whether the prolonged coagulation time is caused by a deficiency of one or more clotting proteins and to determine whether the abnormality can be corrected by plasma. If the medical history and list of current medications is not informative, the most efficient way to make this assessment is to perform an in vitro assay called a mixing study. In this test, patient plasma is mixed with normal control plasma in a 1:1 ratio. The test is then repeated with the mixture immediately after mixing and after incubation at 37°C for 2 hours. When factor deficiency is present, addition of 50% normal plasma to the patient's plasma will shorten the patient's coagulation time, usually bringing it into the normal range. This correction is maintained after incubation. If the prolonged coagulation test is not corrected by the addition of 50% normal plasma, or if it corrects immediately after mixing but becomes prolonged again after incubation, an inhibitor to a coagulation factor is likely to be present. Many inhibitors are autoantibodies to coagulation factors. In dysproteinemias, the abnormal immunoglobulin may nonspecifically inhibit several coagulation factors in in vitro assays.

When the prolonged coagulation time is corrected, one should measure the activity of the individual coagulation proteins involved in the screening test. When an inhibitor is suspected, a hematologist should be consulted to guide the laboratory evaluation and to help plan treatment.

3. What are the most common intraoperative coagulopathies?

The common intraoperative coagulopathies are listed in Table 50.2. They include dilutional coagulopathies secondary to massive transfusion, disseminated intravascular coagulation (DIC), fibrinolysis, acquired platelet dysfunction, acquired inhibitors, heparin excess, vitamin K deficiency, and thrombosis.

Dilutional coagulopathy secondary to massive transfusion is the most common intraoperative coagulopathy. Massive transfusion may be defined as the transfusion of greater than 10 units of blood, replacement of 50% of the circulating blood volume in 3 hours, or replacement of one blood volume in 24 hours. During surgery, maintenance of blood volume by appropriate administration of crystalloids and colloids is essential. Red blood cells (RBCs) are transfused as needed to provide oxygen carrying capacity. Whole blood is virtually unavailable because all donor units collected are used for component preparation. As a consequence, packed RBCs or RBCs in adenine/saline preservative solution are the primary products used. RBC products contain no viable platelets. Most platelets are removed from the unit during the preparation of platelet concentrate; the rest are inactivated after storage at 1–6°C for 24 hours. At a minimum, 48–72 hours is needed to complete the required infectious disease testing. Thus, platelets in RBC products and platelets in whole blood that may have been collected for a special procedure are invariably inactivated. RBC products also contain little plasma. Conventional packed RBCs contain a small amount of residual plasma. However, most RBCs are prepared in adenine/saline preservative solution to extend the shelf life to 42 days. After centrifugation of a unit of whole blood, as much plasma as possible is removed and replaced with 100–110 mL of the preservative solution.

The hematocrit of adenine/saline RBCs is 55–65%, whereas the hematocrit of conventional packed cells is 70–80%. The transfusion of crystalloid and/or colloid solutions with RBCs creates a dilutional coagulopathy manifested by thrombocytopenia and prolongation of coagulation tests. Abnormal bleeding does not invariably occur when these laboratory abnormalities are present. During massive transfusion, hemostasis should be routinely monitored with point-of-care testing. When excessive bleeding occurs, the results of coagulation tests should be used to guide replacement therapy. Excessive microvascular bleeding appears to be more common with platelet counts less than 50,000/μL and fibrinogen levels below 50 mg/dL.

DIC is a syndrome characterized by primary intravascular activation of the coagulation system with secondary activation of fibrinolytic pathways. Although the mechanism of activation may vary, proinflammatory cytokines (interleukin-6, interleukin-1β, and tumor necrosis factor-α) and thrombin generation through the tissue factor/VIIa extrinsic factor pathway are major factors in the development of DIC. Activation of the coagulation cascade leads to the formation of intravascular thrombi and consumption of platelets, clotting factors, and anticoagulant proteins (protein C, protein S, antithrombin III). Although there

TABLE 50.2   **Intraoperative Coagulopathies**

Type	Etiology	Laboratory Tests	Treatment
Dilutional coagulopathy	Massive transfusion	Thrombocytopenia ↑ PT, ↑ aPTT, ↓ fibrinogen	Platelets FFP, cryoprecipitate if fibrinogen <100 mg/dL
Disseminated intravascular coagulation (DIC)	Acidosis Aortic aneurysms Hypoxemia Hemolytic transfusion reaction Obstetric emergencies Malignancies Sepsis Shock	Thrombocytopenia ↑ PT, ↑aPTT, ↓ fibrinogen ↑ D-dimer, ↑ fibrin–fibrinogen degradation products	Platelets FFP, cryoprecipitate Antithrombin III Activated protein C
Fibrinolysis	DIC with fibrinolysis Prostate surgery Neurosurgery Eye trauma Malignancies Thrombolytic therapy Liver disease Liver transplantation	↑ PT, ↑ aPTT Decreased clot lysis time	FFP ε-aminocaproic acid Aprotinin
Acquired platelet dysfunction	Cardiopulmonary bypass Membrane oxygenators Medication Liver failure Renal disease	Abnormal platelet function tests	Platelets Desmopressin Cryoprecipitate
Acquired inhibitors	Autoimmune disease Exposure to bovine thrombin Alloimmunization	↑ PT or ↑ aPTT or both that do not correct with mixing Decreased levels of specific factors	Inhibitor bypassing products Immunosuppression Tolerance induction
Heparin excess	Heparin administration Failure to neutralize heparin	↑ Activated whole blood clotting time ↑ aPTT	Discontinue heparin Administer protamine based on heparin titration/heparin level
Vitamin K deficiency	Coumadin Inflammatory bowel disease Pancreatic/biliary disease Antibiotics	↑ PT	Vitamin K if time permits FFP if surgery urgently needed
Thrombosis	DIC Thrombophilia (deficiency or abnormal anti-coagulant protein) Anti-fibrinolytic drugs Acquired inhibitor to anticoagulant protein	Shortened clotting times	Hemodynamic support Thrombectomy Discontinue anti-fibrinolytic therapy Fibrinolytic therapy Replacement of deficient anticoagulant protein

PT, prothrombin time; aPTT, activated partial thromboplastin time; FFP, fresh frozen plasma.

is secondary activation of the fibrinolytic pathway, there may be impaired fibrin degradation because circulating levels of plasminogen activator inhibitor-type 1 are increased. In the intraoperative setting, bleeding may be the presenting symptom because of consumption of platelets and coagulation proteins. However, occlusion of small and medium-sized vessels may cause multisystem organ dysfunction and failure. Laboratory studies demonstrate a prolonged PT, aPTT, decreased fibrinogen levels, increased D-dimer, and increased fibrin-fibrinogen degradation products. Antithrombin III and protein C levels are also decreased.

DIC may complicate many clinical conditions. It may be clinically silent and compensated or it may be uncompensated and flagrant. DIC occurs in sepsis, aortic aneurysms, massive trauma, placental abruption, eclampsia, amniotic fluid embolism, fetal death in utero, and with brain injuries. Patients with solid tumors and hematologic malignancies may also have DIC. In the patient with normal hemostasis prior to surgery, shock, acidosis, hypoxia, or endotoxemia may trigger DIC. The entry of brain tissue, fat or tumor into the circulation may also activate coagulation.

The treatment of DIC is controversial, particularly in the surgical setting. There is general agreement that control of the underlying disease is essential. When hemorrhagic symptoms predominate, transfusion of platelets, plasma, and cryoprecipitate is indicated. Since levels of anticoagulant proteins are also low, the use of antithrombin III (ATIII) and activated protein C should be considered. ATIII concentrates have been used in congenital antithrombin deficiency, in obstetric emergencies, to treat heparin resistance, and in DIC associated with sepsis. The results in sepsis have been variable but many obstetricians believe that ATIII is invaluable in certain clinical settings. Unfortunately, ATIII concentrate has been in very short supply recently because of decreased production and FFP is the only alternative product.

Recombinant activated protein C was recently licensed in the United States to treat severe sepsis. In clinical trials it decreased levels of D-dimer and interleukin-6 and reduced mortality. Activated protein C has also been used to manage DIC in obstetric patients in Japan. Post-marketing studies may identify other clinical conditions with DIC in which use of this product decreases morbidity and reduces mortality. Clinical trials are also under way to evaluate tissue factor pathway inhibitor in sepsis.

Fibrinolysis occurs when massive activation of plasminogen overwhelms the fibrinolytic inhibitor system. Urologic surgery, pulmonary and cardiovascular surgery, brain trauma, and eye injury may cause such activation. Epsilon-aminocaproic acid and aprotinin are effective antifibrinolytic drugs in these circumstances. Fibrinolysis may also be iatrogenic resulting from thrombolytic therapy. Secondary fibrinolysis in DIC may contribute to intraoperative bleeding.

Patients with severe liver disease who need surgery may also have problems with fibrinolysis. Thrombocytopenia and multiple coagulation deficiencies are present in severe liver disease. Patients often have dysfibrinogenemias and decreased hepatic clearance of fibrin degradation products causing poor clot formation. Delayed clearance of plasminogen activator and reduced hepatic synthesis of inhibitor proteins such as α2-antiplasmin and histidine-rich glycoprotein increase fibrinolytic activity.

The coagulopathy of liver transplantation is also associated with massive fibrinolysis. Shortly after the donor liver is reperfused, massive fibrinolysis is caused by release of tissue-type plasminogen activator from the donor liver. Both ε-aminocaproic acid and aprotinin have been used in this setting.

Acquired platelet dysfunction is relatively common. Usually it is caused by medications that inhibit platelet function and that are not discontinued prior to surgery. Many of these drugs are medications used in cardiovascular disease. Abciximab, tirofiban, epitifibatide, and clopidogrel are prominent because of the frequency with which they are used. Also, because of their frequent exposure to heparin, patients with cardiovascular disease may also have heparin-induced thrombocytopenia and associated platelet dysfunction. Many other medications can cause platelet dysfunction. Volume expanders such as dextran and hydroxyethyl starch and high doses of penicillin and cephalosporins may contribute to surgical bleeding. Finally, in cardiac surgery, bypass produces defective platelet function, probably related to platelet activation and fragmentation.

Acquired inhibitors are infrequent but dramatic causes of intraoperative coagulopathy. Most inhibitors occur in severe hemophilia where antibody develops following exposure to factor VIII or IX when concentrate is used for prophylaxis or therapy. These patients are invariably identified in the preoperative screening process and appropriate plans for treatment and monitoring planned well in advance. The development of recombinant activated factor VIIa to treat such patients has reduced mortality and morbidity in this group of patients. Acquired inhibitors may develop in individuals with no history of abnormal bleeding. These inhibitors are autoantibodies to autologous coagulation proteins. The most commonly reported acquired inhibitors are to factor VIII, although inhibitors to other clotting factors have been reported. These inhibitors may occur in pregnancy, postpartum, in autoimmune diseases such as lupus, with solid tumors, hematologic malignancies, and in the elderly. Recently there has been an alarming increase in reports of acquired inhibitors to factor V in patients exposed to bovine thrombin preparations when "homemade" fibrin sealants were made from cryoprecipitate. Most of these patients have had neurosurgery or cardiovascular surgery, but fibrin sealant is useful in many procedures. The commercially available fibrin sealant (Tisseel) does not use bovine thrombin and is an alternative and preferred product.

Screening coagulation tests are abnormal with acquired inhibitors. However, when a patient urgently requires surgery and there is no history of abnormal bleeding, they are sometimes taken to surgery under the assumption that FFP will correct the abnormality.

If the inhibitor is identified prior to surgery the procedure should be postponed if possible. Some inhibitors spontaneously disappear, while others respond to immunosuppressive treatment. If surgery is urgently needed, plasma exchange or immunoadsorption to reduce the titer of the inhibitor in combination with replacement therapy and/or factor bypassing products such as rVIIa and FEIBA may be helpful.

4. Which blood products are used to treat intraoperative coagulopathies?

Traditional blood components used to treat coagulopathies are presented in Table 50.3 and derivatives are presented in Table 50.4.

Solvent/detergent-treated plasma (SD-plasma) and donor retested plasma are the only additions to the list of components. Both products were developed to identify safer types of plasma for use in clinical conditions that require multiple and long-term exposure to plasma (i.e., therapeutic plasma exchange, replacement of congenital factor deficiencies where concentrates are unavailable). SD-plasma is a pooled plasma product containing plasma from many donors. The plasma is pooled by ABO type and treated with a solvent/detergent process that inactivates enveloped viruses. There is virtually no risk of transmission of HIV or hepatitis B and C. However, because this is a pooled product, the risk of transmission of parvovirus B19 and other non-enveloped viruses is increased. SD-plasma is just as efficacious as FFP in most clinical situations. However, unexpected thrombosis reported in several cases of liver transplantation resulted in a warning from the US Food and Drugs Administration about the use of SD-plasma in liver transplantation. SD-plasma has lower levels of protein S and anti-plasmin than FFP.

TABLE 50.3	Blood Products to Treat Coagulopathies			
Product	**Description**	**Indication**	**Dosage**	**Comment**
Platelet concentrate	Prepared from single unit of whole blood Contains ≥5.5 × 10^{10} platelets in 40–70 mL of plasma	Thrombocytopenia	1 unit of platelets will increase count of 70 kg adult by 5,000–10,000/μL Usual adult dose 4–8 units, often pooled for convenience of infusion	Pooled product expires 4 hours after preparation
Plateletpheresis (single-donor platelets)	Harvested from a single donor using apheresis technology Contains ≥3 × 10^{11} platelets in 100–500 mL plasma	Functionally abnormal platelets	One plateletpheresis (one single donor platelet)	Patients refractory to random platelets may benefit from plateletpheresis products that are either HLA-matched or selected by crossmatching Platelets may be leukoreduced to prevent immunization to HLA or to prevent febrile reactions

Continued

TABLE 50.3	Blood Products to Treat Coagulopathies—cont'd			
Product	**Description**	**Indication**	**Dosage**	**Comment**
Fresh frozen plasma (FFP)

Donor retested (similar to FFP except donor is tested twice at least 112 days apart)

Plasma 24 (frozen between 8 and 24 hours after collection)
Liquid thawed plasma | The fluid portion of a unit of blood frozen within 6–8 hours of collection
Contains all the procoagulant and anticoagulant plasma proteins
Volume 180–225 mL
Assume 1 u activity/mL when estimating replacement
Has lower levels of factors V and VIII than FFP | Management of bleeding patients with deficiencies of coagulation factors
Urgent correction of coumadin effect or vitamin K deficiency | Based on clinical indication, patient size and laboratory assays
Initial dose used often 15 mL/kg | Approximately 15–20 minutes required to thaw a unit of FFP
Plasma for FFP may be obtained by apheresis; this FFP product may have volume of 600 mL and is called jumbo plasma |
| Solvent/detergent plasma | Pooled plasma product treated with solvent/detergent process to inactivate enveloped viruses
Contains normal levels of coagulant protein; has lower level of protein S, antiplasmin and antitrypsin than FFP
Volume 200 mL | Same as FFP; is considered the preferred product for patients with isolated congenital deficiency of procoagulant or anticoagulant protein where concentrate is not available | Same as FFP | Has been associated with thrombosis in liver transplantation |
| Cryoprecipitate | Prepared from a single unit of FFP allowed to thaw between 1°–6°C and recovering precipitate
Each unit contains ≥150 mg fibrinogen, factor XIII, VIII, fibronectin in 15 mL of plasma | Concentrated source of fibrinogen, factor VIII, vWF, and factor XIII | Depends on patient size and laboratory data | Usually provided as pooled product average pool size for an adult in 7–10 units |

Two recombinant coagulation products, recombinant factor VIIa (Novo-7) and recombinant activated protein C, are relatively new. Although recombinant factor VIIa (rFVIIa) was developed for use in patients with hemophilia, it has been used in other clinical situations where thrombin production is impaired. A hemostatic effect of rFVIIa has been reported in thrombocytopathies such as Glanzman thrombasthenia and Bernard-Soulier syndrome and in severe thrombocytopenia. The product has also been used when profuse bleeding has occurred in trauma and extensive surgery. These case reports suggest the need for controlled clinical trials.

Recombinant activated protein C was licensed for use in severe sepsis, and many patients at risk of bleeding were

TABLE 50.4	Blood Derivatives and Biologicals Used in Coagulation Deficiencies		
Product	**Description**	**Example**	**Primary Indication**
Factor VIII	Plasma-derived Intermediate purity product containing factor VIII C and factor VIII vWF	Humate P	von Willebrand disease
	Highly purified plasma-derived factor VIII C		Hemophilia A
	Recombinant FVIII C (with albumin and albumin free)		Hemophilia A (infants and children never exposed to plasma)
Factor IX	Highly purified plasma-derived factor IX		Hemophilia B
	Recombinant factor IX	Benefix	Hemophilia B
Activated prothrombin complex	Activated factors II, VII, IX, X	FEIBA	Hemophilia A or B and inhibitors
Porcine factor VIII	Porcine factor VIII	Hyate C	Hemophilia A and inhibitor, patients with acquired inhibitors to FVIII
Activated recombinant factor VIIa	Recombinant VIIa	Novo-7	Inhibitors-acquired or occurring with congenital factor deficiency

excluded from the initial trials. Because it is an extremely expensive product, off-label use will undoubtedly be limited. However, studies from Japan have demonstrated the product to be useful in managing placental abruption. Post-marketing studies may identify other clinical indications.

SUGGESTED READINGS

American Association of Blood Banks: Technical Manual, 13th edition. pp. 161–191. Bethesda, MD, 1999

Bernard GR, Vincent JL, Laterre PF, et al.: Efficacy and safety of recombinant human activated protein C for severe sepsis. N Engl J Med 344:699–709, 2001

de Jonge E, van der Poll T, Kesecioglu J, et al.: Anticoagulant factor concentrates in disseminated intravascular coagulation: rationale for use and clinical experience. Semin Thromb Hemost: 27:667–674, 2001

Godreuil S, Navarro R, Quittet P, et al.: Acquired haemophilia in the elderly is a severe disease: report of five new cases. Haemophilia 7:428–433, 2001

Gologorsky E, De Wolf AM, Scott V, et al.: Intracardiac thrombus formation and pulmonary thromboembolism immediately after graft reperfusion in 7 patients undergoing liver transplantation. Liver Transpl 7:783–789, 2001

Hedner U, Erhardtsen E: Potential role for rFVIIa in transfusion medicine. Transfusion 42:114–124, 2002

Ozier Y, Steib A, Ickx B, et al.: Hemostatic disorders during liver transplantation. Eur J Anaesth 18: 208–218, 2001

Shattil SJ, Abrams CS, Bennet JS: Acquired qualitative platelet disorders due to diseases, drugs and food. pp. 1583–1602. Beutler E, et al. (eds): Williams Hematology, 6th edition. McGraw-Hill, New York, 2001

Streiff MB, Ness PM: Acquired FV inhibitors: a needless iatrogenic complication of bovine thrombin exposure. Transfusion 42:18–26, 2002

Uhl L, Kruskall M: Complications of massive transfusion. pp. 339–357. In Popovsky MA (ed): Transfusion Reactions, 2nd edition. AABB Press, Bethesda, MD, 2001

51 BLOOD REPLACEMENT

Mark Gettes, MD

A 55-year-old, 70 kg man is scheduled for revision of a total hip prosthesis. He is otherwise in good health. The starting hemoglobin (Hb) and hematocrit (Hct) are 13 g/dL and 40% respectively. He has predonated 2 units of his own blood and stated that he wishes only his own blood to be used during surgery.

QUESTIONS

1. How is oxygen transported by the circulatory system?
2. Describe compensatory mechanisms that take place in response to blood loss.
3. What is the minimum acceptable hemoglobin concentration (transfusion trigger)?
4. List the potential sources of autologous blood.
5. Explain acute isovolemic hemodilution (AIHD).
6. Outline the physiologic response to AIHD.
7. How is AIHD accomplished?
8. Which patients are suitable candidates for AIHD?
9. What is intraoperative cell salvage and how do modern cell salvage devices work?
10. Outline the characteristics of blood obtained by cell salvage.
11. Describe the indications for use of intraoperative cell salvage.
12. Explain the controversies and contraindications involving intraoperative cell salvage.
13. What is a preoperative autologous blood donation (PABD)?
14. Who is eligible and what are the contraindications for PABD?
15. Outline the disadvantages and risks of PABD.
16. Describe postoperative blood salvage.
17. Explain the advantages and disadvantages of different autologous blood sources.

1. How is oxygen transported by the circulatory system?

One of the circulation's major functions is to carry oxygen to tissues for use in metabolism. Oxygen delivery (oxygen transport or $\dot{D}O_2$) is the product of two factors: blood flow or cardiac output (CO) and the amount of oxygen carried in the blood, or arterial oxygen content (CaO_2).

$$\dot{D}O_2 = CO \times CaO_2$$

As the oxygen content of blood decreases, oxygen delivery can be maintained by a proportionate increase in CO.

Oxygen is present in the blood in two forms. It is bound by Hb and dissolved in plasma. The oxygen content of 100 mL of blood is described by the equation:

$$CaO_2 = (Hb \times 1.34 \times SaO_2) + (PaO_2 \times 0.0031)$$

where

CaO_2 = arterial oxygen content in milliliters of oxygen per 100 mL of blood

SaO_2 = percent of Hb saturated with oxygen

PaO_2 = partial pressure of arterial oxygen.

Under normal conditions (e.g., absence of pulmonary disease, normal Hb, physiologic shunt of 2–3%), the oxyhemoglobin saturation is approximately 97%, and the partial pressure of dissolved oxygen is approximately 100 mmHg. CaO_2 can then be calculated as follows:

$$CaO_2 = (15 \text{ g/dL} \times 1.34 \times 0.97) + (100 \text{ mmHg} \times 0.0031)$$
$$= 19.5 + 0.31$$
$$= 20 \text{ mL O}_2/100 \text{ mL blood}$$

This calculation demonstrates that the amount of oxygen dissolved in plasma (0.31 mL/100 mL blood) is negligible compared with the amount carried by Hb (19.5 mL/100 mL blood).

Furthermore, because the oxyhemoglobin binding factor (1.34) and the SaO_2 (0.97) are constant under normal conditions, it can be seen that CaO_2 varies almost linearly with Hb concentration. Under abnormal conditions, such as obesity and term pregnancy, rapid falls in SaO_2 during induction of anesthesia result in immediate decreases in CaO_2. The consequent tachycardia may or may not be sufficient to maintain normal $\dot{D}O_2$.

2. Describe compensatory mechanisms that take place in response to blood loss.

When blood loss occurs during surgery, there is loss of intravascular volume and reduction in oxygen-carrying capacity because of the loss of Hb.

As intravascular volume decreases, compensatory vasoconstriction and tachycardia occur in an attempt to preserve CO. Continuing volume loss results in decreased CO, causing a reduction in oxygen delivery to tissues. Restoration of intravascular volume by infusion of either colloid solution in a 1:1 ratio to blood loss or crystalloid solution in a 3:1 ratio allows normalization of CO and maintenance of hemodynamic stability.

Several mechanisms are available to respond to the loss of oxygen-carrying capacity. First, with restoration of intravascular volume CO may actually increase, maintaining or even increasing oxygen delivery. Second, at the tissue level, oxygen extraction may increase. Normal mixed venous oxygen saturation is approximately 75%. This indicates that only 25% of available oxygen is being extracted. Therefore, a substantial reserve of oxygen is available to the tissues, which can be used simply by increasing the amount extracted.

3. What is the minimum acceptable hemoglobin concentration (transfusion trigger)?

If blood loss continues during surgery, even if intravascular volume is maintained, oxygen-carrying capacity will eventually fall too low to meet metabolic demands, and red cell transfusion will be required. The minimum safe level of Hb, or transfusion trigger, is a question on which much attention has been focused. Awareness of acquired immunodeficiency syndrome (AIDS) and other transfusion-related diseases has led to the desire to withhold blood transfusion until absolutely necessary.

From animal models, and from experience with otherwise healthy Jehovah's Witnesses, it is known that survival is possible down to a Hct of 5–6% (Hb 2 g/dL) if normovolemia is maintained. Experience with other chronically anemic patients, such as renal failure patients, has shown that Hcts in the low 20s are routinely tolerated. From these data, it is apparent that previously recommended transfusion triggers of Hb 10 g/dL and a Hct of 30% are unnecessarily restrictive.

A theoretical model has been developed to determine the critical Hct, below which oxygen delivery is inadequate to meet metabolic needs. In conditions of normal systemic oxygen consumption in an otherwise healthy patient, the critical Hct is 14% (Hb 4.7 g/dL). Increasing systemic oxygen consumption by a factor of 3, which is typical for the postsurgical patient, increases the critical Hct to 21%. Based on such data, as well as clinical studies, the current US National Institutes of Health recommended trigger for transfusion is a Hb of 7 g/dL (Hct approximately 21%). Many clinicians will accept Hcts in the low 20s in otherwise healthy patients.

The transfusion trigger may differ in patients with cardiac disease. Maximal stress on oxygen delivery occurs in the heart, where 70% of available oxygen is normally extracted, as opposed to 25% for the body as a whole. If CaO_2 drops, the reserve for increased extraction is low. The only available compensatory mechanism is to increase coronary blood flow.

In patients with coronary artery disease, ability to increase coronary blood flow may be compromised, and the critical Hct level may be much higher. Therefore, patients with coronary artery disease should probably receive blood to maintain the Hct at approximately 30%. Similarly, patients with significant valvular heart disease or poor ventricular function, as well as those in whom CaO_2 is limited by pulmonary disease or who are in hypermetabolic states with large oxygen extractions, should have high transfusion triggers.

In summary, although it may not be possible to determine with certainty the minimum safe Hb level for a given patient, there are guidelines on which to base transfusion therapy. Healthy patients seem to tolerate Hcts in the low 20s. Patients with cardiopulmonary disease may require Hcts of 30%. Other criteria, such as overall medical condition or likelihood of continued blood loss, may be used to modify the transfusion trigger. Transfusion of red blood cells should be undertaken only to increase the oxygen-carrying capacity and never for volume expansion alone. As with other medical procedures, the benefits of transfusion should always be weighed against the risks.

4. List the potential sources of autologous blood.

Physician awareness of the dangers associated with homologous blood transfusions, as well as increased pressure from the public to avoid transfusions, has properly led to an increased use of autologous blood sources. These sources are:

- Preoperative autologous blood donation
- Acute isovolemic hemodilution (AIHD)
- Intraoperative cell salvage
- Postoperative cell salvage

Each has a role to play in avoidance of homologous transfusion.

5. Explain acute isovolemic hemodilution (AIHD).

AIHD is a procedure in which whole blood is removed during the perioperative period, while intravascular volume is maintained at a normal level by simultaneous infusion of crystalloid or colloid solutions. The blood, which is withdrawn into standard blood bags containing anticoagulant, is available for transfusion to the patient either during the operation or in the postoperative period. In this way, autologous whole blood containing red cells, clotting factors, and platelets is available. Its advantages are summarized in Table 51.1.

6. Outline the physiologic response to AIHD.

To understand how AIHD may be safely accomplished, it is necessary to understand the physiologic response to its use.

As previously discussed, $\dot{D}O_2$ is the product of CO and CaO_2. As isovolemic hemodilution occurs and red cells are removed from the circulation, CaO_2 of blood decreases. It might be expected that $\dot{D}O_2$ would therefore decrease. Surprisingly, as the Hct decreases to 30%, $\dot{D}O_2$ actually *increases* over baseline. This is because hemodilution alters the rheologic properties of blood. Blood viscosity is decreased by hemodilution, which effectively lowers systemic vascular resistance (SVR). An increase in venous return results in an increased stroke volume. CO increases proportionally more than CaO_2 decreases, and $\dot{D}O_2$ rises.

TABLE 51.1	Advantages of Acute Isovolemic Hemodilution

Red blood cell loss is reduced with each milliliter of surgical hemorrhage

It provides fresh whole blood for transfusion when required

Tissue perfusion is improved as viscosity diminishes

Furthermore, the rise in CO is accomplished without an increase in heart rate, if intravascular volume is maintained. Hemodilution to a Hct of 30% causes a 30–50% increase in CO. $\dot{D}O_2$ does not fall to control values until a Hct of approximately 20% is reached. Additionally, during isovolemic hemodilution, local tissue oxygenation is preserved and even enhanced by a more homogeneous distribution of capillary blood flow. Studies with tissue electrodes have shown that hypoxic microareas do not occur during isovolemic hemodilution.

7. How is AIHD accomplished?

AIHD is accomplished early in the perioperative period, usually just after the induction of anesthesia. Blood is removed from the patient via a large-bore intravenous catheter and stored in standard blood bags containing anticoagulant. An arterial catheter may be used for collecting autologous blood, but we have found this to be less satisfactory. Simultaneously, crystalloid, in a 3:1 ratio, or colloid (albumin, hydroxymethyl starch, or dextran) in a 1:1 ratio is infused through another large-bore intravenous catheter. The amount of blood to be removed can be calculated by any of the formulas used to calculate allowable blood loss. We typically use the following formula:

$$\text{Volume to be removed mL} = \frac{(Hct_A \times Hct_B \times EBV)}{(Hct_A + Hct_B/2)}$$

where

Hct_A = starting hematocrit

Hct_B = target hematocrit for hemodilution

EBV = estimated blood volume.

Typically, a target Hct in the mid to upper 20s (25–27%) is used; this allows for substantial hemodilution yet allows some margin of safety when blood loss begins to occur during surgery. In this instance, Hct_A = 40%, EBV = 70 kg × 70 mL/kg = 4,900 mL, and we will choose a Hct_B = 27%. The formula then yields:

$$(40 - 27 \times 4,900)/(40 + 27/2) = 1,900 \text{ mL}$$

Thus, 3–4 units of the patient's blood could be removed for later retransfusion. As units of blood are removed, they

Physiologic Response to Acute Isovolemic Hemodilution

$\dot{D}O_2$ remains constant or may increase

    CaO_2 falls as red blood cells are removed

    CO increases because of lowered SVR and improved venous return without an increase in heart rate

    Beneficial redistribution of capillary blood flow

Performance of Acute Isovolemic Hemodilution

Monitoring
>   +/− Invasive monitoring
>   Urinary catheter
>   Serial hematocrits
>   Tachycardia is a warning sign

Technique for removal
>   Two large-bore intravenous catheters (may substitute one intravenous with an arterial catheter)
>   Simultaneous administration of crystalloid (3:1) or colloid (1:1)

Technique for retransfusion
>   Retransfuse units in reverse order of collection

TABLE 51.2	Selection of Patients for Acute Isovolemic Hemodilution

Indications
>   Anticipated blood loss >1,000 mL
>   Starting Hct >36%

Contraindications
>   Anemia
>   Coronary artery disease
>   Left ventricular dysfunction
>   Valvular heart disease
>   Renal disease
>   Pulmonary disease
>   Carotid stenosis

are labeled and numbered consecutively. Blood is retransfused in reverse order of collection. The first unit removed is the least dilute and the richest in red cells, plasma factors, and platelets; therefore, it should be the last unit retransfused.

Blood removed during hemodilution may be stored in the operating room at room temperature for a maximum of 6 hours. Autologous blood remaining after surgery may be stored in a blood bank refrigerator for further use.

Invasive hemodynamic monitoring (arterial catheter, central venous catheter) is not mandatory during isovolemic hemodilution, but it facilitates serial Hct measurements and provides a guide to fluid replacement. Because CO rises in AIHD without an increase in heart rate, development of intraoperative tachycardia may indicate hypovolemia and the need for retransfusion. A urinary catheter to monitor urine output as a gauge of intravascular volume may be helpful. Also, replacing autologous blood with 3 times the volume of crystalloid initiates a diuresis.

8. Which patients are suitable candidates for AIHD?

The indications and contraindications for AIHD are listed in Table 51.2.

The essential criteria are an anticipated blood loss greater than 1,000 mL and a starting Hct of 36% or greater. Routine use of AIHD has been described for a wide variety of cases, including major urologic surgery, orthopedics, gynecologic surgery, plastic and reconstructive surgery, neurosurgery (brain and tumor resection), and cardiothoracic surgery. Reduction in homologous blood usage has been reported to vary from 18% to 90%. Age per se is not a contraindication to hemodilution, and its use has been described in both the elderly and pediatric populations.

Because the major compensatory mechanism for hemodilution is an ability to increase blood flow, isovolemic hemodilution is contraindicated in those whose ability to increase either systemic or coronary blood flow might be compromised. Thus, AIHD is contraindicated in patients with anemia, carotid artery stenosis, coronary artery disease, left ventricular dysfunction, and aortic or mitral valve stenosis. Because of the fluid shifts involved, AIHD is contraindicated in patients with renal or pulmonary disease.

Significant pre-existing myocardial or brain disease represents a contraindication to isovolemic hemodilution because myocardial ischemia and cerebral hypoxia are its major associated complications. Coagulopathies emanating from reduced factor levels may be exacerbated by dilutional effects.

9. What is intraoperative cell salvage and how do modern cell salvage devices work?

Intraoperative cell salvage refers to a procedure in which blood lost during surgery is collected and made available for transfusion back to the same patient. Modern cell-saving devices function by a four-step process:

- *Collection:* Blood is suctioned from the surgical field and mixed in the suction tubing with an anticoagulant containing either heparin or citrate. The suction pressures used in cell salvage systems are low, below 100 mmHg, to avoid hemolysis of collected blood. The blood is then passed through a filter to remove debris and stored in a canister until a sufficient volume is present for further processing.
- *Concentration:* The mixture of blood, anticoagulant, and irrigating solution collected by the suction is passed into a centrifuge bowl, where the heavier red cells are retained and the lighter elements are spun off and discarded.

- *Washing:* A large volume of saline is passed through the centrifuge bowl, further removing the noncellular elements and debris, leaving the red cells suspended in saline.
- *Reinfusion:* The red cell/saline mixture is pumped from the centrifuge into a standard plastic infusion bag, which is then available for transfusion back to the patient.

Modern cell salvage devices can process and return a unit of blood every 3 minutes in the face of rapid bleeding.

10. Outline the characteristics of blood obtained by cell salvage.

Salvaged autologous blood differs from banked blood and other sources of autologous blood in many ways. Salvaged autologous blood is basically a suspension of red cells in saline. The Hct of salvaged blood may vary depending on the amount of blood collected from the field but is typically in the 50–60% range. Once processed, salvaged blood contains essentially no clotting factors or platelets. If large volumes of salvaged blood are used to replace surgical blood loss, dilutional thrombocytopenia and low levels of clotting factors may result. Salvaged blood does not exhibit the storage lesion that is present in banked blood (Table 51.3). The 2,3-diphosphoglycerate (2,3-DPG) level of salvaged blood is normal, and it does not exhibit the low pH, elevated potassium, and microaggregate formation found in banked blood. Chromium-labeling studies have shown that salvaged red cells have normal survival times in the body once they are reinfused. Furthermore, indices of red cell viability, such as resistance to osmotic stress, are superior in salvaged blood compared with banked blood.

11. Describe the indications for use of intraoperative cell salvage.

Intraoperative cell salvage has been used in a variety of surgical settings, and its ability to reduce homologous blood use is well documented. Intraoperative cell salvage is indicated in cases for which blood loss is expected to exceed 1,000 mL.

Many, though not all, Jehovah's Witnesses will accept cell salvage, and it may be used in cases where obtaining homologous blood is difficult because of rare blood types or multiple antibodies. Cases ideally suited for cell salvage are those where surgical bleeding is confined to a discrete area. Blood loss occurring slowly over a wide area is difficult to collect. Typically, because of losses from the surgical field and those occurring during processing, approximately 50% of shed blood is returned to the patient. Recovery may be higher in some cases, such as abdominal aortic aneurysm resection, where blood loss is well localized. Use of intraoperative cell salvage has had a great impact in vascular surgery, orthopedic surgery, and cardiac surgery. It has also been commonly used in urologic, trauma, transplantation, and neurosurgical procedures. Not only has the average homologous blood requirement decreased, but the percentage of patients requiring *no* homologous blood products has sharply increased, from 4% to 68% in one study involving vascular surgery patients. Another study from a major center demonstrated that 17% of the total institutional red cell requirement was obtained by intraoperative cell salvage.

12. Explain the controversies and contraindications involving intraoperative cell salvage.

The major controversies regarding intraoperative cell salvage involve its use in oncologic surgery, and in contaminated trauma cases. In both situations, questions arise concerning the possibility of intravascular dissemination of unwanted material—in one case tumor cells, in the other case bacteria—by the use of cell salvage.

It has been demonstrated that during oncologic surgery tumor cells may survive processing and be suspended, along with red cells, for transfusion back to the patient. Thus, some experts feel that intraoperative cell salvage

TABLE 51.3	Characteristics of Salvaged Autologous Blood Compared with Banked Blood	

Salvaged Autologous Blood	Banked Blood
Normal 2,3-DPG	Decreased 2,3-DPG
Normal K$^+$	Increased K$^+$
Normal pH	Decreased pH
No microaggregate formation	Microaggregate formation
Normal resistance to osmotic stress	Decreased resistance to osmotic stress

Indications for Intraoperative Cell Salvage

Anticipated blood loss >1,000 mL
Jehovah's Witnesses: not all will accept it
Homologous blood difficult to obtain
    Rare blood type
    Multiple antibodies
Blood loss confined to a discrete area
    Vascular surgery
    Orthopedic surgery
    Trauma surgery
    Cardiac surgery

should not be used during oncologic surgery. However, it has not been demonstrated that transfusion of malignant cells results in dissemination of the tumor. In many forms of cancer, tumor cells may be recovered from blood despite the fact that blood-borne spread does not occur. There is particular reason for wishing to avoid the use of homologous transfusion in oncologic surgery. Homologous transfusions have been shown to produce an immunosuppressive effect, resulting in earlier tumor recurrence and decreased survival times in patients with some forms of cancer. Intraoperative cell salvage may be advantageous in such cases. One group of studies has looked at outcome of cell salvage in patients undergoing major urologic oncologic procedures. No evidence of blood-borne dissemination or high tumor recurrence rates was found in these patients. Use of cell salvage in such cases has been recommended by some. It is possible to compromise by using the cell salvage suction during dissection of tumor-free areas, while employing a separate suction to collect and discard material during actual tumor dissection. Nonetheless, more clinical studies will be necessary to fully resolve this issue.

In abdominal trauma, shed blood is frequently contaminated by intestinal contents. Because of red cell binding, bacteria survive processing by cell salvage equipment and can be transfused back to the patient. Whether transfusion of such contaminated blood contributes to the morbidity is questionable. Many experts feel that such patients are exposed to a bacterial load by the nature of their injuries. Prophylactic antibiotics significantly reduce the risk of sepsis. Consequently, there is little additional danger from bacteria in salvaged blood, and patients are spared the dangers associated with homologous blood. Some authors feel that salvaged contaminated blood should be used only as a lifesaving measure when no other blood is available. A definitive answer to this question awaits further clinical trials.

Cell salvage should not be used in the presence of topical hemostatic agents, povidone-iodine, polymyxin, bacitracin, or other topical antibiotics used with irrigation solutions. Its use is presently contraindicated if shed blood is contaminated by amniotic fluid.

Present cell salvage technology requires specially trained personnel to operate the equipment. These individuals should be free from other activities during processing. Consequently, someone other than the anesthesiologist caring for the patient should receive this responsibility.

13. What is preoperative autologous blood donation (PABD)?

PABD refers to the donation by a patient of their own blood before an operation for storage and possible transfusion intraoperatively or postoperatively. A national multicenter study in 1987 revealed that as much as 10% of all blood transfused for elective surgery could be obtained by PABD. Clearly, the driving force behind the increased interest in PABD at this time was fear of transfusion transmission of viruses, particularly human immunodeficiency virus (HIV). Use of PABD peaked in 1992, when it provided 8.5% of all units of blood collected in the United States. Use of PABD has declined in recent years. In 1999, 4.7% of all units collected, and 3% of all units of red blood cells transfused, were provided by PABD. PABD has clearly been shown to reduce patient exposure to homologous blood.

14. Who is eligible and what are the contraindications for PABD?

PABD is limited to cases where there is a reasonable likelihood that red cell transfusion will be required during the perioperative period. A surgical blood loss of 1,000 mL or more should be anticipated. The surgical blood schedule serves as a guide to whether or not transfusion is likely. Patients should not be encouraged to donate blood for procedures in which there is little chance of significant blood loss.

Criteria for donation of autologous blood are less stringent than those for volunteer donation. Autologous donors need a predonation Hb of 11 g/dL or higher or Hct of 33% or higher. Age is not a criterion for predonation, which has been used in the elderly and the pediatric populations. In patients weighing more than 50 kg, 450 mL of whole blood are donated at each visit. In patients weighing less than 50 kg, the volume of blood removed is proportional to weight, using the formula:

$$\frac{\text{Volume of the blood donated (mL)}}{450 \text{ mL}} = \frac{\text{donor weight (kg)}}{50 \text{ kg}}$$

PABD requires a suitable interval between the decision to undertake surgery and the actual date of the operation. The storage life of blood is 35 days. Consequently, there is no point in donating blood more than 5 weeks preoperatively. A unit of blood may be banked every 3 days depending on the donor's Hct, but donations are usually made every 7 days. Units can be stored for up to 3 days preoperatively. In the event that surgery is postponed blood may be frozen to prevent outdating if necessary.

In rare cases where collection of large numbers of autologous units is required, blood may be frozen and stored over long periods of time. Patients should be started on oral iron therapy once the decision to predonate blood is made. Use of recombinant erythropoietin to increase the amount of blood available for predonation and to decrease the interval between donations has been described and may be beneficial in patients who are anemic, who require large numbers of autologous units, or where the presurgical intervals are short. Erythropoietin therapy as described is expensive and remains experimental as of this writing.

There are several contraindications to PABD. Because bacteria may proliferate during blood storage, bacteremia is an absolute contraindication to predonation. Lack of intravenous access may also prohibit predonation.

Patients who are positive for HIV or hepatitis B surface antigen (HB$_s$Ag) may predonate blood. Such units must be labeled and segregated to protect other patients who might erroneously receive the unit, as well as workers handling it. Retransfusing this blood requires a special order from the patient's physician.

As in other aspects of transfusion medicine, patients with cardiac disease represent a gray area in terms of risk. Most centers exclude patients with unstable angina, aortic stenosis, or left main coronary artery disease but will accept donors with stable coronary artery disease. Some investigators have advocated monitoring (blood pressure, electrocardiograph, pulse, and oxygen saturation), simultaneous fluid administration, and physician supervision of high-risk patients making autologous donations. Precise delineation of risk in these patients awaits the outcome of future studies.

In contrast to homologous blood donation, a history of malignancy does not contraindicate PABD.

15. Outline the disadvantages and risks of PABD.

First, it should be noted that some of the risks associated with blood transfusions—ABO incompatibility due to clinical/administrative error and bacterial contamination—are not eliminated by use of PABD. For this reason, it is generally argued that the criteria for transfusing a unit of autologous blood (i.e., transfusion trigger) should be the same as for a unit of homologous origin. Others argue that, as the risks associated with autologous blood are decreased relative to homologous blood, then the risk/benefit ratio is altered, and the criteria for transfusion of autologous blood should be liberalized.

Paradoxically, use of PABD can result in a lower Hct, on average, of discharged patients. This is because many patients who predonate blood do not have adequate time, in the interval before surgery, to fully regenerate the amount of blood they have donated. Thus, they are essentially hemodiluted at the time of surgery. If they do not then receive a blood transfusion (because of low intraoperative blood loss), their discharge Hct will be lower then if they had not predonated.

Similarly, in an era of cost-effectiveness analysis, the use of PABD has been challenged. In certain surgical settings (i.e., total joint replacement), the use of PABD decreases by approximately 70% the likelihood that a patient will require homologous transfusion. In other settings (i.e., hysterectomy), many fewer patients will require transfusion, and a higher percentage of the units collected by PABD are discarded. Factors that increase the cost-effectiveness of PABD include appropriate case selection (cases where there is a high likelihood that the units will be transfused) and providing a long enough time interval between donation and surgery to allow regenerative erythropoiesis to occur. The use of erythropoietin therapy in conjunction with PABD makes logical sense and is being investigated.

From the patient's standpoint, multiple trips to the hospital or blood center to donate blood are inconvenient, and repeated needle sticks are uncomfortable. Vasovagal reactions occur in 2–5% of patients, of whom 0.3% will lose consciousness and 0.03% will convulse. In one study, 1:16,783 autologous donations led to an adverse event requiring hospitalization, a rate higher than that reported in normal volunteers.

Preoperative Autologous Blood Donation

Indications
 Blood loss >1,000 mL

Patient criteria
 Hb ≥11 g/dL
 Hct ≥33%
 Age is *not* a criterion

Contraindications
 Bacteremia
 Lack of intravenous access
 Cardiac disease
  Unstable angina
  Aortic stenosis
  Left main coronary artery disease
 HIV and HB$_s$Ag are *not* contraindications

PABD Disadvantages and Risks

Donor-related
 Vasovagal reaction
  Loss of consciousness
  Convulsion
 Inconvenience
  Multiple trips
  Repeated needle sticks
 Anemia following multiple donations

Transfusion
 Transfusion reactions
  Clerical/administrative errors
 Sepsis from bacterial contamination
 Congestive heart failure from volume
  overload

Blood collected for autologous use is subjected to the same tests as homologous blood. If not used, it is not "crossed over" into the general blood pool, but is discarded, as it is not felt that patients donating blood for autologous use are truly volunteer donors.

16. Describe postoperative blood salvage.

Currently, postoperative blood salvage systems are simple, inexpensive, and have been shown to be highly effective in decreasing patient requirements for homologous blood products. The systems consist of a container that is attached to drains placed in a surgical wound. Blood collected in this manner is defibrinogenated and will not clot, even in the absence of anticoagulant. When enough blood has been collected, the containers are hung, and the blood passes through a filter to a conventional blood administration set. Though the returned blood is high in fibrin-degradation products, its use seems to be safe and is not associated with development of disseminated intravascular coagulation (DIC). Recently, however, machines have been introduced that, like intraoperative salvage devices, wash the blood before returning it to the patient. Postoperative blood salvage systems have been used most commonly in cardiac and major orthopedic surgery.

17. Explain the advantages and disadvantages of different autologous blood sources.

Much controversy, and little consensus, exists in the literature about the "best" way to utilize autologous blood, with some experts advocating one method and others another. If it is not clear which method is superior, it is clear that each has something to offer, with the relative strengths and weaknesses of each method dependent on the clinical circumstances (Table 51.4).

PABD has the disadvantages of being relatively expensive, subjecting patients to some of the same risks as homologous transfusion (administrative error, storage lesion), and requiring a substantial time interval between harvesting the blood and the date of surgery. If blood is donated too close to the date of surgery, with insufficient time for the resynthesis of red cells to compensate for the amount removed, patients can be relatively anemic at the time of surgery and tend to leave the hospital with a lower Hct compared with controls. However, if blood is collected at a suitable interval before surgery, so that substantive erythropoiesis can occur, PABD can be a highly effective method of preventing exposure to homologous blood. A survey of 1,000 hospitals recently found that PABD is the most commonly practiced method of blood conservation. Its use is widely accepted by patients, and in some states in

---

TABLE 51.4   Comparison of Available Types of Autologous Blood

	Requires Days–Weeks Preoperatively	Acceptance by Jehovah's Witnesses	Expenses	Likely Available for Urgent or Emergent Surgery	Applicability to Oncologic Surgery	Provision of Platelets and Clotting Factors	Amount of Blood Provided
Predeposited autologous	Yes	No	High	Unlikely	Yes	Yes	Limited to amount donated
Acute isovolemic hemodilution	No	Possibly	Low	Likely	Yes	Yes	Limited by initial hematocrit (generally 2–3 U)
Intraoperative cell salvage	No	Possibly	High	Unlikely	?	No	Limited by amount salvaged
Postoperative cell salvage	No	Possibly	Low	Likely	?	Defibrinogenated	Limited to preoperative collection

the United States (California), discussion of PABD is mandatory as part of informed consent for any operation in which blood transfusion is likely.

AIHD has the advantage of being inexpensive, and is a "point-of-care" intervention. It obviates the need for weeks-in-advance planning and eliminates the risk of administrative error associated with stored blood. A number of clinical studies purport to show that it is of comparable efficiency, with less cost, to PABD or cell salvage. However, other studies, as well as mathematical models, have shown that the amount of red blood cells saved by AIHD is quite small and usually clinically insignificant. For AIHD to be clinically useful, both low Hct and large surgical blood losses must be safely tolerated. A number of authors have raised concerns about the iatrogenic introduction of risk in patients with previously unappreciated cardiac disease from moderate or profound hemodilution. Because of such concerns, the use of AIHD is probably of limited benefit to older patients. Its use is probably least controversial, and of greatest benefit, in pediatric or young adult patients with a low likelihood of unappreciated cardiac disease, who are not anemic, and who are having surgeries with large anticipated blood loss.

Intraoperative cell salvage is a widely used and highly effective method of reducing patients' exposure to homologous blood, and in cases involving large amounts of bleeding this procedure can rapidly provide autologous blood for return. Its use has been criticized largely on the grounds of cost-effectiveness, with the "break-even" point being 2 units of blood. However, by initially setting up only the collection (suction) part of the apparatus, and setting up the remainder, and more costly portion, of the machine only if a sufficient amount of blood has been collected, unnecessary costs associated with cell salvage can be decreased. Though there has been theoretical concern about the use of cell salvage in cases involving possible contamination of the blood with malignant cells or bacteria, clinical studies and experience have not shown an increase in either metastatic tumor spread or infection rates. Intraoperative cell salvage is an essential part of blood conservation programs.

Scientific advances over the past decade have greatly decreased the likelihood of transmission of viral diseases such as HIV and hepatitis C via blood transfusion. Nonetheless, avoidance of blood transfusion remains a significant concern on the part of the public, and has been identified as one of the most important factors in a patient's decision as to where to seek medical care. Furthermore, the potential impact of emerging diseases as West Nile virus, severe acute respiratory syndrome (SARS), and spongiform encephalopathies on the safety of the blood supply is of concern to both the public and the medical community. Spurred by such factors, the popularity of so-called bloodless surgery programs, designed to reduce or minimize exposure to homologous blood, has increased, and such programs are offered by approximately 100 centers in the United States.

A comprehensive program to decrease homologous blood exposure utilizes all of the techniques discussed in this chapter. Additional factors in attempting to decrease blood loss include careful surgical techniques, maintenance of normothermia, use of regional anesthesia, and in select patients, use of hypotensive general anesthesia. When combined with the use of an appropriate transfusion trigger, these techniques all contribute to minimizing patient exposure to homologous blood.

An Integrated Program of Blood Conservation

PABD

AIHD
    Intraoperative cell salvage
    Postoperative cell salvage
    Hypotensive anesthetic techniques
    Regional anesthesia when appropriate
    Appropriate transfusion trigger

SUGGESTED READINGS

Brecher ME, Goodnough LT: The rise and fall of preoperative autologous blood donation. Transfusion 41:1459–1462, 2001

Gillon J: Controversies in transfusion medicine—acute normovolemic hemodilution in elective major surgery: con. Transfusion 34:270–271, 1994

Goodnough LT: Risks of blood transfusion. Crit Care Med 31:S678–S686, 2003

Goodnough LT: The role of recombinant growth factor in transfusion medicine. Br J Anaesth 70:80–86, 1993

Klinberg IW: Autotransfusion and blood conservation in urologic oncology. Semin Surg Oncol 5:286–292, 1989

Murray DF, Gress E, Weinstein SL: Coagulation after reinfusion of autologous scavenged red blood cells. Anesth Analg 75:125–129, 1992

Pomper GJ, Wu YY, Snydre EL: Risks of transfusion-transmitted infections: 2003. Curr Opin Hematol 10:412–418, 2003

Rossi EC, Simon TL, Moss GS (eds): Principles of Transfusion Medicine, 2nd edition. Lippincott, Williams & Wilkins, Philadelphia, 1995

Shan H, Zhang P: Viral attacks on the blood supply: the impact of severe acute respiratory syndrome in Beijing. Transfusion 44:467–469, 2004

Shander A: Surgery without blood. Crit Care Med 31:S708–S714, 2003

Simpson P: Perioperative blood loss and its reduction: the role of the anaesthetist. Br J Anaesth 69:498–507, 1992

Stehling LC, Zauder HL: Acute normovolemic hemodilution. Transfusion 31:857–868, 1991

Toy PT, Strauss RG, Stehling LC, et al: Predeposited autologous blood for elective surgery. A national multicenter study. N Engl J Med 316:517–520, 1987

Williamson KR, Taswell HF: Intraoperative blood salvage: a review. Transfusion 31:663–675, 1991

52

THE JEHOVAH'S WITNESS PATIENT

Cheryl K. Gooden, MD

A 13-year-old girl with idiopathic scoliosis is scheduled for posterior spinal fusion with instrumentation. The patient's past medical history is otherwise unremarkable. She has no prior surgical history. The patient is a Jehovah's Witness.

QUESTIONS

1. What is scoliosis?
2. How is scoliosis classified?
3. How is the curvature assessed in the patient with scoliosis?
4. On the issue of blood, what will a Jehovah's Witness (JW) refuse and accept?
5. What are the medicolegal issues concerning blood transfusion in the JW who is a minor?
6. Describe the preoperative evaluation of the patient with scoliosis.
7. Describe the intraoperative anesthetic considerations for posterior spinal fusion surgery.
8. What is the "wake-up test"?
9. Describe the postoperative anesthetic concerns following scoliosis repair.
10. What blood substitutes are available?

1. What is scoliosis?

Scoliosis is characterized by one or more lateral curvatures of the spine. The lateral curvatures are associated with rotation of the vertebrae and can result in a deformity of the rib cage. The curves are classified as structural or nonstructural. In structural scoliosis the curve fails to correct (improve) with side bending toward the convex side. In nonstructural scoliosis the curve is flexible and corrects with side bending toward the convex side.

2. How is scoliosis classified?

Idiopathic scoliosis is the most common form of scoliosis. There may be a genetic component involved but, as the name implies, the cause is unknown. Idiopathic scoliosis can be divided into three different types: infantile, juvenile, and adolescent.

Infantile idiopathic scoliosis is diagnosed between birth and 3 years of age and has a higher incidence among boys. The majority of these curves will resolve spontaneously without treatment. The curves of infantile idiopathic scoliosis are thought to be secondary to molding in utero.

Juvenile idiopathic scoliosis is diagnosed between the ages of 4 and 10 years and is more evenly distributed between males and females.

TABLE 52.1	Classification of Scoliosis

Congenital
   Myelomeningocele
   Hemivertebrae
Idiopathic
Neuromuscular diseases
  Neuropathic
    Poliomyelitis
    Cerebral palsy
    Spinal cord tumors
  Myopathic
    Muscular dystrophies
Neurofibromatosis
Connective tissue disorders
  Marfan's syndrome
  Ehlers-Danlos syndrome
  Rheumatoid arthritis
  Osteogenesis imperfecta
Trauma
  Fracture
  Post-rib resection

Adolescent idiopathic scoliosis occurs between the age of 10 years and skeletal maturity, and is more commonly seen in females.

There are many causes and associated conditions in which scoliosis may occur. A classification of scoliosis is shown in Table 52.1.

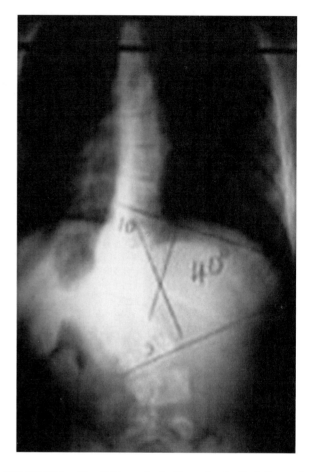

FIGURE 52.1 The Cobb method. (From the Scoliosis Research Society, 2003, with permission.)

3. How is the curvature assessed in the patient with scoliosis?

The Cobb method is the most common method used for measuring the curvature of scoliosis. In the Cobb method, parallel lines are drawn at the uppermost border of the curvature and at the lowermost border of the curvature. Perpendicular lines are then drawn from the two parallel lines, and the point of intersection of the perpendicular lines is the degree of curvature. Cobb's method for determining the degree of curvature is shown in Figure 52.1.

4. On the issue of blood, what will a JW refuse and accept?

The Watchtower Bible and Tract Society's (WTS) policy with regard to blood is based on the JW elders' interpretation of several biblical passages. It was determined that the use of a blood transfusion was a violation of God's law. JWs believe that blood removed from the body must be discarded. Therefore, they will not accept autologous or homologous blood transfusions.

The WTS's current policy prohibits blood components including red blood cells, white blood cells, platelets, plasma, and hemoglobin solutions.

The WTS's policy considers some blood components and procedures acceptable, including clotting factors, albumin, cell saver, and hemodilution. The latter two options are acceptable only if a continuous circuit is maintained. The list of acceptable blood components and procedures is limited to those that are more commonly associated with use in the operating room. A preoperative agreement should be established concerning the use of any of these components or procedures. Each JW patient must decide whether or not there is an objection to the use of these components or procedures.

In 1996, a group within the JW known as the Associated Jehovah's Witness for Reform on Blood (AJWRB) was established. This group has engaged in discussion regarding their difference of opinion towards the blood policy.

5. What are the medicolegal issues concerning blood transfusion in the JW who is a minor?

In circumstances in which the life of the JW minor patient is in danger, the courts have intervened to permit blood transfusions even though it directly opposes the religious beliefs of the parents. The procedure for obtaining consent to transfuse a JW minor patient involves a petition to the judge to declare that the minor is a "neglected child," and the court appoints a guardian. Medical necessity for the blood transfusion is presented by the physician. The appointed guardian can then consent to the blood transfusion.

However, the court's position has varied with respect to elective surgical procedures and blood transfusion in a JW minor. On the basis of religious grounds held by JW parents, some of the court rulings have been in favor of their beliefs, while others have not been. Currently, there is no consensus when it comes to elective procedures and blood transfusion. The decision to transfuse or not to transfuse a JW minor for elective surgery continues to be determined on a case-by-case basis.

6. Describe the preoperative evaluation of the patient with scoliosis.

A complete history and physical examination is a necessary part of the preoperative evaluation. Primarily, the preoperative evaluation should focus on the cause and the implications of the scoliosis for anesthetic management. The evaluation should include the degree of spinal curvature, any cardiovascular impairment, and the presence of coexisting disease(s). Table 52.2 lists the studies that may be performed as part of the preoperative evaluation. Some or all of these studies will be ordered, depending on the severity of the scoliosis.

Pulmonary function tests play a major role in determining the anesthetic management of the patient for posterior spinal fusion surgery. Restrictive lung disease is the most common pulmonary abnormality observed with scoliosis. It is of particular note if the vital capacity is 30% or less of predicted, as this will often indicate the probable need for postoperative ventilation. If obstructive disease is present, it is important to know its response to bronchodilators.

Cardiovascular impairment is not uncommon in the patient with scoliosis. Mitral valve prolapse is the most common cardiovascular abnormality seen in these patients. Pulmonary dysfunction may cause changes in the pulmonary vasculature leading to pulmonary hypertension. The end result of pulmonary hypertension on the cardiovascular system is the development of right ventricular failure or cor pulmonale. Clinical findings of cor pulmonale include an S_4 heart sound, jugular venous distention, hepatomegaly, pedal edema, and a left parasternal lift.

If a wake-up test is planned, then the procedure and what is expected of the patient must be explained and comprehended.

In the majority of patients, preoperative sedation is acceptable. However, it should be kept in mind that some patients with scoliosis will have a significant degree of respiratory dysfunction and preoperative sedation may be contraindicated. The resulting respiratory depression can cause hypoxemia, hypercarbia, and acidosis.

7. Describe the intraoperative anesthetic considerations for posterior spinal fusion surgery.

An inhalation or intravenous induction is acceptable. Any of the nondepolarizing muscle relaxants can be used for this procedure. A balanced technique of nitrous oxide, oxygen, volatile agent, neuromuscular blocker, and an opioid should be considered for the maintenance anesthetic. If somatosensory and/or motor evoked potential monitoring are to be used, then it is recommended that the concentration of the volatile agent be 0.2% or less. An opioid infusion rather than bolus injections is the preferred anesthetic technique, particularly in the presence of evoked potential monitoring.

TABLE 52.2	Preoperative Evaluation for the Patient with Scoliosis

Etiology/implications of the scoliosis
Cobb's angle
Complete blood count, platelet count
Blood type and crossmatching
PT/PTT, INR
Chest radiograph
Electrocardiogram
Pulmonary function tests (in the presence of restrictive or obstructive lung disease)
  Spirometry (FVC, FEV_1, FEV_1/FVC)
  Lung volumes (TLC, FRC, RV, FRC/TLC, RV/TLC)
Arterial blood gas
Assessment for cardiovascular impairment
Coexisting disease(s)

PT, prothrombin time; PTT, partial thromboplastin time; INR, international normalized ratio; FVC, forced vital capacity; FEV_1, forced expiratory volume in 1 second; TLC, total lung capacity; FRC, functional residual capacity; RV, residual volume.

In addition to the standard intraoperative monitors, an arterial catheter, central venous catheter, and a urinary catheter should be placed. The arterial catheter allows for monitoring of arterial blood pressure on a beat-to-beat basis and also facilitates blood sampling. Most anesthesiologists will opt for placement of a central venous catheter to monitor central filling pressures and volume status. Depending on the severity of cardiopulmonary disease, a pulmonary artery catheter may be warranted.

Turning and positioning the patient prone requires extreme care. It is important to avoid pressure on the eyes, which can result in retinal artery occlusion and blindness. It is also necessary to avoid pressure necrosis of the ears, nose, and forehead. The head should be in proper alignment and positioned in such a way that allows for easy inspection of the face. The chest, abdomen, and pelvic areas should rest on properly positioned parallel rolls or other devices that avoid pressure on the axilla, breasts and genitalia. The arms should rest at the sides with the elbows flexed and the shoulders abducted no greater than 90° to avoid stretching the brachial plexus. Appropriate padding should also be present.

A considerable decrease in body temperature can occur during spinal surgery on account of the large body surface area exposed. Precautions should be taken to avoid intraoperative hypothermia. These include using a forced-air warming blanket, an intravenous fluid warming system, and adjustment of the operating room temperature.

Significant blood loss is not uncommon during this surgery. Predonation of autologous blood is efficacious and recommended for spinal fusion surgery. There are several techniques designed to minimize blood loss and the need for homologous blood transfusion (Table 52.3). More specifically, the intraoperative techniques are acute normovolemic hemodilution, cell salvage, hypotensive anesthesia, surgical technique, and local infiltration with an epinephrine-containing solution. The latter technique helps to reduce bleeding at the site of infiltration, but the overall reduction in surgical blood loss is minimal.

A review of each hypotensive anesthetic technique (Table 52.4) is beyond the scope of this chapter. There are a number of excellent resources available for review of these techniques. However, there are several key points to keep in mind when using hypotensive anesthesia. The mean arterial pressure (MAP) should be maintained above 50 mmHg to ensure adequate spinal cord perfusion and cerebral blood flow. In general, a MAP of 50–60 mmHg is ideal. In addition, the arterial blood gases should be monitored during the procedure.

Contraindications to the use of controlled hypotension include pre-existing major end-organ dysfunction, hemoglobinopathies, polycythemia, and elevated intracranial pressure. The clinician must have a thorough understanding of the technique and also be competent with the use of the technique chosen.

TABLE 52.3	Strategies for Avoidance of Homologous Blood Transfusions

Preoperative use of erythropoietin
Predonation of autologous blood
Acute normovolemic hemodilution
Pharmacologic therapy (e.g., aprotinin and tranexamic acid)
Intraoperative cell salvage with retransfusion
Anesthetic technique
Surgical technique

8. What is the "wake-up test"?

A preoperative discussion should occur with the patient concerning the details of the wake-up test and to dispel any fears of awakening during the surgery and/or experiencing pain.

The wake-up test is used to assess the anterior spinal cord (motor) pathway. This test is not reflective of the posterior spinal cord (sensory) pathway. The wake-up test is performed intraoperatively following spine instrumentation. Adequate notice should be given to the anesthesiologist by the surgeon, so as to coordinate the timing of "lightening the anesthesia" to an appropriate level so that the patient can follow commands. The wake-up test can present a challenge for the anesthesiologist, with regard to the balance that must be maintained between the patient performing some level of activity but without excessive movement.

The wake-up test begins by assessing the level of the patient's comprehension by asking the patient to squeeze the anesthesiologist's hand. If the response is acceptable, then the patient is asked to move their feet. If the patient is unable to move their feet, the amount of spinal distraction must be decreased and the test is repeated. Excessive distraction can compromise spinal cord blood flow leading to ischemia and may result in postoperative paraplegia. Following completion of the wake-up test, anesthesia is deepened with an intravenous hypnotic agent, benzodiazepine, and the anesthesiologist's neuromuscular blocking agent of choice.

The wake-up test has its limitations. It evaluates the patient's motor function at only one point in time. It has no bearing on the time following the performance of the test, when spinal cord injury remains a possibility. The wake-up test is not appropriate for young children or the cognitively impaired patient. Excessive patient movement may promote self-extubation, bleeding, air embolus, or disruption of the spinal instrumentation. Somatosensory evoked potential (SSEP) monitoring can be used as an adjunct to the wake-up test. SSEP offers the advantage of continuous monitoring.

TABLE 52.4	Controlled Hypotensive Anesthesia	
Category	**Drug**	**Recommendations**
Volatile anesthetics	Isoflurane	Most commonly used of the volatile agents, due to its ability to maintain cerebral blood flow while reducing cerebral metabolic rate for oxygen
α_2-Adrenergic agonists	Clonidine	Administered orally 1 hour prior to surgery. May work well on its own as a hypotensive agent or may need to be combined with another agent
β-Adrenergic antagonists	Esmolol	Its rapid onset, titratable action, and short duration are features that make it a good agent
	Propranolol	Compared with esmolol, used in situations when a slow onset and long duration of action are acceptable
Vasodilators	Sodium nitroprusside	Good agent to choose due to its rapid onset, titratability, and quick offset after infusion is discontinued
Calcium channel blockers	Nicardipine	Used in situations when rapid onset and intermediate duration of action are desired

9. Describe the postoperative anesthetic concerns following scoliosis repair.

In the majority of patients, the goal at the end of scoliosis repair will be to awaken and extubate in the operating room. In some patients, extubation may be delayed and the factors leading to it can be the same as those associated with any general anesthesia case. Additionally, factors more specifically related to the patient with scoliosis include possible underlying pulmonary dysfunction, persistent muscle weakness, or issues related to any coexisting disease(s).

Postoperative anesthetic concerns focus on known complications following posterior spinal fusion surgery and these include bleeding, pneumothorax, atelectasis, respiratory distress, and neurologic deficit. Another area of concern in the postoperative anesthetic care is pain management. Pain control in the initial postoperative period can be treated by intravenous (IV) patient-controlled analgesia (PCA) with opioids. In young children or cognitively impaired patients, a continuous IV opioid infusion is suggested. Most patients are cared for in an intensive care unit following scoliosis repair.

10. What blood substitutes are available?

Blood substitutes are substances that are characterized by their ability for oxygen transport, volume expansion, and lack of red cell mass. These products include perfluorocarbons and hemoglobin solutions. Some of these products are currently undergoing clinical trials, and their utility remains controversial. A comparison of blood and blood substitutes is shown in Table 52.5.

TABLE 52.5	Blood Versus Blood Substitutes		
Feature	**Blood**	**Perfluorocarbons**	**Hemoglobin solutions**
Size	7 μm/cell	0.2 μm	<0.007 μm
Type and crossmatching	Required	Not required	Not required
Storage life	42 days	2 years	2–3 years
Storage	Refrigeration	Room temperature	Room temperature
Associated risks	Bloodborne disease	Transient thrombocytopenia	Renal damage, systemic toxicity. transient increase in systemic and pulmonary artery pressures

Perfluorocarbons are synthetic substances that have a high oxygen solubility. The emulsified form of perfluorocarbons is surrounded by surfactant, and is administered by the IV route to patients in the presence of high levels of inspired oxygen. The oxygen-carrying emulsion is capable of unloading oxygen to the tissues. Problems encountered with the first-generation perfluorocarbons (e.g., Fluosol DA-20) included a short half-life, pulmonary toxicity, and complement activation. The second-generation perfluorocarbons have a greater oxygen-carrying capacity. Clinical trials with these compounds are in progress.

Hemoglobin solutions have been developed from human, animal, and recombinant sources. Problems associated with these solutions include renal damage, systemic toxicity, short half-life, and increases in mean arterial and pulmonary artery pressures. A group of hemoglobin solutions, referred to as stroma-free hemoglobin, have emerged and have fewer side-effects reported. The stroma-free hemoglobin solutions contain a modified hemoglobin molecule that results in a longer half-life, larger molecule size, and less filtration by the kidneys compared with earlier hemoglobin solutions. Some of these solutions are in clinical trials, and issues remain concerning their safety and efficacy.

SUGGESTED READINGS

Associated Jehovah's Witnesses for Reform on Blood. New Light on Blood. Available at: http://www.ajwrb.org/forbidden.shtml. Accessed March 16, 2003

Benson K: The Jehovah's Witness patient: considerations for the anesthesiologist. Anesth Analg 69:647–655, 1989

Dietz N, Joyner M, Warner M: Blood substitutes: fluids, drugs, or miracle solutions? Anesth Analg 82:390–405, 1996

Dixon J, Smalley M: Jehovah's Witnesses the surgical/ethical challenge. JAMA 246:2471–2472, 1981

Goodnough L, Monk T, Andriole G: Erythropoietin therapy. N Engl J Med 336:933–938, 1997

Grundy B: Intraoperative monitoring of sensory-evoked potentials. Anesthesiology 58:72–87, 1983

Nash C, Brown R: Spinal cord monitoring. J Bone Joint Surg Am 71:627–629, 1989

Spence R, McCoy S, Costablie J, et al.: Fluosol DA-20 in the treatment of severe anemia: randomized, controlled study of 46 patients. Crit Care Med 18:1227–1230, 1990

Testa L, Tobias J: Techniques of blood conservation. II. Autologous transfusion, intraoperative blood salvage, pharmacologic agents, and cost issues. Am J Anesthesiol 23:63–72, 1996

53

HEMOPHILIA A

JoAnne Betta, MD

Neeta Moonka, MD

Aryeh Shander, MD

A 25-year-old man with acute appendicitis presents to the operating room for a laparoscopic appendectomy. His parents state that he has hemophilia A.

QUESTIONS

1. What is the primary deficiency in hemophilia A?
2. How does the disease present and what are the laboratory findings?
3. What is the role of factor VIII in the coagulation process?
4. Describe the treatment options.
5. Discuss von Willebrand disease as another important cause of surgical bleeding.

1. What is the primary deficiency in hemophilia A?

Hemophilia A, the commonest hereditary bleeding disorder, is due to a genetic deficiency of plasma factor VIII. Although the inheritance is X-linked recessive, approximately 30% of those with the disease acquire it through a spontaneous mutation and, therefore, will present with no family history of hemophilia. Regardless of how the disease is acquired, it is primarily a disease of males.

Its incidence approaches 1 in 5,000 male births. This "classical hemophilia A" should be considered in any male who presents with unexplained and uncontrolled bleeding.

The plasma factor VIII concentration correlates strongly with the degree of bleeding seen. Patients with severe hemophilia have factor VIII levels 1% or less compared with normal. Those with factor levels 2–5% of normal have moderate hemophilia, while patients with factor levels 6–30% of normal have mild disease. It is important to quantify the plasma levels of factor VIII prior to surgery to assess the risk of bleeding. Patients with mild hemophilia will usually bleed excessively only after trauma or during surgery, whereas severe hemophiliacs can bleed spontaneously 20–30 times a year, usually into joints and muscle.

2. How does the disease present and what are the laboratory findings?

The most common clinical presentation of hemophilia A is hemarthroses. Typically in infants, as ambulation begins, bleeding into joints and muscles occurs even after minor trauma. Up to 90% of patients with severe disease demonstrate evidence of bleeding by 1 year of life. Of note is the fact that although factor VIII does not cross the placenta, newborns will often not exhibit symptoms.

Bleeding associated with hemophilia A can occur virtually anywhere in the body and give rise to secondary complications. Bleeding in the neck or pharynx may cause airway obstruction. Central nervous system hemorrhages, although uncommon, may be life-threatening and are a common cause of death.

Prolonged and excessive bleeding associated with even minor surgery is common and can be present in mild disease where there may be no history of previous spontaneous or surgical bleeding. The importance of identifying the severity of the deficient factor is therefore underscored. In fact, the diagnosis should be suspected in any male with unusual bleeding. The laboratory data consistent with the diagnosis are a prolonged activated partial thromboplastin time (PTT), a normal platelet count, and normal prothrombin time (PT). Specific assay for factor VIII activity confirms and quantifies the disease.

3. What is the role of factor VIII in the coagulation process?

Blood clot formation with coagulation factors is the body's second line of defense against bleeding after initial platelet plug formation. It occurs through a series of enzyme reactions involving plasma protein cofactors. Factors V and VIII play essential roles in this process. Factor VIII accelerates the rate of cleavage of factor X by activated factor IX. This reaction takes place on a phospholipid surface where factor VIII increases the velocity of the reaction by several thousand-fold.

Factor VIII cannot, however, become part of the reaction, which includes a calcium-dependent complex of factor VIIIa, factor IXa, and phospholipid, until it is released from the von Willebrand factor that binds it. Factor VIII exists in the plasma as a complex with von Willebrand factor and as such cannot bind to phospholipid surfaces. However, the complex will concentrate itself at sites of vascular injury because von Willebrand factor itself binds to subendothelial matrix proteins and platelet aggregates. Thrombin or factor Xa cleaves factor VIII from this complex, freeing it to bind to the phospholipid surfaces of damaged cells and activated platelets.

4. Describe the treatment options.

Hemophilia A is treated by replacement therapy with factor VIII. The infusion of 1 U of factor VIII per kilogram of body weight increases the plasma level by 0.02 U/mL. Mild bleeding episodes can be controlled by a level of 0.3 U/mL, whereas severe bleeding requires 0.5 U/mL for control. Normal plasma levels must be maintained during major surgery or life-threatening bleeding. This can be accomplished either by the administration of repeated doses of factor or by continuous infusion. The half-life of factor VIII in the plasma is approximately 8 hours.

The process of obtaining, concentrating and purifying factor VIII has occurred over the past 30 years. Until plasma cryoprecipitate was discovered in 1964, frozen plasma was the only source of factor VIII available. Elective surgery was thus not feasible due to the large volumes of plasma that would be needed. Currently, highly purified factor VIII concentrates are available which provide rapid reversal or prevention of bleeding. Many patients lead nearly normal life-styles with home treatment or even self-treatment.

In the early 1990s, two preparations of recombinant factor VIII were licensed. Clinical studies have confirmed excellent efficacy and a high correlation between the dose given and the resultant plasma level. This recombinant therapy is not associated with antibody formation or transmission of blood-borne diseases such as human immunodeficiency virus (HIV). It is, however, 2–3 times more expensive than plasma-derived factor, and its availability can be limited by production capacity. In the United States, approximately 60% of severe hemophiliacs use recombinant factor VIII.

One drawback to the use of recombinant factor VIII is its formulation with human albumin and other animal proteins. Several new preparations are in clinical trials and are made without human albumin and other antigenic foreign proteins.

A newly approved product, recombinant activated factor VII, has been licensed in the United States and is intended for home use in patients with inhibitors. This agent provides hemostasis by binding directly or in complex with tissue factors to negatively charged phospholipids exposed on the surface of activated platelets. Recombinant activated factor VIII stops spontaneous and surgically induced bleeding in 70–75% of patients with inhibitors.

Desmopressin (1-deamino-8D arginine vasopressin or DDAVP) can be used to treat mild to moderate hemophilia A. An intravenous dose of 0.3 µg/kg can increase the factor VIII level 3–5 times above baseline. Nasal DDAVP allows for home use.

Hemophilia A as a genetic disease lends itself well to the development of gene therapy since it is caused by the lack of a single gene product. Also, this product is needed in only minute amounts in the plasma. Gene therapy trials are currently under way and offer a future "cure" for all patients with hemophilia A.

5. Discuss von Willebrand disease as another important cause of surgical bleeding.

von Willebrand disease is not as common as hemophilia A but is more common than the other types of hemophilia. It occurs in both males and females with an autosomal dominant pattern in Type 1 and Type II diseases.

TABLE 53.1	Hemophilia A and von Willebrand Disease	
	Hemophilia A	**von Willebrand Disease**
Inheritance pattern	X-linked recessive	Autosomal dominant
Genetic defect	Low to absent factor VIII plasma level	Low von Willebrand factor level or activity, low factor VIII activity
Laboratory findings	Low factor VIII coagulant activity, prolonged PTT	Reduced plasma level of von Willebrand protein, mildly prolonged PTT
Treatment	Plasma-derived factor VIII concentrates	DDAVP
	Recombinant factor VIII	Cryoprecipitate
	DDAVP (helpful in mild disease)	
	Recombinant activated factor VII	
	Future: Gene therapy	

Patients with this disease often have frequent mucosal bleeding and females may have excessive menses and postpartum bleeding. Unlike hemophilia A, spontaneous hemarthroses are uncommon. von Willebrand disease, like hemophilia A, has a broad spectrum of clinical features seen within the same family members afflicted by this disease. All types of von Willebrand disease are associated with the laboratory finding of a prolonged bleeding time (not seen with hemophilia A), a decrease in factor VIII levels, and a mild to moderate prolonged PTT. Platelet count and PT are normal. Type I patients, with classic von Willebrand disease, have reduced plasma levels of von Willebrand protein, von Willebrand factor activity and factor VIII activity. Absent or diminished platelet aggregation occurs in the presence of ristocetin.

Cryoprecipitate is rich in factor VIII and von Willebrand factor and, therefore, corrects both deficiencies. Factor VIII concentrates lack sufficient amounts of von Willebrand factor and are not considered effective treatment. Patients with mild to moderate disease with minor trauma or scheduled for surgery and/or dental extraction should receive DDAVP. As noted above, DDAVP increases factor VIII levels (Table 53.1).

SUGGESTED READINGS

Hoyer LW: Hemophilia A. N Engl J Med 330:38, 1994

Mannucci PM, Tuddenham EGD: The hemophilias – from royal genes to gene therapy. N Engl J Med 344:1773, 2001

Montgomery RR, Scott JP: Hereditary clotting factor deficiencies (bleeding disorders). p. 1508. In Behrman RE, Kliegman RM, Jenson HB (eds): Nelson Textbook of Pediatrics, 16th edition. WB Saunders, Philadelphia, 2000

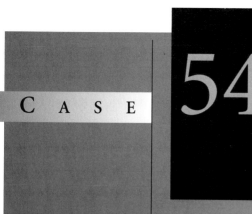

Dan A. Kaufman, MD

CASE 54 — TOTAL HIP REPLACEMENT

A 57-year-old woman presents for a primary total hip arthroplasty. Past medical history is significant for rheumatoid arthritis.

QUESTIONS

1. Briefly describe rheumatoid arthritis and its treatment.
2. What are the anesthetic considerations for the rheumatoid arthritis patient?
3. How is the rheumatoid arthritis patient evaluated for anesthesia?
4. Discuss the options for induction of anesthesia in a primary hip arthroplasty.
5. Several hours into the case the surgeon complains that he is operating on a moving target. How would you manage this situation?
6. Discuss the causes and management of fat embolus syndrome.
7. Discuss thromboembolism prophylaxis and the placement of neuraxial anesthesia.
8. Discuss the options for postoperative pain control after total hip arthroplasty. Discuss the use of a lumbar plexus block.

1. Briefly describe rheumatoid arthritis and its treatment.

Rheumatoid arthritis (RA) is an autoimmune disease affecting primarily women and is present in up to 1% of the population. This chronic and systemic inflammatory condition targets mainly the synovial tissue of the joints. Diagnostic criteria which are indicative of RA, though not specific for it, include morning stiffness, arthritis of three or more joints, arthritis of the hand joints, symmetric distribution, rheumatoid nodules, elevated levels of rheumatoid factor, and radiographic changes. Patients may develop cricoarytenoid arthritis which may make tracheal intubation difficult. Extra-articular manifestations of the disease can present in the heart, lungs, kidneys, and in the blood.

While the diagnosis of RA can be somewhat elusive, it has been shown that the prompt initiation of therapy can delay the course of the disease. Medications used to treat RA are generally divided into three main categories: disease-modifying anti-rheumatic drugs (DMARDs), corticosteroids, and nonsteroidal anti-inflammatory drugs (NSAIDs). Recently the use of Cox-2 inhibitors has also been instituted by many physicians.

DMARDs, as the epithet indicates, alter the course of RA. There are many different drugs in this category, which include methotrexate, sulfasalazine, azathioprine, and cyclosporine. Corticosteroids, which alter the inflammatory response of RA, are used arbitrarily by different physicians. Corticosteroids may be prescribed in a low dose for chronic use or as a steroid taper for exacerbations. NSAIDs are commonly prescribed to provide relief from pain and stiffness; however, they do not alter the course of the disease.

2. What are the anesthetic considerations for the rheumatoid arthritis patient?

Airway

The RA patient may have atlantoaxial instability of the cervical spine. Excessive manipulation of the neck during endotracheal intubation or while positioning the patient can result in devastating consequences such as atlantoaxial subluxation. Cricoarytenoid arthritis presents with hoarseness, pain on swallowing, dyspnea, stridor, and tenderness over the larynx. Erythema and edema of the vocal cords may result in a narrowed glottic opening. Temporomandibular joint arthritis may limit mouth opening.

Cardiac

Though common, cardiac complications rarely necessitate intervention prior to the induction of anesthesia.

Rheumatoid Arthritis

Diagnostic criteria
    Morning stiffness
    Involvement of three or more joints
    Involvement of hand joints
    Symmetric distribution
    Rheumatoid nodules
    Elevated levels of rheumatoid factor
    Radiographic findings

Extra-articular involvement
    Pulmonary
        Pleuritis
        Effusion
        Fibrosis
    Cardiac
        Effusion
        Aortic regurgitation
        Conduction abnormalities

Treatment
    DMARDs – alter the course of the disease
    NSAIDs – relieve pain and stiffness
    Corticosteroids – alter the inflammatory
        response

Many patients develop pericarditis and/or pericardial effusion, which may progress to cardiac tamponade. Valvular abnormalities develop secondary to rheumatoid nodules. Rheumatoid nodules may be present in the conduction system of the heart resulting in dysrhythmias and various degrees of conduction blockade.

Pulmonary

The most common pulmonary symptom is pleuritis or pleural effusion. Rheumatoid nodules can be seen on pleural biopsy. Interstitial pneumonitis can be present and can ultimately progress to pulmonary fibrosis. Small airway disease and emphysema can also occur in the rheumatoid patient. Many DMARDs, including methotrexate, gold, and cyclophosphamide, can cause interstitial lung disease.

Renal

Renal problems are rare in RA patients and are usually related to treatment with NSAIDs or DMARDs. Amyloidosis may occur secondary to long-standing inflammation.

Hematologic

Normochromic, normocytic anemia of chronic disease is usually present. Patients may also have B_{12} and folic acid deficiency.

Other systems

Vasculitis and cutaneous and ocular manifestations may also be present. Peripheral neuropathy may be significant due to local compression from synovial inflammation.

3. How is the rheumatoid arthritis patient evaluated for anesthesia?

A thorough history and physical examination should be conducted with particular attention to the above systems. These patients commonly have concomitant illnesses such as hypertension, coronary artery disease, and chronic obstructive pulmonary disease.

A thorough airway examination is necessary in the RA patient, including evaluation of Mallampati classification, thyromental distance, mouth opening, and neck movement. Since these patients may be limited in activity a focused cardiac examination may reveal limited information, but should be done nonetheless. Auscultation of the chest should be performed to assess for murmurs, rubs, or gallops. An electrocardiogram should be done to assess any conduction delays. A history of shortness of breath may warrant an echocardiogram and/or stress test and possibly a complete cardiology evaluation. Chest pain may be related to coronary artery disease or pleuritis.

Auscultation of the lungs should be performed looking for any areas of decreased breath sounds. A chest radiograph will show the presence of pulmonary fibrosis or emphysema. Pulmonary function tests, while an excellent indicator of the progression of rheumatoid obstructive and restrictive pulmonary disease, are useful preoperatively only in the severely affected patient.

Hematocrit should be performed to assess the degree of anemia. Basic electrolytes including sodium, potassium, BUN, and creatinine will reveal the extent of renal dysfunction. A history of medication use is of course necessary. Many drugs used to treat RA have side-effects that need to be considered; for example, DMARDs cause myelosuppression. The patient taking steroids may need perioperative stress doses.

Though commonly neglected by the anesthesiologist, it is necessary to ask the patient how comfortable he or she will be in the lateral decubitus position, which is used for total hip arthroplasty. The RA patient may suffer from stiffness not allowing maximum flexibility as required by the surgeon. One must ask the patient whether the upper and lower extremities and back need to be padded to provide for comfort. During a regional anesthetic, the awake patient can help in the positioning. However, during a general anesthetic the anesthesiologist will need to ensure that the patient is appropriately positioned.

4. Discuss the options for induction of anesthesia in a primary hip arthroplasty.

General anesthesia or neuraxial anesthesia can be performed for total hip arthroplasty. Neuraxial anesthesia includes spinal, epidural, or combined spinal/epidural anesthesia. When deciding on an anesthetic technique, the advantages and disadvantages need to be considered for each patient.

For general anesthesia, some of the advantages include a secured airway, excellent muscle relaxation, and the ability to extend the anesthetic for as long as the surgery takes. Disadvantages include a high incidence of postoperative nausea and vomiting, hemodynamic changes, and poor postoperative pain control. The advantages of neuraxial anesthesia include good postoperative pain control, decreased incidence of deep vein thrombosis, less nausea and vomiting, and decreased blood loss. Disadvantages include hemodynamic changes, possibility of postdural puncture headache, and possible airway management difficulty if excessive sedation is used or if there is a need to convert to general anesthesia in the middle of the procedure.

When planning any general anesthetic, options for securing the airway must be carefully considered. If there is no history of cervical arthritis, routine endotracheal intubation may be performed. However, it may be prudent to use a depolarizing muscle relaxant because of the possibility of an unrecognized difficult intubation secondary to cricoarytenoid arthritis. If there is a history of cervical arthritis, endotracheal intubation with in-line cervical stabilization may be warranted. Fiberoptic intubation, either with the patient awake or after induction of anesthesia, may be the wisest option in selected patients. As in all potential difficult airway situations, it is imperative that the anesthesiologist be prepared with alternative methods of securing the airway should the initial plan fail.

Neuraxial anesthesia can also be performed safely but there are several considerations that need to be addressed:

- *Duration of block:* Spinal anesthesia, though quick and easy to perform, has a finite duration of action determined by the local anesthetic used. Since there is no indwelling catheter, the duration of the block cannot be extended once the effects begin to wear off. An epidural in this setting has the advantage of the ability to prolong the effect of the block by the presence of a catheter that enables subsequent dosing. Though a combined spinal/epidural anesthetic is commonly used, it has the disadvantage that the epidural catheter's efficacy will not be tested until the spinal anesthetic has begun to wear off during the procedure. If the catheter is not functioning, the anesthesiologist will be faced with a patient in the lateral decubitus position requiring conversion to a general anesthetic. In the patient with a difficult airway, it is probably prudent to perform an epidural (without a spinal) from the onset to ensure its efficacy. This is not completely fail-safe because despite initial success, epidurals occasionally become non-functional.
- *Patient comfort:* The lateral decubitus position is uncomfortable for most patients and it is usually necessary to provide sedation. As the procedure progresses, patients tend to become restless despite sedation and it may be necessary to increase the sedation to the point where airway obstruction may occur.
- *Thromboembolism prophylaxis:* The placement of neuraxial anesthesia and removal of an epidural catheter needs to be coordinated with the surgeon's plan for thromboembolism prophylaxis (see below).
- *Length of procedure:* Many anesthesiologists will have their own threshold for deciding whether to do general versus neuraxial anesthesia. A reasonable plan would be to do general anesthesia if the procedure is expected to last for more than 3–4 hours. This commonly occurs for revision hip arthroplasties as opposed to primary hip replacements. The length of the procedure will also depend on the surgeon.

5. Several hours into the case the surgeon complains that he is operating on a moving target. How would you manage this situation?

This situation presents a unique challenge for the anesthesiologist. It is important to assess the patient for all causes of agitation. The presence of hypoxia, hypercarbia, myocardial ischemia, hypotension, and hypertension must be assessed first and treated accordingly. Methylmethacrylate cement toxicity should be considered in this setting as well, since it can cause any of the above findings. Only after the above differential is ruled out should dissipation of the spinal block be considered.

If inadequate anesthesia is the cause of the agitation, one must first determine the remaining operative time so that an appropriate action can be taken. If the surgeon is already closing, administration of midazolam, fentanyl, propofol and/or ketamine while assuring a patent airway may be all that is needed. If there is still a significant amount of operative time left, then conversion to a general anesthetic may be necessary and the airway should be secured. Ideally, this can be done without disrupting the surgery. It would be advisable to call for help at this time. A reasonable option at this time would be the placement of a laryngeal mask airway (LMA). In most cases, the LMA can be placed safely even in the lateral decubitus position. The LMA will allow for the use of volatile agents and opioids.

If an LMA is deemed not safe, such as in the morbidly obese patient, an endotracheal intubation will be necessary. Since the patient is in the left lateral decubitus position, it will be necessary to position the operating room table so that the patient is somewhat supine. This is accomplished by turning the bed laterally in the direction opposite to that in which the patient is facing. For example, if the patient is in the right lateral decubitus position, the table should be moved toward the left. Although this position is not ideal, it can result in the patient as close to the supine position as possible without disrupting the surgical field. If this maneuver does not provide reasonable intubating conditions, then the surgery should be stopped and the patient positioned supine for intubation. Although a hip infection can be devastating, airway management should always take precedence. Another possible approach to securing the airway would be to perform a fiberoptic intubation in the lateral decubitus position.

6. Discuss the causes and management of fat embolus syndrome.

Microscopic fat emboli are very common in patients who sustain long bone fractures or who undergo total joint replacement. Less commonly fat embolus syndrome (FES) may present. It should be suspected during total joint replacement surgery if the patient develops hypoxia or agitation. FES is present in 0.1% of patients having a total hip arthroplasty and 7% of patients having a total knee arthroplasty. It may also occur during liposuction, osteomyelitis, sickle cell anemia, and burns.

The diagnostic criteria for FES were described by Gurd (Table 54.1). In order to make the diagnosis, the patient must have one major and four minor criteria.

Management of Agitation

Differential diagnosis
  Hypoxia
  Hypercarbia
  Hypotension
  Hypertension
  Methylmethacrylate cement toxicity
  Inadequate anesthesia

Securing the airway
  LMA
  Endotracheal intubation
    Turn operating room table laterally
    Turn patient supine
    Fiberoptic intubation

There are two theories to describe the development of FES. One theory postulates a mechanical phenomenon. Fat cells released into the venous circulation secondary to long bone trauma are transported to the pulmonary circulation where they act as microemboli. The second theory postulates a biochemical phenomenon. Free fatty acids released during trauma may directly cause pulmonary damage and adult respiratory distress syndrome. In addition, the release of stress catecholamines during trauma results in further free fatty acid release.

There is no definitive treatment for FES. Many drugs, such as heparin, albumin, and hypertonic glucose, have been used without success. Steroids may be beneficial in certain high-risk patients. Currently, supportive measures

---

TABLE 54.1	Criteria for fat embolus syndrome (FES)

Major
Petechiae—axillary/subconjunctival
Hypoxemia
Central nervous system depression
Pulmonary edema
Minor
Fever
Tachycardia
Jaundice
Fat globules in urine or sputum
Retinal fat emboli
Decreased hematocrit/platelets
Increased erythrocyte sedimentation rate

to maintain hemodynamic stability and optimal oxygenation and ventilation are the only options available. FES usually resolves in 3–5 days.

7. Discuss thromboembolism prophylaxis and the placement of neuraxial anesthesia.

It is common practice for orthopedists to anticoagulate patients after total joint surgery to prevent thromboembolic events. This is accomplished with a multitude of medications such as unfractionated heparin, low-molecular-weight heparin (LMWH), warfarin, and newer agents such as thrombin inhibitors and fondaparinux. All these medications can place the patient at risk for epidural hematoma if a neuraxial anesthetic is performed.

The American Society of Regional Anesthesia (ASRA) published guidelines in 2002 regarding neuraxial anesthesia in the anticoagulated patient. Patients who receive subcutaneous heparin can safely receive neuraxial anesthesia, although it is probably better to delay heparin administration until after the block is performed. In addition, if the patient has received subcutaneous heparin for 4 or more days, a platelet count should be done prior to performing a neuraxial anesthetic and before catheter removal.

Patients on LMWH should not have neuraxial anesthesia performed until 12 hours after the last dose. For those who receive twice-daily dosing, LMWH should not be administered until 24 hours after surgery. Epidural

---

Thromboembolism Prophylaxis and Neuraxial Anesthesia

Subcutaneous heparin
  Safe to perform neuraxial anesthesia
  Preferable to delay administration until after
    the block is performed
  If on treatment for >4 days, obtain platelet
    count before block is performed

LMWH
  Perform neuraxial anesthesia 12 hours after last
    dose
  Once-daily dosing
    Catheter can remain postoperatively
    Start LMWH 6–8 hours postoperatively
  Twice-daily dosing
    Catheter should be removed postoperatively
    Start LMWH 24 hours postoperatively
  Catheter removal
    12 hours after last dose of LMWH
    Subsequent dose >2 hours after removal

---

catheters should not remain in these patients and LMWH should not be administered until 2 hours after catheter removal. Those who receive single daily dosing can have a catheter safely maintained, and the first dose should begin 6–8 hours postoperatively. Catheters should not be removed until 12 hours after the last LMWH dose and the subsequent dose should not be given until 2 hours after catheter removal.

Those patients who will be initiating warfarin therapy more than 24 hours prior to surgery should have their International Normalized Ratio (INR) assessed. There are no guidelines given by the ASRA for an actual INR ratio below which neuraxial anesthesia can be safely performed, but 1.4 is a commonly agreed upon number. Those patients on chronic warfarin therapy should stop this medication 4–5 days prior to the procedure.

The ASRA guidelines comment that chronic NSAID use is not known to increase the incidence of epidural hematoma after neuraxial anesthesia.

There are no guidelines for the newer anticoagulating agents, such as thrombin inhibitors and fondaparinux, as these have not been time-tested yet. The ASRA recommends that the use of neuraxial anesthesia in this setting should be done only in the course of clinical trials.

8. Discuss the options for postoperative pain control after total hip arthroplasty. Discuss the use of a lumbar plexus block.

Patient-controlled analgesia with morphine sulfate or fentanyl is always a good option in the patient who received general anesthesia. For those who are to receive a spinal anesthetic, the addition of long-acting morphine can provide up to 24 hours of pain relief. This requires appropriate monitoring for delayed respiratory depression. An epidural catheter allows for excellent pain relief with an infusion of an opioid either with or without local anesthetic. The latter should be discontinued prior to the initiation of physical therapy.

Lumbar plexus blocks may be performed to provide postoperative comfort. The lower portion of the lumbar plexus consists of the femoral, obturator, and lateral cutaneous femoral nerves. The lateral cutaneous femoral nerve provides sensation to the area of the skin incision.

The lumbar plexus block is performed prior to the initiation of anesthesia with the patient in the lateral decubitus position, in a fetal posture, and with the side to be blocked facing upward. A 10 cm insulated needle attached to a nerve stimulator is inserted approximately 4 cm lateral to the spinous process of L_4 until movement of the quadriceps muscle is elicited. Injection of local anesthetic should only be done when the quadriceps muscle still responds between 0.5 and 1.0 milliamps. Response above a current of 1.0 milliamp may indicate needle placement too far from the plexus and below 0.5 milliamp may represent epidural or intrathecal placement. A test dose of local anesthetic is administered to assess for those possibilities. Either a long-acting local anesthetic, such as ropivacaine with epinephrine, can be injected through the needle or a catheter can be inserted for long-term use.

SUGGESTED READINGS

Bernstein RL, Rosenberg, AD: Manual of Orthopedic Anesthesia and Related Pain Syndromes, Churchill Livingstone, New York, 1993

Brown DL: Regional Anesthesia and Analgesia, WB Saunders, Philadelphia, 1996

Consensus Conference of the American Society of Regional Anesthesia and Pain Medicine: Regional Anesthesia in the Anticoagulated Patient – Defining the Risks. Chicago, Illinois, April 25–28, 2002

O'Dell JR: Therapeutic strategies for rheumatoid arthritis. N Engl J Med 350:25, 2004

Stoelting RK, Dierdorf SF: Skin and musculoskeletal diseases. pp. 528–532. In Stoelting RK, Dierdorf SF (eds): Anesthesia and Co-existing Disease, 4th edition. Churchill Livingstone, New York, 2002

Williams EA, Fye KH: Rheumatoid arthritis: targeted interventions can minimize joint destruction. Postgrad Med 114:5, 2003

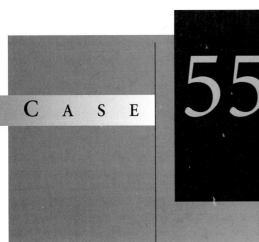

LOCAL ANESTHETICS

Isabelle deLeon, MD

Allan P. Reed, MD

A 35-year-old woman presents for bunionectomy. She is in good general health and has never received general anesthesia. Her dentist told her that she had an allergy to Novocain, and her surgeon told her that he always performs this operation under ankle block.

QUESTIONS

1. Describe the chemistry of local anesthetics.
2. Describe the mechanism of action of local anesthetics.
3. What factors affect the potency, onset, and duration of action of local anesthetics?
4. Discuss the sequence of clinical anesthesia following neural blockade.
5. What are the clinical differences between the ester and amide local anesthetics?
6. Describe the pharmacokinetics of local anesthetics.
7. How do factors such as dosage of local anesthetic, addition of vasoconstrictors, carbonation and pH adjustment, mixtures of local anesthetics, and pregnancy influence local anesthetic blockade?
8. Which local anesthetics are appropriate for the various regional anesthetic procedures?
9. Describe the toxic effects of local anesthetics.
10. How is systemic local anesthetic toxicity treated?

11. Is it prudent to use regional anesthesia in a patient who reports a Novocain allergy?
12. What is the treatment for local anesthetic allergic reactions?

1. Describe the chemistry of local anesthetics.

Local anesthetics are drugs that produce transient sensory, motor, and autonomic nervous system blockade following regional anesthesia. Local anesthetics are weak bases that consist of a lipophilic group (usually a benzene ring) and a hydrophilic group (usually a tertiary amine) separated by a connecting hydrocarbon chain. Most local anesthetics have an ester or an amide bond that links the hydrocarbon chain to the lipophilic group. The nature of this bond is the basis for classifying them as ester or amide local anesthetics. Examples of the ester group are cocaine, procaine (Novocain), chloroprocaine (Nesacaine), benzocaine (Americaine), and tetracaine (Pontocaine). Lidocaine (Xylocaine), mepivacaine (Carbocaine), bupivacaine (Marcaine, Sensorcaine), etidocaine (Duranest), prilocaine (Citanest), and ropivacaine (Naropin) are examples of the amide local anesthetics. Mepivacaine, bupivacaine, and ropivacaine have an asymmetric carbon atom resulting in levoisomers and dextroisomers. Commercial preparations of mepivacaine and bupivacaine consist of racemic mixtures, whereas the recently developed ropivacaine and levo-bupivacaine consist of the pure levoisomers.

Local anesthetics in aqueous solution exist in dynamic equilibrium between the nonionized lipid-soluble form and the ionized water-soluble form. The pH at which there are equal amounts of nonionized and ionized molecules is known as the pKa of that drug. Local anesthetics have pKa values somewhat above physiologic pH and, as a result, less than 50% of the drug will exist in the lipid-soluble nonionized form.

2. Describe the mechanism of action of local anesthetics.

Local anesthetics produce conduction blockade of neural impulses by impairing propagation of the action potential in axons. They interact directly with sodium (Na⁺) channels in nerve membranes and inhibit the passage of Na⁺. This does not alter the resting transmembrane potential or threshold potential, but it slows the rate of depolarization such that the threshold potential is not reached and an action potential is not propagated. However, the exact mechanism of how these drugs inhibit Na⁺ ion influx is still unknown.

Local anesthetic bases are marketed most often as water-soluble hydrochloride salts because they are otherwise poorly soluble in water. The pKa of the drug and the tissue pH determine the amount of drug that exists in solution as free base (lipid-soluble) or as positively charged cation (water-soluble) when injected into tissues. The free base form penetrates across the neural sheath and nerve membrane to reach the nerve axon, where the positively charged cation acts on the Na⁺ channel.

During onset and recovery from local-anesthetic-induced conduction blockade, some nerve fibers exist in a partially blocked state. Impulse transmission through these fibers is inhibited by repetitive stimulation, which fosters further local anesthetic binding to Na⁺ channels. This is known as use-dependent binding to Na⁺ channels. The clinically observed rates of onset and recovery from conduction blockade are primarily dependent on slow diffusion of local anesthetic molecules into and out of the nerve.

3. What factors affect the potency, onset, and duration of action of local anesthetics?

Anesthetic potency correlates with lipid solubility as lipophilic local anesthetics more easily cross nerve membranes. In general, lengthening the connecting hydrocarbon chain or increasing the number of carbon atoms on the tertiary amine or aromatic ring often results in a more potent drug. For example, adding a halide to the aromatic ring (2-chloroprocaine vs. procaine), an ester linkage (tetracaine vs. lidocaine), and large alkyl groups on the tertiary amine (tetracaine vs. procaine) increases potency.

Onset of action of local anesthetics depends primarily on the pKa of the drug. Drugs with a lower pKa or pKa closer to physiologic pH will have a higher concentration of the nonionized, lipophilic form which easily diffuses across nerve membranes and thus have a faster onset. Likewise, the addition of a small amount of sodium bicarbonate to the local anesthetic solution may speed onset and improve quality of blockade by increasing the amount of the nonionized form of the drug. However, lower tissue pH, as seen in infected tissue, results in delayed onset of action because of a decreased proportion of the nonionized form.

Duration of action is associated with plasma α_1-acid lipoprotein binding. A high degree of this protein binding results in prolonged duration of effect. Bupivacaine, etidocaine, and prilocaine are more highly protein-bound than most other agents and thus have a longer duration of action. The addition of vasoconstrictors, such as epinephrine, also prolongs duration of action by decreasing local blood flow and consequently decreasing drug absorption. This enhances neuronal uptake leading to a greater degree and duration of blockade.

4. Discuss the sequence of clinical anesthesia following neural blockade.

Nerve fibers are classified according to their fiber diameter, whether they are myelinated or unmyelinated, and their function. Generally, the small-diameter fibers are more easily blocked than large-diameter fibers. However, larger myelinated fibers are more readily blocked than the

Classification of Local Anesthetics

Esters:	Amides:
Cocaine	Lidocaine
Procaine	Mepivacaine
Chloroprocaine	Bupivacaine
Benzocaine	Levobupivacaine
Tetracaine	Etidocaine
	Prilocaine
	Ropivacaine

Correlation Characteristics of Local Anesthetics

Potency:	lipid solubility
Onset of action:	pKa
Duration of action:	degree of protein binding
	addition of vasoconstrictor

smaller unmyelinated fibers. Preganglionic B fibers are more readily blocked than any fiber, even though their fibers are larger than the smallest type C, presumably because of the presence of myelin. Thus, sympathetic blockade with peripheral vasodilation and skin temperature elevation occurs first following neural blockade. This is sequentially followed by loss of pain and temperature sensation, loss of proprioception, loss of touch and pressure sensation, and finally motor paralysis (largest myelinated A-α fibers).

5. What are the clinical differences between the ester and amide local anesthetics?

The important differences between ester and amide local anesthetics relate to the mechanisms by which they are metabolized and their potential to produce allergic reactions.

Ester local anesthetics undergo rapid hydrolysis by plasma pseudocholinesterases and to a lesser extent in the liver with resulting pharmacologically inactive metabolites. However, para-aminobenzoic acid is one of the metabolites that has been associated with allergic reactions in a small percentage of patients. Cerebrospinal fluid lacks the pseudocholinesterase enzyme, so ester local anesthetics administered intrathecally will persist until they have been absorbed by the bloodstream. Patients with atypical plasma pseudocholinesterase are at increased risk for toxic side-effects because of impaired metabolism. Plasma pseudocholinesterase activity may also be decreased in patients with liver disease or those taking certain chemotherapeutic drugs. Cocaine is the only ester local anesthetic not metabolized in the plasma; rather it undergoes significant liver metabolism.

Amide local anesthetics undergo enzymatic degradation in the liver, which in general is much slower than ester hydrolysis. Patients with decreased liver function (e.g., liver cirrhosis) or decreased liver blood flow (e.g., congestive heart failure) are predisposed to systemic toxicity from impaired metabolism. The amide local anesthetics are not metabolized to para-aminobenzoic acid, and allergic reactions are extremely rare. However, solutions of these drugs may contain preservatives (paraben family, whose structure is similar to para-aminobenzoic acid) or additives (sodium bisulfite) that are the frequent culprits of adverse reactions.

6. Describe the pharmacokinetics of local anesthetics.

The blood concentration of local anesthetics is determined by the following: the amount injected, the rate of absorption from the site of injection, the rate of tissue distribution, and the rate of biotransformation and excretion of the drug. Local absorption is a function of the site selected, dose injected, and blood flowing through the area. Of all the traditional locations, absorption of local anesthetics is most rapid following application to airway epithelium (especially alveoli). Other types of blockade have been assessed with regard to associated blood levels of local anesthetic. In decreasing order of associated local anesthetic blood concentrations, they are intrapleural, intercostal, lumbar epidural, brachial plexus, and subcutaneous. Consequently, local anesthetic administered into the airway is more likely to result in dangerously high blood levels than the same dose injected subcutaneously. Absorption is, also, dependent on perfusion of the injection site. As blood flow past the area is diminished, absorption of local anesthetic is decreased. For this reason, vasoconstrictors are often added to local anesthetic solutions. Epinephrine, 5 μg/ml (1:200,000), is frequently mixed with lidocaine or mepivacaine regardless of the site of injection. Although epinephrine will reduce absorption of bupivacaine and etidocaine during major nerve blocks, it does not significantly alter plasma concentrations following lumbar epidural blockade.

Absorbed local anesthetics are distributed first to highly perfused tissues, such as lung, brain, and heart. This is the α-elimination phase. A short α-elimination phase indicates rapid distribution from blood to tissues. Residual local anesthetics in plasma are next distributed to poorly perfused areas (β-elimination phase) as well as being metabolized and excreted (γ-elimination phase).

Ester local anesthetics are hydrolyzed by plasma pseudocholinesterases. Qualitative or quantitative pseudocholinesterase deficiencies may impair ester local anesthetic metabolism. Para-aminobenzoic acid is an important ester degradation product because it is a highly allergenic molecule. Amides are metabolized in the liver to a variety of by-products. Sources of impaired hepatic function such as extremes of age, congestive heart failure, and hepatitis will decrease amide biotransformation.

7. How do factors such as dosage of local anesthetic, addition of vasoconstrictors, carbonation and pH adjustment, mixtures of local anesthetics, and pregnancy influence local anesthetic blockade?

Dose of Local Anesthetics   As the dosage of local anesthetics is increased, by administration of either a larger volume or a more concentrated solution, the probability and duration of satisfactory anesthesia increases and the time to onset of blockade is shortened.

Addition of Vasoconstrictors   Epinephrine, norepinephrine, and phenylephrine are the vasoconstrictors frequently added to local anesthetic solutions. Of these, epinephrine is the most frequently used. Vasoconstrictors decrease local blood flow and thereby impair uptake of the drug, which allows more molecules to remain at the nerve to act on it. In this way, the degree and duration of blockade are enhanced. Lidocaine with 1:200,000 epinephrine is optimal for epidural and intercostal blockade. Although epinephrine extends the duration of action of local anesthetics when employed for peripheral nerve blocks and infiltration anesthesia, it does not significantly prolong the duration of epidural anesthesia produced by bupivacaine or etidocaine. The high lipid solubility of bupivacaine and etidocaine allow for storage by, and extended release of drug from, adipose tissue, thereby prolonging the block beyond the influence of the vasoconstrictor mechanism.

Carbonation and pH Adjustment   Sodium bicarbonate may be added to local anesthetic solutions in an attempt to decrease the onset time. Alkalinizing an anesthetic solution increases the amount of drug in the free base form, which increases diffusion of the drug through nerve sheaths and membranes. The latency of both lidocaine and bupivacaine can be decreased in this way. This method has proven to be successful in the epidural space, but has met with varying results when applied to brachial plexus blockade.

Local Anesthetic Mixtures   The use of mixtures of local anesthetic solutions for regional anesthesia has become popular in recent years, especially for ambulatory procedures. Mixtures of local anesthetic solutions such as chloroprocaine and bupivacaine offer theoretical clinical advantages, owing to the rapid onset and low systemic toxicity of chloroprocaine and the long latency of action of bupivacaine. Anesthesiologists should be aware, however, that there are no existing data that show that local anesthetic toxicities are independent of each other. Mixtures of local anesthetics should be considered to have roughly additive toxic effects.

Pregnancy   The spread of epidural and spinal anesthesia has been reported to be greater in pregnant women than nonpregnant women. This was originally attributed to mechanical factors, such as engorged epidural veins. A study by Moller et al. (1992) has demonstrated a more rapid onset of action and an increased sensitivity to local anesthetics during pregnancy. Such studies suggest that hormonal changes may result in increased sensitivity of nerve to local anesthetics. Thus the dosage of local anesthetics should be reduced in patients in all stages of pregnancy.

8. Which local anesthetics are appropriate for the various regional anesthetic procedures?

Regional anesthesia may be divided into infiltration, intravenous regional, peripheral nerve blocks, central neural blocks, and topical. Widely utilized by plastic surgeons, tumescent anesthesia is another form of local anesthetic injection.

Infiltration Anesthesia   Any local anesthetic may be utilized for infiltration anesthesia. The choice of drug depends primarily on the desired duration of action, as the onset of action for most of the local anesthetics is almost immediate following injection. The addition of vasoconstrictors, such as epinephrine, markedly prolongs the effect of the drug, especially with lidocaine.

Intravenous Regional Anesthesia   The Bier block involves intravenous injection of a large volume of local anesthetic solution into a tourniquet-occluded limb. This technique can be used for a variety of short surgical procedures, primarily involving the hand and forearm. It has also been used for foot procedures with a calf tourniquet. All the common local anesthetic agents have been used for intravenous regional anesthesia. However, lidocaine 0.5%, preservative free and without epinephrine, and prilocaine are the drugs most frequently used. Chloroprocaine is no longer used because of its association with thrombophlebitis. Bupivacaine is also not being utilized because of its cardiac toxicity profile. However, ropivacaine has been safely used for this technique.

Peripheral Nerve Blocks   These blocks, whether involving blocking a single nerve entity (e.g., ulnar or radial nerve) or blocking two or more distinct nerves or a nerve plexus (e.g., brachial plexus), are used for anesthesia, postoperative analgesia, and diagnosis and treatment of chronic pain syndromes. Most local anesthetics can be used for peripheral nerve blocks. The choice of drug to be utilized depends primarily on the desired duration of anesthesia, as the onset of block is rapid with most of the drugs. Lower concentrations of local anesthetics (e.g., lidocaine 1% or bupivacaine 0.25–0.5%) are commonly used because of concerns regarding local and systemic toxicity, since large volumes of anesthetic solutions are often required to achieve adequate anesthesia. The addition of a vasoconstrictor to most local anesthetic solutions prolongs their duration of action. However, it has not been shown to predictably prolong the duration of action produced by bupivacaine or ropivacaine.

Central Neural Blockade (Spinal or Epidural Anesthesia)
Local anesthetic is injected into the subarachnoid space for spinal anesthesia and into the epidural space for epidural anesthesia.

Spinal Anesthesia: Drugs commonly used for spinal anesthesia include tetracaine, bupivacaine, ropivacaine, lidocaine, and procaine.

■ The *baricity* of the local anesthetic plays an integral part in choosing the drug appropriate for spinal anesthesia. Local anesthetics are characterized as hyperbaric, hypobaric, or isobaric compared with cerebrospinal fluid. Hyperbaric solutions such as tetracaine 0.5% (obtained by mixing equal volumes of 1% tetracaine and 10% glucose), lidocaine 5%, and bupivacaine 0.75% (both commercially premixed with glucose) settle to the most dependent aspect of the subarachnoid space, which is dependent on the patient's position from the time of and immediately after spinal anesthesia placement. The solution gravitates to the thoracic kyphosis in supine patients, providing adequate spinal anesthetic levels for intra-abdominal surgery. However, in the sitting position, hyperbaric solutions provide "saddle block" anesthesia or low sensory levels, appropriate for vaginal or anorectal surgeries. Hypobaric solutions, on the other hand, will tend to move away from the dependent area. Tetracaine is the most commonly used agent for the hypobaric technique and is obtained by mixing it with sterile water. Patients undergoing anorectal surgery, such as hemorrhoidectomy, may be positioned in the jackknife position during spinal anesthesia placement. The injected anesthetic solution will float to the non-dependent area, in this case, the sacral area, resulting in the blockade of the sacral dermatomes. Isobaric solutions will stay at about the same level where they are injected, irrespective of the patient's position. They are produced by mixing the local anesthetic with cerebrospinal fluid or are commonly formulated with sodium chloride. Tetracaine, bupivacaine, ropivacaine, and lidocaine are commonly used as isobaric local anesthetics.

- The *desired duration* of spinal anesthesia is another determinant factor in choosing which local anesthetic is appropriate. Local anesthetics differ in their length of action. Tetracaine, bupivacaine, and ropivacaine provide a long duration of spinal anesthesia, whereas lidocaine and procaine provide a short duration. However, onset of action is more rapid with lidocaine relative to the other agents.

Epidural Anesthesia: The choice of drug for epidural anesthesia depends on the *desired onset and duration of blockade, degree of sensory or motor blockade, and postoperative analgesia requirements.* Chloroprocaine is characterized as a rapid-onset and short-acting agent providing up to 90 minutes of surgical anesthesia, and is suitable for outpatient surgical procedures. Lidocaine and mepivacaine are considered to have an intermediate onset of action and duration. However, mepivacaine lasts from 15 to 30 minutes longer than lidocaine at equivalent dosages. Lidocaine provides surgical anesthesia that lasts from 60 to 100 minutes. The addition of epinephrine to any of these three agents significantly prolongs the duration of blockade. Bupivacaine is the most widely used long-acting anesthetic (with slow onset of action) for epidural anesthesia, providing between 120 and 240 minutes of epidural anesthesia. The addition of epinephrine, however, does not reliably prolong its duration of action. Ropivacaine is another long-acting anesthetic being used for epidural anesthesia. Its duration of action and intensity of motor block are slightly less than those of bupivacaine. However, it does have a more favorable cardiac toxicity profile than bupivacaine.

Topical Anesthesia Anesthesia of the mucous membranes of the nose, oral cavity, tracheobronchial tree, esophagus, or genitourinary tract can be achieved by topical placement of local anesthetic on these areas. Lidocaine, either applied topically or nebulized, is commonly used to provide topical anesthesia to the upper or lower respiratory tract prior to fiberoptic tracheal intubation. Tetracaine is also an effective topical anesthetic used during bronchoscopy. Clinicians must be aware, however, that both drugs undergo significant systemic absorption after topical placement on the tracheobronchial mucosa.

Tumescent Anesthesia This method is commonly employed by plastic surgeons during liposuction procedures and involves subcutaneous injection of large volumes of dilute local anesthetic in combination with epinephrine and other agents. The most commonly used drug, lidocaine, with total doses ranging from 35 to 55 mg/kg, has been reported to produce a safe plasma concentration.

9. Describe the toxic effects of local anesthetics.

Systemic toxicity of local anesthetics is the result of the effect of excess plasma concentrations of these drugs on the central nervous system and cardiovascular system. Most often, excess plasma concentration of local anesthetic solution is due to accidental intravascular injection. Less frequently, it may result from absorption of local anesthetic solution from tissue injection sites. As blood levels increase, the central nervous system is affected first. Central nervous system manifestations of local anesthetic toxicity are both excitatory and inhibitory in nature. Increasing concentrations of local anesthetics in the blood initially depress inhibitory neurons in the cerebral cortex allowing facilitatory neurons to discharge without the normal negative input. Consequently, excitatory pathways function in an unopposed manner, leading to signs and symptoms of central nervous system excitation (Table 55.1). Further increases in local anesthetic blood levels depress excitatory neuronal activity, producing signs and symptoms of central nervous system depression.

Acid–base status may also affect seizure threshold. Respiratory acidosis tends to decrease the local anesthetic blood concentration required to produce seizures. Elevated arterial carbon dioxide tension ($PaCO_2$) levels will increase cerebral blood flow, thereby delivering additional local anesthetic to neurons. Diffusion of carbon dioxide into neurons predisposes patients to intracellular acidosis and cationic trapping. Positively charged forms of the local anesthetic tend to concentrate within the neuron, thereby exerting a greater effect than would otherwise have been expected at a particular blood concentration.

The cardiovascular system is not as vulnerable to local anesthetic toxicity as the central nervous system. Local anesthetics act directly on the heart by blocking cardiac Na^+ channels, to produce both electrophysiologic and

TABLE 55.1	Clinical Manifestations and Management of Local Anesthetic Systemic Toxicity

System	Signs and Symptoms	Treatment
Central nervous system		
Excitatory phase		
Cerebral cortex	Circumoral tingling Tinnitus Metallic taste Olfactory stimulation Disorientation Excitement	Augmented FiO_2 Benzodiazepine and barbiturate optional
	Muscle twitching, shivering, tremors Generalized tonic-clonic seizures	Diazepam 0.1–0.3 mg/kg IV or Barbiturate 2 mg/kg IV
Medulla	Tachycardia Hypertension Tachypnea Other respiratory rhythm alterations	As above
	Nausea and vomiting	Suction, intubation, bronchoscopy as required
Depressive phase		
Cerebral cortex	Drowsiness Light-headedness Slurring of speech Slowing of mentation Loss of consciousness	As above
Medulla	Bradypnea Apnea	Positive-pressure ventilation
	Bradycardia Hypotension Cardiac arrest	Atropine, epinephrine IV fluids, phenylephrine, dopamine Cardiopulmonary resuscitation
Cardiovascular system		
Excitatory phase	Supraventricular tachycardia ?CNS stimulation?	Specific therapy
	Ventricular fibrillation, especially with bupivacaine	Epinephrine
Depressive phase	Bradycardia Sinus arrest Hypotension	Atropine, epinephrine Epinephrine IV fluids, phenylephrine, dopamine

mechanical effects. They decrease the rate of depolarization in Purkinje fibers and ventricular muscle. Consequently, heart rate decreases as automaticity and conduction slow, manifesting on the electrocardiogram as P-R interval prolongation and QRS complex widening. Profound hypotension from arteriolar vascular smooth muscle relaxation and direct myocardial depression can occur. Ventricular dysrhythmias, including ventricular fibrillation, may also manifest. Local anesthetics differ in their ability to produce cardiac toxicity. The most potent local anesthetics, bupivacaine, etidocaine, and tetracaine, affect rhythm and contractility at lower

blood concentrations than less potent agents. Bupivacaine has a greater tendency to produce cardiac toxicity (selective cardiac toxicity) compared with other agents because of the slow dissociation of highly lipid-soluble bupivacaine from cardiac Na^+ channels. This results in an exaggerated and persistent depressant effect of bupivacaine on cardiac function. The dextroisomer of bupivacaine is believed to be responsible for the anesthetic's systemic toxic effects. Thus, ropivacaine and levobupivacaine, both pure levoisomers, are less cardiotoxic than bupivacaine. Bupivacaine seems to be more cardiotoxic in pregnant patients. Resuscitation from bupivacaine-induced cardiac arrest requires massive doses of epinephrine and atropine.

Direct effects of local anesthetics on the peripheral vasculature are variable. Central nervous system effects generally predominate over direct vasodilating or vasoconstricting influences.

Cocaine is unique among all local anesthetics because it impairs reuptake of norepinephrine. The norepinephrine that is not returned to storage granules produces vasoconstriction. Use of 10% cocaine has been associated with coronary artery constriction and dysrhythmias. Four percent cocaine functions well as a local vasoconstrictor without these side-effects.

Prilocaine and benzocaine have been reported to produce methemoglobinemia. Prilocaine at doses higher than 600 mg may result in the accumulation of ortho-toluidine and nitro-toluidine, both of which are capable of causing methemoglobin formation. Patients with methemoglobinemia may appear cyanotic and their blood may be chocolate-colored because of the impaired oxygen transport. Treatment of significant methemoglobinemia requires intravenous administration of methylene blue.

In addition to systemic toxicity, the use of local anesthetics for spinal and epidural anesthesia may result in transient radicular irritation or overt neurotoxicity as manifested by the cauda equina syndrome. Transient radicular irritation, the majority of cases occurring in the lumbar and sacral areas, produces moderate to severe pain in the lower back, buttocks, and posterior thighs that occurs within 24 hours after complete recovery from spinal anesthesia. Full neurologic recovery usually occurs within a week. Lidocaine, with concentrations ranging from 0.5% to 5%, seems to be associated with a higher incidence of transient radicular irritation compared with bupivacaine or tetracaine. Furthermore, the incidence seems to be increased when the lithotomy position is used during surgery. Though the etiology of the radicular irritation is still unknown, use of lidocaine doses greater than 80–100 mg for spinal anesthesia has been questioned.

Cauda equina syndrome has been reported following cases that are believed to have concentrated subarachnoid lidocaine and/or bupivacaine at the cauda equina. This syndrome was reported as a complication of continuous spinal anesthesia with lidocaine 5% and the usage of small microcatheters. Pooling of very high local anesthetic concentration on dependent nerves is thought to be contributory. For this reason, microcatheters were removed from the market. However, rare occurrences of this syndrome continue to be reported despite the absence of microcatheters. They may be due to the accidental subarachnoid injection of the intended epidural dose, repeat administration of local anesthetic after a failed spinal anesthetic, or the use of large doses of local anesthetic during continuous spinal anesthesia without the use of microcatheters. The syndrome presents with varying degrees of sensory anesthesia, bowel and bladder sphincter dysfunction, and paraplegia.

10. How is systemic local anesthetic toxicity treated?

The first step in the treatment of systemic local anesthetic toxicity is to stop the further administration of the offending agent into the central circulation. In the case of continuous intravenous infusion, for the treatment of premature ventricular contractions, cessation of administration of local anesthetic is simple to accomplish. Tourniquet leak or premature deflation of the tourniquet during intravenous regional anesthesia requires tourniquet adjustment to prevent further loss of local anesthetic into the circulation.

The initial manifestations of local anesthetic toxicity are those of central nervous excitation. As neurons discharge at rapid rates, they consume oxygen and glucose. Consequently, oxygen should be administered early (though supplemental oxygen should already have been supplied to the patient), because the triad of hypoxemia, acidosis, and hypercarbia develops rapidly, due to the previously described respiratory and cardiovascular impairments. When positive-pressure ventilation is initiated, hyperventilation is preferred to prevent and treat hypercarbia. Once consciousness is lost, the patient is at increased risk for aspiration pneumonitis, thus the airway should be protected with a cuffed endotracheal tube. Diazepam, 0.1–0.3 mg/kg intravenously, suppresses seizure activity with little or no adverse cardiovascular effect. Although rapid-acting barbiturates are also effective for seizure control, their use can be complicated by cardiovascular depression. Because local anesthetic toxicity is fraught with dysrhythmias, depressed contractility, and vasodilation, the addition of another source of cardiovascular depression, a barbiturate, is best avoided. Tonic-clonic seizure activity may prevent adequate ventilation with positive pressure and succinylcholine may need to be administered in order to facilitate oxygenation and ventilation. Although succinylcholine stops the major muscle manifestations of seizure activity, it does not treat the central nervous system source. Uncontrolled rapid neuronal discharge persists, with huge cerebral requirements for oxygen and glucose. During this period, oxygen delivery assumes an even greater importance than it normally does.

Cardiovascular toxicity manifests as hypotension, which is treated with intravenous fluids, the Trendelenburg position, and phenylephrine. Left ventricular dysfunction is managed with an inotropic agent such as dopamine or amrinone. Cardiac dysrhythmias may require large doses of epinephrine and atropine.

11. Is it prudent to use regional anesthesia in a patient who reports a Novocain allergy?

Details of the patient's previous reaction are critical to the decision process. Many patients reporting a Novocain allergy received local anesthesia for a dental procedure. The term Novocain is frequently used by laymen to refer to all local anesthetics. Novocain is the trade name for procaine, an ester-type local anesthetic. Most dentists today use lidocaine, mepivacaine, or bupivacaine, with or without epinephrine. Although true allergic reactions to local anesthetics are uncommon, when they occur, episodes are usually the result of exposure to the ester-type local anesthetics. These agents are metabolized to para-aminobenzoic acid, a known allergen. The agents most often used by dentists are amides. Allergic reactions are mediated by antibodies and/or complement activation and are characterized by urticaria, pruritus, angioneurotic edema, hypotension, and/or bronchospasm. Frequently, patients reporting adverse reactions from local anesthetics actually experienced the effects of high blood levels of local anesthetics or epinephrine rather than true allergic reactions. Elevated blood levels of local anesthetics often lead to circumoral numbness, dizziness, tinnitus, blurred vision, drowsiness, or frank seizures. Tachycardia, hypertension, and hypotension may also occur as side-effects. Differentiation between an allergic reaction and the recognized side-effects of high blood levels becomes critical. Allergy skin testing has met with inconsistent results and remains an unreliable technique. Cross allergenicity between ester and amide local anesthetics does not seem to exist.

Although amide local anesthetics rarely produce true allergic reactions, the preservative methylparaben may be detrimental in some patients. Methylparaben is an allergen similar to para-aminobenzoic acid and may also produce allergic reactions. Therefore, it is advisable to use preservative-free solutions whenever possible.

12. What is the treatment for local anesthetic allergic reactions?

Mast cell degranulation liberates histamine, leukotrienes, prostaglandins, platelet-activating factor, and kinins that produce adverse systemic effects. Table 55.2 summarizes the clinical manifestations of allergic reactions and notes specific therapy for potentially lethal reactions. Management of allergic reactions requires immediate identification of the offending agent and cessation of its administration. Cutaneous manifestations such as itching, burning, urticaria, or flushing can be treated with diphenhydramine, 0.5–1.0 mg/kg intravenously. Respiratory signs, including coughing and wheezing, are indications for supplemental oxygen and bronchodilators. The inhaled β-2-selective agents, such as albuterol, are the preferred bronchodilators. Severe cases may require epinephrine or isoproterenol. Laryngeal edema, pulmonary edema, and other signs of respiratory distress require endotracheal intubation and positive pressure ventilation. Mild hypotension is treated with intravenous fluids. Profound hypotension requires therapy with fluids and epinephrine. Epinephrine 0.5–1.0 mg is administered for cardiovascular collapse. Hydrocortisone or methylprednisolone helps prevent future reactions but probably does little for the acute situation. When endotracheal intubation is performed for airway edema, extubation should be preceded by a deflation test. To perform this test, deflate the endotracheal

TABLE 55.2	Clinical Manifestations and Treatment of Allergic Reactions	
System	**Manifestations**	**Treatment**
Cutaneous	Urticaria Flushing Facial edema	Diphenhydramine 0.5–1.0 mg/kg
Pulmonary	Coughing Wheezing	Oxygen Albuterol inhalation Epinephrine 2–4 µg/min Isoproterenol 0.5–1.0 µg/min
	Laryngeal edema Pulmonary edema Respiratory distress	Endotracheal intubation
Cardiac	Hypotension	Intravenous fluids Epinephrine 4–8 µg
	Tachycardia Dysrhythmias	Specific therapy
	Cardiac arrest	ACLS protocol

tube's cuff, administer positive-pressure ventilation, and listen for gas escaping between the tube and the airway. The absence of gas escaping from the outside the endotracheal tube suggests persistent airway edema.

SUGGESTED READINGS

Berde CB, Strichartz GR: Local anesthetics. pp. 491–517. In Miller RD (ed): Anesthesia, 5th edition. Churchill Livingstone, Philadelphia, 2000

Brown DL, Ransom DM, Hall JA, et al: Regional anesthesia and local anesthetic-induced systemic toxicity: Seizure frequency and accompanying cardiovascular changes. Anesth Analg 81:321–328, 1995

Bonica JJ, Buckley FP: Regional anesthesia with local anesthetics. pp. 1883–1966. In Bonica JJ (ed): The Management of Pain, 2nd edition. Lea & Febiger, Philadelphia, 1990

Butterworth JF, Strichartz GR: Molecular mechanisms of local anesthesia: A review. Anesthesiology 72:722–734, 1990

Cox CR, Faccenda KA, Gilhasly C, et al: Extradural S(–)-bupivacaine: comparison with racemic RS-bupivacaine. Br J Anaesth 80:289–293, 1998

Drasner K: Lidocaine spinal anesthesia: a vanishing therapeutic index? Anesthesiology 87:467–472, 1997

Freedman J, Li D, Drasner K, et al: Transient neurologic symptoms after spinal anesthesia. An epidemiologic study of 1863 patients. Anesthesiology 89:633–641, 1998

McClure JH: Ropivacaine. Br J Anaesth 76:300–307, 1996

Mitchell ME: Local anesthetic toxic effects in complications. pp. 249–253. In Atlee JL (ed) Anesthesia. WB Saunders, Philadelphia, 1999

Moller RA, Covino BG: Cardiac electrophysiologic properties of bupivacaine and lidocaine compared with those of ropivacaine, a new amide local anesthetic. Anesthesiology 72:322–329, 1990

Moller RA, Datta S, Fox J, et al: Effects of progesterone on the cardiac electrophysiologic action of bupivacaine and lidocaine. Anesthesiology 76:604–608, 1992

56

SPINAL ANESTHESIA

Isabelle deLeon, MD

Allan P. Reed, MD

An 80-year-old-man with prostatic carcinoma is admitted for open prostatectomy. He had a myocardial infarction 5 years prior to admission but has not reported experiencing angina or palpitations since that time. He is maintained on digoxin 0.25 mg/day. Examination of the back reveals flattening of the lumbar lordosis, with inability to flex or extend the vertebral column.

QUESTIONS

1. Other than the spinal kit, what equipment must be immediately available while performing spinal anesthesia?
2. When arranging the spinal tray, where is the antiseptic placed in relation to the tray's other constituents?
3. What are the advantages of the lateral decubitus position for placing a subarachnoid block?
4. What are the advantages of the sitting position for placing a subarachnoid block?
5. Describe a technique for placing a spinal anesthesia.
6. Describe alternative approaches to the subarachnoid space.
7. What factors affect the spread of anesthetic within the subarachnoid space?

8. What agents are commonly used for subarachnoid block?
9. Besides local anesthetics, what other agents are administered in the subarachnoid space?
10. What are the advantages of adding a vasoconstrictor to the spinal anesthetic solution?
11. What are the recognized complications of spinal anesthesia?
12. What are the contraindications to spinal anesthesia?
13. Describe the advantages of spinal anesthesia over general anesthesia.
14. Explain the advantages of spinal anesthesia over epidural anesthesia.
15. Outline the advantages and disadvantages of catheter (continuous) spinal anesthesia.

1. Other than the spinal kit, what equipment must be immediately available while performing spinal anesthesia?

Spinal anesthesia, like other types of anesthesia, is associated with significant physiologic trespass. Potential exists for significant cardiovascular and respiratory side-effects, including cardiopulmonary arrest. Resuscitative equipment and drugs must be readily available during spinal anesthesia. Electrocardiographic (ECG) monitoring, blood pressure, pulse oximetry, and intravenous fluid loading should precede the subarachnoid block. A means of administering 100% oxygen under positive pressure is essential, and vasopressors must be handy. Laryngoscopes, endotracheal tubes, and rapid-acting muscle relaxants are frequently useful.

2. When arranging the spinal tray, where is the antiseptic placed in relation to the tray's other constituents?

The spinal tray should conform to a design devised to prevent contamination of needles and drugs. This is usually achieved in one of two ways. The tray can be arranged so that the antiseptic is held in the corner closest to the patient and away from the other contents. Alternatively, a double-decker setup with the preparation solution and sponges placed on the upper level can be used. The aim is to prevent dripping antiseptic onto needles or into drugs that, on introduction into the subarachnoid space, may produce neurolysis or arachnoiditis.

3. What are the advantages of the lateral decubitus position for placing a subarachnoid block?

In the United States, the lateral decubitus position is used most commonly for several reasons. Some patients, depending on their medical condition, may be unable to sit up. The heavily sedated patient may be at risk of falling if in the sitting position. Also, the lateral decubitus position reduces the potential for dural puncture syncope, which is a loss of consciousness during dural penetration.

4. What are the advantages of the sitting position for placing a subarachnoid block?

In the sitting position, patients generally find it easier to flex the spine and thereby enlarge the interlaminar space. This position helps prevent rotation or distortion of the vertebral bodies. In obese patients, the midline is not obscured by fat pads rolling over it, as occurs in the lateral decubitus position.

5. Describe a technique for placing a spinal anesthesia.

After placing the patient in either the lateral decubitus or sitting position, the skin is prepared with antiseptic solution and draped in a sterile fashion. Dural puncture can be performed anywhere along the spinal column, but the risk of spinal cord trauma can be minimized by inserting the spinal needle at a point below which the spinal cord terminates. In most patients, the spinal cord ends at the second lumbar vertebral body. Therefore, the spinal needle is inserted just below this, usually at the L_3–L_4 interlaminar space. The iliac crest, which usually lies at the level of the L_4 spinous process, provides an excellent landmark. A small intradermal wheal of local anesthetic is placed at the level

of the selected interlaminar space using a 25-gauge needle. A 19-gauge, 1.5-inch introducer needle is placed through the anesthetized skin and into the interspinous ligament. The 25-gauge spinal needle is then inserted through the introducer needle. Twenty-two-gauge spinal needles do not require passage through an introducer needle. The needle's bevel should be aligned with the longitudinal fibers of the dura in an effort to separate the fibers rather than cut them. It is postulated that lacerating the fibers may retard closure of the dural hole, predisposing patients to headaches. Resistance to needle passage frequently results from encountering bone or calcified ligaments. The cooperative patient can frequently help differentiate the two. Calcified ligaments do not usually hurt when the needle impinges upon them. Encountering bone is often painful owing to periosteal trauma.

The posterior aspect of the vertebral lamina is curved, so that the inferior portion is more superficial than the superior part. Therefore, if the spinal needle encounters bone superficially, it is probably abutting the inferior aspect of the vertebra above. If the needle encounters bone at a deeper location, then it is probably abutting the superior aspect of the lamina below. The spinal needle is then advanced through the increased resistance of the ligamentum flavum, and a loss of resistance is often appreciated as the needle tip enters the epidural space. A characteristic "pop" is obtained as the needle pierces the dura and enters the subarachnoid space. The distance from the skin to the ligamentum flavum is usually between 3.5 and 5.0 cm.

The spinal needle stylet is removed and cerebrospinal fluid (CSF) allowed to escape by gravity drainage or with gentle aspiration. Insertion of the needle too far within the subarachnoid space may place its tip against the vertebral body or intervertebral disc, thereby preventing CSF flow through the needle. This problem is easily corrected by withdrawing the needle slightly and observing the hub for fluid. Flow should be obtained in all four quadrants to ensure proper placement of the bevel within the subarachnoid space. Levy et al. (1985) and Machikanti et al. (1987) have debated the importance of free-flowing CSF as a prognosticator of a successful block. When obtained, CSF should be clear and colorless. Bleeding that does not readily stop requires repositioning of the needle. The properly placed needle should be held securely while bracing your hand against the patient's back. The syringe is attached to the spinal needle hub sufficiently well so that local anesthetic cannot leak during injection. About 0.2 mL of CSF should be aspirated, observing the resulting change in optical density within the syringe, to confirm that you are still in the subarachnoid space. The local anesthetic is injected, and the syringe aspirated once again to confirm that the needle has not been dislodged from the subarachnoid space. The spinal needle is removed at this point. The patient can now be repositioned at any time.

Frequent blood pressure determinations are required to detect hypotension.

6. Describe alternative approaches to the subarachnoid space.

In the United States, the most popular approach to the subarachnoid space is the median approach. With the lumbar spine flexed, the spinal needle is inserted through a point approximately midway between the upper and lower vertebral spines. The spinal needle should be maintained at a 90° angle to the back at the point of entry. It is frequently necessary to reinsert the spinal needle through a point somewhat closer to the inferior spine. The median approached is the most commonly taught in medical school and, therefore, is most comfortable to many physicians.

The lateral or paramedian approach is especially useful in patients with calcified supraspinous and interspinous ligaments, which might prevent passage of a fine spinal needle. This technique is, also, particularly useful in patients who are unable to flex their spines because of arthritis or ankylosing spondylitis. Flexion of the lumbar spine is useful but not necessary. The spinal needle is inserted approximately 2 cm lateral to the supraspinous ligament, which lies in the midline, and level with the upper quarter of the inferior vertebral spine. The needle is passed in a superomedial direction to pierce the ligamentum flavum in the middle of the interlaminar space. In the event that bone is encountered, the spinal needle is "walked off" the lamina until it encounters the interlaminar space. The distance between the skin and subarachnoid space varies considerably from patient to patient, but is usually between 3.5 and 5 cm.

The major advantages of the lateral or paramedian approach are that the calcified interspinous ligament is avoided and the needle traverses the widest portion of the interlaminar space.

The Taylor approach involves placing a spinal needle through the skin 1 cm medial and 1 cm cephalad to the posterior superior iliac spine and directing the needle in a mediocephalad direction. This places the spinal needle through the L_5–S_1 interlaminar space. The Taylor approach provides the patient with maximal comfort by using the largest interlaminar space. The overriding L_5 spinous process is avoided. The modified Taylor approach involves placing the needle 1.5 cm lateral to the midpoint of the L_5–S_1 space and directing it toward the midline at a 25° angle. The caudal approach uses a 10-cm spinal needle, which is introduced into the caudal canal and advanced superiorly until it pierces the dura at approximately the S_2 level.

7. What factors affect the spread of anesthetic within the subarachnoid space?

Specific gravity greatly influences the local anesthetic's spread within the subarachnoid space. The specific gravity of CSF ranges between 1.003 and 1.008. Local anesthetics with lower specific gravities, i.e., hypobaric solutions, tend to float toward the nondependent areas. Hypobaric solutions have been used for patients with fractured hips, placing the injured extremity above as the patient lies in the lateral decubitus position. Hypobaric solutions are created by dissolving local anesthetic in distilled water. Local anesthetic solutions with specific gravities above 1.008 are hyperbaric. Hyperbaric solutions tend to migrate toward dependent areas. They are the local anesthetic preparations most commonly used for spinal anesthesia in the United States. Hyperbaric solutions are readily adaptable to most spinal anesthetic needs and are particularly valuable for anesthetizing lower thoracic nerve roots and for "selectively" anesthetizing sacral nerve roots (saddle blocks). Hyperbaric solutions are created by mixing a local anesthetic with 10% dextrose in water. Level of the dural puncture and patient position also affect anesthetic spread.

The spinal column contains a natural lumbar lordosis as well as a thoracic and sacral kyphosis. L_4 resides at the peak of the lumbar lordosis, and T_5 lies at the nadir of the thoracic kyphosis (Fig. 56.1). After local anesthetic is injected at the L_4 level and the patient is turned to the supine position, hyperbaric solutions tend to pool in the sacral and thoracic kyphoses. In other words, hyperbaric solutions run downhill, providing maximal anesthesia of the sacral and midthoracic nerve roots. Middle lumbar spinal roots may be exposed to minimal amounts of local anesthetic, thereby providing poor sensory block to these dermatomes whenever inadequate local anesthetic is administered. Raising the legs into the lithotomy position will flatten the lumbar lordosis and help prevent large unanesthetized windows. Pooling of solution in the thoracic kyphosis tends to prevent anesthesia rising above the T_4 dermatome, preventing a "total spinal". Using excessively large volumes of anesthetic may overcome the lumbar lordosis problem but it may also spread the anesthetic above T_4. To avoid both excessively high levels and inadequate levels, the process of selecting the proper dose of local anesthetic for subarachnoid injection has, in the past, taken into account innumerable variables. Height, weight, age, increased abdominal pressure, position, site of injection, volume of injectate, concentration of local anesthetic, amount of local anesthetic, and baricity represent only some of the factors that were traditionally thought to significantly affect anesthetic spread. With these criteria in mind, a myriad of guidelines for spinal anesthesia dosing have been presented over the years. Table 56.1 lists one of the many possible dosing schedules for hyperbaric tetracaine spinal anesthetics. It has generally been recommended to reduce amounts by 2 mg for patients 5 feet (152 cm) tall and to increase amounts by 2 mg for patients 6 feet (183 cm) tall. Despite rigorous adherence to such dosing schedules, spinal anesthesia has frequently been inadequate to provide satisfactory patient comfort during surgery.

SPINAL COLUMM CONTOUR

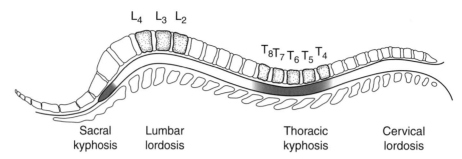

FIGURE 56.1 Pooling of hyperbaric local anesthetic in the sacral and thoracic kyphoses.

Recognizing the high frequency of inappropriately low anesthesia levels, Norris (1988) conducted a study that has revolutionized spinal anesthesia dosing regimens. Evaluation of term parturients receiving 12 mg of hyperbaric bupivacaine demonstrated no correlation between the spread of anesthesia and the subject's height, weight, or body mass index. Although peak analgesic levels ranged from $T_7–C_8$, most patients attained levels between T_4 and T_1. Extrapolating these results to the nonpregnant patient, several authors revised the recommended dosing schedules for subarachnoid block. Adult patients, placed in the supine position, can receive 15 mg of hyperbaric bupivacaine or hyperbaric tetracaine. These solutions will eventually migrate to the T_5 nerve roots, producing profound and reliable anesthesia below this level. This technique is especially useful for surgery on structures innervated below T_8. The newer recommendations calling for significantly larger local anesthetic doses provide more intense blockade for longer durations without significantly extending the spread of anesthesia. Tuominen and colleagues (1992) have

suggested that unpredictable individual anatomic variations may play an important role in subarachnoid spread of local anesthetics.

To prevent local anesthetic spread to thoracic levels when only lumbosacral anesthesia is required, isobaric lidocaine 2.0% or isobaric bupivacaine 0.5% without preservatives represent an excellent choice. Isobaric solutions tend to remain in the lumbosacral area into which they are injected. These local anesthetics do not migrate significantly, providing for maintenance of adequate anesthetic concentrations bathing the lumbosacral nerve roots. The benefits include more intense analgesia, greater duration of action, and reduced potential for hypotension and respiratory depression.

Speed of anesthetic injection should approximate 0.5 mL/sec. Significantly more rapid injection rates tend to push the anesthetic toward higher dermatome levels.

8. What agents are commonly used for subarachnoid block?

The most frequently used agent for spinal anesthesia is hyperbaric tetracaine. Tetracaine is usually supplied as a 1% solution, which is made hyperbaric by addition of an equal volume of 10% dextrose in water. Anticipated duration of anesthesia is usually 1.5–2.5 hours. The addition of epinephrine (0.2–0.4 mg) will generally provide a duration of action between 2.5 and 4 hours.

Hyperbaric lidocaine is usually supplied as a 5% solution and does not require mixing. Its duration of action is 0.5–1.5 hours. Adding 0.2 mg of epinephrine extends the duration of action to 1–2 hours.

Spinal bupivacaine has gained popularity and is commercially available as a 0.75% solution with dextrose. Its duration of action is similar to that of tetracaine. The addition of epinephrine only minimally prolongs bupivacaine's duration of action. Spinal bupivacaine provides a

TABLE 56.1	Traditional Subarachnoid Tetracaine Doses for Patients 5 Feet 6 Inches (168 cm) Tall	

Region	Dermatome	Hyperbaric Tetracaine (mg)
Rectal	S_1	5.5
Lower extremities	L_1	10.5
Inguinal area	T_8	14.0
Urinary bladder	T_8	14.0
Lower abdomen	T_6	14.0
Upper abdomen	T_4	16.0

Operations Appropriate for Isobaric Spinal Anesthetics

Lower extremity
  Hip, femur, tibia, fibula, metatarsals

Genitourinary
  Prostate, bladder, urethra, scrotum

Perineum
  Anus, rectum

dense sensory block, but its motor block is less profound than that of tetracaine.

Lidocaine 2.0%, and bupivacaine 0.5%, are commonly employed isobaric preparations. Their use requires a solution free of preservatives and antioxidants. Methylparaben, sodium bisulfite, or sodium metabisulfite may be neurotoxic and are contraindicated for injection into the subarachnoid space. A large experience with isobaric preservative-free solutions of both agents has found them to be safe and effective subarachnoid medications.

Hypobaric tetracaine is prepared from the standard 1% solution, which is mixed with a large volume of distilled water. Tetracaine, 5–10 mg, is usually diluted with 5–10 mL of distilled water to form a very hypobaric solution. Dibucaine, 0.066%, an alternative to hypobaric tetracaine, is no longer available in the United States. Hypobaric and isobaric solutions are not commonly employed in the United States. However, they do provide excellent anesthesia when used properly.

9. Besides local anesthetics, what other agents are administered in the subarachnoid space?

Opioids are another class of agents that may be administered into the subarachnoid space. Intrathecal opioids work via opiate receptors within the second and third laminae of the substantia gelatinosa in the dorsal horn of the spinal cord to produce intense visceral analgesia without sympathetic nervous system denervation, skeletal muscle weakness, or loss of proprioception. Commonly used intrathecal opioids are the lipophilic agents such as fentanyl and sufentanil, and the hydrophilic agents such as morphine. The lipophilic agents have a much more localized effect, a rapid onset of action, and a duration of about 2–8 hours. The hydrophilic agent, morphine, has a greater spread of action and can last anywhere from 6 to 24 hours. Intrathecal opioids are also used as adjuncts to local anesthetics during spinal anesthesia. They may

prolong the sensory blockade of the local anesthetic without increasing the postoperative duration of the motor blockade or time to voiding. Side-effects associated with the use of intrathecal opioids include nausea and vomiting, urinary retention, pruritus, and respiratory depression. Opioid antagonists or agonist/antagonist agents are useful in treating these side-effects.

Other types of agents that have been administered intrathecally are the α_2-agonist clonidine and the centrally acting muscle relaxant baclofen. Clonidine administered into the subarachnoid or epidural space produces intense analgesia, presumably by activating α_2-receptors in the substantia gelatinosa of the spinal cord. Unlike intrathecal opioids, clonidine does not produce nausea and vomiting, urinary retention, pruritus, or respiratory depression. The combination of local anesthetics and clonidine during a neuraxial blockade produces a longer duration of sensory and motor blockade compared with local anesthetics alone. This combination produces a greater drop in diastolic blood pressure, necessitating preloading these patients with intravenous fluids.

Baclofen is a gamma-aminobutyric acid (GABA) analog used to treat spasticity resulting from spinal cord disease such as multiple sclerosis or spinal cord injury. Patients who have not responded effectively to oral administration of baclofen may benefit from intrathecal administration. Baclofen has been shown to have spinal analgesic effects without increased muscle tone, both in animal models and in cancer patients who are resistant or tolerant to opioids. However, the use of baclofen is limited by its side-effects, which include skeletal muscle weakness, sedation, and confusion. Toxicity to baclofen results in coma, respiratory depression, and seizures.

10. What are the advantages of adding a vasoconstrictor to the spinal anesthetic solution?

The goal of adding vasoconstrictors to local anesthetics is usually to decrease local anesthetic uptake secondary to diminished blood flow. Nerves are bathed in the local anesthetic longer, and the duration of blockade is frequently prolonged. Although 0.2–0.4 mg of epinephrine prolongs the effects of isobaric solutions and hyperbaric tetracaine, it does not increase the duration of blockade produced by hyperbaric bupivacaine. Nevertheless, vasoconstrictors do seem to provide other beneficial effects for spinal anesthesia. α-Agonists such as epinephrine and phenylephrine, when applied to the spinal cord, demonstrate analgesic properties. It is postulated that the vasoconstrictors' independent spinal cord actions add to those of the local anesthetics to improve intensity of anesthesia.

Fear that vasoconstrictors might impair spinal cord blood flow to the point of neuronal damage has been dispelled. Lidocaine and tetracaine increase spinal cord blood flow, which is minimally offset by the addition of epinephrine. The addition of vasoconstrictors to subarachnoid local anesthetics has not proven to be deleterious.

Clonidine, a centrally acting α_2-agonist, has also been shown to prolong the duration of action of spinal tetracaine. This has been achieved with intrathecal injection and oral premedication administration.

11. What are the recognized complications of spinal anesthesia?

The single most common complication of spinal anesthesia is probably hypotension. Postganglionic autonomic nerves, which are small, unmyelinated C fibers, are exquisitely sensitive to spinal blockade. The greater the extent of anesthesia, the greater the sympathectomy. Interruption of sympathetic stimuli to the capacitance vessels markedly increases peripheral venous pooling, resulting in decreased venous return to the heart. Consequently, cardiac output falls. The usual compensatory response to reduced cardiac output is an increase in heart rate. Sudden tachycardic responses are mediated through the cardiac accelerator nerves, which receives contributions from spinal nerves $T_1–T_4$. Blockade of the upper thoracic nerve roots not only prevents acute increases in heart but also allows for unopposed vagal influence, thereby slowing heart rate. Therefore, cardiac output is impaired by two mechanisms: peripheral venous pooling and bradycardia.

Before administration of spinal anesthesia, fluid loading with approximately 500 mL of a balanced salt solution helps to prevent the state of relative hypovolemia induced by venous dilatation. Most cases of spinal-induced hypotension respond favorably to altering the patient's position into $10°$ of Trendelenburg, lithotomy, or left lateral uterine displacement. Intravenous volume infusion is frequently required to restore blood pressure toward its normal range. Hypotension unresponsive to fluid administration requires immediate treatment and usually responds to ephedrine, 5–10 mg, intravenously. Ephedrine works by stimulating both α- and β-receptors causing an increase in the heart rate, contractility, and peripheral resistance, which are frequently sufficient to correct hypotension. Hypotension, dysrhythmias, and myocardial ischemia are associated untoward effects. Ephedrine causes little or no alteration in uterine blood flow. Alternatively, a continuous infusion of phenylephrine may return vascular tone toward normal. The solution is frequently prepared by adding 10 mg of phenylephrine to 250 or 500 mL of 5% dextrose in water. Phenylephrine acts as an α-adrenergic agonist. Its side-effects include hypertension, bradycardia, and uterine vasoconstriction. It is not the first choice for treating hypotension in the pregnant patient. Bradycardia is effectively treated with atropine 0.4 mg intravenously, or ephedrine in small doses.

Ventilatory impairment frequently results from hypotension leading to impaired medullary blood flow and hypoxia of the respiratory center. Blockade of the phrenic nerve, composed of contributions from $C_3–C_5$, leading to impaired diaphragmatic movement, is highly unusual. Motor blockade of the intercostal and abdominal muscles may prevent effective coughing. Loss of the intercostal muscle's proprioception frequently prevents the patient from appreciating chest expansion, thereby creating a subjective feeling of difficulty breathing.

Nausea and vomiting accompanying spinal anesthesia often result from parasympathetic imbalance, hypotension, or hypoxemia. Treatment with atropine, vasopressors, or oxygen usually provides relief. Retching, apprehension, agitation, and shortness of breath may also be secondary to hypotension or hypoxemia. Treatment requires increasing the blood pressure, oxygen administration, and assisted or controlled ventilation.

Post-dural puncture headache (PDPH) remains the most commonly encountered postanesthetic side-effect of spinal anesthesia. The frequency of PDPH following dural puncture with a 17-gauge Tuohy needle has been reported to be as high as 75%. The incidence of PDPH is lower in the elderly and in those whose dura is punctured by a pencil-point or a fine needle. PDPH following the use of a 26-gauge needle may be as low as 2.5%. In an ambulatory setting, Kang et al. (1992) noted a PDPH rate of 9.6% and 1.5% associated with 26- and 27-gauge needles, respectively. Aligning the needle bevel parallel to the dural fibers seems to markedly reduce the incidence of PDPH. This approach tends to separate rather than cut the longitudinal dural fibers, resulting in a smaller, more readily repairable hole.

PDPH following subarachnoid block emanates from traction on the meninges and vascular structures, as CSF leaks through the dura. Symptomatic treatment requires mild analgesics, bed rest, and fluid administration. Injection of morphine into the subarachnoid space along with a local anesthetic does not decrease the incidence of PDPH. In patients with severe incapacitating headaches, or headaches of several days' duration, an epidural blood patch is indicated. An epidural blood patch is performed by placing a needle in the epidural space at the suspected level of dural puncture. Fifteen to twenty milliliters of the patient's own blood, drawn under sterile conditions, are injected through the newly placed epidural needle. This maneuver is highly successful, but risk of re-puncturing the dura exists. Slight elevations in temperature are occasionally seen for 1 or 2 days following this procedure. Low back pain and neck discomfort have also been reported following epidural blood patching. Caffeine, a cerebral vasoconstrictor, may also provide beneficial effects. Other causes of PDPH, such as septic or aseptic meningitis and arachnoiditis, are extremely rare. Urinary retention

Signs and Symptoms of Post-Dural Puncture Headache

Character of pain
    Constant
    Dull
    Throbbing

Location of pain
    Occipital
    Frontal
    Global

Factors improving pain
    Supine position
    Analgesic

Factors exacerbating pain
    Sitting position
    Standing position

Associated findings
    Vertigo
    Tinnitus
    Photophobia
    Scotomata

epidural hemorrhage exist in anticoagulated patients. Current American Society of Regional Anesthesia and Pain Medicine (ASRA) recommendations concerning the use of spinal or epidural anesthesia in patients on antiplatelet drugs are as follows. Nonsteroidal anti-inflammatory drugs and aspirin do not present an increased risk for intraspinal bleeding when used as a single agent. Use of spinal or epidural anesthesia is at the discretion of the anesthesiologist. However, there is the known risk of a hemorrhagic complication when these drugs are concurrently given with other antiplatelet drugs such as heparin, low-molecular-weight heparin, warfarin, ticlopidine (Ticlid), or clopidogrel (Plavix). If spinal or epidural anesthesia is considered, there should be careful documentation of the lack of therapeutic effect (normal coagulation tests) of the second drug. Regarding the new antiplatelet drugs, ticlopidine and clopidogrel, which are drugs prescribed for prevention of myocardial infarction, stroke, and vaso-occlusive disorders, there are no current studies to establish the safety of performing regional anesthesia during their use.

Causes of Major Neurologic Sequelae Following Spinal Anesthesia

Hematoma
    Usually associated with a major clotting diathesis

Abscess

Septic meningitis
    Bacterial contamination of local anesthetic or needle

Aseptic meningitis
    Antiseptic, detergent, or powder contamination of local anesthetic needle

Direct neurotoxicity
    Preservatives in the local anesthetic

Mechanical neurotrauma
    Needles, catheters

Spinal cord ischemia
    Systemic hypotension, aortic cross-clamping

Transient Radicular Irritation
    Greatest incidence with lidocaine although reported with other local anesthetics

that is due to prolonged blockade has also been associated with spinal techniques.

Backache occurs frequently following spinal anesthesia but is usually short-lived and of only mild-to-moderate intensity. Its causes generally include lumbar ligamentum strain, paraspinous muscle spasm, and muscle hematoma formation. Severe back pain requires immediate neurologic investigation.

The incidence of major neurologic sequelae following spinal anesthesia approaches 0.5%. If exacerbations of pre-existing neurologic diseases are eliminated from this figure, the probability of encountering neurologic damage following spinal anesthesia diminishes even further. Transient radicular irritation (TRI) consists of pain, and/or dysesthesia in the legs or buttocks. This occurred more frequently with lidocaine, but has been seen with tetracaine and bupivacaine. Other factors that contribute to the incidence of TRI are the lithotomy position, ambulatory patients, and obesity. TRI usually resolves within 72 hours but may take as long as 6 months.

Hematoma or abscess formation producing a cauda equina syndrome is potentially identifiable and remediable. Numerous cases of spontaneous subarachnoid and

There are also no data regarding their interaction with other anticoagulant drugs. Thus, ASRA guidelines recommend discontinuing ticlopidine for 10–14 days and clopidogrel for 7 days prior to performing a spinal or epidural anesthetic.

Direct neurotoxicity of commonly used local anesthetic solutions is almost nonexistent. Chloroprocaine, however, represents a notable exception. Although apparently free of direct neurotoxicity in the epidural space, chloroprocaine possesses neurolytic properties in the subarachnoid space. Sodium bisulfite, a preservative, has been identified as the causative agent. Sodium bisulfite has been eliminated from many currently available preparations. At present, chloroprocaine is not recommended for use in the subarachnoid space. Cauda equina syndrome has been reported following administration of hyperbaric local anesthetics through subarachnoid catheters. Septic and aseptic meningitis has been attributed to contamination of drugs and needles with bacteria, detergents, and powder. Single-use, disposable equipment has almost eliminated this problem. Direct neural trauma may theoretically occur from needles or catheters but should be relegated to a practical improbability in most cases. Spinal cord ischemia has been associated with systemic hypotension and cross-clamping of the aorta. Pre-existing neurologic disease, improper patient positioning, or pressure from retractors on the fetal head may also predispose the patient to neurologic defects following spinal anesthesia and are unrelated to the spinal anesthetic.

Failure of spinal anesthesia to provide adequate analgesia remains another commonly encountered complication. Prospective studies have estimated the rate of failed spinals to be 4–16%. A study by Munhall et al. (1988) demonstrated that only 25% of spinal failures were due to factors such as inability to identify the subarachnoid space and lack of free-flowing CSF before, as well as after, injection of local anesthetic. Most inadequate spinal anesthetics were due to faulty selection of local anesthetic, dose, vasoconstrictor, baricity, position, interspace, or single-injection versus catheter technique. An example of such a judgment error is the selection of tetracaine 0.5% over bupivacaine 0.5% to block tourniquet pain.

Long-term follow-up studies of patients receiving large numbers of spinal anesthetics have shown spinal anesthesia to be a safe technique (e.g., Vandam and Dripps 1960).

12. What are the contraindications to spinal anesthesia?

Patients with increased intracranial pressure run a risk of brainstem herniation after dural puncture, as CSF pressure within the vertebral column is released. Passage of the spinal needle through areas of infected tissue may seed the subarachnoid space with microorganisms. Septicemia has been questioned as a potential source of contamination of the subarachnoid space. In 1992, Carp and Bailey noted that dural puncture in bacteremic rats was associated with the development of meningitis. Antibiotic treatment before dural puncture appeared to eliminate the risk of post-dural puncture meningitis.

Inability to obtain consent for spinal anesthesia from the patient is an absolute contraindication to the technique. Patients with documented allergies to local anesthetics should not receive a drug from the class of anesthetics to which they have reacted. Hypovolemia increases the risk of hypotension following sympathectomy and should be corrected before the initiation of spinal anesthesia. Clotting abnormalities increase the risk of epidural or even subarachnoid hematoma formation, with subsequent compression of neural structures. Pre-existing neurologic disease had been considered a relatively strong contraindication to spinal anesthesia at one time. Experience with subarachnoid blocks in such patients has not demonstrated exacerbation of peripheral neuropathies or low back pain. Progressive neurologic abnormalities, such as multiple sclerosis and amyotrophic lateral sclerosis, may present with increased symptomatology following spinal anesthesia, but this probably represents the natural course of the disease and not an adverse effect of the spinal anesthetic.

13. Describe the advantages of spinal anesthesia over general anesthesia.

Although general anesthesia frequently provides airway control for the anesthesiologist, spinal anesthesia offers many advantages over general anesthesia. Both orthopedic and vascular surgeries on the lower extremities are associated with diminished blood loss under spinal anesthesia compared with general anesthesia. The inference, which has been proven to be true, is that patients undergoing these procedures with spinal anesthesia receive less transfused blood. The risk of receiving the human immunodeficiency virus (HIV) and other communicable diseases through blood transfusion is therefore reduced also (Table 56.2).

Metabolic alterations associated with general anesthesia and surgery are well described. Increases in energy-liberating hormones, such as epinephrine, norepinephrine, cortisol, and growth hormone occur. Glucose levels may also increase in patients undergoing surgery and general anesthesia. Spinal anesthesia to the upper thoracic levels is associated with decreased epinephrine and norepinephrine concentrations, while lower thoracic levels allow epinephrine and norepinephrine levels to remain essentially unchanged. Surgery under spinal anesthesia is associated with depressed levels of cortisol, insulin, and free fatty acids. Glucose concentrations under spinal anesthesia increase slightly and then tend to fall slightly.

It is postulated that spinal anesthesia prevents increases in metabolic hormone concentrations by afferent and efferent neural blockade. Inhibition of adrenal medullary catecholamine release is probably secondary to efferent autonomic blockade. Inhibition of pituitary hormone release is probably due to afferent pathway interruption.

TABLE 56.2	Advantages of Spinal Anesthesia Over General Anesthesia
Criteria	**Advantages of Spinal Anesthesia**
Blood loss	Diminished bleeding during lower extremity surgery
Risk of HIV transmission	Decreased requirement for blood transfusion reduces the risk of transmitting HIV
Metabolic alterations	Decreased concentrations of glucose, insulin, free fatty acids, and cortisol
	Decreased epinephrine and norepinephrine concentrations associated with upper thoracic spinal levels
	Essentially normal epinephrine and norepinephrine concentrations associated with lower thoracic spinal levels
Postoperative deep vein thrombosis	Incidence reduced
	?Decreased incidence of pulmonary emboli
Mortality	Improved short-term mortality
	No change in long-term survival

Ablation of the hyperglycemic response seen under spinal anesthesia may be secondary to efferent sympathetic blockade to the liver as well as inhibition of catecholamine release from the adrenal medulla.

The incidence of deep vein thrombosis following lower extremity orthopedic surgery is reduced under spinal anesthesia compared with general anesthesia. Although one would anticipate the incidence of pulmonary emboli to be reduced following spinal anesthesia, this has not been documented.

Elderly patients undergoing surgery for femoral neck fractures under spinal anesthesia demonstrate an improved short-term survival rate. Interestingly, the long-term survival rate of patients undergoing similar surgery under spinal anesthesia is approximately the same as that for patients who had undergone general anesthesia. Pulmonary embolism was a frequent cause of death for those who received general anesthesia and who died within 1 month of surgery.

14. Explain the advantages of spinal anesthesia over epidural anesthesia.

Although major similarities exist between spinal anesthesia and epidural anesthesia, significant differences are noted (Table 56.3). Spinal anesthesia is usually accomplished with a 26- or 22-gauge needle, which is technically easier to manipulate between bony prominences than the typical 17-gauge epidural needle. CSF flowing through the needle is a more reliable indicator of proper needle placement than subtle movement of a liquid drop or even loss of resistance as used in epidural techniques. Spinal anesthesia requires minute amounts of local anesthetic which, if injected intravascularly, often might not manifest central nervous system alterations. Epidural techniques require such large amounts of local anesthetic that the risk of toxicity from absorption is markedly increased. Direct intravascular injection is almost certain to result in profound central nervous system and cardiovascular collapse. Although spinal techniques are infamous for their potential to produce headaches, the intensity of the discomfort is often less severe than that associated with unintentional dural puncture with the standard 17-gauge epidural needle. Epidural anesthesia offers a lower risk of headache but frequently produces a more severe, incapacitating headache. The incidence of significant neurologic complications other than headache is extremely low for both techniques. Spinal anesthesia tends to provide far more profound analgesia than do epidural techniques. The incidence of patchy block is very low with spinal anesthesia but considerably more frequent with epidural anesthesia. Spread of anesthesia is more predictable with spinal techniques using varying baricities and positions. Spread of anesthesia associated with epidural techniques is less predictable and cannot be adjusted by position or baricity of the injected anesthetic. The onset of spinal anesthesia is rapid and that of epidural anesthesia tends to be slower. The duration of both techniques is virtually limitless when using catheters. It is debatable whether hemodynamic alterations and hypotension are more pronounced with spinal anesthesia than with epidural anesthesia.

15. Outline the advantages and disadvantages of catheter (continuous) spinal anesthesia.

In one form or another, catheter spinal anesthesia techniques have provided excellent anesthesia for approximately 100 years. They offer all the benefits of single-injection spinal anesthesia plus limitless duration of action. Continuous spinal anesthesia lapsed into disuse with the

TABLE 56.3	Comparison of Spinal Anesthesia and Epidural Anesthesia	
	Spinal	**Epidural**
Needle placement	Smaller-gauge needle is easier to place	Larger-gauge needle is more difficult to place
	Cerebrospinal fluid flowing through the needle is a more reliable endpoint	Movement of a fluid drop or loss of resistance are more subtle endpoints
Potential for local anesthetic toxicity	Negligible	Considerable
Potential for headache	Higher incidence, but headache often less severe	Lower incidence, but headache often more severe
Incidence of neurologic complications	Very low	Very low
Intensity of anesthesia	Profound	Less profound
Incidence of patchy block	Very low	More frequent
Spread of anesthesia	Highly predictable	Less predictable
Onset of anesthesia	Rapid	Slow
Duration of action	Variable based on agents selected	Limitless using catheter technique
Hemodynamic alterations	More pronounced	Less pronounced

advent of continuous epidural anesthesia, which offered relief from the high incidence of PDPH. The relatively recent development of smaller catheters designed for use in the subarachnoid space has led to renewed interest in catheter spinal anesthesia. It may be selected over single-injection spinal anesthesia for basically two reasons. Catheter spinal anesthesia offers the option for slow incremental dosing intended to minimize hemodynamic changes. It also extends the duration of anesthesia for operations expected to outlast the course of single-dose methods.

Advances in technology and pharmacology have brought us to the present state of the art. In the past, catheter spinal anesthesia was performed with large-bore needles and catheters designed for epidural use. Presently there are catheters ranging in size from 24- to 32-gauge. These catheters are intended for insertion through 20- to 27-gauge needles in an attempt to reduce the incidence of PDPH. Establishment of continuous spinal anesthesia is usually simple. A needle is placed in the subarachnoid space, and the difference from skin to the space is estimated by subtracting the length of the exposed needle from the needle's total length. The catheter is passed through the needle until its tip resides at the needle bevel. This is usually a distance of 10 cm. The catheter is then advanced 3 cm into the subarachnoid space. Inability to thread the catheter beyond the needle bevel generally results from obstruction by one of several anatomic structures. Combinations of needle manipulation, such as rotation and/or advancement and/or withdrawal, generally allow for passage into the space. If these maneuvers fail, the procedure is repeated at another interspace.

With the catheter properly inserted into the subarachnoid space, slowly withdraw the needle over the catheter with one hand as the other hand applies slight pressure in the opposite direction. Recall the distance from the skin to the space and add 3 cm, this being the length of the catheter which should be inserted into the patient's back. Gently aspirate CSF through the catheter to confirm proper placement.

The recognized complications of continuous spinal anesthesia include all those attributed to single-injection methods plus those summarized below.

One of the most frequent and frustrating complications of catheter techniques is the inability to pass a catheter into the proper location. The incidence of inability to thread spinal catheters approximates 8%. The potential causes of this problem are numerous and poorly defined for any individual patient.

Complications Specific to Catheter Spinal Anesthesia

Inability to thread the catheter
Breakage
Cauda equina syndrome
Knotting
Trapping by neural structures
Migration into a blood vessel
Dislocation from the subarachnoid space

Experience with epidural catheters has shown occasional breakage during insertion and removal. Spinal catheter breakage during attempted insertion generally occurs when catheters are withdrawn through the needle. An entire catheter segment may be sheared off by this maneuver. Even a partial cut in the catheter could reduce its tensile strength, predisposing to breakage during removal in the postoperative period. Inability to pass a catheter must result in simultaneous removal of both needle and catheter from the back. The procedure is then repeated at the same interspace or another one.

Catheter breakage during removal from the back is generally heralded by catheter elongation. Stretching can be considered a warning sign of imminent danger. Break strengths of one presently available 24-gauge spinal catheter and a commonly used 20-gauge epidural catheter are 3.55 lb (1.6 kg) and 6.35 lb (2.9 kg), respectively. This is a very narrow range, placing most catheters at risk of snapping during removal. Consequently, removal must take place with the vertebrae flexed to the same degree as they were during insertion. This maneuver attempts to realign the various ligaments, minimizing their grip on the catheter.

Catheter breakage is a difficult problem to deal with. If breakage occurs close to the skin, then superficial dissection under local anesthesia may allow for isolation of the catheter. It can be grasped with a clamp and gently removed. If the catheter is severed in deep tissues, it may be left in situ. The risk of infection is small, because it is placed under strictly sterile conditions. General anesthesia and laminectomy to retrieve the catheter may place the patient at higher risk for associated complications than leaving it in place. A moral and ethical obligation exists to inform the patient of this complication in the rare event of its occurrence.

Another theoretical problem is a small segment of catheter floating freely within the subarachnoid space, which could migrate cephalad and produce significant complications. This situation may present a more compelling reason for surgical removal than a catheter which is held firmly by ligaments.

Another unusual but noteworthy complication of catheter spinal anesthesia is cauda equina syndrome. In 1991, Rigler et al. reported 4 cases of cauda equina syndrome occurring after catheter spinal anesthesia. Evidence of subarachnoid block was achieved in all cases, and additional doses were administered to raise the level of analgesia. The total initial dose of local anesthetic was generally greater than that administered in a single bolus dose through a spinal needle. The authors speculate that pooling of large doses of local anesthetic resulted in neurotoxicity.

Later in 1991, Lambert and Hurley described a model that demonstrated hyperbaric and isobaric lidocaine loculation in the sacral and lower lumbar regions. In the event of inadequate local anesthetic spread following injection of 2% isobaric lidocaine (40 mg) they suggest the addition of 1–2 mL of hypobaric 0.375% bupivacaine.

Hypobaric 0.375% bupivacaine is readily prepared by dilution of 0.75% plain bupivacaine with an equal volume of distilled water. This technique should allow spread of local anesthetic into the upper lumbar area while limiting local anesthetic exposure to only 40 mg of lidocaine and 7.5 mg of bupivacaine. Such low doses of anesthetic would be expected to place patients at low risk for cauda equina syndrome. This combination of isobaric and hypobaric solutions is logical, based on observed subarachnoid spread of these solutions.

Catheters can curl on themselves and tighten into knots when withdrawn. Such occurrence could prevent withdrawal postoperatively, because the knot would be too large to fit through the dural hole. A worse circumstance could occur if a nerve were entrapped by the knot. In this case, one would expect radicular pain during attempted catheter removal. Catheter curling is most likely to happen if excessive lengths are inserted into the subarachnoid space. To prevent this, never advance more than 3 cm of catheter beyond the needle tip.

Migration into a blood vessel is generally of little consequence. The usual doses of local anesthetic delivered for spinal anesthesia (approximately 50 mg of lidocaine) are less than those purposefully administered intravenously for the treatment of premature ventricular contractions (approximately 100 mg of lidocaine).

Dislocation from the subarachnoid space will result in epidural placement. The small doses of local anesthetic generally employed for spinal anesthesia will yield minimal or no blockade following administration into the epidural space. It is theoretically possible, although highly unlikely, that a catheter intended for the subarachnoid space could lodge in the subdural space. The subsequent delivery of local anesthetic would then cause either segmental anesthesia or massive sympathetic, sensory, and motor blockade, depending on the dose administered into the subdural space.

A century of spinal anesthesia has witnessed advances in pharmacology and technology culminating in the use of small catheters for placement in the subarachnoid space. Although spinal anesthesia, like general anesthesia, is fraught with potential problems, its judicious application has benefited innumerable patients. Continuous spinal anesthesia represents a double-edged sword. It offers advantages over general anesthesia and catheter epidural anesthesia but is associated with its own potential complications. With knowledge of these potential problems and careful application of the procedure, catheter spinal anesthesia remains a safe and desirable technique.

SUGGESTED READINGS

Abboud TK, Miller H, Afrasiabi A, et al: Effect of subarachnoid morphine on the incidence of spinal headache. Reg Anesth 17:34, 1992

Bernards CM, Hymas NJ: Progression of first degree heart block to high-grade second degree heart block during spinal anesthesia. Can J Anaesth 39:173, 1992

Carp H, Bailey S: The association between meningitis and dural puncture in bacteremic rats. Anesthesiology 76:739, 1992

Concepcion MA, Lambert DH, Welch KA: Tourniquet pain during spinal anesthesia: a comparison of plain solution of tetracaine and bupivacaine. Anesth Analg 67:828, 1988

Denny N, Masters R, Pearson D, et al: Postdural puncture headache after continuous spinal anesthesia. Anesth Analg 66:791, 1987

Freedman JM, Li DK, Drasner K, et al: Transient neurologic symptoms after spinal anesthesia: An epidemiologic study of 1,863 patients. Anesthesiology 89:533, 1998

Kang SB, Goodnough DE, Lee YK, et al: Comparison of 26- and 27-g needles for spinal anesthesia for ambulatory surgery patients. Anesthesiology 76:734, 1992

Lambert DH, Hurley RJ: Cauda equina syndrome and continuous spinal anesthesia. Anesth Analg 72:817, 1991

Levy JA, Islos JA, Ghia JN, et al: A retrospective study of the incidence and causes of failed spinal anesthetics in a university hospital. Anesth Analg 64:705, 1985

Machikanti L, Hadley C, Markwell SJ: A retrospective analysis of failed spinal anesthetic attempts in a community hospital. Anesth Analg 66:363, 1987

Mihic DN: Postspinal headache and relationship of needle bevel to longitudinal dural fibers. Reg Anesth 10:76, 1985

Munhall RJ, Sukhani R, Winnie AP: Incidence of etiology of failed spinal anesthetics in a university hospital: a prospective study. Anesth Analg 67:843, 1988

Norris MC: Height, weight, and the spread of subarachnoid hyperbaric bupivacaine in the term parturient. Anesth Analg 67: 555, 1988

Ota K, Namiki A, Ujike Y, Takashi I: Prolongation of tetracaine spinal anesthesia by oral clonidine. Anesth Analg 75: 262, 1992

Reed AP, Atlin N, Kreitzer JM: Inability to pass continuous spinal catheters: explanations and recommendations. Anesth Rev 18:44, 1991

Rigler ML, Drasner K, Krejcie TC, et al: Cauda equina syndrome after continuous spinal anesthesia. Anesth Analg 72:275, 1991

Ross BK, Chadwick HS, Mancuso JJ, Benedetti C: Sprotte needle for obstetric anesthesia: decreased incidence of post-dural puncture headache. Reg Anesth 17:29, 1992

Tuominen M, Pitkanen M, Taivainen T, Rosenberg PH: Prediction of the spread of repeated spinal anesthesia with bupivacaine. Br J Anesth 68:136, 1992

Vandam LD, Dripps RD: Long-term follow-up of patients who received 10,098 spinal anesthetics. JAMA 172:1483, 1960

BRACHIAL PLEXUS ANESTHESIA

Jodi L.W. Reiss, MD

A 54-year-old man with a left rotator cuff tear presents for shoulder arthroscopy. His past medical history is significant for chronic obstructive pulmonary disease. After a previous general anesthetic, he remained intubated overnight and would now prefer to have regional anesthesia. Performance of the regional anesthetic proceeds uneventfully, but 45 minutes into the procedure the patient becomes profoundly hypotensive and develops bradycardia.

QUESTIONS

1. Describe the anatomic course of the brachial plexus.
2. What structures of the upper extremity do the terminal branches of the brachial plexus innervate?
3. What are the anatomic landmarks of the axilla?
4. What are the major approaches to blocking the brachial plexus and their indications for use?
5. Describe the interscalene approach to blocking the brachial plexus.
6. Describe the supraclavicular approach to blocking the brachial plexus.
7. Describe the infraclavicular approach to blocking the brachial plexus.
8. Describe the axillary approach to blocking the brachial plexus.
9. What complications can arise from upper extremity blocks?
10. What is the Bezold-Jarisch reflex?
11. What local anesthetics are appropriate for blocks of the brachial plexus and in what doses?
12. Is chronic obstructive pulmonary disease (COPD) a contraindication to performing an interscalene block?

1. Describe the anatomic course of the brachial plexus.

The brachial plexus is composed of the ventral rami of C_{5-8} and T_1, and at times includes C_4 and T_2. These nerve roots combine to form three trunks – the superior (C_{5-6}), the middle (C_7), and the inferior (C_8–T_1) – after passing between the anterior and middle scalene muscles. The plexus continues its course under the clavicle and over the first rib. At the lateral border of the first rib, each trunk divides into an anterior and a posterior division. In the axilla these divisions form three cords. The anterior divisions of the superior and middle trunks form the lateral cord. The posterior divisions of all three trunks form the posterior cord. The anterior division of the inferior cord continues as the medial cord. The cords acquire their names from their anatomic relationship to the axillary artery. Finally, at the lateral border of the pectoralis minor muscle in the axilla, the cords give rise to the terminal branches of the brachial plexus. The posterior cord terminates as the axillary and radial nerves. The lateral cord splits to form the musculocutaneous nerve and with the medial cord forms the median nerve. The medial cord also terminates as the ulnar nerve.

2. What structures of the upper extremity do the terminal branches of the brachial plexus innervate?

Table 57.1 shows the structures of the upper extremity that the brachial plexus innervates.

3. What are the anatomic landmarks of the axilla?

The axilla is a pyramidal structure consisting of an apex and base and surrounded on all four sides by different anatomic landmarks. The clavicle makes up the apex of the axilla, and its base is the concave armpit. The anterior wall consists of the pectoralis muscles. The posterior wall embodies the scapula and scapular muscles, the subscapularis, and teres major. The median wall is made up of the serratus anterior muscle and the humerus comprises the lateral wall, along with its surrounding muscles and tendons.

4. What are the major approaches to blocking the brachial plexus and their indications for use?

There are four major approaches to blocking the brachial plexus:

- The interscalene approach is performed at the level of the nerve roots and is ideal for surgical procedures of the shoulder and upper arm.
- The supraclavicular block, which produces a fast onset of anesthesia because of the compact nature of the

divisions in the plexus, is also appropriate for surgical procedures of the upper arm.
- The infraclavicular approach is indicated for surgeries that include the elbow and hand. It is ideal for patients who are unable to abduct and extend their arms in order to perform an axillary block. This approach is also exemplary for continuous postoperative analgesia because of the ease of catheter stabilization on the chest wall.
- The axillary block is performed at the level of the terminal branches and is ideal for surgeries distal to the elbow. Frequently, the musculocutaneous nerve is missed during this block.

To avoid nerve injury during performance of peripheral blocks, they should not be performed while the patient is under general anesthesia.

5. Describe the interscalene approach to blocking the brachial plexus.

The interscalene block can be achieved by either a paresthesia or nerve stimulator technique. With the patient in the supine position, arms at the side and head turned to the contralateral side, the landmarks are identified. At the level of C_6, the lateral border of the clavicular head of the sternocleidomastoid muscle is palpated. The fingers are then rolled posteriorly onto the belly of the anterior scalene muscle. The interscalene groove is located posterior to the anterior scalene muscle, between the anterior and middle scalene muscles, and is the point of needle insertion.

TABLE 57.1		Innervation of the Nerves of the Brachial Plexus	
Nerve	**Branch**	**Motor Supply**	**Sensory Supply**
Ulnar	C_8–T_1	Interosseous muscles of the hand Flexor muscles of the hand	Medial half of the hand Medial half of the 4th finger 5th finger
Median	C_5–T_1	Flexor muscles of the hand	Palmar surface of the hand Digits 1–3, and lateral fourth of the 4th finger
Radial	C_5–T_1	Triceps Brachioradialis Extensor muscles of thumb and fingers	Posterior forearm Posterior hand
Axillary	C_5–C_6	Deltoid	Posterior shoulder Posterior arm
Musculocutaneous	C_5–C_7	Biceps Coracobrachialis Brachialis	Lateral forearm

Using a 22G 2-inch *insulated* needle attached to a nerve stimulator, the skin is pierced at a 45° angle aiming toward the sternal notch. Proper positioning of the needle is determined by the detection of twitches of the triceps muscle and/or wrist movements when the nerve stimulator is at or below 0.4 mA. The local anesthetic preparation is injected, aspirating every 5 cc to avoid intravascular injection of large amounts of local anesthetic. This block usually requires a volume of 40 cc of local anesthetic to be successful. A 1:1 mixture of mepivacaine 1.5% and bupivacaine 0.5% provides a quick onset of anesthesia and a block of long duration.

6. Describe the supraclavicular approach to blocking the brachial plexus.

With the patient supine, arms at the side, and head turned to the contralateral side, the midpoint of the clavicle is identified. At the superior border, a 22G 4-inch *insulated* needle is inserted, directed caudally in the plane of the patient. Making contact with the first rib, one then walks off the rib posteriorly until a paresthesia is achieved. After a negative aspiration, a volume of 40 cc of local anesthetic is injected. The same preparation as used for the interscalene block can also be used here. It is important to be aware that the subclavian artery is in close proximity to this area and, if punctured, it would be very difficult to provide adequate compression. This block has a high incidence of pneumothorax.

7. Describe the infraclavicular approach to blocking the brachial plexus.

There are several different approaches to the infraclavicular block. One effective technique uses the coracoid process as the major landmark. With the patient supine, head turned to the contralateral side, and arms at the side, the coracoid process is identified. One then measures 2 cm caudad and 2 cm medial to the coracoid. Using a 22G 4-inch *insulated* needle attached to a nerve stimulator, the needle is aimed posteriorly and laterally. When forearm and hand twitches are elicited at or below 0.4 mA, the local anesthetic is injected, making sure to aspirate after every 5 cc. A catheter can be inserted for postoperative pain relief. For a long-acting block, 40 cc of bupivacaine 0.5% is effective.

8. Describe the axillary approach to blocking the brachial plexus.

There are four different methods for ascertaining the correct position of the needle: paresthesia, transarterial, nerve stimulator, or blunt needle through the sheath method. This block requires the patient to lie supine with the arm abducted to a 90° angle.

The transarterial method is the method most commonly used. With this method, the axillary artery is palpated in the axilla and stabilized between two fingers. A 23G 1½-inch blunt-tipped needle is advanced toward the pulsations. A pop is usually appreciated as the needle enters the fascial sheath. As arterial blood is aspirated, the needle is slowly advanced until blood is no longer aspirated. The needle will now be posterior to the artery. Half of the local anesthetic preparation is injected, gently aspirating after every 5 cc. Then, the needle is retracted slowly until it is anterior to the artery (when no arterial blood is aspirated). The remainder of the local anesthetic preparation is injected at this site. Pressure should be held over the injection site for approximately 10 minutes to prevent hematoma formation. For short procedures, 40 cc of lidocaine 1.5% or mepivacaine 1.5% may be used. If a longer-duration block is required, a 1:1 solution of either of the above can be mixed with bupivacaine 0.5%.

9. What complications can arise from upper extremity blocks?

The complications that can arise from upper extremity blocks are shown in Table 57.2.

10. What is the Bezold-Jarisch reflex?

Mechanoreceptors in the left ventricle activate inhibitory vagal afferents to increase sympathetic tone and guard the body against hypotension. This protective physiologic response occurs during times of severe stress, such as hemorrhage. The Bezold-Jarisch reflex is a paradoxical activation of these left ventricular receptors by a decrease in venous return, causing a decrease in sympathetic tone with an increase in vagal outflow. This produces severe bradycardia and hypotension, which can lead to asystole.

Patients undergoing shoulder repair are at risk for activating this reflex. The "beach chair" position causing pooling of blood in the lower extremities, patient anxiety and the addition of epinephrine to the arthroscopy infusate are all factors contributing to this phenomenon.

Ephedrine is the treatment of choice because it has a direct action on the heart and peripheral activation of catecholamines. Fluid resuscitation is important to prevent further stimulation of these receptors. If progression to asystole occurs, epinephrine is essential. Atropine will not adequately treat this event, should it occur.

11. What local anesthetics are used for blocks of the brachial plexus and in what doses?

Local anesthetics are sodium channel blockers that inhibit the progression of the action potential across the

TABLE 57.2	Complications of upper extremity blocks

Interscalene	Supraclavicular	Infraclavicular	Axillary
Vertebral artery injection	Pneumothorax	Pneumothorax	Nerve injury
Epidural injection	Subclavian artery injection	Nerve injury	Axillary hematoma
Total spinal	Recurrent laryngeal nerve block	Seizure	Seizure
Subdural injection	Nerve injury		
Pneumothorax	Seizure		
Nerve injury			
Seizure			
Side-effects			
Recurrent laryngeal nerve block			
Ipsilateral diaphragmatic paralysis			
Horner's syndrome			

membrane. Therefore, nerve impulses are interrupted. There are two main groups of local anesthetics: esters and amides. Both consist of a hydrophilic hydrocarbon chain and a lipophilic aromatic ring. The ester anesthetics have an ester bond (-CO-), whereas the amides have an amide bond (-NHC-) linking the two groups.

The amide local anesthetics used for brachial plexus anesthesia are lidocaine, mepivacaine, bupivacaine, levobupivacaine, and ropivacaine. Each differs in its duration of onset, action, and toxicity (Table 57.3). The surgical procedure and need for postoperative analgesia must be considered when choosing an appropriate drug. Lidocaine and/or mepivacaine can be used for surgical procedures of short duration, such as carpal tunnel repair or bone manipulations. Surgeries of much longer duration, such as joint replacements, benefit from bupivacaine, ropivacaine, or levobupivacaine. When postoperative pain control is needed, a mixture of a short- and a long-acting anesthetic is optimal. The newer local anesthetics, levobupivacaine and ropivacaine, are less cardiotoxic than bupivacaine, and therefore may be safer to use.

12. Is chronic obstructive pulmonary disease (COPD) a contraindication to performing an interscalene block?

COPD is a relative contraindication to performing an interscalene block. Ipsilateral phrenic nerve paralysis occurs in all patients who receive an interscalene block, which will result in a 25% decrease in pulmonary function. Therefore, patients who cannot tolerate a 25% decrease in pulmonary function should not be considered for this block.

Other contraindications to regional anesthesia include: patient refusal, infection at the site of needle insertion, anatomic anomalies, allergies to local anesthetics used, and severe coagulopathies.

TABLE 57.3	Local Anesthetics

Local Anesthetic	Onset	Duration (minutes)	Maximum Dose (mg/kg)	Concentration (%)
Lidocaine	Fast	60–120	4–5 7 (w/epinephrine)	0.5–2
Mepivacaine	Intermediate	90–180	5–6	1.5
Bupivacaine	Slow	240–480	1–3	0.5
Levobupivacaine	Slow	240–480	1–3	0.5
Ropivacaine	Slow	240–480	1–3	0.5

SUGGESTED READINGS

Borgeat A, Edatodramis G, Kalberar F, Benz C: Acute and non-acute complications associated with interscalene block and shoulder surgery. Anesthesiology 95:875–880, 2001

Brown DL: Atlas of Regional Anesthesia, 2nd edition. WB Saunders, Philadelphia, 1999

Brown AR: Regional anesthesia for shoulder surgery. Techniques in Regional Anesthesia and Pain Management 3:64–78, 1999

Campagna JA, Carter C: Clinical relevance of the Bezold-Jarisch reflex. Anesthesiology 98:1250–1260, 2003

de Jong R: Local anesthetic pharmacology. pp.124–142. In Brown DL (ed): Regional Anesthesia and Analgesia, 1st edition. WB Saunders, Philadelphia, 1996

Kinsella SM, Tuckey JP: Perioperative bradycardia and asystole: relationship to vasovagal syncope and the Bezold-Jarisch reflex. Br J Anesth 86:859–868, 2001

Pollock JE: Regional anesthesia for hand surgery. Techniques in Regional Anesthesia and Pain Management 3:79–84, 1999

Stoelting RK: Local anesthetics. pp.158–181. In Stoelting RK (ed): Pharmacology and Physiology in Anesthetic Practice, 3rd edition. Lippincott-Raven, New York, 1999

Urmey WF: Upper extremity blocks. p. 254. In Brown DL (ed): Regional Anesthesia and Analgesia, 1st edition. WB Saunders, Philadelphia 1996

Wilson JL, Brown DL, Wong GY, Ehman RL, Cahill DR: Infraclavicular brachial plexus block: parasagittal anatomy important to coracoid technique. Anesth Analg 87:870–873, 1998

58

LOWER EXTREMITY ANESTHESIA

Dan A. Kaufman, MD

A 62-year-old former professional football player presents for a total knee arthroplasty. He is in otherwise excellent health.

QUESTIONS

1. What are the anesthetic options for this patient?
2. What are the advantages and disadvantages of the various anesthetic options?
3. Describe the innervation of the lower extremity.
4. Why is a sciatic nerve block necessary for adequate anesthesia for a total knee arthroplasty?
5. How are femoral and sciatic nerve blocks performed? Which local anesthetic agents would you use?
6. Would you sedate the patient for the performance of the femoral and sciatic nerve blocks and/or during the procedure?
7. After performing the block and starting a propofol infusion, the patient begins to flail about upon surgical incision. Should you induce general anesthesia?
8. Describe the use of the tourniquet in a total knee arthroplasty and its hemodynamic consequences.
9. What are the options for postoperative pain control?

1. What are the anesthetic options for this patient?

A total knee arthroplasty allows for several different types of anesthesia and all of the following are acceptable choices:

- General anesthesia
- Neuraxial anesthesia
  Spinal
  Epidural
  Combined spinal/epidural (CSE)
- Regional anesthesia
  Femoral nerve block (psoas compartment block) in combination with a sciatic nerve block
- Combinations of the above
  e.g., general anesthesia and femoral nerve block.

The type of anesthesia chosen will depend on the anesthesiologist's evaluation of the patient's condition and personal preference, the surgeon's needs, and the patient's preference.

2. What are the advantages and disadvantages of the various anesthetic options?

General anesthesia allows for excellent muscle relaxation and a secure airway. Also, the anesthetic can be continued for as long as the procedure lasts. However, it necessitates multiple drugs and may foster hemodynamic instability. There is also a strong possibility of the patient incurring postoperative nausea and vomiting from volatile agents, opioids, and reversal agents, and a sore throat if tracheal intubation is performed.

Spinal anesthesia also provides excellent muscle relaxation, but like general anesthesia may cause hemodynamic instability. While general anesthesia can continue indefinitely, a spinal anesthetic will only last a finite amount of time (as spinal catheters are not utilized currently) and may wear off in the middle of a case, necessitating conversion to a general anesthetic. Intrathecal morphine can provide excellent postoperative pain relief but requires appropriate monitoring. Other complications associated with spinal anesthesia include but are not limited to postdural puncture headache, back pain, transient neuropathies, and the rare but devastating consequence of epidural abscess and hematoma.

Epidural anesthesia can be titrated to allow for better hemodynamic stability. If a catheter is placed, the anesthetic can be prolonged for an indefinite period of time. A catheter can also be utilized for postoperative pain control. Onset is significantly slower than for spinal anesthesia and at times muscle relaxation may not be adequate, especially when there is a "patchy" block. An epidural, like a spinal, carries the risk of neurologic complications, headache, back pain, infection, and hematoma.

Both spinal and epidural anesthesia seem to decrease the risk of deep vein thrombosis in the lower extremity.

A combined spinal/epidural technique provides the excellent muscle relaxation and quick onset of spinal anesthesia and the ability to provide anesthesia indefinitely by placement of the epidural catheter. A disadvantage of this technique, however, is that the efficacy of the epidural catheter cannot be tested until the spinal anesthetic has begun to recede. If the catheter is non-functional, this would necessitate converting to a general anesthetic in the middle of the surgical procedure.

Femoral and sciatic nerve blocks, while somewhat time-consuming to perform, in experienced hands probably take as long as the performance of a difficult spinal anesthetic. These nerve blocks, like neuraxial anesthetics, obviate the need for the polypharmacy associated with general anesthesia and at the same time allow for greater hemodynamic stability compared with neuraxial anesthesia. The placement of femoral and sciatic nerve catheters allow for the provision of excellent postoperative pain control.

3. Describe the innervation of the lower extremity.

The lower extremity is innervated by the lumbar plexus and the sciatic plexus.

The lumbar plexus consists of six nerves:

- The upper part consists of three nerves: ilioinguinal, genitofemoral, and iliohypogastric. These nerves supply parts of the anterior abdominal wall, buttocks, and perineum. The lower part consists of three nerves: femoral, lateral cutaneous nerve of the thigh, and obturator. The femoral is the main nerve of concern in a total knee arthroplasty. It supplies innervation to the anterior

Advantages and Disadvantages of Anesthetic Techniques

General Anesthesia
    Advantages
        Secure airway
        Excellent muscle relaxation
        Length of procedure not a factor
    Disadvantages
        Possible hemodynamic instability
        Postoperative nausea and vomiting
        Sore throat, hoarseness

Spinal anesthesia
    Advantages
        Excellent muscle relaxation
        Decreases the incidence of deep vein thrombosis
        Quick onset
    Disadvantages
        Possible hemodynamic instability
        Length of procedure a factor due to finite time of anesthesia
        Postdural puncture headache

Epidural anesthesia
    Advantages
        Better hemodynamic control as able to titrate anesthetic level
        Length of procedure not a factor
        Ability to use catheter for postoperative pain control
        Decreased incidence of deep vein thrombosis
    Disadvantages
        Slower onset than spinal anesthesia
        Muscle relaxation may not be adequate
        Postdural puncture headache

Combined spinal/epidural anesthesia
    Advantages
        Quick onset
        Excellent muscle relaxation (during spinal portion)
        Decreased incidence of deep vein thrombosis
    Disadvantages
        Unknown whether epidural catheter effective until later during surgery

Continued

portion of the thigh and knee and to the quadriceps, sartorius, pectineal, and vastus muscles. It continues as the saphenous nerve below the knee and provides sensory innervation to the medial aspect of the leg in this region. The lateral femoral cutaneous nerve provides sensory innervation to the lateral aspect of the thigh, and the obturator nerve provides innervation to the adductors of the thigh and sensory innervation to the medial aspect of the thigh.

Innervation of the Lower Extremity

Lumbar plexus
    Femoral nerve
        Sensory – anterior portion of the thigh and
            knee
        Motor – quadriceps, sartorius, and pectineal
            muscles
    Saphenous nerve
        Sensory – medial aspect of the leg below the
            knee
    Lateral femoral cutaneous nerve
        Sensory – lateral aspect of the thigh
    Obturator nerve
        Sensory – medial aspect of the thigh
        Motor – adductor muscles of the thigh

Sciatic plexus
    Sciatic nerve
        Motor – hamstring muscles
    Common peroneal and posterior tibial nerves
        Sensory – leg below the knee except for the
            medial aspect
        Motor – all muscles below the knee
    Posterior cutaneous nerve
        Sensory – posterior aspect of the thigh

The sciatic plexus consists of the sciatic and the posterior cutaneous nerves of the thigh. The sciatic nerve provides innervation to the hamstring muscles. At the popliteal fossa the sciatic nerve splits into the common peroneal and posterior tibial nerves, which together provide all the motor innervation to the leg below the knee and sensory innervation to this area except for the medial part of the leg below the knee, which is provided by the saphenous nerve. The posterior cutaneous nerve provides sensory innervation to the posterior aspect of the thigh.

4. Why is a sciatic nerve block necessary for adequate anesthesia for a total knee arthroplasty?

Firstly, most orthopedists utilize a thigh tourniquet for the total knee arthroplasty to minimize blood loss. Without the sciatic nerve block, the posterior thigh would not be anesthetized. Secondly, although there is a trend in the orthopedic world to minimize the incision for a total knee arthroplasty, it may still extend into an area below the knee that is not innervated by the femoral or saphenous nerves. Thirdly, drilling into the anterior knee may reach posterior portions of the knee which are not innervated by the femoral nerve.

5. How are femoral and sciatic nerve blocks performed? Which local anesthetic agents would you use?

There is no one way to perform these blocks. There are variations in all the parameters and how a block is performed is usually user-dependent. The reader is directed to the suggested reading list for more details about these blocks. The following is this author's preferred method for performing these blocks.

Femoral Nerve Block

With the patient in the supine position, the femoral artery is palpated. Approximately 1–2 cm below the inguinal ligament and lateral to the artery a 2 inch needle attached to a nerve stimulator set at 1.5 milliamps is inserted. The needle is slowly advanced until a quadriceps twitch or a "patella snap" is elicited. The nerve stimulator is lowered to 0.4 milliamps and if the "patella snap" is still present, local anesthetic is injected.

Sciatic Nerve Block

With the patient in the lateral decubitus position (operative side up), a line is drawn between the greater trochanter and posterior superior iliac spine. A 5 cm line is drawn perpendicularly caudad from the midpoint of this line. At this point, a 4 or 6 inch needle attached to a nerve stimulator set at 1.5 milliamps is inserted and is advanced until a hamstring twitch or any motor movement in the foot is elicited. Local anesthetic is injected when the twitch is still present at less than 0.4 milliamps.

The choice of local anesthetic will be dependent on the length of the procedure, the quickness of the surgeon, whether a catheter will be placed, the toxicity of each local anesthetic, and the user's preference. One option for either of the above-described blocks is to use 30 cc of ropivacaine 0.5% with epinephrine 1:200,000. This provides for a long duration of anesthesia and, while the onset may not be as quick as with mepivacaine, there is usually sufficient time from when the block is performed to surgical incision for the anesthetic to take effect.

6. Would you sedate the patient for the performance of the femoral and sciatic nerve blocks and/or during the procedure?

This is controversial and depends on many factors. Many patients do not want to have any awareness of the operating room and will only agree to regional anesthesia if they are convinced that this will be the case. In most instances, sedation facilitates a smoother induction of a regional anesthetic. Midazolam, fentanyl, or small doses of propofol is appropriate in this setting. The disadvantages of sedating the patient during performance of the block are that paresthesias and/or symptoms of local anesthetic toxicity (e.g., metallic taste, seizure) will go unnoticed. Sometimes, patients become disinhibited with sedation, which will interfere with performance of the block as well.

During the procedure, a propofol infusion provides adequate sedation. However, the anesthesiologist should be prepared to treat the negative respiratory and hemodynamic effects of this drug.

7. After performing the block and starting a propofol infusion, the patient begins to flail about upon surgical incision. Should you induce general anesthesia?

The first consideration in the agitated patient is hypoxia from respiratory compromise. In addition, hemodynamic instability, such as from a myocardial infarction, should be addressed as well. Another cause of agitation in this setting might be local anesthetic toxicity. Once these more serious causes are ruled out, one needs to consider the adequacy of the block(s) and other related causes. Patient movement from surgical incision does not necessarily mean that the block is inadequate. Some things to consider are:

- Was there enough time for the local anesthetic to take complete effect?
- Is the patient responding to pain or pressure?
- Is the propofol infusion causing burning in his arm?
- Is the patient disinhibited from the propofol infusion?

The skin is usually the last organ to be anesthetized and local infiltration by the surgeon will usually overcome this deficit. Of course any block, even in the best of hands, may fail and an alternative anesthetic will need to be instituted. Usually this means that general anesthesia is induced.

8. Describe the use of the tourniquet in a total knee arthroplasty and its hemodynamic consequences.

The use of a tourniquet in a total knee arthroplasty is standard and is used to minimize blood loss. Inflation of the tourniquet can be quite painful and therefore, needs to be considered in the anesthetic plan. General, neuraxial, and regional anesthesia provide excellent relief from tourniquet pain. The tourniquet is usually set to an inflation pressure above the patient's blood pressure, commonly 350 mmHg for the lower extremity. The inflation time is usually limited to 2 hours of continuous use. Longer tourniquet times can result in a metabolic acidosis and ischemic changes in the operative limb.

The release of the tourniquet results in a transient systemic metabolic acidosis and increase in arterial carbon dioxide. A small increase in heart rate, drop in blood pressure, and rise in serum potassium may also be noted. It is prudent to administer a fluid bolus prior to tourniquet release. Usually these changes result in no adverse effects to the patient.

9. What are the options for postoperative pain control?

Patient-controlled analgesia (PCA) with opioids, such as morphine sulfate or fentanyl, is an appropriate choice for postoperative pain control in the absence of indwelling catheters (epidural or femoral-sciatic). While PCA provides patients with better control of their pain, it is associated with nausea and vomiting that may need treatment. In addition, older patients may be more sensitive to the effects of the opioid and may become heavily sedated and ultimately apneic. Appropriate PCA settings and monitoring are necessary for the safe administration of a PCA in these patients.

The placement of an epidural catheter has the advantage in that it allows for the administration of an opioid and/or local anesthetic. However, nausea, vomiting, and itching may occur. In addition, the use of anticoagulation and antiplatelet medications in the postoperative period has to be coordinated with removal of the epidural catheter.

Intrathecal opioids can provide excellent pain control but they only last up to 24 hours. Nausea, vomiting, and itching may occur as well with this modality.

Femoral and sciatic catheters provide excellent pain control but their use needs to be coordinated with the patient's physical therapy program. Otherwise, the patient may not have adequate motor function at a time when it is important to be able to move the operative extremity.

SUGGESTED READINGS

Bernstein RL, Rosenberg AD: Manual of Orthopedic Anesthesia and Related Pain Syndromes. Churchill Livingstone, New York, 1993

Boezaart AP: Regional Anesthesia Study Center of Iowa Workshop Course Material. CD ROM. University of Iowa, 2003

New York School of Regional Anesthesia Website: www. nysora.com

Rogers JN, Ramamurthy S: Lower extremity blocks. Chapter 17. In Brown DL (ed): Regional Anesthesia and Analgesia. WB Saunders, Philadelphia, 1996

59

LABOR AND DELIVERY

Yaakov Beilin, MD

A 27-year-old woman presents to the delivery suite in labor after an uncomplicated pregnancy. A lumbar epidural catheter is placed at the L_4–L_5 interspace to facilitate analgesia. After an adequate trial of labor, the obstetricians elect to perform a cesarean section for cephalopelvic disproportion. A T_4 level of anesthesia is achieved via the epidural catheter and the cesarean section is initiated. Immediately after delivery of the baby, maternal hemorrhage becomes severe.

QUESTIONS

1. What options are available to the mother for labor analgesia?
2. Explain the advantages and disadvantages of various regional anesthetic techniques for labor and delivery.
3. What is a "walking epidural"?
4. Describe the regional anesthetic techniques that can be employed for cesarean section.
5. Outline the treatment for postdural puncture headache.
6. What are the advantages and disadvantages of general anesthesia for cesarean section?
7. Describe the elements of placental drug transfer.
8. What techniques can be used for post-cesarean pain relief?

9. Outline the differential diagnosis of postpartum hemorrhage.
10. Explain the risk factors, presentation, and treatment of uterine atony.
11. Describe the presentation and treatment of retained placenta.

1. What options are available to the mother for labor analgesia?

Many techniques have been utilized to reduce the perception of pain during labor. In addition to systemic medications, inhalation agents, and regional anesthesia, hypnosis, psychoprophylaxis, acupuncture, and transcutaneous electrical nerve stimulation (TENS) have been used.

Systemic opioids can be used to attenuate labor pains; however, low-dose opioids do not completely eliminate the pain. Meperidine is the most frequently used opioid for labor analgesia. Intravenous meperidine peaks in about 10 minutes and lasts approximately 3–4 hours. Neonates born within 2 hours of maternal administration of meperidine are at risk for respiratory depression. Morphine is rarely used during labor because neonates are extremely sensitive to its respiratory depressant effect. Remifentanil can be used as part of patient-controlled analgesia (PCA) during labor. The advantage of remifentanil is that its onset and duration of action are shorter than those of meperidine. However, it is also more potent and close maternal respiratory monitoring is required, preferably with pulse oximetry.

The goal of inhalation analgesia during labor is to achieve analgesia without depressing airway reflexes. Typically, at the beginning of each contraction the mother, using a hand-held device, self-administers the anesthetic agents. The most commonly used vapors are nitrous oxide and enflurane. Although this technique provides moderately good analgesia, it is not commonly used because of the risk of maternal aspiration with deep levels of anesthesia.

Regional anesthesia, epidural or combined spinal-epidural, have become popular modalities for labor analgesia because of their safety and efficacy profile.

2. Explain the advantages and disadvantages of various regional anesthetic techniques for labor and delivery.

Rational use of regional anesthesia necessitates an understanding of the pain pathways involved during labor. Labor is traditionally divided into three distinct stages:

- First stage: begins with the onset of regular contractions and ends with complete cervical dilation.
- Second stage: begins when the cervix is completely dilated and ends with delivery of the fetus.
- Third stage: begins after delivery of the fetus and concludes with delivery of the placenta.

The first stage of labor is associated with uterine and cervical pain mediated by spinal segments T_{10}–L_1 (Fig. 59.1). Local anesthetics administered to the epidural, spinal, or caudal spaces readily anesthetize these pain pathways. In addition, subarachnoid opioids and paracervical blocks can be used for pain relief during the first stage of labor.

Caudal anesthesia is rarely used because of the risk of inadvertent fetal scalp penetration and the associated high fetal levels of local anesthetic.

The second stage of labor is associated with perineal and vaginal distention mediated by spinal segments S_2–S_4. Epidural, spinal, and caudal anesthetics are also effective during the second stage of labor. In addition, pudendal nerve blocks can be used for second-stage analgesia.

Epidural analgesia is the most popular technique for the relief of labor pain. Its popularity is first and foremost related to its efficacy. Women can obtain almost complete relief from the pain of labor. From the anesthesiologist's perspective, because a catheter is threaded into the epidural space, it is also a versatile technique. During the earlier stages of labor, dilute solutions of local anesthetic can be used to achieve analgesia. As labor progresses, a more concentrated solution of local anesthetic may be necessary or an adjunct, such as an opioid, may be needed. Additionally, the epidural catheter can be utilized to maintain a low dermatomal level of anesthesia for labor (T_{10}–L_1) and, when needed, the dermatomal level can be raised to T_4 for cesarean section.

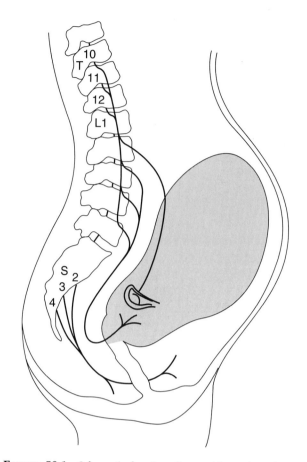

FIGURE 59.1   Schematic drawing of parturition pain pathways. First-stage labor pain is due to uterine contraction and cervical dilatation. Afferent pain fibers from the uterus and cervix accompany sympathetic fibers and enter the spinal cord from T_{10} to L_1. Second-stage labor pain originates from the vagina and perineum. Afferent pain fibers from the vagina and perineum course with the pudendal nerves, S_2–S_4. (From Stoelting RK, Miller RD: Basics of Anesthesia, 3rd edition. Churchill Livingston, New York, 1994, p. 364, with permission.)

Patient-controlled epidural analgesia (PCEA) is a technique that allows the patient to self-medicate, thereby controlling her own analgesia. Compared with continuous infusion or intermittent bolus techniques, PCEA is associated with a lower total dose of local anesthetic, less motor blockade, and fewer interventions by anesthesiologists. Although maternal satisfaction may be greater with PCEA, the above-stated advantages have not been documented in all studies. Therefore, this technique is not routinely offered.

A commonly used PCEA regimen is bupivacaine 0.0625% with fentanyl 2 µg/mL with the following PCEA settings: basal rate of 10 mL/hr, bolus dose of 5 mL,

10 minute lockout, and a 30 mL/hr maximum limit. A basal rate is not always used because it may be associated with a greater total milligram dose of local anesthetic when compared with the total milligram dose when a basal rate is used. Theoretical risks of PCEA, such as high dermatomal levels or overdose, have been described in the general surgical patient. Overdose occurs because of catheter migration into the subarachnoid space or from excessive administration by the patient or a helpful family member. To date, these complications have not been reported in the parturient during labor.

There are a number of disadvantages with labor epidural analgesia that have prompted the search for alternative techniques. One disadvantage is the time it takes to provide analgesia to the patient. The time from epidural catheter placement until the patient is comfortable is variable, but depending on the local anesthetic used can take up to 30 minutes. Other disadvantages of labor epidural analgesia include: maternal hypotension, inadequate analgesia (15–20% of cases), and motor blockade, even with the very dilute local anesthetic solutions.

Subarachnoid opioids offer rapid, intense analgesia with minimal changes in blood pressure or motor function. Most patients can, if desired, ambulate with this technique. The opioid is usually administered as part of a combined spinal-epidural (CSE) technique where a spinal and an epidural are performed at the same time. After locating the epidural space in the usual manner, a long small-gauge spinal needle is inserted through the epidural needle into the subarachnoid space. An opioid (usually fentanyl 25 μg or sufentanil 5 μg), either alone or in combination with a local anesthetic, is administered through the spinal needle. The spinal needle is removed and an epidural catheter is inserted for future use. Analgesia begins within 3–5 minutes and lasts 1–1.5 hours.

There are several advantages to the CSE technique. The primary advantage is the rapid (3–5 min) onset of analgesia. There is also less motor blockade. Because of these advantages there is greater satisfaction by women who receive a CSE than those who receive the "standard" epidural technique of bupivacaine 0.25%.

There are some concerns about CSE, most of which are only theoretical but have not been documented. There is no increased risk of subarachnoid catheter migration of the epidural catheter. Metallic particles are not produced as a result of passing one needle through another. The incidence of postdural puncture headache is not increased by the intentional dural puncture. Fetal bradycardia in association with a hypertonic uterus may occur immediately or shortly after induction of either epidural or subarachnoid labor analgesia. There does not appear to be any difference in the incidence of fetal heart rate decelerations or emergent cesarean section following labor epidural or spinal anesthesia. One proposed theory for increased uterine tone after CSE is related to the rapid decrease in maternal catecholamines associated with the rapid onset of pain relief. The decrease in circulating β-adrenergic agonists results in a predominance of α activity, which causes uterine contractions. If this should occur, treatment is with subcutaneous terbutaline or intravenous nitroglycerin.

3. What is a "walking epidural"?

The term "walking epidural" has become popular, especially in the lay community. The term refers to any epidural

Stages of Labor

	Begins	Ends	Innervation	Anesthesia
First	Regular contractions	Complete cervical dilation	T_{10}–L_1	E, S, C Subarachnoid opioids Paracervical block
Second	Complete cervical dilation	Delivery of the fetus	S_2–S_4	E, S, C Pudendal block
Third	Delivery of the fetus	Delivery of the placenta		

Note: caudal analgesia is rarely used.
E, epidural; S, spinal; C, caudal.

or spinal technique that allows the parturient to ambulate. Some initial retrospective data had suggested that ambulating or the upright position is associated with a shorter first stage of labor, less pain in early labor, and decreased analgesia requirements. However, prospective and randomized studies have not been able to document any medical benefit of ambulating, in terms of either duration of labor or mode of delivery.

Although few patients really want to ambulate, using a technique that produces minimal motor blockade will improve maternal satisfaction. Both epidural analgesia using dilute local anesthetic/opioid solutions or a CSE technique can achieve this goal. However, several precautions should be taken before allowing a parturient to walk after receiving epidural or CSE analgesia. First, it should be determined whether she is a candidate for intermittent fetal heart rate monitoring. Blood pressure and fetal heart rate should be monitored for 30–60 minutes after induction of analgesia and reassessed at least every 30 minutes thereafter. Because even small doses of subarachnoid and epidural local anesthetics can produce motor deficits, motor function should be assessed. This is accomplished by asking the parturient to perform a modified deep knee bend or step up and down on a stool. She must have an escort at all times.

4. Describe the regional anesthetic techniques that can be employed for cesarean section.

Regional anesthetic techniques include spinal and epidural anesthesia. During regional anesthesia the mother remains awake during the delivery, thereby significantly decreasing the risk of maternal aspiration associated with general anesthesia. Regional anesthesia also minimizes the potential for depression of the neonate from maternal drug administration. Because regional anesthesia is safer than general anesthesia for both the mother and the fetus, it should be used for all elective cesarean deliveries.

Relatively few absolute contraindications exist to regional anesthesia. These include infection at the injection site, severe hypovolemia, raised intracranial pressure, patient refusal, and coagulation abnormalities. Relative contraindications include neurologic disease such as multiple sclerosis, history of back surgery or back pain, and systemic infection.

Regional Anesthesia for Cesarean Section

Advantages
   Decreased risk of maternal aspiration
   Minimizes neonatal depression from maternal
      drug administration

Absolute contraindications
   Infection at site
   Severe hypovolemia
   Increased intracranial pressure
   Patient refusal
   Coagulation abnormalities

Relative contraindications
   Neurologic disease (e.g., multiple sclerosis)
   History of back surgery
   History of back pain
   Systemic infection

Spinal Versus Epidural Anesthesia

	Spinal	Epidural
Advantages	Reliable and rapid onset	Better control of spread Mitigates precipitous drop in blood pressure Unlimited duration
Disadvantages	Potential for hypotension Inability to control spread Limited duration PDPH	Time to achieve adequate surgical anesthesia Local anesthetic toxicity

PDPH, postdural puncture headache.

A Suggested Technique for Performing Regional Anesthesia for Cesarean Section

1. Check the anesthesia machine. Prepare resuscitative equipment and drugs including endotracheal tubes of different sizes, laryngoscopes, airways, suction, thiobarbiturate, succinylcholine, ephedrine or phenylephrine.

2. Transport to the operating room with left uterine displacement.

3. Administer a nonparticulate antacid by mouth.

4. Rapidly prehydrate with 1000–1500 mL of a crystalloid solution.

5. Place routine monitors including blood pressure cuff, electrocardiogram, and pulse oximeter. Administer oxygen via nasal cannula or facemask.

6. *Epidural*: After placing an epidural catheter, administer 3 cc of 2% lidocaine as a test dose. Wait 5 minutes, observing for signs of either intravascular or subarachnoid injection. After confirming catheter position, inject 2% lidocaine with epinephrine 1:200,000, 3% chloroprocaine, or 0.5% bupivacaine in aliquots of 5 mL no more frequently than every 5 minutes until a T4 level of anesthesia is achieved.

   Spinal: Use a small-gauge pencil-point spinal needle. Administer 1.5–2.0 mL of 0.75% hyperbaric bupivacaine.

7. Monitor vital signs every 2 minutes for the first 20 minutes, and then every 5 minutes thereafter, if stable.

8. If hypotension occurs, administer 250–500 mL boluses of crystalloid and ephedrine in 5 mg or phenylephrine in 50 μg increments, until the blood pressure returns to normal.

Spinal anesthesia provides reliable and rapid anesthesia. In certain urgent situations, spinal anesthesia can even be used in place of general anesthesia. Disadvantages of spinal anesthesia include a potential for hypotension, inability to control the spread of anesthesia, limited duration and possibility of postdural puncture headache.

Continuous epidural anesthesia allows for multiple repeat doses of local anesthetic, which offers better control over anesthetic spread, mitigates against precipitous drops in blood pressure, and allows almost unlimited duration of anesthesia. Epidural anesthesia can be used for both labor and cesarean delivery. Compared with spinal anesthesia, the major disadvantages of epidural anesthesia are the time required to place a needle or catheter and the potential for local anesthetic toxicity.

5. Outline the treatment for postdural puncture headache.

Postdural puncture headache (PDPH) can occur any time the dura is punctured. Persistent cerebrospinal fluid (CSF) leak decreases the amount of fluid available to cushion the brain. In the absence of an adequate fluid buffer, the brain shifts within the calvarium, placing tension on pain-sensitive blood vessels. Risk factors for PDPH include increasing size of needle, type of needle (lower with pencil-point needles), bevel perpendicular to dural fibers (for non-pencil-point needles), female gender, pregnancy, and increasing number of attempts.

The headache is classically located over the occipital or frontal regions. It is frequently accompanied by neck tension, tinnitus, diplopia, photophobia, nausea, and vomiting. The most diagnostic feature of PDPH is that it changes with position. The symptoms improve in the supine position and are exacerbated in the erect position (sitting or standing).

Treatment is divided into noninvasive and invasive measures. Noninvasive therapy includes analgesics, hydration, and caffeine. Invasive therapy involves placing an epidural blood patch. This is accomplished by sterilely injecting 20 mL of autologous blood into the epidural space. The success rate is 70–75%. A second blood patch is needed occasionally. Prophylactic blood patching or prophylactic epidural saline infusions to reduce the incidence of PDPH are controversial.

6. What are the advantages and disadvantages of general anesthesia for cesarean section?

The major advantages of general anesthesia over regional anesthesia are the shorter preoperative preparatory time and the freedom from sympathectomy.

The disadvantages of general anesthesia include maternal aspiration and neonatal depression. In addition, general anesthesia precludes immediate maternal bonding.

Aspiration pneumonia is a leading cause of morbidity and mortality in the parturient undergoing general anesthesia, thus general anesthesia should be reserved for the emergent situation. Before induction of general anesthesia, a careful evaluation of the airway should be performed and a nonparticulate antacid administered. Antacids increase gastric pH resulting in a decreased incidence and severity of pneumonitis should aspiration occur. Defasciculating doses of nondepolarizing muscle relaxants are avoided prior to induction because they may produce profound weakness predisposing to aspiration and may delay the onset time of succinylcholine.

After preoxygenation, induction of anesthesia can proceed with essentially any of the available induction agents and application of cricoid pressure. There are some data indicating that Apgar scores and neurobehavioral scores are depressed when propofol is used, but these are controversial. A thiobarbiturate is often chosen for patients who are hemodynamically stable, whereas ketamine is frequently selected when there is hemodynamic instability or severe bronchospasm. Although thiamylal crosses the placenta, doses less than 7 mg/kg do not adversely affect the fetus. This is because the small amount of drug reaching the fetus is diluted by fetal blood returning from the lower half of the body before it reaches the central nervous system.

Muscle relaxation for endotracheal intubation is achieved with succinylcholine because it provides the most rapid onset amongst relaxants currently available. Succinylcholine's duration of action may be prolonged, due to abnormally low levels of pseudocholinesterase, when compared with the nonpregnant state. The extended duration of action generally does not exceed 15 minutes and is, therefore, clinically insignificant. Muscle relaxants do not cross the placenta because they are highly ionized and have a large molecular weight.

Anesthesia is maintained with 50% nitrous oxide (N_2O) in O_2 and either isoflurane 0.3–0.5% or enflurane 0.5–0.7%. N_2O does cross the placenta but due to fetal tissue uptake it does not cause significant fetal depression if the induction to delivery time is less than 20 minutes. Sub-MAC concentrations of the potent inhaled anesthetic agents administered prior to delivery protect from maternal recall without causing fetal depression or uterine relaxation. After delivery of the fetus, N_2O concentrations are increased and opioids administered to supplement the anesthetic.

Extubation of the trachea follows classic full stomach precautions. The residual muscle relaxation is antagonized with an anticholinesterase and vagolytic agents and the patient must be fully awake.

7. Describe the elements of placental drug transfer.

Placental drug transfer occurs by diffusion. Fick's equation describes the factors governing the transfer of drugs across the placenta.

$$Q_d = K_d \times A \times [P_d(m) - P_d(f)]/b$$

A Suggested Method of Performing General Anesthesia for Cesarean Section

1. Check the anesthesia machine. Prepare resuscitative equipment and drugs including endotracheal tubes of different sizes, laryngoscopes, airways, suction, thiamylal, succinylcholine, ephedrine or phenylephrine.

2. Transport to the operating room with left uterine displacement.

3. Administer a nonparticulate antacid by mouth.

4. Prehydrate with 1000–1500 mL of crystalloid.

5. Place routine monitors including blood pressure cuff, electrocardiogram, and pulse oximeter. Administer oxygen by facemask or nasal cannula.

6. After denitrogenation with 100% oxygen for 3–5 minutes, induce anesthesia with thiamylal 4 mg/kg or ketamine 1–2 mg/kg followed by succinylcholine 100 mg and apply cricoid pressure. Do NOT use a defasciculating dose of a nondepolarizing agent.

7. Maintain anesthesia with 50% N_2O/O_2, and isoflurane 0.3–0.5% or enflurane 0.5–0.7% until the baby is delivered.

8. After delivery of the baby, administer fentanyl 100 µg and increase the N_2O concentration to 70%. Keep the concentration of the halogenated agent below 0.5 MAC to avoid uterine relaxation.

9. At completion of the procedure, administer neostigmine 0.07 mg/kg and glycopyrrolate 0.01 mg/kg to antagonize residual neuromuscular blockade.

10. Extubate the trachea when the patient is fully awake.

---

where:

Q_d = quantity of drug transferred per unit time
K_d = diffusion constant for the drug
A = surface area of the placenta

$P_d(m)$ = mean drug concentration of maternal blood in the intervillous space

$P_d(f)$ = mean drug concentration of fetal blood in the intervillous space

b = thickness of the placenta.

Factors over which the anesthesiologist has control are limited to the specific drug administered and the amount used. Other factors, such as the surface area and thickness of the placenta, are clearly not under our control. In order to minimize the amount of drug reaching the placenta, the quantity of maternally administered drug needs to be reduced.

Diffusion constants, which vary from one drug to another, are determined by four main properties: molecular weight, lipid solubility, protein binding, and electrical charge. Placental transfer of drug is facilitated by a molecular weight of less than 500, high lipid solubility, minimal maternal protein binding, and a low degree of ionization. Thus, fentanyl, a non-ionized, highly lipid-soluble molecule with a low molecular weight, crosses the placenta easily. In contrast, succinylcholine, a highly ionized molecule, does not cross the placenta readily.

8. What techniques can be used for post-cesarean pain relief?

Intravenous (IV), intramuscular (IM), and neuraxial opioids can be administered for post-cesarean pain relief. Women who receive epidural morphine sulfate complain of less pain than women who receive IV or IM morphine sulfate. Morphine sulfate in either the subarachnoid or epidural space provides analgesia for up to 24 hours. The dose of epidural morphine is 3–4 mg and of subarachnoid morphine is 0.1–0.25 mg.

9. Outline the differential diagnosis of postpartum hemorrhage.

The most common cause of postpartum hemorrhage is uterine atony, which occurs in 2–5% of all deliveries. Other causes of postpartum hemorrhage include retained placenta, placenta accreta, cervical and vaginal lacerations, inverted uterus, and conditions associated with coagulopathy such as amniotic fluid embolism and preeclampsia. Treatment of postpartum hemorrhage is etiology-specific. Coagulopathies often respond to therapy for their specific cause.

10. Explain the risk factors, presentation, and treatment of uterine atony.

Any condition associated with overdistention of the uterus, such as multiple births, polyhydramnios, or a large baby, is a risk factor for uterine atony. Other risk factors include multiparity, retained placenta, prolonged labor, previous tocolysis, β-agonists, prolonged general anesthesia with potent inhaled anesthetic agents, ruptured uterus, and chorioamnionitis.

Uterine atony presents as continued painless vaginal bleeding after delivery. The noncontracting uterus appears boggy and large. Obstetric management is aimed at increasing myometrial tone. Massaging the uterus through the abdominal wall or directly via the vagina is initially attempted to induce contractions. If massaging does not work, oxytocin and ergot derivatives are administered intravenously as well as prostaglandin $F_{2\alpha}$ directly into the uterus to induce contractions.

Anesthetic management is initially aimed at maternal resuscitation. Intravascular volume is restored with crystalloid, colloid, and/or blood. Massive blood loss may lead to shock. Coagulation factor replacement may be required. Vaginal examination and suturing in attempts to stop the bleeding require anesthesia; however, conduction techniques are hazardous in the face of hypovolemia. Intravenous sedation with small amounts of fentanyl, ketamine, and/or midazolam generally suffices. If sedation is inadequate, a rapid sequence induction of general anesthesia with endotracheal intubation is required to reduce the risk of maternal aspiration.

Continued hemorrhage may require hypogastric artery ligation or hysterectomy, which necessitate general anesthesia. Anesthetic management for these procedures is the same as for placenta previa. Pelvic artery embolization, usually performed in the radiology suite, can sometimes reduce the bleeding and prevent the need for a hysterectomy. Although general anesthesia is not required, maternal fluid resuscitation must be continued during embolization.

Differential Diagnosis of Postpartum Bleeding

Uterine atony

Retained products of conception

Placenta accreta

Cervical and vaginal lacerations

Inverted uterus

Coagulopathy
  Preeclampsia
  Amniotic fluid embolus

Frequent vital sign monitoring is required and resuscitative equipment must be available.

Successful intraoperative cell salvage (cell saver) have been reported in obstetrics. The major concern with its usage is that the amniotic fluid will not be completely removed during the centrifuging and cleansing process leading to iatrogenic amniotic fluid embolism. Recommendations for its use include discarding all surgical field fluids before collecting blood with the cell saver device. Use of this technique should be reserved for situations where there is no other blood available or the patient refuses autologous blood transfusion (Jehovah's witness).

11. Describe the presentation and treatment of retained placenta.

Retained placenta occurs in about 1 in 300 deliveries and is characterized by painless vaginal bleeding following delivery. Treatment goals focus on manually removing the placenta, which prevents uterine contractions. Dilatation and curettage may be required to evacuate the uterus.

Abnormal implantation in the uterus, such as placenta accreta, placenta increta, or placenta percreta, may make removal of the placenta impossible. Hysterectomy, hypogastric artery ligation, or arterial embolization may be lifesaving maneuvers.

For the anesthesiologist, maternal resuscitation is the first priority. Intravenous sedation usually suffices for evacuation of the uterus. Hysterectomy or hypogastric artery ligation requires general anesthesia, the management of which is similar to that described above.

SUGGESTED READINGS

Ackerman WE, Colclough GW: Prophylactic epidural blood patch: the controversy continues. Anesth Analg 66:913–917, 1987

Finster M, Mark LC, Morishima HO, et al.: Plasma thiopental concentrations in the newborn following delivery under thiopental–nitrous oxide anesthesia. Am J Obstet Gynecol 95:621–629, 1966

Heubert WN, Cefalo RC. Management of postpartum hemorrhage. Clin Obstet Gynecol 27:139–150, 1984

Marx GF, Joshi CW, Louis RO: Placental transmission of nitrous oxide. Anesthesiology 32:429–432, 1970

Nageotte MP, Larson D, Rumney PJ, et al.: Epidural analgesia compared with combined spinal-epidural analgesia during labor in nulliparous women. N Engl J Med 337:1715–1719, 1997

Pais SO, Glickman M, Schwartz P, et al.: Embolization of pelvic arteries for control of postpartum hemorrhage. Obstet Gynecol 55:754–758, 1980

Reisnner LS, Lin D: Anesthesia for cesarean section. pp. 465–492. In Chestnut DH (ed): Obstetric Anesthesia, Principles and Practice, 2nd edition. Mosby, St. Louis, 1999

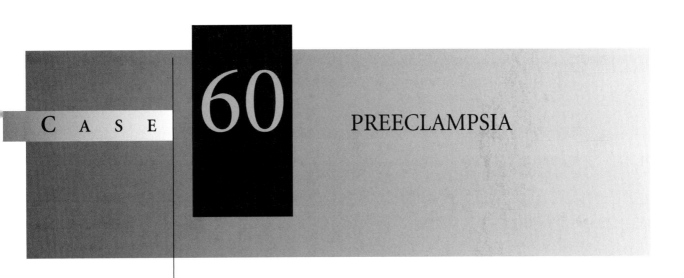

PREECLAMPSIA

Yaakov Beilin, MD
Celeste Telfeyan, DO

A 15-year-old nulliparous woman presents to the labor and delivery suite at the 35th week of her pregnancy. Her chief complaint is headache. Her blood pressure is 145/95 mmHg, and she appears edematous.

QUESTIONS

1. Classify the hypertensive disorders of pregnancy.
2. What are the incidence and risk factors of preeclampsia?
3. Explain the etiology of preeclampsia.
4. Describe the pathophysiology of preeclampsia.
5. Outline the obstetric management of preeclampsia.
6. How is preeclampsia prevented from degenerating into eclampsia?
7. Explain the management of preeclampsia-related hypertension.
8. What are the potential consequences of epidural anesthesia in the patient with preeclampsia?
9. Describe the anesthetic options for cesarean section for the preeclamptic patient.
10. Outline the anticipated postpartum problems associated with preeclampsia.

1. Classify the hypertensive disorders of pregnancy.

The hypertensive disorders of pregnancy are classified into four groups by the American College of Obstetricians and Gynecologists: chronic hypertension, preeclampsia-eclampsia, chronic hypertension with superimposed preeclampsia, and gestational hypertension.

Hypertension is defined as:

- Systolic blood pressure: >140 mmHg or 30 mmHg above baseline
- Diastolic blood pressure: >90 mmHg or 15 mmHg above baseline
- Mean arterial blood pressure: >105 mmHg or 20 mmHg above baseline

Blood pressures should be measured at rest with left uterine displacement and should be reproducible at least 6 hours later.

Chronic hypertension is diagnosed when the blood pressure is elevated prior to the 20th week of pregnancy. Chronic hypertension is a disease state that predates pregnancy. Since blood pressure normally decreases during pregnancy, any parturient with a diastolic blood pressure greater than 80 mmHg is suspected of having chronic hypertension.

Preeclampsia-eclampsia is a hypertensive disorder unique to pregnancy. The triad of hypertension, proteinuria,

TABLE 60.1		Signs and Symptoms of Preeclampsia	
		Mild Preeclampsia	**Severe Preeclampsia**
Hypertension	Systolic pressure	>140 mmHg >30 mmHg above baseline	>160 mmHg
	Diastolic pressure	>90 mmHg >15 mmHg above baseline	>110 mmHg
	Mean pressure	>105 mmHg >20 mmHg above baseline	>120 mmHg
Proteinuria		1–2+ by dipstick >1 g/24 hr	3–4+ by dipstick >5 g/24 hr
Edema		Generalized	Generalized
Patient symptoms			Headache Visual disturbances Epigastric pain Cyanosis

and edema characterizes preeclampsia. Except in association with hydatidiform mole, preeclamptic hypertension does not manifest prior to the 20th week of gestation. Proteinuria is defined as the excretion of greater than 0.3 grams of protein in a 24-hour urine collection or 1+ on dipstick analysis. Edema must be generalized and not confined to dependent areas of the body. Preeclampsia is classified as either mild or severe depending on the degree of hypertension, extent of proteinuria, or patient complaints. Preeclampsia degenerates into eclampsia when generalized seizures occur (Table 60.1).

Gestational hypertension is defined as hypertension occurring after the 20th week of pregnancy in the absence of other signs of preeclampsia. Gestational hypertension is frequently essential hypertension that is unmasked by pregnancy.

2. What are the incidence and risk factors of preeclampsia?

Preeclampsia occurs in approximately 5–10% of pregnancies and eclampsia manifests in 0.2–0.7% of pregnancies. The young primigravida with poor prenatal care is at highest risk for preeclampsia. Preeclampsia is associated with rapid uterine enlargement such as occurs with hydatidiform mole, diabetes mellitus, and multiple gestations. There is a 33% probability of preeclampsia recurring with subsequent pregnancies.

3. Explain the etiology of preeclampsia.

Although the etiologies of preeclampsia are unknown, uteroplacental ischemia appears to be a common factor. Beer (1978) suggested that uteroplacental ischemia may result from altered immunity such as graft-versus-host reaction.

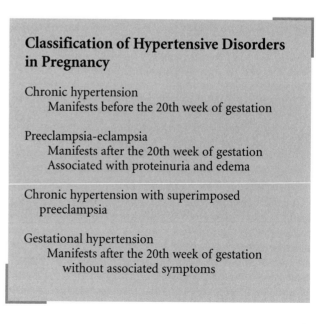

Classification of Hypertensive Disorders in Pregnancy

Chronic hypertension
  Manifests before the 20th week of gestation

Preeclampsia-eclampsia
  Manifests after the 20th week of gestation
  Associated with proteinuria and edema

Chronic hypertension with superimposed
  preeclampsia

Gestational hypertension
  Manifests after the 20th week of gestation
    without associated symptoms

It is also possible that placental prostaglandin imbalance between thromboxane and prostacyclin leads to preeclampsia. In the normal pregnancy, prostacyclin and thromboxane are produced in equal amounts by the placenta. In the pregnancy complicated by preeclampsia, there is a relative increase in thromboxane production. Thromboxane causes increased vasoconstriction, platelet aggregation, and uterine activity as well as a simultaneous decrease in uteroplacental blood flow. These effects are observed in preeclampsia.

Uteroplacental ischemia leads to the production of substances similar to renin and thromboplastin. Renin causes release of angiotensin and aldosterone, which result in hypertension and edema. Thromboplastin can initiate coagulopathies such as disseminated intravascular coagulation (DIC).

4. Describe the pathophysiology of preeclampsia.

The hallmark of preeclampsia is vasospasm that occurs secondary to increased circulating levels of renin, aldosterone, angiotensin, and catecholamines. Aldosterone also causes sodium and water retention, which leads to generalized edema. Since almost every organ system is affected in the parturient with preeclampsia, it is best to take a systematic approach when discussing the changes seen in preeclampsia.

Central Nervous System   Cerebral edema and cerebral vasospasm lead to the central nervous system effects of preeclampsia. Intracranial pressure increases in some cases but cerebral blood flow and oxygen consumption remain normal. Clinical findings related to the above changes include headache, hyperreflexia, blurred vision, vertigo, blindness, seizures, and coma. Cerebral hemorrhage is the leading cause of death in the preeclamptic patient.

Pulmonary   Intubation may be exceedingly difficult secondary to laryngeal and upper airway edema. Increased secretions and airway congestion predispose the mother to upper airway infections. Pulmonary capillary leak into the interstitium accounts for intrapulmonary shunting and a deteriorating alveolar to arterial (A-a) oxygen gradient.

Cardiovascular   Generalized vasoconstriction produces hypertension, impaired tissue perfusion, and cellular hypoxia. Translocated fluid from the vascular compartment to the interstitium leads to generalized edema, hypovolemia, and hemoconcentration. An inverse relationship exists between the intravascular volume and the degree of hypertension. Hemoconcentration leads to increased blood viscosity, which further exacerbates tissue hypoxia. Although the hematocrit is typically elevated, a relative anemia usually exists and blood loss is poorly tolerated. Vasospasm leads to an increase in systemic vascular resistance (SVR), which increases cardiac work. The already hyperdynamic cardiovascular system becomes stressed further and cardiac output rises. Over time, left ventricular hypertrophy occurs leading to left ventricular dysfunction. Cotton and colleagues (1985) have shown that central venous pressure does not necessarily correlate with pulmonary capillary wedge pressure and left ventricular end diastolic volume in preeclampsia. Consequently, pulmonary artery catheters may be necessary in some preeclamptic patients.

Renal   Renal blood flow is reduced leading to a decrease in the glomerular filtration rate and creatinine clearance. Almost all renal function tests are impaired. An increasing uric acid level correlates with the severity of disease. Damaged glomeruli allow for renal loss of proteins.

Hepatic   Vasospasm leads to hepatic periportal hemorrhages and hepatocellular damage. Swelling of the liver capsule from subcapsular hematomas may produce abdominal pain. Hepatic rupture has been reported in severe cases. Elevated liver enzymes occur with deteriorating hepatic function.

Hematologic   Coagulation abnormalities also occur. The most common finding is thrombocytopenia that can occur with or without other coagulopathies. A syndrome of *h*emolysis, *e*levated *l*iver function tests and *l*ow *p*latelet count (acronym HELLP) has been described. There is also frequently a qualitative platelet abnormality even without a quantitative problem. The prothrombin time, thrombin time and partial thromboplastin time can also be elevated. Fibrinogen levels can decrease and frank DIC can occur.

Uteroplacental   Intervillous blood flow is decreased 2- to 3-fold and is a major contributing factor of fetal morbidity and mortality. The incidence of premature labor is high due to placental hypoperfusion. Because of decreased uteroplacental blood flow, the placenta is often small and shows signs of premature aging. The uterus is also hyperactive and markedly sensitive to oxytocin. The parturient with preeclampsia is at an increased risk for placental abruption.

5. Outline the obstetric management of preeclampsia.

Obstetric management of the patient with preeclampsia is aimed at controlling the disease and preventing its progression. The patient should be on complete bed rest with left uterine displacement. Serial determinations of blood pressure, weight gain, renal and coagulation function, and central nervous system irritability should be done. Oral fluid and sodium intake should not be restricted. The routine use of diuretics to control edema is no longer recommended.

Pathophysiologic Changes in Preeclampsia

Central nervous system
    Cerebral edema and vasospasm
        Headache
        Hyperreflexia
        Blurry vision
        Blindness
        Seizures
        Coma
    Cerebral hemorrhage

Pulmonary
    Upper airway/laryngeal edema
        Difficult intubation
    Predisposition to upper respiratory infections
    Pulmonary capillary leak
        Increased A-a gradient

Cardiovascular
    Vasoconstriction
        Hypertension
        Impaired tissue perfusion
        Cellular hypoxia
        Increased cardiac work
    Fluid translocation
        Generalized edema
        Hypovolemia
        Hemoconcentration
    Increased blood viscosity
    Left ventricular hypertrophy and dysfunction

Renal
    Decreased renal blood flow
    Decreased glomerular filtration rate
    Decreased creatinine clearance
    Proteinuria
    Increased uric acid levels correlate with severity of
        disease

Hepatic
    Periportal hemorrhage
    Subcapsular hematomas
    Abnormal liver function tests

Hematologic
    Decreased platelet count
    Qualitative platelet abnormality
    Abnormal coagulation profile
    Disseminated intravascular coagulation
    HELLP—Hemolysis, Elevated Liver function tests,
        and Low Platelet count

Uteroplacental
    Decrease in intervillous blood flow
    Premature labor
    Small placenta
    Uterine hyperactivity
    Uterine sensitivity to oxytocin
    Placental abruption

Fetal well-being should be monitored via a non-stress test, oxytocin challenge, or biophysical profile. Delivery of the fetus and placenta is considered the definitive treatment of preeclampsia and should be done for either fetal or maternal reasons. Fetal indications include evidence of fetal distress or cessation of fetal maturation. Maternal indications include worsening preeclampsia that cannot be controlled medically.

6. How is preeclampsia prevented from degenerating into eclampsia?

Magnesium sulfate ($MgSO_4$), a central nervous system depressant and anticonvulsant, is the first-line drug in the United States for the prevention of eclampsia. One of the many sites of action of $MgSO_4$ is at the myoneural junction.

The decrease in hyperreflexia seen with the administration of $MgSO_4$ is secondary to the inhibition of acetylcholine release at the neuromuscular junction, decreased sensitivity of the motor endplate to acetylcholine, and the decreased excitability of the muscle membrane. $MgSO_4$ is also a mild vasodilator and decreases uterine hyperactivity, which results in an increase in uterine blood flow. It also causes vasodilation at the renal and liver beds thus improving their function.

Therapeutic levels of magnesium are between 4 and 8 mEq/L. Above this level, magnesium has both maternal and neonatal side-effects. Magnesium can lead to electrocardiographic changes and ultimately cardiac and respiratory arrest. These severe side-effects, however, do not occur until after the loss of deep tendon reflexes (Table 60.2). Therefore, by monitoring serum magnesium

Magnesium Plasma Levels (mEq/L)	Systemic Effects
1.5–2	Normal plasma levels
4–8	Therapeutic range
5–10	ECG changes: prolonged PR interval widened QRS
10	Decreased deep tendon reflexes Respiratory depression
15	Respiratory arrest Sinoatrial and atrioventricular conduction defects
25	Cardiac arrest

TABLE 60.2 Effects of Magnesium at Different Plasma Levels

levels and deep tendon reflexes catastrophic side-effects may be avoided. Magnesium, because of its actions at the neuromuscular junction, increases the sensitivity of the mother to both depolarizing and nondepolarizing muscle relaxants.

Since magnesium crosses the placenta, the neonate can also exhibit signs of magnesium toxicity. Signs of magnesium toxicity in the newborn include respiratory depression, apnea, and decreased muscle tone. Magnesium toxicity in the newborn and the mother can be reversed with the administration of calcium.

$MgSO_4$ is administered intravenously with a loading dose of 2–4 grams over 15 minutes, followed by an infusion of

Magnesium Sulfate Properties

Central nervous system depressant
Anticonvulsant

Myoneural junction
    Inhibits release of acetylcholine
    Decreases acetylcholine sensitivity of motor
        endplate
    Decreases excitability of muscle membrane

Mild vasodilator
Decreases uterine hyperactivity
Crosses the placenta
Toxicity treated with calcium administration

1–3 grams per hour. $MgSO_4$ is primarily excreted by the kidneys. Therefore, renal function must be carefully monitored and the magnesium dose decreased accordingly in the face of renal insufficiency.

7. Explain the management of preeclampsia-related hypertension.

Control of hypertension in the parturient with preeclampsia is imperative since acute elevations of blood pressure can lead to cerebral hemorrhage, the leading cause of mortality. The patient's blood pressure should be neither acutely decreased nor decreased to levels considered normal for other parturients since a low blood pressure could compromise uteroplacental blood flow. Although $MgSO_4$ causes vasodilation, it does not treat hypertension adequately and an alternative antihypertensive drug is usually needed. Also, as in any patient with hypertension, responses to both antihypertensive and pressor agents are exaggerated. Therefore, reduced doses of these agents should be used initially and the response noted prior to increasing the dose.

The most frequently used antihypertensive agent is hydralazine, which not only decreases blood pressure but also increases renal and uteroplacental blood flow. The tachycardia that occurs with the use of hydralazine can be treated with propranolol. Hydralazine is not the agent of choice in the acute situation since it takes 10–15 minutes before an effect is seen.

Nitroprusside, a potent arterial vasodilator, is often used when immediate control of blood pressure is required. It is administered by infusion making it easy to titrate to effect. Nitroprusside, however, crosses the placenta and cyanide toxicity has been described in the neonate after prolonged infusion in the mother. Trimethaphan, a ganglionic blocker, has also been used with good success in the emergent situation.

Nitroglycerin, a venous dilator, is useful when tight control of blood pressure is required for prolonged periods. Nitroglycerin is not as potent as nitroprusside but is easy to titrate and has minimal effect on the fetus.

Propranolol, diazoxide, methyldopa, and captopril are generally not used in the patient with preeclampsia because of their adverse side-effects (Table 60.3).

8. What are the potential consequences of epidural anesthesia in the patient with preeclampsia?

Epidural anesthesia can be beneficial for the patient with preeclampsia. Decreasing or eliminating the sensation of pain will reduce hyperventilation, decrease catecholamine release, decrease anxiety, and increase uteroplacental blood flow. A regional anesthetic will also obviate the need for a general anesthetic with its inherent risk

TABLE 60.3	Antihypertensive Treatment in Toxemia of Pregnancy		
Drug	**Mechanism of Action**	**Advantage**	**Disadvantages**
Hydralazine	Vasodilator	Onset of action approximately 10 min Increased renal blood flow Duration of action approximately 2 hr Hypotension usually responds to volume administration	Tachycardia
Propranolol	β-Blocker	Augments antihypertensive action of hydralazine	Fetal bradycardia Fetal hyopoglycemia
Sodium nitroprusside	Direct smooth muscle relaxation	Onset of action = 1 minute, Duration of action = 1–10 minutes	Fetal cyanide toxicity Increases maternal intracranial pressure
Nitroglycerin	Direct smooth muscle relaxation	Onset of action = 1–2 minutes Duration of action = 10 minutes Improves uterine blood flow	Increased maternal intracranial pressure
Methyldopa	α_2-Agonist	Good maintenance drug due to prolonged duration of action	Neonatal tremors
Labetalol	α- and β- antagonist	As effective as methyldopa for maintenance	Not recommended with bronchoconstrictive disease
Captopril	Angiotensin-converting enzyme inhibitor	Not recommended	Fetal death
Diuretics	Sodium and water excretion	Generally not recommended	Hypotension
Nifedipine	Calcium channel blocker	Uterine relaxation Increased renal blood flow	Hypotension in combination with magnesium
Clonidine	α_2-Agonist	Insufficient data	Fetal hypoxia Increased uterine tone (Decreased uterine blood flow in animals) Generally not recommended

of aspiration. However, prior to administering the epidural catheter the blood pressure must be controlled, the intravascular volume replete, and the coagulation profile normal.

The diastolic blood pressure should be less than 110 mmHg before beginning a neuraxial anesthetic. Frequent blood pressure measurements will be needed during the anesthetic. An arterial line may be necessary if the blood pressure is labile.

The parturient with hypertensive disease is usually fluid-depleted and unless the fluid level is restored toward normal, the patient will be subject to profound drops in blood pressure. Urine output is monitored to guide fluid administration. If urine output is diminished, a fluid challenge of 500–1000 mL of an isotonic crystalloid should be given depending on the clinical scenario. If urine output does not increase, central venous pressure monitoring should be instituted. Severe preeclampsia may require

pulmonary artery pressure rather than central venous pressure monitoring, since these patients may have left ventricular dysfunction and congestive heart failure.

Fluid replacement should be with either an isotonic crystalloid or colloid solution. Dextrose in water should not be administered because of the risk for water intoxication, especially in the presence of oxytocin. There is also the risk for neonatal hypoglycemia.

Platelet consumption is a component of preeclampsia that can lead to factor consumption and DIC. Therefore, a platelet count and coagulation profile must be checked prior to administering the anesthetic. Generally, the platelet count decreases before other indices of coagulation are prolonged. Therefore, it is acceptable to first check the platelet count and, if it is less than 100,000 mm^{-3}, to then check the prothrombin time (PT), partial thromboplastin time (PTT), and fibrinogen. Since preeclampsia is a dynamic process, the coagulation parameters should be checked as close to the time of administering the block as possible.

9. Describe the anesthetic options for cesarean section for the preeclamptic patient.

Once the blood pressure is controlled and the fluid status and coagulation parameters normalized, cesarean section can be safely performed under epidural, spinal or general anesthesia. The advantage of an epidural anesthetic over a spinal anesthetic is that the hemodynamic changes are minimized because the anesthetic level can be raised slowly. Although a spinal anesthetic is technically easier to perform and has a quicker onset than an epidural anesthetic, the hemodynamic alterations may be more profound.

General anesthesia is often required for an emergency cesarean section. Even in the presence of fetal distress, time should be taken to adequately control the blood pressure prior to induction. This is because laryngoscopy may cause a significant increase in blood pressure, which can lead to cerebral hemorrhage. After preoxygenation, a rapid sequence induction with thiopental, succinylcholine, and cricoid pressure is performed. If the patient is on $MgSO_4$, succinylcholine and the nondepolarizing muscle relaxants may have a prolonged duration of action. However, the dose of succinylcholine should not be reduced since a fast onset of paralysis is needed. A neuromuscular monitor should be used to guide subsequent doses of muscle relaxants. An array of laryngoscopes, endotracheal tubes, combitubes, and laryngeal mask airways should be available to deal with a potentially difficult airway.

10. Outline the anticipated postpartum problems associated with preeclampsia.

Although delivery of the fetus and placenta are considered the definitive treatment for preeclampsia, it can take hours to days for the symptoms to resolve completely. The patient is still at risk for convulsions. Therefore, the blood pressure should be monitored and the $MgSO_4$ infusion continued for at least 24 hours after delivery.

SUGGESTED READINGS

Beer AE: Possible immunologic bases of preeclampsia/eclampsia. Semin Perinatol 2:39–59, 1978

Cotton DB, Gonik B, Dorman K, Harrist R: Cardiovascular alterations in severe pregnancy-induced hypertension: relationship of central venous pressure to pulmonary capillary wedge pressure. Am J Obstet Gynecol 151:762–764, 1985

Gaiser RR, Gutsche BB, Cheek TG: Anesthetic considerations for the hypertensive disorders of pregnancy. pp. 297–321. In Hughes SC, Levinson G, Rosen MA (eds): Shnider and Levinson's Anesthesia for Obstetrics, 4th edition. Lippincott Williams and Wilkins, Philadelphia, 2002

James MF: Clinical use of magnesium infusions in anesthesia. Anesth Analg 74:129–136, 1992

Jouppila P, Jouppila R, Hollmen A, Koivula A: Lumbar epidural analgesia to improve intervillous blood flow during labor in severe preeclampsia. Obstet Gynecol 59:158–161, 1982

61

ABRUPTIO PLACENTA AND PLACENTA PREVIA

Howard H. Bernstein, MD

Yaakov Beilin, MD

A 25-year-old woman at 37 weeks gestation presents to the labor floor complaining of abdominal pain accompanied by vaginal bleeding. Her blood pressure on admission is 110/60 mmHg with a pulse of 90 beats per minute. She is contracting every 5 minutes and is 3 cm dilated. Fetal heart rate (FHR) monitoring demonstrates a reactive tracing.

QUESTIONS

1. Summarize the major causes of third-trimester bleeding.
2. What is abruptio placenta and what are its risk factors?
3. What are the presenting signs and symptoms of abruptio placenta and how is the diagnosis made?
4. Describe the obstetric management of abruptio placenta.
5. Describe the effects of pregnancy on coagulation.
6. What is disseminated intravascular coagulopathy and how is it managed?
7. How is fetal distress diagnosed?
8. The patient is given a trial of labor, and the obstetrician requests a consult for labor analgesia. What are your concerns and how would you proceed?
9. Three hours into labor, the obstetrician notes a significant increase in the vaginal bleeding and a fall in maternal blood pressure to 80/40 mmHg with a pulse of 120 beats per minute. Late decelerations are noted on the FHR monitor. Assuming the patient has *not* yet received an epidural for regional analgesia, how would you anesthetize this patient for an emergency cesarean section?
10. What is placenta previa?
11. What is the clinical presentation of placenta previa and how is the diagnosis made?
12. What is the obstetric management of placenta previa?
13. How would you anesthetize the patient with placenta previa for cesarean section?

1. Summarize the major causes of third-trimester bleeding.

A "bloody show" is the most common cause of bleeding during the third trimester. This occurs during labor and is due to effacement and dilatation of the cervix. Placental problems are responsible for most pathologic third-trimester bleeding, of which placental abruption and placenta previa account for the majority. Cervical bleeding due to polyps and carcinoma is much less common. Vasa previa, umbilical cord vessels traveling within the placental membranes and covering the cervical os, is a rare cause of third-trimester bleeding. Other rare causes of third-trimester bleeding are maternal coagulopathy, due to preeclampsia, and intrauterine fetal demise (Table 61.1).

TABLE 61.1   Differential Diagnosis of Third-Trimester Bleeding

Bloody show
Abruptio placenta
Placenta previa
Vasa previa
Uterine rupture
Cervical pathology
   Polyps
   Carcinoma
   Varicosities
Maternal coagulopathy
   Preeclampsia
   Intrauterine demise
   Other causes of coagulopathy

2. What is abruptio placenta and what are its risk factors?

Abruptio placenta refers to premature separation of the placenta, i.e., before delivery of the fetus. It occurs in about 1/100 to 1/150 deliveries and carries a perinatal mortality rate of approximately 20%. The incidence of abruption increases with age and is more common in African-American women. Abruption is associated with hypertension, either chronic or pregnancy-induced, multiparity, cigarette smoking, and cocaine abuse. In women who have experienced a prior abruption, the risk of recurrence is 10 times higher than that of the general population.

3. What are the presenting signs and symptoms of abruptio placenta and how is the diagnosis made?

Classically, abruptio placenta is described as painful bleeding. The patient may experience a sudden "tearing" pain in the abdomen, followed by the onset of vaginal bleeding and labor pains. A tumultuous labor pattern follows, with frequent contractions and an increase in base tone of the uterus. The patient may state that it feels as though the contraction never ends. The amount of vaginal bleeding is variable and does not always correlate with the degree of placental separation. If the abruption is central, then little vaginal bleeding may be noted, as most of the bleeding will be retroplacental; however, an increase in uterine fundal height may occur as up to 2 liters of blood may collect behind the placenta. Blood extravasation into the myometrium causes the purple-colored Couvelaire uterus. Severe hemorrhage may lead to maternal hypovolemic shock, fetal distress, or fetal demise. Disseminated intravascular coagulopathy (DIC) may also occur in the face of a severe abruption. Pritchard and Brekke (1967) were the first

to demonstrate that the retroplacental clot could not account for the degree of systemic hypofibrinogenemia seen in abruptio placenta. Gilabert and colleagues (1985) explained how open venous sinuses beneath the abrupted placenta could allow thromboplastic material to enter the maternal circulation and initiate DIC.

Diagnosis of abruption is initially made by clinical evaluation. Ultrasound evaluation of the placenta may identify a retroplacental clot and separation of the placenta from the uterine wall. After delivery, examination of the placenta may demonstrate an adherent clot; however, the placenta may appear normal.

4. Describe the obstetric management of abruptio placenta.

Obstetric management consists of vigorous maternal resuscitation with fluids and blood replacement and delivery of the fetus. In the presence of a small abruption and in the absence of fetal distress a vaginal delivery may be attempted. In the presence of life-threatening hemorrhage or fetal compromise, cesarean section is the most expeditious route of delivery. Preventing and treating coagulopathy requires evacuation of the uterus as well as transfusion of coagulation factors and platelets, as indicated.

5. Describe the effects of pregnancy on coagulation.

Pregnancy is commonly referred to as a hypercoagulable state and is associated with an increased incidence of thrombotic disease. Pregnancy is characterized by an increase in the level of clotting factors, in particular fibrinogen. There is an increase in fibrinogen catabolism by thrombin, as marked by increased levels of fibrinopeptide A. Platelet count may fall or remain normal in pregnancy. Rolbin et al. (1988) demonstrated no statistically significant change in platelet count during pregnancy; however, 104 of 2,000 patients had platelet counts of under 150×10^9 per liter. Fay et al. (1983) found a fall in platelet count due to increased platelet consumption in the last 8 weeks of gestation. In addition, there is a dramatic short-term increase in coagulability immediately following delivery as manifested by an increase in factor V and VIII activity, a fall in fibrinogen levels, and a decrease in partial thromboplastin time (Table 61.2).

6. What is disseminated intravascular coagulopathy and how is it managed?

DIC is characterized by activation of systemic coagulation leading to consumption of clotting factors and activation of secondary fibrinolysis. This will result in hypofibrinogenemia, thrombocytopenia, and the production of fibrin degradation products. The clinical presentation is marked by hemorrhage, lack of clot formation, and bleeding from all puncture sites, such as intravenous

TABLE 61.2	Coagulation Changes in Pregnancy

Increased factor levels
    Fibrinogen
    Factor V
    Factor VII
    Factor VIII
    Factor IX
    Factor X
    Factor XII
    Fibrin split products
    von Willebrand factor

No change
    Factor XI
    Antithrombin III
    Antifactor Xa
    Platelet count

Decrease
    Factor XIII
    Platelet count
    PT
    PTT

TABLE 61.3	Diagnosis of Disseminated Intravascular Coagulopathy

Clinical suspicion
    Pregnancy
    Non-clotting blood
    Inability to control hemorrhage
Laboratory
    Prolonged PT/PTT
    Low fibrinogen levels
    Low platelet count
    Presence of fibrin degradation products

insertion sites. Abnormal laboratory values include elevation in prothrombin time (PT), partial thromboplastin time (PTT), low platelet count, and fibrinogen level (Table 61.3).

Successful treatment of DIC requires removal of the source, i.e., delivery of the fetus and placenta. In addition to delivery, treatment of the coagulopathy with fresh frozen plasma, cryoprecipitate, for fibrinogen replacement, and platelets will be necessary until the process begins to reverse.

7. How is fetal distress diagnosed?

Continuous electronic FHR monitoring was developed, in the 1960s, to assess fetal well-being during labor. FHR monitoring can be performed directly by placing an electrode on the fetal scalp or indirectly by placing an ultrasound probe on the maternal abdomen. Characteristics of FHR patterns are divided into baseline and periodic features. Baseline features include heart rate as well as variability. In normal labor, the FHR is determined by a balance between the sympathetic and parasympathetic innervation of the fetal heart. Normal FHR is between 110 and 160 beats per minute (bpm). Variability of the FHR is very important in determining fetal well-being. In normal labor there is beat-to-beat variability (R-R interval) of about 3–5 bpm, and long-term periodic accelerations of 10–15 bpm lasting 10–15 seconds, occurring 3 or more times per 20 minute window (Figure 61.1). FHR tracings demonstrating good beat-to-beat and long-term variability are referred to as reactive tracings and imply normal neonatal acid–base status, as assessed by a normal scalp pH (7.25–7.35). This is associated with the delivery of a healthy and vigorous neonate, with Apgar score ≥7 at 5 minutes. The absence of long-term and beat-to-beat variability may indicate fetal hypoxia (Figure 61.2).

The presence of good variability is the most sensitive indicator of fetal well-being. However, poor FHR variability is not always due to fetal hypoxia. Non-rapid eye movement fetal sleep cycles, lasting about 20 minutes, are the most common cause of poor variability. Congenital fetal heart disease, such as heart block, and fetal anencephaly are associated with poor FHR variability. Iatrogenic causes include the maternal administration of opioids, local anesthetics, and atropine.

Periodic decelerations, early, late and variable, have been described. They are classified according to their occurrence relative to the beginning of a contraction. Early decelerations begin with the onset of a contraction, late decelerations after the contraction begins, and variable decelerations are variable in onset relative to a contraction.

Early decelerations occur with the onset of the contraction and appear as a mirror image of the contraction. They are thought to occur secondary to fetal head compression. They are accompanied by good variability and are not associated with fetal hypoxia or acidosis.

Late decelerations are always associated with fetal hypoxemia (Figure 61.3). In the presence of uteroplacental insufficiency there is a significant decrease in fetal pO_2 resulting in a vagal-mediated slowing of the FHR. In interpreting the significance of a late deceleration, FHR variability must be assessed. In the presence of good variability significant neonatal cerebral hypoxia has not yet occurred and a good neonatal outcome can be expected. If late decelerations occur with poor FHR variability, the tracing is more ominous. Fetal scalp blood sampling to assess neonatal acid–base status or immediate delivery is indicated.

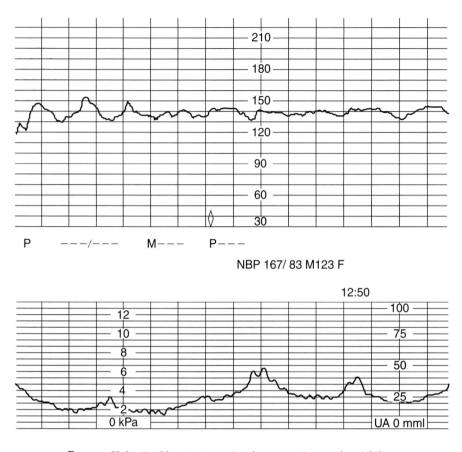

FIGURE 61.1   Fetal heart rate tracing demonstrating good variability.

Variable decelerations are unrelated to the time of onset of the uterine contraction (Figure 61.4). Variable decelerations are due to a vagal-mediated reflex stimulated by umbilical cord compression. Variable decelerations are considered severe if they last for more than 30 seconds with a nadir FHR of 60 bpm or less. Mild to moderate variable decelerations are rarely associated with fetal hypoxia. However, severe and recurrent decelerations may lead to the development of fetal hypoxia and acidosis. In that case, the FHR tracing will also demonstrate loss of variability. Fetal scalp blood sampling or immediate delivery may be indicated.

Fetal scalp blood sampling is performed when the FHR tracing is indicative of fetal hypoxia and delivery is not imminent. Scalp pH <7.20 is considered ominous and necessitates immediate delivery. Fetal scalp stimulation, by digital examination, may also be used to assess fetal well-being. The presence of fetal heart rate acceleration after scalp stimulation is associated with a scalp pH above 7.20.

Intrapartum fetal pulse oximetry is a new technology that may offer advantages over traditional monitoring techniques, but is currently not widely used.

When a non-reassuring FHR tracing is identified, in utero fetal resuscitation should commence. Correctable causes include maternal hypotension, hyperstimulation of the uterus by pitocin, and umbilical cord compression. Fetal well-being may be enhanced by administering oxygen to the mother, improving left uterine displacement, and increasing maternal blood pressure with either fluids or vasopressors.

8. The patient is given a trial of labor, and the obstetrician requests a consult for labor analgesia. What are your concerns and how would you proceed?

The clinical presentation, painful vaginal bleeding, is consistent with the diagnosis of a placental abruption. Before a regional anesthetic is initiated, the patient's intravascular volume, blood count, and coagulation status require careful evaluation. Initial laboratory evaluation should include a hemoglobin, hematocrit, platelet count, PT/PTT, fibrinogen level, and fibrin split products to evaluate the degree of hemorrhage and to rule out the development of DIC. Volume repletion should be with crystalloid, colloid, or packed red blood cells, as indicated.

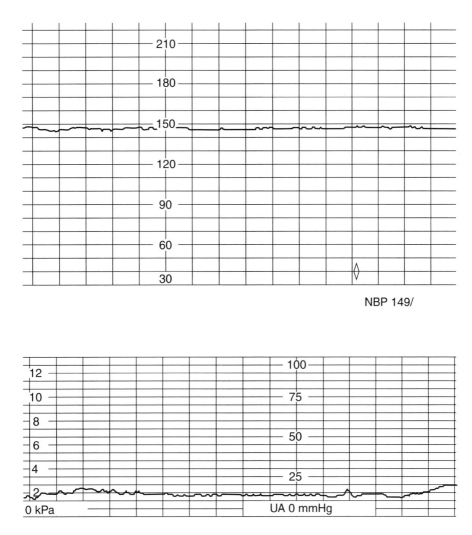

NBP 149/

FIGURE 61.2 Fetal heart rate tracing demonstrating poor variability.

Fetal Heart Rate Monitoring

Baseline
Beat-to-beat variability

Heart rate	110–160 bpm
R-R interval	3–5 bpm

Long-term periodic accelerations
    10–15 bpm for 10–15 seconds
    Occurs ≥3× per 20 minutes

Fetal Heart Rate Decelerations

Type	Relation to Contraction	Significance
Early	Onset	Fetal head compression
Late	After the onset	Fetal hypoxemia secondary to uteroplacental insufficiency
Variable	Variable	Vagal-mediated secondary to umbilical cord compression

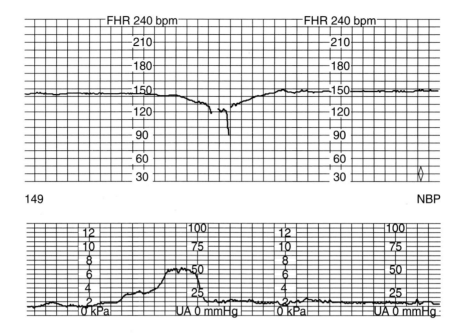

149   NBP

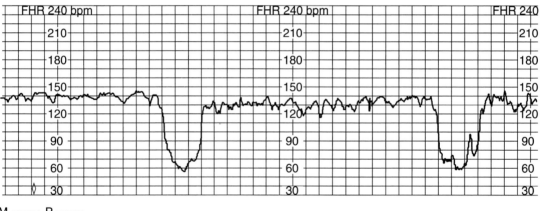

FIGURE 61.3   Fetal heart rate tracing demonstrating a late deceleration.

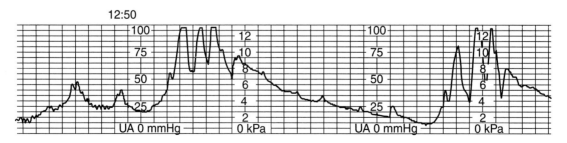

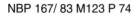

M − − −, P − − −

NBP 167/ 83 M123 P 74

12:50

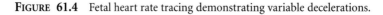

FIGURE 61.4   Fetal heart rate tracing demonstrating variable decelerations.

Cesarean Section for Abruptio Placenta

Laboratory testing
  Type and crossmatch
  Hematocrit
  Platelet count
  PT/PTT
  Fibrinogen level
  Fibrin degradation products

Adequate intravenous access

Fluid resuscitation
  Crystalloids
  Colloids
  Blood products as indicated

Anesthetic choice
  Regional anesthesia contraindicated in the
    presence of coagulopathy or hypovolemia
  General anesthesia preferable

Induction agents
  Etomidate 0.1–0.2 mg/kg IV
  Ketamine 1 mg/kg IV

Rapid sequence induction

If significant hemorrhage has not occurred and there is no laboratory evidence of DIC, epidural analgesia may be instituted.

9. Three hours into labor, the obstetrician notes a significant increase in the vaginal bleeding and a fall in maternal blood pressure to 80/40 mm Hg with a pulse of 120 beats per minute. Late decelerations are noted on the FHR monitor. Assuming the patient has *not* yet received an epidural for regional analgesia, how would you anesthetize this patient for an emergency cesarean section?

To decide upon an anesthetic plan, both maternal and fetal condition must be evaluated. The maternal and fetal conditions have deteriorated since admission and are consistent with a worsening abruption complicated by significant blood loss and fetal distress. It should be remembered that the amount of vaginal bleeding may underestimate the true blood loss as a significant volume of blood may be concealed behind the placenta. The hemoglobin concentration should be determined to guide blood transfusion therapy. Maternal coagulopathy, such as DIC, secondary to the placental abruption must also be ruled out. If maternal and/or fetal instability exist, cesarean delivery may be performed before the laboratory assessment is obtained.

Although spinal anesthesia can be rapidly established to provide surgical anesthesia for an emergency cesarean section, the presence of maternal coagulopathy and hypovolemia due to hemorrhage are contraindications to the placement of a regional anesthetic. For these reasons, regional anesthesia should be avoided and the cesarean section should be performed under general anesthesia.

Prior to the induction of general anesthesia adequate intravenous access must be established. Blood should be drawn and sent for typing and crossmatching, hematocrit level, platelet count, PT/PTT, fibrinogen level, and for the presence of fibrin degradation products. Fluid resuscitation should also begin immediately. Because the pregnant patient is considered to have a full stomach, a rapid sequence induction with cricoid pressure must be performed. In the hypovolemic patient, etomidate 0.1–0.2 mg/kg or ketamine 1 mg/kg intravenously should be considered as induction agents. Propofol and thiopental should probably be avoided as they are associated with more hypotension than ketamine or etomidate after induction. Succinylcholine should be utilized to facilitate tracheal intubation.

10. What is placenta previa?

Placenta previa is a condition where a low-lying placenta covers the internal cervical os; it occurs in about 1/200 deliveries. Predisposing factors include multiparity, advanced maternal age, and prior cesarean section.

The previa may be marginal, partial, or complete. With a complete placenta previa, the placenta covers the entire cervical os, thereby preventing vaginal delivery of the fetus. Incomplete coverage of the cervical os is referred to as a partial placenta previa. A marginal previa is a partial placenta previa associated with a low-lying placenta and minimal placental coverage of the cervix. In a low-lying placenta, the placenta is implanted in the lower uterine segment but does not cover the internal cervical os.

11. What is the clinical presentation of placenta previa and how is the diagnosis made?

Bleeding associated with a placenta previa is not associated with abdominal pain and may be sudden in onset. The amount of bleeding may range from very mild and intermittent to profuse and life-threatening.

TABLE 61.4	Placenta Previa Versus Abruptio Placenta	
	Placenta Previa	**Abruptio Placenta**
Pain	Painless bleeding	Painful bleeding
Blood	Bright red	Port wine
Clotting	Yes	No
Blood loss	Obvious	Concealed behind the placenta
DIC	Rare	Possibility
Diagnosis	Confirmed by ultrasound	Clinical and ultrasound

Diagnosis is usually made by ultrasonic evaluation of the position of the placenta relative to the internal cervical os. If the diagnosis cannot be made by ultrasound then a vaginal examination will be performed in the operating room. The patient is brought to the operating room and prepared for emergency induction of general anesthesia and cesarean section in the event of profuse hemorrhage after vaginal examination. This is referred to as a "double set-up" (Table 61.4).

12. What is the obstetric management of placenta previa?

Management of placenta previa depends on the amount of blood loss; the presence or absence of further bleeding; the type of previa, and the gestational age of the fetus. If bleeding has stopped and both the mother and fetus are stable, then a conservative approach is elected. Bed rest with fetal monitoring is prescribed to allow further maturation of the fetus. Additional bleeding episodes or signs of fetal distress indicate the need for an immediate cesarean section.

13. How would you anesthetize the patient with placenta previa for cesarean section?

As with a placental abruption, both the fetal and maternal condition must be evaluated. Most women with a placenta previa have an uneventful prenatal course. As the placenta covers the cervical os, cesarean delivery will be needed. In the absence of maternal hemorrhage, a regional anesthetic, spinal or epidural, may be performed in the usual fashion. Adequate intravenous access should be obtained prior to placement of the spinal anesthetic and the patient should have crossmatched blood available should unexpected hemorrhage occur. The anesthesia team must also be prepared to convert to general anesthesia should significant hemorrhage and maternal hemodynamic instability develop.

In the presence of significant hemorrhage, regional anesthesia is contraindicated and a general anesthetic should be performed. Adequate intravenous access should be obtained prior to induction and appropriate monitoring (e.g., arterial line) should be placed. Induction of anesthesia would follow the same guidelines as for a placental abruption.

SUGGESTED READINGS

Beard RW, Filshie GM, Knight CA, Roberts GM: The significance of the changes in the continuous fetal heart rate in the first stage of labour. J Obstet Gynaecol Br Commonw 78: 865-881, 1971

Cunningham GA, MacDonald PC, Gant NF, Leveno KJ, Gilstrap III, LC, Hankins GDV, Clark SL: Willams Obstetrics, 20th edition. Appleton & Lange, Stamford, CT, 1997

Fay RA, Hughes AO, Farron NT: Platelets in pregnancy: hyperdestruction in pregnancy. Obstet Gynecol 61:238-240, 1983

Gilabert J, Estelles A, Aznar J, Galbis M: Abruptio placentae and disseminated intravascular coagulation. Acta Obstet Gynecol Scand 64:35-39, 1985

Pritchard JA, Brekke AL: Clinical and laboratory studies on severe abruption placentae. Am J Obstet Gynecol 97: 681-700, 1967

Rolbin SH, Abbott D, Musclow F, Papsin F, Lie LM, Freedman J: Epidural anesthesia in pregnant patients with low platelet counts. Obstet Gynecol 71:918-920, 1988

Salamalekis E, Vitoratos N, Loghis C, et al.: Evaluation of fetal heart rate patterns during the second stage of labor through fetal oximetry. Gynecol Obstet Invest 48:151-154, 1999

ANESTHESIA FOR NONOBSTETRIC SURGERY DURING PREGNANCY

Yaakov Beilin, MD

A 32-year-old woman presents to the emergency room complaining of abdominal pain, nausea, and vomiting. After physical examination, a presumptive diagnosis of appendicitis is made and an emergency appendectomy is scheduled. The patient is also 17 weeks pregnant.

QUESTIONS

1. What is the incidence of nonobstetric surgery in the pregnant patient?
2. What are the anesthetic concerns when anesthetizing a pregnant patient?
3. What are the physiologic changes during pregnancy and how do they impact on anesthesia?
4. What is a teratogen and which anesthetic agents are known teratogens?
5. What precautions should be taken to avoid intrauterine fetal asphyxia?
6. How is preterm labor prevented?
7. What monitors should be used when anesthetizing the pregnant patient?
8. What are the special considerations for laparoscopic surgery?
9. What general recommendations can be made when anesthetizing the pregnant patient for nonobstetric surgery?

1. What is the incidence of nonobstetric surgery in the pregnant patient?

The incidence of nonobstetric surgery during pregnancy is between 0.3% and 2%. There are approximately 3.5 million deliveries per year in the United States, which means that between 10,000 and 70,000 pregnant patients will require surgery. This may be an underestimate due to surgery performed prior to clinical recognition of pregnancy. Appendectomy is the most common nonobstetric operation during pregnancy. However, almost every type of surgical procedure has been successfully performed in the pregnant patient, including open-heart procedures with cardiopulmonary bypass, neurosurgical procedures requiring hypotensive techniques and hypothermia, and liver transplantation.

2. What are the anesthetic concerns when anesthetizing a pregnant patient?

Anesthetizing the pregnant patient is one of the only times an anesthesiologist must consider two patients simultaneously. Maternal considerations result from the physiologic changes of pregnancy that affect almost every organ system (Table 62.1). In order to provide safe anesthesia to the pregnant patient, one must not only understand the physiologic changes but also when they occur during the gestational period and how they impact on the administration of anesthesia. Fetal concerns include the possible teratogenic effects of anesthetic agents, avoidance of intrauterine fetal asphyxia, and prevention of premature labor.

TABLE 62.1	Physiologic Changes of Pregnancy		

Respiratory		Gastrointestinal	
Minute ventilation	Increases by 50%	Motility	Decreases
Tidal volume	Increases by 40%	Stomach position	More cephalad and
Respiratory rate	Increases by 10%		horizontal
Oxygen consumption	Increases by 20%	Transaminases	Increases
PaO_2	Increases by 10 mmHg	Alkaline phosphatase	Increases
Dead space	No change	Pseudocholinesterase	Decreases by 20%
Alveolar ventilation	Increases by 70%	Hematologic	
$PaCO_2$	Decreases by 10 mmHg	Hemoglobin	Decreases
Arterial pH	No change	Coagulation factors	Increase
Serum HCO_3^-	Decreases by 4 mEq/L	Platelet count	Decreases by 20%
Functional residual capacity	Decreases by 20%	Lymphocyte function	Decreases
Expiratory reserve volume	Decreases by 20%	Renal	
Residual volume	Decreases by 20%	Renal blood flow	Increases
Vital capacity	No change	Glomerular filtration rate	Increases
		Serum creatinine and BUN	Decrease
Cardiovascular		Creatinine clearance	Increases
Cardiac output	Increases by 30–40%	Glucosuria	1–10 g/day
Heart rate	Increases by 15%	Proteinuria	300 mg/day
Stroke volume	Increases by 30%	Nervous system	
Total peripheral resistance	Decreases by 15%	MAC	Decreases by 40%
Femoral venous pressure	Increases by 15%	Endorphin levels	Increase
Central venous pressure	No change		
Systolic blood pressure	Decreases by 0–15%		
Diastolic blood pressure	Decreases by 10–20%		
Intravascular volume	Increases by 35%		
Plasma volume	Increases by 45%		
Red blood cell volume	Increases by 20%		

3. What are the physiologic changes during pregnancy and how do they impact on anesthesia?

Respiratory System

Due to increased progesterone levels during the first trimester, minute ventilation is increased by almost 50% and remains at this level for the remainder of the pregnancy. The increase in minute ventilation leads to a decrease in arterial carbon dioxide tension ($PaCO_2$) to approximately 30 mmHg. Arterial pH remains unchanged because of a compensatory increase in renal excretion of bicarbonate ions. At term, alveolar ventilation is increased by 70% because anatomic dead space does not change significantly during pregnancy. After the fifth month of pregnancy, the functional residual capacity, expiratory reserve volume, and residual volume are all decreased by about 20% because of the gravid uterus pushing on the diaphragm. Vital capacity is not appreciably changed from prepregnancy levels.

Anesthetic Implications Increased alveolar ventilation and decreased functional residual capacity lead to a more rapid uptake and excretion of inhaled anesthetics.

The decrease in functional residual capacity in conjunction with increases in cardiac output, metabolic rate, and oxygen consumption make the pregnant patient more susceptible to arterial hypoxemia during periods of apnea or airway obstruction.

Edema, weight gain, and increase in breast size may make intubation of the trachea technically difficult. An array of laryngoscope blades and handles and other emergency airway management equipment should be available. Capillary engorgement of the mucosal lining of the upper airway accompanies pregnancy. This mandates extreme care during manipulation of the airway and the use of a smaller-than-normal tracheal tube. The use of a nasal airway and nasotracheal intubation should be avoided.

Cardiovascular System

Cardiac output is increased by 30–40% during the first trimester. This is primarily related to an increase in stroke volume (30%) and secondarily related to an increase in heart rate (15%). Cardiac output increases slightly further during the second trimester and lasts throughout the pregnancy.

Blood pressure normally decreases during pregnancy because of a 15% decrease in systemic vascular resistance. Near term, 10–15% of patients have a dramatic reduction in blood pressure in the supine position, often associated with diaphoresis, nausea, vomiting, pallor, and changes in cerebration. This is the "supine hypotensive syndrome" and is caused by compression of the inferior vena cava and aorta by the gravid uterus. Other manifestations of the syndrome are decreases in renal and uteroplacental blood flow from compression of the aorta. Displacing the uterus by tilting the patient on her left side can alleviate the symptoms of this syndrome.

Intravascular volume is increased by 35% during pregnancy. Because plasma volume increases by a greater percentage than red blood cell volume (45% and 20% respectively) there is a relative anemia during pregnancy. Nevertheless, a hemoglobin concentration of less than 11 g/dL is considered abnormal.

Anesthetic Implications   Increases in cardiac output will hasten the speed of intravenous inductions.

Gastrointestinal System

Due to increased progesterone levels, gastrointestinal tract motility is decreased by the end of the first trimester. The stomach, displaced upward by the enlarging uterus, eventually assumes a horizontal position further slowing stomach emptying. This also results in a change in position and function of the gastroesophageal sphincter. Anxiety, pain, and administration of opioids and anticholinergics will further slow gastric emptying. Gastrin production is increased during pregnancy (because the placenta produces gastrin) leading to an increase in acid production.

Anesthetic Implications   The above changes in the gastrointestinal system, by the end of the first trimester, place the pregnant patient at increased risk for aspiration of gastric contents. A nonparticulate antacid, H_2 receptor blocker, and metoclopramide should be used to decrease the acidity and volume of the gastric contents. After the first trimester, all general anesthetics should be conducted with a rapid sequence induction, cricoid pressure, and tracheal intubation.

Hepatic System

Tests of liver function (serum glutamic-oxaloacetic transaminase, lactic acid dehydrogenase, alkaline phosphatase, and cholesterol) are commonly increased during pregnancy. These increases do not necessarily indicate abnormal liver function. Pseudocholinesterase activity declines by as much as 20% during the first trimester and remains fairly stable during the remainder of the pregnancy.

Anesthetic Implications   Prolonged apnea is rarely a problem following a standard dose of succinylcholine. Similarly, prolonged activity of ester-linked local anesthetics has not been a problem.

Hematologic System and Blood Constituents

Pregnancy does not significantly alter the lymphocyte count, but lymphocyte function is depressed, which can decrease maternal resistance to infection. The risk of upper respiratory infections is increased, which may complicate airway management during general anesthesia.

The platelet count decreases by about 20% during pregnancy but is usually of no clinical significance. Circulating levels of coagulation factors increase significantly during pregnancy leading to the hypercoagulable state of pregnancy.

Anesthetic Implications   The increased risk of upper airway infections may complicate airway management during general anesthesia. Increased coagulability may predispose the pregnant patient to thromboembolic events including pulmonary embolism.

Renal System

Renal blood flow (RBF) and glomerular filtration rate (GFR) are increased during the first trimester, leading to a rise in creatinine clearance and a fall in serum creatinine. During the third trimester, RBF and GFR decrease toward prepregnant levels because of compression of the aorta by the enlarging uterus. Due to progesterone, renal calyces and pelves dilate during the third month of pregnancy. During the third trimester, they dilate further because of ureteral compression. This dilatation may lead to stasis and urinary tract infections.

Anesthetic Implications   Care should be taken not to overhydrate the patient because urinary retention is common during spinal or epidural anesthesia, which may necessitate bladder catheterization and further predispose the patient to urinary tract infections.

Central Nervous System

The minimum alveolar concentration (MAC) for inhaled anesthetics is decreased by up to 40% during pregnancy. This is related to a progesterone and endorphin effect. Compression of the inferior vena cava by the gravid uterus leads to dilatation of the azygos system and the epidural veins. Epidural venous engorgement decreases the size of the epidural and intrathecal spaces.

Anesthetic Implications   The decrease in MAC along with an increase in alveolar ventilation places the pregnant patient at risk for anesthetic overdose. The decreased size of the epidural and intrathecal spaces as a result of epidural venous engorgement explains why the doses of drugs used during a major conduction block must be decreased. An alternative explanation is that progesterone may increase the sensitivity of nerve cells to local anesthetics since neuraxial drug requirements decrease prior to uterine enlargement.

4. What is a teratogen and which anesthetic agents are known teratogens?

A teratogen is a substance that produces an increase in the incidence of a particular defect that cannot be attributed to chance. In order to produce a defect, the teratogen must be administered in a sufficient dose at a critical point in development. In humans, this critical point is during organogenesis, which extends from 15 days to approximately 60 days gestational age. However, the central nervous system does not fully develop until after birth; therefore the critical time for this system may extend beyond gestation.

Three approaches have been utilized to study the effects of anesthetic agents or anesthesia in the pregnant patient: (1) animal studies, (2) studies of operating room personnel chronically exposed to trace concentrations of inhaled anesthetics, and (3) studies of women who underwent surgery while pregnant.

The results of animal studies are of limited value because of (1) species variation, (2) the fact that the doses of anesthetic agents used in animal studies were usually far greater than those used clinically, and (3) other factors such as hypercarbia, hypothermia, and hypoxemia (known teratogens) were either not measured or not controlled. Species variation is particularly important. Thalidomide has no known teratogenic effects on rats and was approved

by the United States Food and Drug Administration (FDA) for use in humans. It is now known that thalidomide is teratogenic in humans.

The FDA has established a risk classification system to assist physicians in weighing the risks and benefits when choosing therapeutic agents for the pregnant woman (Table 62.2). Most anesthetic agents, including the intravenous induction agents, local anesthetics, opioids, and neuromuscular blocking drugs have been assigned a Category B or C classification (Table 62.3).

The use of two commonly used agents, benzodiazepines and nitrous oxide, are controversial. Some investigators, in retrospective studies, noted an association between diazepam taken in the first 6 weeks of pregnancy and cleft palate. Although this finding has been questioned by the results of a prospective study, diazepam and other benzodiazepines are classified by the FDA as Category D drugs (i.e., positive evidence of risk) and, therefore, should be avoided.

Nitrous oxide is a known teratogen in mammals. The presumption was that the teratogenicity of nitrous oxide in animals is related to its oxidation of vitamin B_{12}, which then cannot function as a cofactor for the enzyme methionine synthetase. Methionine synthetase is needed for the formation of thymidine, a subunit of DNA. However, pretreatment of rats exposed to nitrous oxide with folinic acid, which bypasses the methionine synthetase step in DNA synthesis, does not prevent congenital abnormalities. In addition, suppression of methionine synthetase occurs at low concentrations of nitrous oxide – concentrations found safe in animal studies. Despite these theoretical concerns, nitrous oxide has not been found to be associated with congenital abnormalities in humans. Interestingly, the FDA has not given nitrous oxide a category classification because it is a medical gas and not directly regulated by the FDA.

TABLE 62.2	**United States Food and Drug Administration Category Ratings of Drugs During Pregnancy**
Category A:	Controlled studies demonstrate no risk
	Well-controlled studies in humans have not demonstrated risk to the fetus
Category B:	No evidence of risks in humans
	Either animal studies have found a risk but human studies have not; or animal studies are negative but adequate human studies have not been done
Category C:	Risk cannot be ruled out
	Human studies have not been adequately performed and animal studies are positive or have not been conducted. Potential benefits may justify the risk
Category D:	Potential evidence of risk
	Confirmed evidence of human risk. However, benefits may be acceptable despite the known risk, i.e., no other medication is available to treat a life-threatening situation
Category X:	Contraindicated in pregnancy
	Human or animal studies have shown fetal risk which clearly outweighs any possible benefit to the patient

| TABLE 62.3 | United States Food and Drug Administration Category Ratings of Specific Anesthetic Agents |

Anesthetic Agent	Classification
Induction agents	
Etomidate	C
Ketamine	C
Methohexital	B
Propofol	B
Thiopental	C
Inhaled agents	
Desflurane	B
Enflurane	B
Halothane	C
Isoflurane	C
Sevoflurane	B
Local anesthetics	
2-chloroprocaine	C
Bupivacaine	C
Lidocaine	B
Ropivacaine	B
Tetracaine	C
Cocaine	X
Opioids	
Alfentanil	C
Fentanyl	C
Sufentanil	C
Meperidine	B
Morphine	C
Neuromuscular blocking drugs	
Atracurium	C
Cisatracurium	B
Curare	C
Mivacurium	C
Pancuronium	C
Rocuronium	B
Succinylcholine	C
Vecuronium	C
Benzodiazepines	
Diazepam	D
Midazolam	D

A number of epidemiologic studies have been performed to determine the health hazards, including birth defects and spontaneous abortions, of chronic exposure to anesthetic gases. All the studies found similar results. The authors of the largest study, sponsored by the American Society of Anesthesiologists (1974), sent questionnaires to 73,496 individuals who may have been exposed to anesthetic gases. The study population included the entire membership of the American Society of Anesthesiologists, the American Association of Nurse Anesthetists, the Association of Operating Room Nurses, and the Association of Operating Room Technicians. These personnel (anesthesiologists, nurses, etc.) received questionnaires in the mail designed to gather information about the extent of their exposure and reproductive outcome. They found that operating room personnel had an increased risk of spontaneous abortions and congenital abnormalities. They recommended that a means to scavenge trace anesthetic gases should be mandatory in all operating rooms, which is the current standard. However, all these studies were later criticized for their lack of a control group, low response rate to questionnaires, recall bias, and statistical inaccuracies.

There have also been several retrospective studies of pregnant patients who had undergone surgery to determine whether there is an association between anesthesia and surgery and congenital defects, spontaneous abortions, or fetal demise. All studies have found similar results. In the largest study, Mazze and Kallen (1989) linked the data from three Swedish health registries: the Medical Birth Registry, the Registry of Congenital Malformations, and the Hospital Discharge registry for the 9-year period 1973–1981. They examined the data for four adverse outcomes including congenital defects, stillborn infants, infants born alive but who died within 7 days, and infants with a birth weight <1,500 grams and <2,500 grams. They found 5,405 of 720,000 women had undergone surgery during their pregnancy. In their data set, most procedures were performed during the first trimester (41.6%), and the incidence decreased during the second (34.8%) and third (23.5%) trimesters. There was no increase in babies with congenital abnormalities or stillborn births among those who underwent surgery while pregnant during any trimester. However, the number of babies born with a birth weight <1,500 grams and <2,500 grams, and the number of babies who died within 7 days of birth, was greater in those who underwent surgery while pregnant. This was true during all three trimesters. These risks could not be linked to either the specific anesthetic agents or the anesthetic technique. Most operations (54%) were performed under general anesthesia and nitrous oxide was used in 98% of the general anesthetics. The increased risk to the fetus may be due to the condition that necessitated surgery in the first place, with the highest rate occurring with gynecologic procedures. These data are very important because they clearly demonstrate that anesthetic agents are not teratogenic and that the greatest risk is premature labor with the delivery of a low birth weight baby. Furthermore, the data strongly suggest that the anesthetic agents are not responsible for the major complication of surgery: premature labor and early delivery of the fetus.

5. What precautions should be taken to avoid intrauterine fetal asphyxia?

Intrauterine fetal asphyxia is avoided by maintaining normal maternal arterial oxygen tension (PaO_2), $PaCO_2$, and uterine blood flow. Maternal hypoxemia may lead to fetal hypoxemia and even fetal demise. General anesthesia is a particular risk to the pregnant woman because management of the airway can be difficult and the rate of hemoglobin oxygen desaturation is increased due to the decreased functional residual capacity and increased oxygen consumption. However, care must also be taken during a regional anesthetic because a high segmental level of anesthesia during a major conduction block, a toxic local anesthetic reaction, or oversedation can also lead to a hypoxic event. High inspired oxygen tension does not adversely affect the fetus even if 100% oxygen is administered.

Both maternal hypercapnia and hypocapnia can be detrimental to the fetus. Severe hypocapnia produced by excessive positive pressure ventilation may increase mean intrathoracic pressure, decrease venous return, and lead to a decrease in uterine blood flow. In addition, maternal alkalosis, as produced by hyperventilation, will decrease uterine blood flow by direct vasoconstriction and will decrease oxygen delivery by shifting the maternal oxyhemoglobin dissociation curve to the left. Severe hypercapnia is detrimental because it is associated with fetal acidosis and myocardial depression.

Both drugs and anesthetic procedures affect uterine blood flow. Placental blood flow is directly proportional to the net perfusion pressure across the intervillous space and inversely proportional to the resistance. Perfusion pressure will be decreased by hypotension, which may be due to the use of an epidural or spinal anesthetic, from aortocaval compression in the supine position, or from hemorrhage. Vasoconstriction due to the use of α-adrenergic drugs, decreased $PaCO_2$, or increased catecholamines such as occurs during pain, apprehension, or light anesthesia, will increase vascular resistance and decrease uteroplacental blood flow.

6. How is preterm labor prevented?

Premature labor, preterm delivery, and the delivery of an infant <1,500 grams are the most significant risks to the fetus. Medications that have α-adrenergic agonist properties (e.g., ketamine and phenylephrine) can increase uterine vascular tone and should be avoided, if possible. The potent inhaled anesthetic agents decrease uterine tone and inhibit uterine contractions and may, therefore, be beneficial. No study, however, has ever documented that any particular anesthetic agent or technique is associated with a higher or lower incidence of miscarriage or preterm labor. The greatest risk for preterm labor occurs when there is uterine manipulation, as occurs during gynecologic procedures.

The lowest risk for preterm labor occurs during the second trimester.

7. What monitors should be used when anesthetizing the pregnant patient?

In addition to the routine intraoperative monitors, the fetal heart rate and uterine tone should be monitored, if at all possible. Using a Doppler apparatus, fetal heart rate monitoring becomes feasible after the 16th week of pregnancy. An external tocodynamometer can be used if the uterus is at or above the level of the umbilicus. These monitors may be technically difficult or impossible to use during an intra-abdominal procedure or in an obese patient. It is important that someone proficient in fetal monitoring be present throughout the case to interpret the uterine/fetal tracings. Also, there should be a plan as to how to proceed in the event of fetal distress. Prior to 23–24 weeks gestation when the baby is not viable, optimization of the maternal condition, by increasing the blood pressure or increasing the inspired oxygen concentration, may improve the fetal condition. After 23–24 weeks gestation, in addition to attempts at correcting the intrauterine milieu, emergent cesarean section should be part of the plan. Fetal heart rate and uterine tone monitoring should continue into the postoperative period.

8. What are the special considerations for laparoscopic surgery?

Once considered an absolute contraindication during pregnancy, laparoscopic surgery is now commonly performed during pregnancy. Outcome in those who have surgery laparoscopically and those who undergo a traditional laparotomy is the same. Specific anesthetic considerations during laparoscopy include maintaining normocarbia, because carbon dioxide is commonly used to maintain a pneumoperitoneum. Surgical concerns include caution during placement of the trochars, which can be accomplished as an open technique, and maintaining low pneumoperitoneum pressures (<15 mmHg) so that uterine perfusion is maintained.

9. What general recommendations can be made when anesthetizing the pregnant patient for nonobstetric surgery?

Whenever possible, anesthesia and surgery should be avoided during the first trimester. Prior to initiating any anesthetic, an obstetrician should be consulted and fetal heart rate tones should be documented. Precautions against aspiration should be taken from as early as the 12th week by administering a clear nonparticulate oral antacid, H_2 receptor blocker, and metoclopramide. Apprehension should be allayed by personal reassurance rather than with premedication, if possible. The patient should be informed that there is no known risk to the baby regarding congenital malformations but that there is an increased risk of miscarriage or premature labor. The patient should be transported to the operating room with left uterine displacement to avoid aortocaval compression.

In addition to the routine intraoperative monitors, the fetal heart rate and uterine tone should be monitored, and should continue to be monitored into the postoperative period.

The type of anesthesia is determined by maternal indications, the site and nature of the surgery, and the anesthesiologist's experience. The dose of all anesthetic agents for general or regional anesthesia should be reduced. Unless otherwise contraindicated, local or regional anesthesia may be preferable to general anesthesia to avoid the risk of aspiration and to decrease fetal drug exposure.

If a spinal or an epidural anesthetic is to be conducted then adequate prehydration (at least 1000 cc of a crystalloid solution) should be administered to prevent hypotension. If hypotension does occur, it must be treated immediately with the administration of additional crystalloid or by using a drug with predominantly β-adrenergic effects, such as ephedrine.

General anesthesia should be preceded by careful evaluation of the airway, denitrogenation, and a rapid sequence induction with the application of cricoid pressure. Since tracheal intubation may be technically difficult an array of laryngoscope blades, handles, and other emergency airway management equipment should be available. Extreme care should be taken during manipulation of the airway and a smaller-than-normal tracheal tube should be inserted. The use of a nasal airway and nasotracheal intubation should be avoided. A high concentration of oxygen should be used (at least 50%) and $PaCO_2$ should be maintained at normal pregnancy levels (30–35 mmHg). End-tidal carbon dioxide ($ETCO_2$) is an excellent approximation of $PaCO_2$ in the pregnant patient because the $PaCO_2$–$ETCO_2$ gradient decreases during pregnancy.

Cardiopulmonary bypass, hypothermia, and hypotensive techniques have all been performed successfully during pregnancy and should not be withheld, if necessary.

Epidural or subarachnoid opioids are an excellent choice for pain management because they cause minimal sedation and smaller doses can be utilized compared with the intramuscular or intravenous routes. Nonsteroidal anti-inflammatory drugs should be avoided because they may cause premature closure of the ductus arteriosus.

Regardless of the technique, maintenance of a normal intrauterine physiologic milieu throughout the perioperative period, including the avoidance of hypotension, hypoxemia, hypercarbia, hypocarbia, and hypothermia is the key to a successful outcome.

Recommendation for Anesthetizing the Pregnant Patient for Nonobstetric Surgery

Avoid surgery during the first trimester
Document FHR tones prior to surgery
Monitor uterine tone and FHR tones during and
    after surgery
Avoid premedication
Transport with left uterine displacement
Regional anesthesia is recommended whenever
    possible

Aspiration prophylaxis after the first trimester
    Nonparticulate antacid
    H_2 blocker
    Metoclopramide

If regional anesthesia:
    Fluid preloading
    Treat hypotension with fluid administration
        and/or ephedrine

If general anesthesia:
    Fluid preloading
    Denitrogenate with 100% oxygen
    Rapid sequence with cricoid pressure induction
    Use drugs with history of relative safety
    Adequate oxygenation
    Maintain normocarbia
    Treat hypotension with fluid administration
        and/or ephedrine

SUGGESTED READINGS

American Society of Anesthesiologists Ad Hoc Committee: Occupational disease among operating room personnel: a national study. Anesthesiology 41:321–340, 1974

Brodsky JB, Cohen EN, Brown BW, et al.: Surgery during pregnancy and fetal outcome. Am J Obstet Gynecol 138: 1165–1167, 1980

Fink BR, Shepard TH, Blandau RJ: Teratogenic activity of nitrous oxide. Nature 214:146–148, 1967

Katz JD, Hook R, Barash PG: Fetal heart rate monitoring in pregnant patients undergoing surgery. Am J Obstet Gynecol 125:267–269, 1976

Mazze RI, Kallen B: Reproductive outcome after anesthesia and operation during pregnancy: a registry study of 5,405 cases. Am J Obstet Gynecol 161:1178–1185, 1989

Physician's desk reference, 54th edition. p. 345. Medical Economics Data Production Company, Montvale, 1995

Reedy MB, Kallen B, Kuehl TJ: Laparoscopy during pregnancy: a study of five fetal outcome parameters with use of the Swedish Health Registry. Am J Obstet Gynecol 177:673–679, 1997

Safra MJ, Oakley GP: Association between cleft lip with or without cleft palate and prenatal exposure to diazepam. Lancet ii:478–480, 1975

Society of American Gastrointestinal Endoscopic Surgeons (SAGES): Guidelines for laparoscopic surgery during pregnancy. Surg Endosc 12:189–190, 1998

63

THROMBOCYTOPENIA IN PREGNANCY

Yaakov Beilin, MD

Sharon Abramovitz, MD

A 22-year-old woman presents to the labor and delivery suite at 40 weeks gestation with mild uterine contractions. The obstetricians decide to augment labor with oxytocin and request an epidural anesthetic for labor analgesia. Past medical history is significant for having a miscarriage during a previous pregnancy. Until 2 weeks ago, she has been on lovenox injections 30 mg twice a day. Her laboratory data are within normal limits except for a platelet count of 76,000 mm^{-3}.

QUESTIONS

1. What are the concerns when placing an epidural catheter if the platelet count is low?
2. Who is at risk for developing an epidural hematoma?
3. What is considered a low platelet count from the perspective of epidural catheter placement and why is there controversy regarding choosing a lowest "safe" platelet count?
4. What is the expected platelet count during pregnancy?
5. Describe coagulation and the role platelets play in the process.

6. What are the causes of thrombocytopenia during pregnancy?
7. What tests are available to evaluate platelet function?
8. Describe the bleeding time test and its limitation.
9. Describe the thromboelastogram and its limitations.
10. Describe the platelet function analyzer and its limitations.
11. What is the overall risk of epidural hematoma?
12. Describe the known cases in the literature of epidural hematoma in the parturient.
13. What is the evidence that initiating an epidural anesthetic in a woman with a platelet count <100,000 mm^{-3} may be safe?
14. How do you evaluate the patient who has a platelet count <100,000 mm^{-3}?
15. What are some practical recommendations regarding neuraxial anesthesia in the parturient who presents with a low platelet count?
16. What is low-molecular-weight heparin (LMWH) and how does it compare with and differ from standard heparin?
17. Why do some pregnant women take LMWH?
18. What has been the anesthetic experience with LMWH and neuraxial anesthesia?
19. What are some of the unique recommendations for anesthetizing the parturient on LMWH?

1. What are the concerns when placing an epidural catheter if the platelet count is low?

The concern when placing an epidural catheter in the face of a low platelet count is that either the needle or the catheter will puncture a blood vessel and the blood will not clot, leading to an epidural hematoma.

2. Who is at risk for developing an epidural hematoma?

Anyone who receives a spinal or epidural anesthetic is at risk for developing an epidural hematoma. Epidural hematoma is extremely rare and is generally associated with patients who have disorders of hemostasis. A patient with a clinically active coagulopathy or with a history of easy bruising or bleeding is considered to have an absolute contraindication to regional anesthesia. However, many gray areas exist and this is especially true in patients with thrombocytopenia.

3. What is considered a low platelet count from the perspective of epidural catheter placement and why is there controversy regarding choosing a lowest "safe" platelet count?

An epidural hematoma is a catastrophic complication, which can lead to permanent paralysis. It is, therefore, prudent to practice in a conservative manner and not place an epidural anesthetic if the patient is at any risk of developing this complication. Cousins and Bromage recommended in 1988 that one should not perform an epidural anesthetic if the platelet count is less than 100,000 mm^{-3}. Recently, however, this recommendation has been widely disputed.

Thrombocytopenia is the most common hematologic disorder during pregnancy. Choosing an absolute platelet count below which it is considered too dangerous to place a neuraxial anesthetic may dictate the use of general anesthesia, a riskier technique in the parturient. Hawkins et al. (1997) reviewed pregnancy-related deaths in the United States between 1985 and 1990 and found that the fatality rate for a parturient administered general anesthesia for cesarean section was 32 deaths per million and for neuraxial anesthesia was only 2 deaths per million.

Refraining from administering a neuraxial anesthetic during the labor and delivery process based on a low platelet count commits the patient, at least, to a painful labor. It is possible that later in the course of labor the woman may require a cesarean delivery, perhaps emergently. The anesthesiologist in that situation may then be forced to administer an anesthetic under less than optimal conditions.

4. What is the expected platelet count during pregnancy?

Platelet count decreases by approximately 20% during a normal pregnancy. This decrease does not generally affect the ability to place an epidural anesthetic. However, approximately 7% of all parturients will present with a platelet count <150,000 mm^{-3} and 0.5–1% will present with a platelet count <100,000 mm^{-3}.

5. Describe coagulation and the role that platelets play in the process.

Clotting can be thought of as occurring in two phases: primary and secondary hemostasis. Primary hemostasis is the creation of the initial platelet plug and secondary hemostasis is the creation of the stable fibrin clot. Platelets play an important role in both processes. Generally, blood vessels prevent platelet adhesion by releasing a potent vasodilator, prostacyclin. After vessel wall injury, prostacyclin levels decrease and platelets adhere to the vessel wall. Adhesion leads to activation and degranulation with release of adenosine-5-diphosphate (ADP), serotonin and thromboxane that leads to platelet aggregation. Further aggregation leads to formation of a platelet plug. This plug is unstable and requires fibrin formation, which occurs by activation of the intrinsic and/or extrinsic coagulation system. Platelets provide the phospholipid membrane upon which the coagulation cascade occurs. Platelet abnormalities can be qualitative or quantitative and are the most common hematologic disorders during pregnancy.

6. What are the causes of thrombocytopenia during pregnancy?

Most cases (99%) of thrombocytopenia during pregnancy are related to one of three causes: hypertensive disorders such as preeclampsia, gestational thrombocytopenia, or idiopathic thrombocytopenic purpura (ITP). When evaluating the parturient with thrombocytopenia there are two specific issues to consider. The first concern is whether the disorder is static or dynamic. If the disorder is static, as occurs during gestational thrombocytopenia or ITP, the platelet count is usually stable. If the disorder is dynamic, as occurs during preeclampsia, the platelet count may change rapidly and it is important to obtain serial platelet counts. The second issue is whether platelet function is normal or abnormal. Platelet function is typically normal in gestational thrombocytopenia and ITP and usually abnormal in preeclampsia.

7. What tests are available to evaluate platelet function?

The patient who presents with a platelet disorder is difficult to evaluate with standard laboratory tests because both platelet quantity and quality must be assessed. Tests of platelet function have been criticized for being difficult to perform, lacking reproducibility, and being of questionable clinical relevance. The ideal test would be easy to perform, inexpensive, and would not require specialized equipment,

Thrombocytopenia During Pregnancy

Static disorders
    Gestational thrombocytopenia
    Idiopathic thrombocytopenia purpura

Dynamic disorders
    Preeclampsia

with results that could be reproduced and correlate with outcome. Bedside tests of coagulation include the bleeding time test, thromboelastography (Haemoscope Corporation, Skokie, IL), and newer tests such as the platelet function analyzer, PFA-100 (Dade Behring, Newark, DE).

8. Describe the bleeding time test and its limitation.

The bleeding time test is a simple bedside test that evaluates both the quality and quantity of the platelets. A small skin nick is made with a template on the volar surface of the forearm and the time until the blood clots is measured. A bleeding time of less than 10 minutes is considered normal. Anesthesiologists formerly used the bleeding time test to assess the safety of epidural or spinal anesthesia placement. They would only proceed if the result of the bleeding time test was normal. The bleeding time, however, is no longer recommended for determining the safety of epidural

catheter placement because it does not necessarily reflect the risk of bleeding at other sites and there is wide observer variation. In one study, 12 observers assessed the bleeding time on five separate volunteers. The reliability of the measurements obtained was poor among the 12 observers and the authors concluded that the test is unreliable.

9. Describe the thromboelastogram and its limitations.

The thromboelastogram (TEG) measures all phases of coagulation and fibrinolysis by using less than 1 mL of a whole blood sample to measure the shear elasticity of clotting blood. Blood is placed in a cylindrical cup that oscillates. A pin is suspended in the blood by a torsion wire and is monitored for motion. The torque of the rotating cup only affects the pin after fibrin–platelet bonding has linked the cup and pin together. The strength of the developing clot affects the magnitude of the pin motion such that strong clots move the pin directly in phase with the cup and weak clots do not. The resulting profile is a measure of the time it takes for the first fibrin strand to form, the kinetics of the clot, strength of the clot, and breakdown of the clot (Figure 63.1). The maximum amplitude (MA) has been found to correlate best with platelet function.

Orlikowski et al. (1996) measured platelet counts, TEG parameters, and bleeding times in healthy pregnant women and in those with preeclampsia. They found that the MA remains normal (53 mm) until the platelet count decreases to less than 54,000 mm^{-3} (95% confidence limit 40,000–75,000 mm^{-3}). Based on their study, they suggested that a platelet count of 75,000 mm^{-3} should be associated

Normal TEG

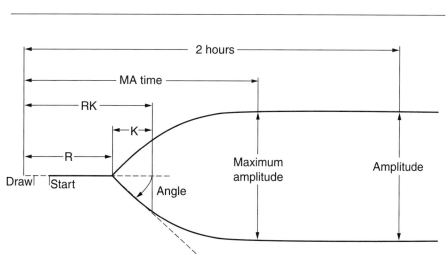

FIGURE 63.1   Thromboelastogram (TEG). R: Time until the onset of clotting. K: Time until the tracing amplitude reaches 20 mm. A: Measures the angle between the tangent line drawn from the curve to the split point and the tracing's horizontal line, in degrees. MA: Measures the maximum amplitude, a measure of clotting strength.

with adequate hemostasis. There is no clinical evidence, however, that a normal MA correlates with safe epidural anesthesia.

10. Describe the platelet function analyzer and its limitations.

The platelet function analyzer (PFA-100) is an intriguing test because it is specific for platelet function, the primary disorder in the parturient. The machine simulates the in vivo hemostatic mechanism of platelet function by accelerating citrated whole blood through a 150 μm aperture cut in a collagen membrane. The collagen membrane is coated with one of two platelet activators: epinephrine or ADP. The cartridges are named for the platelet activator that coats them, CEPI or CADP, respectively. The time taken for the aperture to close is called the closure time (CT). This machine is commonly used by hematologists as a screening tool for patients who present with unknown coagulopathies and is sensitive for the detection of von Willebrand disease. Initial studies in the parturient have focused on defining the expected CT and have found that it may be more sensitive than the MA from the TEG for patients with thrombocytopenia and preeclampsia.

11. What is the overall risk of epidural hematoma?

The overall risk of spinal or epidural hematoma following neuraxial anesthesia is in the range of 1:150,000–250,000. Vandermeulen et al. (1994) reviewed the literature and found 61 cases of anesthesia-related epidural hematoma. This review has better defined the risks of epidural hematoma. Most (68%) occurred in patients with coagulopathies and 75% of all patients had an epidural rather than a spinal anesthetic. Of those who received an epidural anesthetic, 88% had an epidural catheter inserted and almost 50% of those patients developed an epidural hematoma following catheter removal.

12. Describe the known cases in the literature of epidural hematoma in the parturient.

There are 10 reports in the literature of neuraxial (spinal or epidural) hematoma occurring in parturients. The cases are as follows:

- Three cases: The diagnoses were made clinically and the symptoms resolved spontaneously.
- One case: Magnetic resonance imaging (MRI) was performed in a patient with neurofibromatosis to make the diagnosis of epidural hematoma. The symptoms resolved spontaneously.
- One case: Details about the patient were not available but the patient did require surgery to evacuate an epidural hematoma. The patient was reported as "still improving".

- Two cases: Both patients were reportedly healthy but were later found to have a subdural ependymoma, which is an unpredictable event.
- Two cases: Epidural hematomas were reported in patients who had disorders of coagulation, both of whom recovered fully or had only minor residual deficits. One of these patients presented with cholestasis of pregnancy and received labor epidural analgesia. The patient later developed an epidural hematoma and was found to have an elevated prothrombin time (PT 27.7 seconds) and partial thromboplastin time (PTT 59.1 seconds). The second woman presented with preeclampsia and had a history of a lupus anticoagulant. Her preoperative laboratory tests revealed a normal platelet count of 425,000 mm^{-3}, a PT of 10.5 seconds, and a bleeding time of 3 minutes. Her PTT was elevated at 49 seconds but this was attributed to the lupus anticoagulant. The decision was made to proceed with an epidural anesthetic for cesarean delivery. However, in the operating room, the patient had a grand mal seizure after catheter placement and a general anesthetic was performed. The epidural catheter was never used. The next day, the patient complained of leg weakness and an MRI showed an epidural hematoma that was subsequently evacuated.
- One case: A woman with preeclampsia, who had a platelet count of 71,000 mm^{-3} received an epidural anesthetic with 13 mL of bupivacaine 0.5% for cesarean delivery. One hour after the procedure, she had a seizure in the postanesthesia care unit. It was noted that there was no seizure activity in her lower extremities and a computerized tomography (CT) scan revealed an epidural collection. A laminectomy was performed 6 hours after epidural catheter placement, at which time 4 mL of blood was drained from the epidural space. The patient recovered 72 hours later. Whether the 4 mL was sufficient to cause her symptoms is unknown; it is possible that the symptoms were related to residual local anesthetic effects.

13. What is the evidence that initiating an epidural anesthetic in a woman with a platelet count <100,000 mm^{-3} may be safe?

The safety of initiating an epidural anesthetic when the platelet count is less than 100,000 mm^{-3} is supported by the results of three retrospective studies. In the largest study, Beilin et al. (1997) reviewed the medical records of 15,919 consecutive parturients during a 3-year period. They found 80 women who presented with a platelet count less than 100,000 mm^{-3}, 30 of whom received an epidural anesthetic without sequelae. These 30 women had certain characteristics in common. The platelet count did not decrease around the time of epidural catheter placement and there was no clinical evidence of bleeding. In that study, 5 women were denied an epidural anesthetic because of a decreasing platelet count and 2 women because of evidence of bruising.

14. How do you evaluate the patient who has a platelet count <100,000 mm⁻³?

The history and physical examination are key components when deciding whether to proceed with a regional anesthetic in the parturient with thrombocytopenia. If there is any history of easy bruising or the patient has evidence of petechiae or ecchymosis, regional anesthesia should not be offered. If the patient has no bleeding history, it is our practice to obtain at least one additional platelet count as close in time to epidural placement as possible to assure that it not decreasing further. This is especially important in disease processes that are dynamic, such as preeclampsia. We do not obtain any tests of platelet function nor do we have any absolute lower limit for the platelet count. A patient with a stable platelet count of 50,000 mm^{-3} is probably at lower risk of developing an epidural hematoma than one with a platelet count of 75,000 mm^{-3} that has been rapidly decreasing.

15. What are some practical recommendations regarding neuraxial anesthesia in the parturient who presents with a low platelet count?

If the decision is made to proceed with neuraxial anesthesia, a subarachnoid block using a small-caliber spinal needle is preferable to epidural anesthesia. This is not always possible, especially for women in labor who will require repeated doses of local anesthetic. An epidural anesthetic should be placed using a midline technique. The lowest concentration of local anesthetic necessary to produce analgesia while preserving motor function should be used. The patient should be examined every 1–2 hours to assess the extent of the motor block, and these examinations should continue until after the anesthetic has worn off and the catheter has been removed. In this way, if the patient develops a motor block out of proportion to what one would expect, or if the anesthetic has a prolonged duration of action, the patient can be immediately assessed with MRI for the development of an epidural hematoma. Immediate evaluation is necessary because an emergent laminectomy and decompression must be performed within 6–12 hours of diagnosis to preserve neurologic function. If a patient develops a coagulopathy with an epidural catheter already in situ, the catheter should be removed only after the coagulation status is corrected.

16. What is low-molecular-weight heparin (LMWH) and how does it compare with and differ from standard heparin?

Standard, unfractionated heparin (UH) is a mixture of linear polysaccharide chains, with a molecular weight that ranges from 5,000 to 30,000. Heparin acts as an anticoagulant by binding to antithrombin III and potentiates the inhibition of factors IIa (thrombin), IXa, Xa, XIa, and XIIa. A specific pentasaccharide sequence on the heparin chain has a high-affinity binding site for antithrombin III, and only about 30% of the heparin molecule has this sequence. In order to catalyze inhibition of factor Xa, only the pentasaccharide binding sequence is necessary. However, to catalyze inhibition of factor IIa, a heparin molecule must contain both this high-affinity pentasaccharide sequence and an additional chain of at least 13 sugars. UH is highly sulfated and negatively charged. As a result, it has a great affinity for plasma and vascular matrix proteins, and has less than a 30% bioavailability.

LMWH is produced by chemical or enzymatic depolymerization of standard heparin, which produces shorter polysaccharide chains of 13 to 22 sugars and a molecular weight of 4,000 to 6,000. LMWH has the same anti-Xa activity as standard heparin with less anti-IIa (thrombin) activity. The concentration of LMWH is referred to in international standards and expressed as anti-Xa units per millimeter. The reduced molecular size leads to lower binding of plasma and endothelial cell proteins. This results in greater than 90% bioavailability after subcutaneous injection, a longer plasma half-life (4–6 hours versus 0.5–1 hours for standard heparin), and a predictable and reproducible dose response. Laboratory monitoring is not required. The peak LMWH anti-Xa activity occurs 3–4 hours after subcutaneous injection, and 12-hour anti-Xa levels are approximately 50% of peak levels. LMWH excretion is accomplished almost solely by the kidneys. Protamine sulfate is able to neutralize 100% of anti-IIa activity but only 60–70% of anti-Xa activity, and therefore is not effective at neutralizing LMWH effects.

17. Why do some pregnant women take LMWH?

Pregnancy induces a state of hypercoagulability but the risk of thromboembolic complications is rare. However, some parturients require anticoagulant medication during the antepartum period, such as those with disorders of hemostasis, mechanical heart prostheses, or at high risk for venous thromboembolism. Additionally, anticoagulant medication is used in women with a history of fetal loss related to thrombophilia and hypercoagulable syndromes, such as antithrombin III deficiency, antiphospholipid syndrome, and protein C or S deficiency. Warfarin causes abnormal fetal development and congenital malformations during the first trimester, such as nasal hypoplasia and skeletal dysplasias. It also increases the risk of maternal and fetal hemorrhage when given during the peripartum period. Heparin and LMWH do not cross the placenta, are not teratogenic, and are unlikely to cause fetal hemorrhage. LMWH has gained widespread use in pregnancy, and has certain advantages over UH. UH and LMWH have similar hemorrhagic complication rates and antithrombotic efficacy.

However, LMWH, unlike UH, does not require laboratory monitoring. Also, there is less risk of serious complications with LMWH, such as heparin-induced thrombocytopenia and osteoporosis.

18. What has been the anesthetic experience with LMWH and neuraxial anesthesia?

The release of LMWH for general use in the United States in May 1993 sparked a new challenge for anesthesiologists. Previously, a spinal or epidural hematoma was a rather rare occurrence, reportedly less than 1 in 150,000–220,000. Enoxaparin, the first LMWH to be approved by the United States Food and Drug Administration (FDA), had been used for many years in Europe. However, the approved dosing schedule of enoxaparin was 30 mg (3000 U) every 12 hours in the United States as opposed to 40 mg (4000 U) once daily in Europe. Within 1 year of its introduction in the United States, two cases of epidural hematoma were voluntarily reported through the MedWatch system. The warning section of the drug label was revised and a letter from the manufacturer was issued to practitioners to alert them to the risk of spinal hematoma in patients undergoing neuraxial anesthesia while receiving LMWH. Despite these warnings, a total of 40 cases of perioperative neuraxial hematoma in patients on LMWH were voluntarily reported between May 1993 and November 1997. An FDA Health Advisory was issued in December 1997.

The actual risk of spinal or epidural hematoma in patients receiving LMWH while undergoing neuraxial anesthesia is difficult to estimate. There are certainly additional, unreported cases. The reported incidences of spinal or epidural hematoma in patients receiving LMWH may be approximately 1 in 3,000 for continuous epidural anesthesia and 1 in 100,000 for spinal anesthesia. Of the 40 cases of spinal or epidural hematoma associated with LMWH in conjunction with neuraxial anesthesia, two patients received epidural steroid injections, six underwent spinal anesthesia, one of which was continuous spinal anesthesia, 23 had continuous epidural anesthesia, six were unspecified techniques, and three had general anesthesia after attempted or failed neuraxial anesthesia. Also, some patients had additional risk factors for the development of spinal or epidural hematoma, such as difficult needle placement or administration of antiplatelet or anticoagulant medication. None of the patients were pregnant.

19. What are some of the unique recommendations for anesthetizing the parturient taking LMWH?

Neuraxial anesthesia can be safely administered to the patient receiving LMWH if certain guidelines and precautions are met. The American Society of Regional Anesthesia (ASRA) convened a consensus conference on neuraxial anesthesia in association with anticoagulation on May 2–3, 1998.

TABLE 63.1	Summary of the Recommendations of the Consensus Conference Convened by the American Society of Regional Anesthesia and Pain Medicine Regarding Anticoagulants and Neuraxial Anesthesia and Analgesia

1. The decision to perform a neuraxial block when a patient is receiving LMWH must be made on an individual basis by weighing the risk of spinal hematoma with the benefits of regional anesthesia for a specific patient

2. Monitoring of the anti-Xa level is not recommended, because it is not predictive of the risk of bleeding

3. Concomitant medications known to potentiate bleeding, such as antiplatelet agents or oral anticoagulants, create an additional risk for the development of spinal hematoma

4. If blood is seen during needle or catheter placement, the first dose of LMWH should be delayed for 24 hours

5. If a patient is receiving LMWH preoperatively, neuraxial anesthesia should occur at least 10–12 hours after the last LMWH dose. Patients receiving high doses of LMWH, such as enoxaparin 1 mg/kg twice a day, will require waiting longer, such as 24 hours

6. A single-shot spinal technique may be the safest choice for neuraxial anesthesia

7. The first dose of LMWH should be given no sooner than 24 hours after neuraxial anesthesia. Indwelling catheters should be removed prior to initiation of LMWH, and the first dose may be given 2 hours after catheter removal

8. If a patient is receiving LMWH and has an indwelling catheter, the catheter should not be removed for at least 10–12 hours after the last dose of LMWH

A team of clinicians devised recommendations regarding the administration of neuraxial anesthesia to the patient receiving anticoagulation therapy. These are summarized in Table 63.1.

SUGGESTED READINGS

Beilin Y, Zahn J, Comerford M: Safe epidural analgesia in thirty parturients with platelet counts between 69,000 and 98,000 mm⁻³. Anesth Analg 85:385–388, 1997

Cosmi B, Hirsh J: Low molecular weight heparins. Curr Opin Cardiol 9:612–618, 1994

Cousins MJ, Bromage PR: Epidural neural blockade. p. 335. In Cousins MJ, Bridenbaugh PO (eds): Neural Blockade in Clinical

Anesthesia and Management of Pain, 2nd edition. JB Lippincott, Philadelphia, 1988

Hawkins JL, Koonin LM, Palmer SK, Gibbs CP: Anesthesia-related deaths during obstetric delivery in the United States, 1979–1990. Anesthesiology 86:277–284, 1997

Heit JA: Low-molecular-weight heparin: biochemistry, pharmacology, and concurrent drug precautions. Reg Anesth Pain Med 23:135–139, 1998

Horlocker TT: Low molecular weight heparin and neuraxial anesthesia. Thromb Res 101:141–154, 2001

Horlocker TT, Heit JA: Low molecular weight heparin: biochemistry, pharmacology, perioperative prophylaxis regimens, and guidelines for regional anesthetic management. Anesth Analg 85:874–885, 1997

Horlocker TT, Wedel DJ: Neuraxial block and low-molecular-weight heparin: balancing perioperative analgesia and thromboprophylaxis. Reg Anesth Pain Med 23 [Suppl]: 164–177, 1998

Lind SE: The bleeding time does not predict surgical bleeding. Blood 77:2547–2552, 1991

Orlikowski CE, Rocke DA, Murray WB, Gouws E, Moodley J, Kenoyer DG, Byrne S: Thromboelastography changes in preeclampsia and eclampsia. Br J Anaesth 77:157–161, 1996

Scott DB, Hibbard BM: Serious non-fatal complications associated with extradural block in obstetric practice. Br J Anaesth 64:537–541, 1990

Vandermeulen EP, Van Aken H, Vermylen J: Anticoagulants and spinal-epidural anesthesia. Anesth Analg 79:1165–1177, 1994

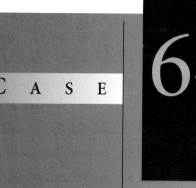

Francine S. Yudkowitz, MD, FAAP

CASE 64 — NEONATAL RESUSCITATION

A 42-year-old woman is in labor. The fetal heart rate (FHR) monitor is showing intermittent variable decelerations with good recovery. The obstetrician ruptures membranes and notes that the amniotic fluid is meconium-stained. Since the FHR monitor shows good beat-to-beat variability the decision is made to allow the mother to continue in labor and deliver vaginally. Two hours later, the baby is delivered vaginally and is noted to be meconium-stained.

QUESTIONS

1. Describe the fetal circulation.
2. What are the physiologic changes that occur at birth?
3. How is neonatal resuscitation managed in the delivery room?
4. What is the Apgar score?

1. Describe the fetal circulation.

The fetal circulation (Figure 64.1) is a parallel circuit in contrast to a series circuit in the adult. In the fetus, gas exchange occurs at the placenta and not the lung. Blood leaving the placenta enters the fetus via the umbilical vein. This relatively well oxygenated blood (pO_2 30–35 mmHg) enters the inferior vena cava, predominantly bypassing the liver via the ductus venosus. Most of this blood upon entering the right atrium is preferentially shunted across the patent foramen ovale to the left side of the heart and out the ascending aorta to the cerebral and coronary circulation. Thus, the brain and heart receive most of the relatively well oxygenated blood. Blood returning from the cerebral circulation via the superior vena cava, which is considerably less oxygenated (pO_2 12–14 mmHg), enters the right side of the heart. This blood is preferentially directed to the right ventricle and exits through the pulmonary artery. Because of the high pulmonary vascular resistance (PVR) that exists in utero, only 10% of this blood enters the pulmonary circulation to provide nutrients for lung growth. The remaining blood is shunted across the ductus arteriosus because of the relatively low systemic vascular resistance (SVR) secondary to the presence of the placenta. Blood enters the descending aorta and supplies the lower fetal body, returning to the placenta via the umbilical arteries.

2. What are the physiologic changes that occur at birth?

When the neonate is delivered, the first breaths expand the lungs with air and alveolar pO_2 increases. These changes lead to a dramatic decrease in PVR. At the same time, the umbilical cord is clamped and the low-resistance placenta is removed from the circulation. This results in an abrupt increase in SVR. These changes lead to:

■ functional closure of the patent foramen ovale because the pressure on the left side of the heart (SVR) is greater than on the right side (PVR);

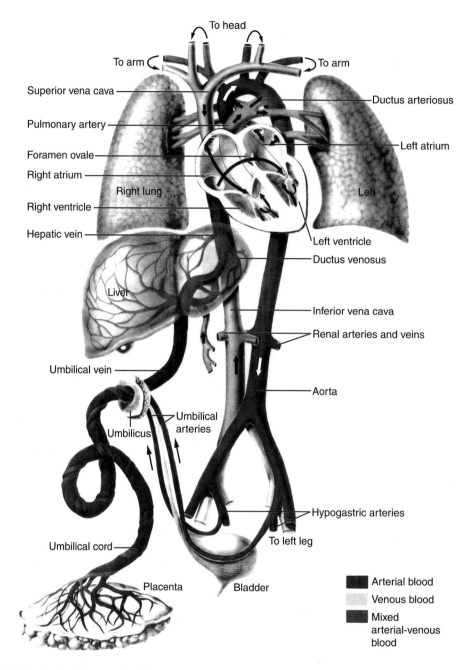

FIGURE 64.1   Fetal circulation. (Reprinted with permission from Miller et al. Anesthesia, 5th edition, p. 1807. Churchill Livingstone, Philadelphia, 2000.)

- functional closure of the ductus arteriosus because of an increase in arterial pO_2. The ductus arteriosus will become the ligamentum arteriosum;
- functional closure of the ductus venosus because of removal of the placenta.

This pattern of circulation closely resembles the adult circulation. However, it is referred to as the transitional circulation because of the reversibility of the above-mentioned changes during adverse events such as hypoxia or acidosis. Any insult that will increase pulmonary vascular resistance will result in reopening of the functionally closed fetal shunts. Factors that will adversely affect PVR are hypoxia, hypercarbia, acidosis, hypothermia, and sympathetic stimulation. Therefore, it is imperative that the initial management of the neonate in the delivery room is to pay meticulous attention to ensuring adequate oxygenation, ventilation, and maintenance of normothermia. Reversion to fetal circulation is referred to as persistent pulmonary hypertension of the newborn (PPHN).

3. How is neonatal resuscitation managed in the delivery room?

Within the first 20 seconds of birth, the neonate should be placed under a radiant warmer and actively dried (Figure 64.2). The mouth and nose should be suctioned. Respiratory effort and adequacy should be assessed within the first 30 seconds of birth. If there are adequate spontaneous respirations, the heart rate should then be assessed. If there is no respiratory effort, inadequate respiratory effort (central cyanosis), or the neonate is gasping, positive-pressure ventilation (PPV) with 100% oxygen should be initiated at a rate of 40–60 breaths per minute with initial peak inspiratory pressures of 30–40 cm H_2O. Endotracheal intubation should be performed if bag-and-mask ventilation is inadequate, a congenital diaphragmatic hernia is suspected, or if there is a need for prolonged intubation.

An endotracheal tube (3.0–3.5 mm ID) may also be placed if a route for administration of resuscitative drugs is needed.

The heart rate should be checked after 15–30 seconds of PPV. If the heart rate is less than 60 beats per minute chest compressions should be started at 120 compressions per minute. Chest compressions can be accomplished in two ways:

1. Place both thumbs on the lower sternum while the other fingers encircle the neonate supporting the back.
2. Place two fingers of one hand on the lower sternum while the other hand supports the back.

The first method is preferred. Compressions should be about one third of the depth of the chest. More importantly, compression depth should be sufficient to produce a palpable pulse. There should be a 3:1 ratio of compressions to ventilations. Heart rate should be reassessed every 30 seconds. Since cardiac depression is usually a result of inadequate respirations, once oxygenation and ventilation is restored the heart will in most cases resume normal function.

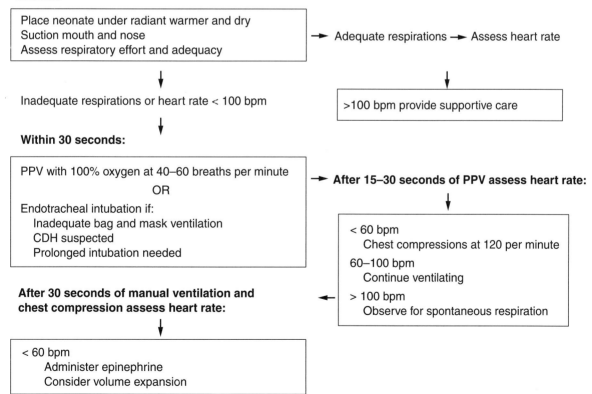

FIGURE 64.2 Neonatal resuscitation in the delivery room. Endotracheal intubation may be performed at any time if circumstances indicate it. PPV, positive-pressure ventilation; bpm, beats per minute.

If after 30 seconds of manual ventilation and chest compressions (90 seconds after birth) the heart rate remains below 60 beats per minute, epinephrine should be administered. Epinephrine 1:10,000 at a dose of 0.01–0.03 mg/kg can be given either intravenously or endotracheally. The epinephrine may be diluted to 1–2 cc with normal saline for endotracheal administration. This should be repeated every 3–5 minutes as indicated (Table 64.1).

Additional resuscitative measures may include volume expansion with an isotonic crystalloid solution or colloids for the hypovolemic infant. Hypovolemia should be suspected in the infant who is not responding to the usual resuscitative measures or whose physical examination is consistent with shock. The initial dose of fluid is 10 cc/kg as a bolus. Additional fluid management should be based on clinical assessment.

Naloxone, a narcotic antagonist, is indicated for the respiratory-depressed neonate born within 4 hours of the mother receiving opioids. The recommended dose is 0.1 mg/kg and may be given by the intravenous, endotracheal, intramuscular, or subcutaneous route. Naloxone is not given to a neonate of a mother who is narcotic-addicted because it may precipitate withdrawal in the neonate. Once naloxone is given, the neonate must be observed for recurrence of apnea because the duration of action of the opioid may exceed the effect of the naloxone.

Sodium bicarbonate should not be used routinely during resuscitation of the neonate. It is indicated only after prolonged resuscitation and documented metabolic acidosis on arterial blood gas. Adequate ventilation and circulation should be established prior to its administration. The recommended dose is 1–2 mEq/kg of a **0.5 mEq** solution.

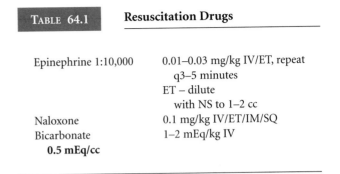

TABLE 64.1	Resuscitation Drugs
Epinephrine 1:10,000	0.01–0.03 mg/kg IV/ET, repeat q3–5 minutes ET – dilute with NS to 1–2 cc
Naloxone	0.1 mg/kg IV/ET/IM/SQ
Bicarbonate **0.5 mEq/cc**	1–2 mEq/kg IV

When meconium is present in the amniotic fluid, specific steps should be taken to limit the risk of meconium aspiration (Figure 64.3). When the head of the neonate is delivered and prior to the neonate's first breath, suctioning of the mouth, pharynx, and nose should be done. Despite this suctioning, there is a subset of neonates who will have meconium in the trachea despite the absence of spontaneous respirations. It is presumed that this occurred in utero. If there is meconium-stained amniotic fluid and the neonate is vigorous after delivery, there is no need to perform tracheal suctioning because it does not improve outcome. In fact, there may be complications associated with tracheal suctioning such as laryngeal trauma. However, if the neonate should develop respiratory or cardiac depression subsequently, suctioning of the trachea should precede PPV. In the neonate who has respiratory and/or cardiac depression (heart rate 60–100 beats per minute) at birth, direct laryngoscopy should be performed to suction the hypopharynx and to intubate the trachea for suctioning of any residual meconium that may be present.

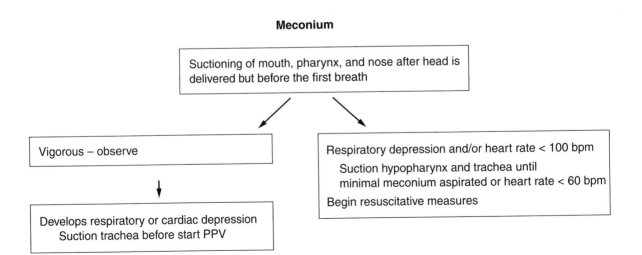

FIGURE 64.3   Neonatal resuscitation in the delivery room in the presence of meconium. Endotracheal intubation may be performed at any time if circumstances indicate it. PPV, positive-pressure ventilation; bpm, beats per minute.

TABLE 64.2	Equipment for Neonatal Resuscitation

Airway
Oxygen source with flowmeter and tubing
Neonatal resuscitation bag with pressure relief valve
Face masks: premature and newborn
Oropharyngeal airways
Laryngoscope handle with extra batteries
Laryngoscope blades: Miller 0 and 1, extra bulbs
Endotracheal tubes: 2.5–4.0 mm ID
Stylet
Bulb syringe
Suction apparatus and catheters 6–10 Fr
Meconium suction device
CO_2 detector (optional)
Laryngeal mask airway (optional)
Adhesive tape

Medications
Epinephrine 1:10,000
Naloxone hydrochloride
Sodium bicarbonate **0.5 mEq/cc**
Dextrose 10%
Intravenous access and fluids
Isotonic crystalloid
24G and 22G angiocatheters
Umbilical catheters: 3.5 Fr, 5 Fr
Alcohol pads
Syringes and needles
Miscellaneous
Gloves
Radiant warmer
Stethoscope
ECG
Pulse oximeter

Repeated intubations and suctioning should be performed until there is minimal meconium recovered or the heart rate is less than 60 beats per minute. During this maneuver, an assistant should be monitoring the heart rate continuously. Even if there is still meconium, once the heart rate is less than 60 beats per minute, resuscitative measures should be initiated immediately.

It is important that all the equipment and pharmacologic agents necessary for resuscitation efforts are available and of the appropriate size (Table 64.2).

4. What is the Apgar score?

Dr. Virginia Apgar, an anesthesiologist, devised a scoring system to assess newborns for their clinical condition and need for medical intervention. The Apgar score (Table 64.3) consists of five parameters that are assessed at 1 and 5 minutes after birth. The five parameters are heart rate, respiratory effort, muscle tone, reflex irritability, and color. A score of 0, 1, or 2 is assigned to each parameter. A score of 8–10 is normal and requires no additional treatment. A score of 5–7 indicates moderate impairment and may only need supplemental oxygen and tactile stimulation. A score of 0–4 indicates the need for immediate resuscitation. The 1 minute score is said to be inversely proportional to the risk of infant mortality, whereas the 5 minute score may relate to the degree of future neurologic impairment.

However, the Apgar score, though still widely performed, is not used to guide resuscitation efforts in the delivery room. One should not wait until 1 minute after birth to begin resuscitative efforts (see discussion above).

TABLE 64.3	Apgar Score

Apgar Score			
	0	**1**	**2**
Heart rate	Absent	<100	>100
Respiratory effort	Absent	Poor	Vigorous
Muscle tone	Limp	Minimal flexion	Active movement
Reflex irritability	Absent	Grimace	Cry
Color	Blue	Extremities blue	Pink

SUGGESTED READINGS

Arkoosh VA: Neonatal resuscitation. pp 675–682. In Norris MC (ed): Obstetric Anesthesia, 2nd edition. Lippincott Williams & Wilkins, Philadelphia, 1999

Bernstein D: The cardiovascular system. pp 1341–1343. In Behrman RE, et al. (ed): Nelson Textbook of Pediatrics, 16th edition. WB Saunders, Philadelphia, 2000

McGowan FX, Steven JM: Cardiac physiology and pharmacology. pp 353–356. In Cote CJ, Todres ID, Goudsouzian NG, Ryan JF (eds): A Practice of Anesthesia for Infants and Children, 3rd edition. WB Saunders, Philadelphia, 2001

Pediatric Working Group of the International Liaison Committee on Resuscitation. Part 11: Neonatal resuscitation. Circulation 102 (Suppl I):I-343–357, 2000

65

GASTROSCHISIS AND OMPHALOCELE

Gregg Lobel, MD

You are informed that a 35-week gestational age infant will be born tomorrow and is being scheduled for closure of an abdominal wall defect. The abdominal wall defect was diagnosed by prenatal ultrasound and the pregnancy has been otherwise uneventful.

QUESTIONS

1. What are the differences between gastroschisis and omphalocele?
2. How is this neonate managed preoperatively?
3. How is the operating room prepared for this newborn?
4. What is the anesthetic plan, and what are the intra-operative and postoperative concerns in this patient?
5. Describe the fluid and blood product management for this neonate intraoperatively.

1. What are the differences between gastroschisis and omphalocele?

The anesthetic management of gastroschisis and omphalocele is very similar but their embryologic origin and associated pathology can vary greatly. Both can be diagnosed during the first trimester of pregnancy by fetal ultrasonography. High levels of α-fetoprotein (AFP) in the mother or in amniotic fluid obtained at amniocentesis raise concerns about the possibility of an abdominal wall defect.

The presence of a peritoneal covering is what distinguishes omphalocele from gastroschisis. Omphalocele results from a failure of the intestinal contents to return to the abdominal cavity at about the 10th week of gestation. It is covered with a membrane that protects the contents and the umbilical cord is usually found near the apex. Gastroschisis develops after the intestinal contents have returned to the abdominal cavity. A defect in the abdominal wall is thought to develop due to a problem with the omphalomesenteric artery and herniation of abdominal contents occurs without a membranous covering. Gastroschisis is associated with a higher incidence of intestinal atresia while omphalocele is more commonly associated with congenital abnormalities outside the gastrointestinal tract. An early amniocentesis is recommended in omphalocele due to the increased incidence of trisomies, while a later amniocentesis may be done with gastroschisis to establish lung maturity. Some believe that if the lungs are mature, an early cesarean section should be done to decrease the changes that occur in the bowel that is extruded in gastroschisis.

2. How is this neonate managed preoperatively?

Immediately after birth, the exposed intra-abdominal contents should be wrapped in a sterile dressing which is then kept warm and moist. Plastic coverings may also help to decrease heat and fluid loss. It is important to monitor and maintain temperature preoperatively. Preoperative preparation should include placement of an intravenous

Gastroschisis Versus Omphalocele

Gastroschisis	Omphalocele
Omphalomesenteric artery occlusion	Failure of the gut to return to the abdominal cavity
No peritoneal membrane	Peritoneal membrane
Protrudes lateral to the umbilicus	Protrudes midline
Intestinal atresia	Associated congenital anomalies

Preoperative Preparation

Fluid replacement with balanced salt solution for third-space losses

Maintenance fluid with glucose (monitor glucose levels)

Temperature maintenance

Wrap defect with warm saline gauze

Avoid trauma to the exposed bowel

Antibiotics only if sepsis develops

catheter for fluid replacement. An arterial catheter may be placed for frequent laboratory analysis, including measurements of blood glucose.

Infants are more susceptible to dehydration because of their increased metabolic rate and water losses. Insensible fluid losses are greater in infants because of their greater surface area/weight ratio and thinner skin. In addition, gastroschisis, omphalocele, pyloric stenosis, intussusception, and many other processes can cause significant electrolyte and fluid imbalances.

Assessment of volume status involves many variables: moistness of mucous membranes, skin turgor, weight, mean arterial pressure, capillary perfusion time, urine output, peripheral pulse quality, and heart rate. Significant fluid deficits and electrolyte imbalances should be corrected preoperatively. Initially a balanced salt solution should be used to increase blood volume and replace third-space losses. Fluid replacement should also include maintenance fluids, with or without glucose, depending on blood glucose analysis. Excess glucose can be detrimental since the neonatal kidney can spill glucose easily, resulting in an osmotic diuresis. As replacement occurs, multiple parameters need to be monitored to assess hydration status, such as vital signs, urine output, clinical examination, and laboratory values.

Maintaining temperature is critical during the perioperative period since hypothermia is a potential risk. Hypothermia causes an increase in the metabolic rate with increased oxygen consumption resulting in hypoxemia, acidosis, and possibly apnea. The neonate attempts to maintain body temperature through nonshivering thermogenesis. This is accomplished by the metabolism of brown fat, which is more abundant in newborns than in adults. Brown fat metabolism is stimulated by norepinephrine released through sympathetic innervation in an attempt to maintain core temperature at a great metabolic cost.

The intestines are susceptible to both morphologic and functional compromise, especially in gastroschisis due to the lack of a protective peritoneal membrane and possible pre-existing fetal peritonitis. Bowel atresia is seen in about 10% of cases. Care should be taken to avoid traumatizing the exposed bowel and to avoid incarceration at the site of extrusion.

Although sepsis may occur, there is no indication for the administration of prophylactic antibiotics.

The neonate should be examined for other associated congenital anomalies, especially those involving the cardiovascular and pulmonary system, which may affect morbidity and mortality. Omphalocele can be a part of the Beckwith-Wiedemann syndrome, which also includes macroglossia, gigantism, organomegaly, and symptomatic hypoglycemia. Neonates with Beckwith-Wiedemann syndrome are known to have a difficult airway due to the macroglossia.

3. How is the operating room prepared for this newborn?

Before any pediatric patient is brought to the operating room, appropriately sized equipment must be prepared for both anesthesia and surgery. Mnemonics may be used to aid in making sure that all critical equipment is available. This has added importance when preparing for a neonate, infant, or child because they will require equipment that is not normally stocked in the operating room, except in a pediatric hospital. A useful mnemonic is MADIMS, which stands for *M*achine, *A*irway, *D*rugs, *I*ntravenous, *M*onitors, and *S*uction.

Machine

Preparing the machine includes following the standard US Food and Drug Administration (FDA) Anesthesia Apparatus Checkout Recommendations, 1993. It is necessary to choose a breathing circuit, either a Mapleson D or a pediatric circle system. The pediatric circle system differs from the adult in that it has hoses that are of lower volume and compliance, which may allow for more constant tidal volumes. Also, heated humidified circuits are available, which can conserve heat and decrease evaporative losses. Some older anesthesia machines have separate pediatric bellows, which may increase the accuracy of delivering very small tidal volumes. Also, the ability to add air to the gas mixture should be assured. This may be necessary for the premature infant, when nitrous oxide cannot be used, in order to avoid high arterial oxygen partial pressures and limit the risk of retinopathy of prematurity.

Airway

Airway equipment is available in all sizes and styles and the anesthesiologist should use the equipment with which he or she is most familiar. The key is to have the appropriate sizes available. This includes masks, oral airways, laryngeal mask airways, endotracheal tubes (ETT), and laryngoscope blades. The best way to be prepared is to have the size that you think you will need and also one size above and below that size. Oral airways are available from size 000 (very small premature neonates) to 9 (large adult). Nasal airways are rarely used in young children due to the risk of adenoidal hemorrhage and the small lumen of the nares. A straight laryngoscope blade (Miller 0 for preterm infants, Miller 0–1 for full-term infants) is often used in neonates and infants.

Uncuffed ETTs have historically been used in infants and children under age 7 years, but a new trend is developing for the use of cuffed tubes in younger age groups. There are many factors to consider when making this decision. In a young child, the narrowest portion of the airway is at the cricoid ring. An ETT should be selected that is neither too small to adequately ventilate the patient nor too large to cause damage to the subglottic area. An important factor, whether the ETT is cuffed or uncuffed, is to have an appropriate air leak, which is <30 cm H_2O in most cases. A general rule for choosing uncuffed tubes in children ages 2 years and above is: [Age + 16]/4.

If a cuffed ETT is chosen, it should be a half-size smaller. Most full-term neonates will have an appropriate leak with a 3.0 uncuffed ETT, and by a few months of age a 3.5 uncuffed ETT can be used (Table 65.1). After placing the correct size ETT, it is critical to secure it well since even the slightest movement of the ETT in a neonate could result in a mainstem intubation or extubation. If a cuffed ETT is used, the cuff should be inflated only if the air leak is less than that needed to provide adequate positive pressure ventilation. A leak at <30 cm H_2O should be present. During the course of the case, the air leak should be checked since the use of nitrous oxide as part of the anesthetic may increase the volume in the cuff. If lung compliance changes

TABLE 65.1	Guidelines for Endotracheal Tubes
Patient Age	**Size (Internal Diameter, mm)[a]**
Premature neonate	2.5–3.0
Full-term to 3 months	3.0–3.5
3 months to 18 months	3.5–4.0
18 months to 2 years	4.5

[a]These are uncuffed endotracheal tube sizes.

during surgery, it may be necessary to add air to the cuff to increase the air leak pressure and improve ventilation.

Drugs

Drugs refer to both the anesthetic and non-anesthetic medications that should be drawn up and immediately available during the anesthetic. These include induction agents, muscle relaxants, and opioids, as well as emergency medications such as atropine and epinephrine. The appropriate dose of these drugs should be determined in advance, based on the weight of the patient, and drawn up in an appropriately sized syringe.

Intravenous

Intravenous fluid and supplies for placing an intravenous line should be available in the operating room. A buretrol should be a part of the set and no more than 10 mL/kg of fluid should be in the buretrol at any time to prevent fluid overload if it accidentally ran in quickly. All air bubbles should be removed from the intravenous tubing because there is a high incidence of patent foramen ovale in neonates.

Monitors

Monitors should include all those set forth by the American Society of Anesthesiologists (ASA) in their Standards for Basic Intraoperative Monitoring, last amended in October 1998. All other monitors will be based on the clinical condition of the patient and the type of surgery planned.

Suction

Suction should be immediately available and within easy reach of the anesthesiologist. A Yankauer is the best for large volumes because of its large holes, but in small infants it may be necessary to use smaller suction catheters.

Methods for maintaining normothermia in the neonate should also be made available. This is best accomplished with a forced-air warming blanket and warming of the operating room.

4. What is the anesthetic plan, and what are the intraoperative and postoperative concerns in this patient?

The patient should be transported to the operating room in a warmed isolette and placed on a forced-air warming blanket. Gastric decompression should be done if it has not already been performed. Monitors should be placed before preoxygenation. The pulse oximeter probe should be placed on the right hand in order to monitor preductal oxygen saturations. If post-ductal oxygen saturations are measured, you may be delivering a higher concentration of oxygen than necessary, increasing the risk of retinopathy of prematurity. Premedication with atropine will help to reduce secretions and prevent the bradycardia sometimes seen in infants during laryngoscopy. A rapid sequence intravenous induction with cricoid pressure followed by endotracheal intubation should be performed. An awake intubation may cause further extrusion of abdominal contents. A mixture of air and oxygen is used, maintaining the oxygen saturation between 90% and 95%. A balanced technique using a volatile anesthetic and intravenous opioid, such as morphine or fentanyl, may be used for the anesthetic maintenance. In order to avoid distention of the gastrointestinal tract, nitrous oxide is avoided. Maximal muscle relaxation should be provided in order to facilitate the surgeon's attempt to replace the bowel in the abdomen.

The decision whether a primary closure will be tolerated or whether a gradual reduction of the hernia will be necessary is determined intraoperatively. A primary closure can lead to multiple organ system dysfunctions, including the pulmonary, circulatory, renal and gastrointestinal systems, if there is excessive intra-abdominal pressure. Intra-abdominal pressures of up to 20 mmHg are usually well tolerated. Visualizing the lower extremities as well as measuring pulse oximetry and blood pressure in the lower extremities may help determine whether primary closure will be tolerated. Monitoring peak airway pressures during the closure will also provide information about the appropriateness of the primary closure. Alternatively, intra-abdominal pressures can be indirectly measured through either the nasogastric tube or the Foley catheter. If central venous pressure is monitored, increases greater than 4 mmHg are associated with compromised venous return and a decrease in cardiac index.

Ventilation and fluid management are the major concerns both intraoperatively and postoperatively. Ventilatory requirements may change during the surgical procedure as the bowel is returned to the abdomen. Large amounts of balanced salt solutions are often necessary to replace losses from the exposed bowel. Peripheral circulation, urine output, blood pressure, and acid-base measurements are helpful in assessing the adequacy of fluid resuscitation.

If a primary closure is performed in a patient with a large defect, the patient is kept intubated and muscle relaxation is continued until the intra-abdominal pressure has decreased to an acceptable level. If a silon chimney is used

for a gradual reduction and closure, the patient's trachea can usually be extubated. A daily reduction is done without anesthesia in the neonatal intensive care unit. The patient is returned to the operating room for final closure of the abdominal defect.

5. Describe the fluid and blood product management for this neonate intraoperatively.

Intraoperative fluid requirements can be divided into three basic areas: maintenance fluid, preoperative fluid deficit replacement, and replacement of third-space and blood losses.

Maintenance Fluid

Maintenance fluid volume is determined based on weight as shown in Table 65.2.

Maintenance requirements for water, electrolytes, and glucose have been standardized using metabolic rates. This has led to D_5 0.2% NS being used as standard maintenance fluid. Several factors including increased temperature and increased metabolic rate can increase maintenance fluid requirements. Balanced salt solutions are standard replacement fluids used in the operating room and in the older infant are used for maintenance also. Glucose-free fluids are generally used in the operating room for several reasons. Most notably, intraoperative hypoglycemia is very rare in older infants and children. Hyperglycemia, on the other hand, is associated with adverse outcomes related to the brain, heart, and intestines during ischemic events. However, neonates and specifically preterm infants are at risk for hypoglycemia and may require glucose infusions during the intraoperative period. In these situations, *only* the maintenance fluids should contain glucose.

Fluid Deficit Replacement

This patient presenting to the operating room would not have a fluid deficit, as it would have already been corrected during the preoperative preparation. Typically, the fluid deficit results from prolonged fasting times. This deficit is determined by multiplying the hourly maintenance fluid

TABLE 65.2	Maintenance Fluid Requirements According to the Patient's Weight
Patient's Weight	**Fluid Requirements**
0–10 kg	4 mL/kg/hr
10–20 kg	40 mL + 2 mL/kg/hr above 10 kg
≥20 kg	60 mL + 1 mL/kg/hr above 20 kg

requirement by the number of hours that the patient has been fasting. The deficit is replaced with a balanced salt solution over a 3-hour period: 50% infused in the first hour and 25% infused the second and third hours.

Third-Space Losses

The magnitude of third-space losses depends on the site and extent of surgical manipulation. The guidelines for third-space loss replacement recommend 8–15 mL/kg/hr during extensive intra-abdominal surgery. A neonate with gastroschisis could potentially require 5–10 times this amount for third-space replacement. Third-space loss should be replaced with a balanced salt solution without glucose. The state of hydration needs to be continually assessed.

Blood Losses

Prior to any procedure where blood loss is expected, the anesthesiologist should determine the approximate blood volume and estimate the allowable blood loss (ABL). It is important to remember that the ABL is an estimate, as many variables are considered when determining the level of anemia that each patient will tolerate. ABL is calculated as follows:

$$ABL = EBV \times \frac{(Hct_i - Hct_p)}{Hct_{av}}$$

where
EBV = estimated blood volume (see Table 65.3)
Hct_i = initial hematocrit
Hct_p = allowable perioperative hematocrit
Hct_{av} = average of Hct_i and Hct_p ($Hct_i + Hct_p/2$).

When determining the estimated allowable perioperative hematocrit, the affinity for oxygen of hemoglobin F must be considered. In the neonate with high levels of hemoglobin F, oxygen delivery at the tissue level is low despite potentially high hemoglobin levels (P_{50} approximately 19 mmHg.)

Replacement of blood and fluid is critical in small neonates since their total blood volume is so small. Blood loss needs to be replaced as it occurs to maintain normovolemia. It can be replaced with crystalloid (3 times the amount of blood loss) or with colloid or blood in equal volumes.

TABLE 65.3	Estimated Blood Volume (EBV) According to Age
Age	**EBV**
Preterm	95 mL/kg
Full-term	90 mL/kg
Infants	80 mL/kg
Children	70 mL/kg

Once a decision is made to transfuse, every effort should be made to limit exposures to multiple donors. In pediatric patients, this means dividing a single donor unit into a "pedi pack" (1 unit divided into multiple 50–100 mL parts) so that the same donor unit can be administered at different times. A general rule is that the increase in hematocrit with red blood cell administration will be approximately the same as the milliliters per kilogram infused.

SUGGESTED READINGS

American Society of Anesthesiologists Task Force on Blood Component Therapy: Practice guidelines for blood component therapy. Anesthesiology 84:732, 1996

Cravero JP, Rice LJ: Pediatric anesthesia. pp.1195–1204. In Barash PG, Cullen BF, Stoelting RK (eds): Clinical Anesthesia, 4th edition. Lippincott Williams and Wilkins, Philadelphia, 2001

Fisher DM: Anesthesia equipment for pediatrics. pp. 191–216. In Gregory GA (ed): Pediatric Anesthesia, 4th edition. Churchill Livingstone, Philadelphia, 2002

Fontana JL, Welborn L, Mongan PD, et al.: Oxygen consumption and cardiovascular function in children during profound intraoperative normovolemic hemodilution. Anesth Analg 80:219, 1994

Holl JW: Anesthesia for abdominal surgery. pp. 567–585. In Gregory GA (ed): Pediatric Anesthesia, 4th edition. Churchill Livingstone, Philadelphia, 2002

Stehling L: Blood transfusion and component therapy. pp. 117–144. In Gregory GA (ed): Pediatric Anesthesia, 4th edition. Churchill Livingstone, Philadelphia, 2002

Francine S. Yudkowitz, MD, FAAP

A full term, 3-kg infant born vaginally is noted to be cyanotic despite blow-by of 100% oxygen and adequate respiratory effort. On closer inspection, you observe that the infant has a scaphoid abdomen. On physical examination there are no breath sounds on the left and the heart sounds are shifted to the right. You intubate the trachea and the neonate is brought to the neonatal intensive care unit for further evaluation and management.

QUESTIONS

1. Describe the embryology and pathophysiology of congenital diaphragmatic hernia (CDH).
2. What are the clinical features of CDH?
3. How is CDH diagnosed?
4. What is the preoperative management of a neonate with CDH?
5. What is permissive hypercapnia?
6. What are the anesthetic considerations for the neonate with CDH?
7. What problems may occur intraoperatively and postoperatively?
8. Describe the techniques for fetal surgery.

1. Describe the embryology and pathophysiology of congenital diaphragmatic hernia (CDH).

The incidence of CDH is 1–2:5,000 live births. There may be associated congenital anomalies of the central nervous, gastrointestinal, genitourinary, and cardiovascular systems. In the fetus, during the first month of life there is a single pleuroperitoneal cavity. During the second month, the pleuroperitoneal membrane begins to form, separating the pleural and peritoneal cavities. The last portion of this membrane to form is the posterolateral portion, the right side closing before the left side. The fetal gut is outside the pleuroperitoneal cavity in the yolk sac during the first month of fetal life and returns to the peritoneal cavity during the second month of development. If the gut returns prior to full closure of the pleuroperitoneal membrane, any or all portions of the gut may migrate up into the pleural cavity. There are three sites where migration of the gut may occur:

- posterolateral (foramen of Bochdalek)
- anteromedial (foramen of Morgagni)
- esophageal hiatus

The most common site of migration (80%) is through the posterolateral portion, the left side more commonly than the right. Approximately 1% of diaphragmatic hernias occur through the anteromedial portion and the remaining cases occur through the esophageal hiatus.

Lung development is impaired by the presence of abdominal contents in the pleural cavity during fetal growth. The degree of impairment of lung development is determined by both the amount of abdominal contents in the pleural cavity and the time of migration. The greater the amount of abdominal contents in the pleural cavity and the earlier the migration, the greater the degree of pulmonary hypoplasia that will be present at birth. Not only is the ipsilateral lung affected but there are developmental changes in the contralateral lung as well. These changes include:

- decreased number of bronchi and alveoli
- smaller pulmonary artery
- inappropriately muscularized pulmonary arteries
- decreased cross-sectional area of pulmonary artery branches

The physiologic changes that occur secondary to the developmental changes in the lung are an increase in pulmonary vascular resistance (PVR) and persistent pulmonary hypertension (PPHN). This is reflected in the neonate as progressive hypoxia and acidosis. These physiologic changes can be divided into two components:

1. *Irreversible:* due to pulmonary hypoplasia and abnormal vasculature.
2. *Reversible:* due to vasoconstriction of the abnormal muscularized arteries.

The greater the irreversible component, the poorer the prognosis. To date, there is no method available to accurately determine which component is predominant.

Although compression of the lung by the presence of abdominal contents in the pleural cavity is detrimental, it does not significantly contribute to the hypoxia and acidosis that may be present. Therefore, CDH is no longer considered a surgical emergency. The initial management of these neonates is directed at improving oxygenation and ventilation. Only after stabilization of the neonate's condition should surgery be entertained.

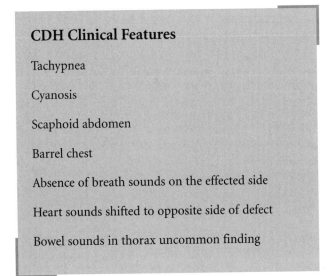

CDH Clinical Features

Tachypnea

Cyanosis

Scaphoid abdomen

Barrel chest

Absence of breath sounds on the effected side

Heart sounds shifted to opposite side of defect

Bowel sounds in thorax uncommon finding

2. What are the clinical features of CDH?

The presenting symptom of CDH is respiratory distress, with tachypnea and cyanosis, in the neonatal period. On visual inspection, the abdomen may appear scaphoid and the thorax barrel-shaped. On physical examination there is an absence of breath sounds on the affected side (most commonly the left side) and the cardiac impulse will be shifted to the opposite side of the defect (most commonly the right side). Bowel sounds on the affected side is an uncommon finding.

The time of onset of the respiratory symptoms correlates well with the degree of lung hypoplasia and therefore with prognosis. The earlier the symptoms present, the greater the degree of lung hypoplasia is present. Those neonates presenting in the first hour of life have the highest mortality.

3. How is CDH diagnosed?

The diagnosis of CDH may be made prenatally or postnatally. With the increased use of ultrasonography in the prenatal period, the prenatal diagnosis of CDH is more common. A poor prognosis can be anticipated if polyhydramnios is present, the fetal stomach is visualized in the thorax, or if the diagnosis is made prior to 20 weeks gestation.

Postnatally, the diagnosis should be considered if the above clinical features are present. The definitive diagnosis is made by chest radiograph showing abdominal contents in the thoracic cavity.

4. What is the preoperative management of CDH?

In the delivery room, once the diagnosis of CDH is suspected, mask ventilation should be avoided to prevent

Types of Diaphragmatic Hernia

Foramen of Bochdalek	Posteromedial	80%
Foramen of Morgagni	Anteromedial	1%
Esophageal hiatus		19%

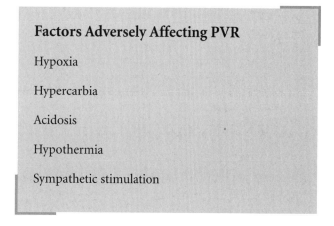

Delivery Room Management

Avoid bag and mask ventilation

Tracheal intubation

Peak inspiratory pressures <40 cm H_2O

Orogastric tube

Transfer to NICU for stabilization

Factors Adversely Affecting PVR

Hypoxia

Hypercarbia

Acidosis

Hypothermia

Sympathetic stimulation

distention of the abdominal organs in the thorax, which would further impair oxygenation and ventilation. The trachea should be intubated and inflation pressures limited to less than 40 cm H_2O to avoid causing a pneumothorax. A pneumothorax will most likely occur in the contralateral lung, which is where most of the gas exchange occurs. An orogastric tube should be inserted to assist in deflation of the stomach. If transfer to the neonatal intensive care unit (NICU) is delayed, an arterial and intravenous catheter should be inserted to guide therapy and for administration of pharmacologic agents. If possible, the arterial line should be placed in the right radial artery so that preductal oxygenation is measured.

Measures to both prevent further increases in PVR and promote a decrease in PVR, thereby increasing pulmonary blood flow, should be instituted. These include increased oxygenation, hypocarbia, alkalosis, avoiding sympathetic stimulation, and normothermia. Pharmacologic vasodilator therapy may be necessary. Tolazoline is most commonly used for this purpose. However, there may be systemic hypotension associated with its use and pharmacologic support of the systemic blood pressure may be necessary. Nitric oxide, a specific pulmonary vasodilator, has been used in these patients with variable results. If these measures do not improve the neonate's condition, extracorporeal membrane oxygenation (ECMO) may be utilized.

5. What is permissive hypercapnia?

Permissive hypercapnia was recently introduced as an alternative modality in the treatment of neonates with CDH. Conventional ventilatory management resulted in barotrauma to the lungs secondary to the high pressures needed to achieve adequate ventilation and oxygenation. In permissive hypercapnia, the arterial carbon dioxide tension ($PaCO_2$) is allowed to rise while maintaining adequate oxygenation and acid-base balance. The goal is to maintain a preductal oxygen saturation of greater than 90%. Acid-base balance is maintained with either bicarbonate or tris(hydroxymethyl) aminomethane (THAM).

6. What are the anesthetic considerations for the neonate with CDH?

Once the patient is stabilized, surgery may be scheduled. A transabdominal approach is the technique preferred by most surgeons. The abdominal organs are reduced and the diaphragm is either repaired primarily or with a synthetic patch. In most cases, the abdomen can be closed primarily but in some instances a Silastic pouch may need to be created.

The anesthetic management of these patients includes the continuation of the measures instituted preoperatively to improve oxygenation and ventilation and to promote a decrease in PVR. This includes hyperventilation to achieve a $PaCO_2$ of 25–30 mmHg, oxygenation so that the arterial oxygen tension (PaO_2) is greater than 80 torr, and a pH greater than 7.5. To decrease the need for excessive ventilator pressures, small tidal volumes and rapid respiratory rates may be necessary. Pharmacologic infusions should be continued. Arterial blood gases should be monitored frequently and any changes in ventilation, oxygenation, and acid–base balance should be treated expeditiously. It is important to avoid hypoxia and acidosis, which would lead to an increase in PVR that would be very difficult to reverse. Measures to prevent hypothermia are also important in the management of these patients.

All anesthetic agents may be used in these neonates with the exception of nitrous oxide. Nitrous oxide may cause intestinal distention, which may further compromise the neonate and impede abdominal closure. However, depending on the cardiovascular stability of the neonate, inhalation agents may not be tolerated well. In most cases, an oxygen-opioid-muscle relaxant combination would be optimal.

7. What problems may occur intraoperatively and postoperatively?

Meticulous attention should be paid to adequate oxygenation and ventilation of these neonates. There is an

Anesthetic Management

Oxygenation: PaO$_2$ >80 torr

Hyperventilation: PaCO$_2$ 25–30 mmHg

Acid–base balance: pH >7.5

Normothermia

Continue pharmacologic infusions

Avoid nitrous oxide

increased risk for pneumothorax, especially on the contralateral side. If this should occur it would be life-threatening. Efforts should be made to avoid using ventilation pressures greater than 40 cm H$_2$O to avoid causing a pneumothorax. No attempt should be made to manually inflate the contralateral lung because of this potential life-threatening risk. A diagnosis of a pneumothorax should be considered when any abrupt change in the condition of the neonate occurs during surgery. When in doubt of the diagnosis, a needle should be inserted into the contralateral chest. This maneuver will both diagnose the presence of a pneumothorax and treat it as well. A chest tube should be placed once the diagnosis is made.

Postoperatively, these neonates may continue to require oxygen and ventilatory support. There may be continued pulmonary hypertension and the patient may continue to deteriorate despite surgical correction. This deterioration is due to the severe degree of pulmonary hypoplasia that existed preoperatively and the change in pulmonary mechanics after surgery.

8. Describe the techniques for fetal surgery.

Two techniques for fetal correction of CDH are currently under investigation. The first technique is surgical correction of the diaphragmatic defect and reduction of the abdominal contents into the abdominal cavity. This could not be performed if the liver was in the thoracic cavity because it resulted in compromised flow through the umbilical vein. The second technique is tracheal occlusion, which has been shown to result in lung development. However, this technique has been fraught with problems and is not widely used.

SUGGESTED READINGS

Katz AL, Wiswell TE, Baumgart S: Contemporary controversies in the management of congenital diaphragmatic hernia. Clin Perinatol 25:219–248,1998

Langer JC: Congenital diaphragmatic hernia. Chest Surg Clin North Am 8:295–314, 1998

Roberts Jr. JD, Cronin JH, Todres ID: Neonatal emergencies. pp. 304–305. In Cote CJ, Todres ID, Goudsouzian NG, Ryan JF (eds): A Practice of Anesthesia for Infants and Children. WB Saunders, Philadelphia, 2001

Ulma G, Geiduschek JM, Zimmerman AA, Morray JP: Anesthesia for thoracic surgery. pp. 434–440. In Gregory GA (ed): Pediatric Anesthesia, 4th edition. Churchill Livingstone, New York, 2002

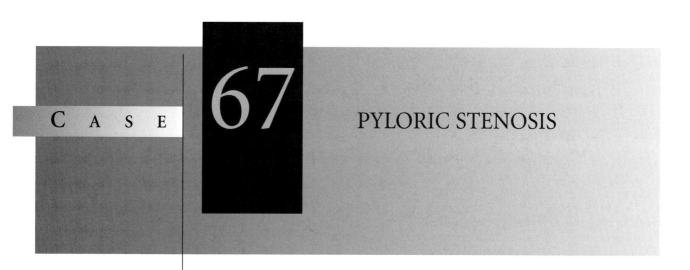

Francine S. Yudkowitz, MD, FAAP

A 4-week-old infant presents for pyloromyotomy. The patient has a 3-day history of nonbilious, projectile vomiting.

QUESTIONS

1. What is pyloric stenosis?
2. What is the clinical presentation of pyloric stenosis?
3. How is the diagnosis made?
4. What are the metabolic derangements and how are they treated?
5. What is the surgical treatment for pyloric stenosis?
6. What are the anesthetic considerations?

1. What is pyloric stenosis?

Pyloric stenosis is caused by hypertrophy of the circular muscular layers of the pylorus causing gastric outlet obstruction. It usually occurs between 2 and 6 weeks of age but has presented earlier. There is a higher incidence in male infants.

2. What is the clinical presentation of pyloric stenosis?

Symptoms may begin with regurgitation which progresses to nonbilious, projectile vomiting. Jaundice may occur in 5% of infants. This is thought to occur because of a deficiency of hepatic gluconyltransferase. The jaundice usually resolves after treatment.

3. How is the diagnosis made?

On physical examination, an olive-like mass can be palpated in the epigastrium just right of the midline. The diagnosis can be confirmed either by ultrasound or by barium swallow. However, a barium swallow adds to the risk of aspiration pneumonitis in the perioperative period.

4. What are the metabolic derangements and how are they treated?

The clinical symptoms of pyloric stenosis usually lead to hypovolemia and a hypochloremic, hypokalemic metabolic alkalosis. Since the vomitus consists only of gastric contents, there is a loss of hydrogen, sodium, potassium, and chloride ions. Initially, the renal response is to maintain acid–base balance. Alkaline urine is excreted because the bicarbonate load presented to the kidney exceeds the absorption capability of the proximal tubules. Therefore, the excess bicarbonate is excreted in the urine. In addition, at the distal tubules aldosterone is secreted which increases sodium reabsorption and potassium excretion. The loss of potassium is further exacerbated by the exchange of hydrogen ions for potassium ions in an effort to maintain acid–base balance.

As the infant becomes more dehydrated the renal response is aimed at maintaining intravascular volume. This is attained by secretion of aldosterone which will result in conservation of sodium ions and further loss of potassium ions. Furthermore, in the distal tubule sodium is conserved at the expense of hydrogen ions and an acidic urine is excreted.

The degree of dehydration should be assessed to guide fluid resuscitation. Sodium chloride is the isotonic fluid of choice for resuscitation. It may be necessary to rapidly correct hypovolemia with 10–20 cc/kg of normal saline if the patient is exhibiting signs of shock. Glucose should be administered as well. These infants may have depleted glycogen stores in the liver leading to the development of hypoglycemia if glucose is not provided.

Hypovolemia and electrolyte and acid–base derangements should be corrected prior to surgical intervention.

5. What is the surgical treatment of pyloric stenosis?

The surgical treatment of pyloric stenosis is a pyloromyotomy in which the circular muscles of the pylorus are spread apart. Occasionally, duodenal perforation may occur, which is easily sutured closed. This complication may slightly delay the start of oral feeds after surgery.

6. What are the anesthetic considerations?

These cases are a medical and not a surgical emergency. Therefore, prior to the start of anesthesia, hypovolemia and electrolyte and acid–base derangements should be completely corrected. Prior to induction, the stomach should be suctioned with a large bore (14Fr) orogastric tube to decrease the risk of regurgitation and aspiration. If a smaller sized orogastric or nasogastric tube is already present, it should be replaced.

Although inhalation induction has been described for these patients, most anesthesiologists would consider these patients as having a "full stomach" and would either do a rapid sequence induction with cricoid pressure or an awake intubation. Maintenance of anesthesia can be accomplished either by inhalation or a balanced technique. Muscle relaxants are not absolutely necessary. The use of opioids may not be necessary because the surgeon usually infiltrates the surgical wound with local anesthetic, which provides adequate analgesia postoperatively. Glucose infusion should be administered during the procedure to avoid hypoglycemia. Extubation should be done only when the infant is awake and protective airway reflexes are re-established.

Depending on the postconceptual age of the infant, apnea monitoring may be necessary postoperatively.

SUGGESTED READINGS

Davis PJ, Hall S, Deshpande JK, Spear RM: Anesthesia for general, urologic, and plastic surgery. pp. 573–574. In Motoyama EK, Davis PJ (eds): Smith's Anesthesia for Infants and Children. Mosby, St. Louis, 1996

Holl JW: Anesthesia for abdominal surgery. pp. 579–580. In Gregory GA (ed): Pediatric Anesthesia, 4th edition. Churchill Livingstone, New York, 2002

Roberts JD Jr., Cronin JH, Todres ID: Neonatal emergencies. pp. 306–307. In Cote CJ, Todres ID, Ryan JF, Goudsouzian NG (eds): A Practice of Anesthesia for Infants and Children, 3rd edition. WB Saunders, Philadelphia, 2001

CASE 68

TRACHEOESOPHAGEAL FISTULA

Michael Chietero, MD

A 1-day-old neonate presents to the operating room for repair of a tracheoesophageal fistula.

QUESTIONS

1. What is a tracheoesophageal fistula (TEF)?
2. How does a patient with a TEF typically present?
3. What are the preoperative concerns in a patient with a TEF?
4. How is the patient with a TEF managed intraoperatively?
5. What are the postoperative concerns in TEF patients?

1. What is a tracheoesophageal fistula (TEF)?

The most common classification system of tracheo-esophageal fistulas, illustrated in Figure 68.1, is that of Gross.

The incidence of esophageal atresia (EA) and TEF is approximately 1 in 3,000 births. Table 68.1 provides a description of the various types of TEF and their approximate incidence.

Embryologically, the trachea and esophagus both originate from the ventral diverticulum of the primitive foregut. They normally become separated by the eso-phagotracheal septum. Since the trachea is situated ante-rior to the esophagus, the fistula is located on the posterior aspect of the trachea and usually just proximal to the carina.

2. How does a patient with a TEF typically present?

In utero, there is often polyhydramnios, as the fetus can-not swallow amniotic fluid secondary to the esophageal atresia. At the time of delivery, an orogastric tube cannot be passed into the stomach. Typically, the orogastric tube will only pass to a distance of approximately 10 cm from the gums. In most cases, the diagnosis is initially suspected at the first feeding, when the neonate presents with coughing, choking and cyanosis (the "three Cs"). Excessive salivation and respiratory distress can also occur.

Confirmation of the diagnosis is made radiographically when a radiopaque orogastric catheter is seen curled in the proximal esophageal pouch. The presence of air in the stomach and intestines on radiography signifies the pres-ence of a fistula between the trachea and distal esophagus.

The "H" type fistula (tracheoesophageal fistula without atresia) usually presents later in life, most commonly with choking during feedings and recurrent pneumonitis.

3. What are the preoperative concerns in a patient with TEF?

There is a 30–50% incidence of associated anomalies in infants with EA and TEF. Particular combinations have been described, termed VATER or, more recently, VACTERL (Table 68.2).

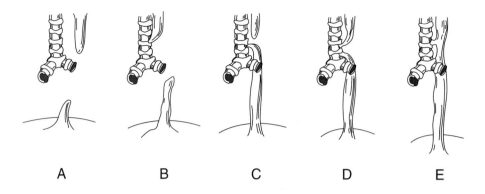

FIGURE 68.1   Gross' classification of tracheoesophageal fistula. (Reproduced with permission from Gregory GA: Pediatric Anesthesia, 4th edition. Churchill Livingstone, New York, 2002.)

The approximate incidence of associated anomalies is shown in Table 68.3.

The management of TEF patients preoperatively primarily involves preventing pulmonary complications until surgery can be performed:

- Cessation of feeding
- Positioning of the infant slightly head-up (30°) to minimize regurgitation of gastric contents through the fistula
- Intermittent suctioning of the proximal esophageal pouch catheter

Atelectasis from gastric distention and aspiration from regurgitation are common pulmonary complications.

There is also an increased incidence of prematurity in patients with TEF, especially in those who have associated anomalies. All the concerns of the premature patient must also be assessed in this situation.

4. How is the patient with a TEF managed intraoperatively?

The optimal surgical management is a one-stage repair, where the fistula is ligated and the proximal and distal ends of the esophagus are primarily anastomosed. The approach is typically through a right thoracotomy incision, with the patient in the left lateral decubitus position. In the presence of a right aortic arch, a left thoracotomy may be performed.

The anesthetic management includes warming of the operating room and the use of a warming blanket and a radiant overhead warmer. Standard monitors are applied. An intravenous catheter is placed prior to induction, if one is not already present. An arterial catheter may be necessary in high-risk infants. A precordial stethoscope should be securely positioned in the left axilla for detection of intraoperative airway obstruction. The esophageal pouch is suctioned and the patient is preoxygenated. Atropine 0.02 mg/kg may be administered intravenously to prevent bradycardia during laryngoscopy.

A gastrostomy tube may be placed to decompress the stomach. However, this may result in a further loss of ventilation through the fistula during positive pressure ventilation, necessitating clamping of the gastrostomy tube. Once a common practice, a gastrostomy tube is usually not placed nowadays, as it may increase the incidence of gastroesophageal reflux later in life. If a gastrostomy is performed, it is usually accomplished under local anesthesia

TABLE 68.1	Type and Incidence of Esophageal Atresia and Tracheoesophageal Fistula

Type	Incidence	Description
A	10%	Esophageal atresia without fistula
B	1%	Esophageal atresia with proximal fistula
C	80%	Esophageal atresia with distal fistula
D	2%	"K" type, esophageal atresia with proximal and distal fistula
E	7%	"H" type, fistula without atresia

TABLE 68.2	VACTERL
V	Vertebral (vertebral malformations, hemivertebrae)
A	Anal (imperforate anus, also midgut malrotation, Meckel's diverticulum)
C	Cardiac (VSD, PDA, TOF, ASD, coarctation of aorta)
T	Trachea (TEF)
E	Esophagus (EA)
R	Renal (renal agenesis, hydronephrosis, renal lobulation)
L	Limb (radial aplasia, polydactyly, wrist anomalies)

VSD, ventricular septal defect; PDA, patent ductus arteriosus; TOF, tetralogy of Fallot; ASD, atrial septal defect; TEF, tracheoesophageal fistula; EA, esophageal atresia.

prior to induction. It can then be used to aid in the placement of the endotracheal tube (ETT). If the gastric distention does not impair ventilation, the surgeon may perform the gastrostomy after induction of general anesthesia.

The optimal anesthetic management of these patients is to maintain spontaneous ventilation until the fistula is ligated. Positive pressure ventilation is avoided because it can result in insufflation of the stomach via the fistula or loss of ventilation through the gastrostomy. Gastric distention may compromise ventilation and may also lead to aspiration of gastric contents via the fistula. However, it is not always feasible to maintain spontaneous ventilation.

Awake intubation is the safest approach. It allows airway reflexes to be maintained and also allows appropriate positioning of the ETT without positive pressure ventilation. The administration of supplemental oxygen during laryngoscopy can be achieved with the use of an oxyscope. Awake intubation, however, may be difficult and traumatic in a vigorous infant. Alternatively, an inhalation or intravenous induction may be performed without muscle relaxation, thus allowing the infant to continue to breathe spontaneously. If a

TABLE 68.3	Incidence of Associated Anomalies

Anomaly	Incidence
Cardiovascular	35%
Musculoskeletal	30%
Gastrointestinal	20%
Genitourinary	10%
Craniofacial	4%

muscle relaxant is used, care must be taken during positive pressure ventilation to avoid excessive insufflation of the stomach via the fistula.

Placement and positioning of the ETT can be tricky. To avoid intubating the fistula, which is located on the posterior aspect of the trachea, the ETT should be inserted with the bevel facing posteriorly. After intubation, the bevel is rotated anteriorly to avoid ventilating the fistula.

Since the fistula is usually located just proximal to the carina, positioning the ETT so that it is above the carina but still occluding the fistula may be difficult. One commonly used method is to insert the ETT (without a Murphy eye) into the right mainstem bronchus and then gradually withdraw it until breath sounds are heard on the left. However, this does not always assure that the endotracheal tube occludes the fistula. If a gastrostomy tube is in place, the distal end is submerged in a beaker of water and if bubbling occurs there is leakage through the fistula. The ETT is then advanced until the bubbling ceases while still maintaining left-sided breath sounds. The gastrostomy tube may be left to water seal during the surgery, which allows for continued monitoring for ventilation through the fistula.

A second method of confirming placement of the ETT is with the use of a fiberoptic bronchoscope. After intubation, the fiberoptic bronchoscope is passed through the ETT and the carina is visualized. Upon withdrawal of the bronchoscope, if the fistula is not visualized then the ETT is appropriately positioned. If the fistula is visualized,

Intraoperative Concerns

Operating room set-up
  Warm room
  Warming blanket
  Overhead warmer
  ?Arterial line

Intubation
  Awake versus after induction
  Maintain spontaneous ventilation
  Positioning of ETT
    proximal to carina, occluding the fistula
    right mainstem intubation and withdrawal
  Confirmation
    fiberoptic bronchoscopy
    gastrostomy to water seal

Occlusion of fistula
  Fogarty catheter via trachea or through
    gastrostomy

the ETT is advanced making sure that its tip remains above the carina.

Sometimes, with a large fistula or one that is located at or distal to the carina, placement of the ETT to avoid ventilating the fistula is not possible. In this situation, the fistula may need to be occluded with a Fogerty balloon catheter placed from above with the help of a bronchoscope or from below through the gastrostomy.

Once positioned, the ETT should be carefully secured. After the patient is positioned in the left lateral decubitus position, reconfirmation of the position of the ETT may be necessary.

Loss of breath sounds and the end-tidal carbon dioxide ($ETCO_2$) tracing commonly occurs during surgery secondary to airway obstruction. This may be due to the accumulation of secretions or blood in the ETT. More often, however, it results from kinking of the trachea during surgical manipulation. The surgeon should immediately be instructed to release the surgical traction.

5. What are the postoperative concerns in TEF patients?

The postoperative management of TEF patients depends upon the degree of pulmonary dysfunction and the presence of associated anomalies. In healthy, vigorous infants, extubation of the trachea at the completion of surgery is not only possible but also desirable, in order to decrease the stress at the surgical anastomosis.

Postoperative pain management may be accomplished by either neuraxial analgesia or intravenous opioids. For neuraxial analgesia, a thoracic epidural catheter is placed via the caudal approach. Position of the catheter should be confirmed radiographically prior to starting an infusion of a local anesthetic and opiate solution.

Postoperative survival in healthy infants approaches 100%, but may be affected by prematurity, severity of pulmonary dysfunction, and associated anomalies.

SUGGESTED READINGS

Bikhazi GB, Davis PJ: Anesthesia for neonates and premature infants. pp. 464–466. In Motoyama EK, Davis PJ (eds): Smith's Anesthesia for Infants and Children, 6th edition. CV Mosby, St. Louis, 1996

Roberts Jr. JD, Cronin JH, Todres ID: Neonatal emergencies. pp. 302–304. In Cote CJ, Todres ID, Goudsouzian NG, Ryan JF (eds): A Practice of Anesthesia for Infants and Children, 3rd edition. WB Saunders, Philadelphia, 2001

Ulma G, Geiduschek JM, Zimmerman AA, Morray JP: Anesthesia for thoracic surgery. pp. 440–443. In Gregory GA (ed): Pediatric Anesthesia, 4th edition. Churchill Livingstone, New York, 2002

A 5-week-old infant is scheduled for bilateral inguinal herniorrhaphy. On preoperative evaluation the baby is noted to be tachypneic and tachycardic. A IV/VI systolic murmur is heard at the left sternal border.

QUESTIONS

1. How are innocent and pathologic systolic murmurs differentiated?
2. What is the incidence of congenital heart disease?
3. What are the general anesthetic considerations for the common cardiac lesions?
4. What should be included in the preoperative assessment?
5. What are the anesthetic implications of intracardiac lesions with left-to-right shunting?
6. What are the common intracardiac left-to-right intracardiac lesions?
7. What are the anesthetic implications of right-to-left shunting lesions?
8. What are the common right-to-left shunting lesions with reduced pulmonary blood flow?
9. How are congenital heart lesions repaired?
10. Discuss the sequelae associated with the repair of specific cardiac lesions.

1. How are innocent and pathologic systolic murmurs differentiated?

Innocent murmurs are soft flow murmurs without physiologic consequences. Pathologic murmurs are loud, pansystolic, or late systolic and associated with a cardiac anomaly. The most common lesion associated with a systolic murmur in the young infant is a ventricular septal defect or patent ductus arteriosus. This infant has signs of mild congestive heart failure (tachypnea and tachycardia) and should undergo a cardiology evaluation prior to surgery. Transthoracic echocardiography is presently the fastest, most accurate, and least invasive diagnostic tool to establish an exact anatomic diagnosis in the majority of patients with congenital heart disease.

2. What is the incidence of congenital heart disease?

The incidence of congenital heart disease is approximately 6–8:1,000 live births. Once considered rare, the incidence of congenital heart disease has increased secondary to increased awareness and improvements in diagnostic testing and medical treatments of the critically ill. This means that 40,000 children are born each year with congenital heart disease. The most common cardiac lesions present with a systolic murmur (Table 69.1). The main consequences of significant congenital heart disease are congestive heart failure and/or cyanosis.

TABLE 69.1	Frequency of the Most Common Congenital Cardiac Lesions	
Lesion		**%**
Ventricular septal defect		25
Atrial septal defect		12
Patent ductus arteriosus		12
Pulmonic stenosis		9
Tetralogy of Fallot		8
Coarctation of the aorta		7
Aortic stenosis		5
Transposition of the great arteries		5

3. What are the general anesthetic considerations for the common cardiac lesions?

Extracardiac Defects

Associated extracardiac defects are present in 5–50% of children with congenital heart disease. In 17–18%, the defect is part of a syndrome or chromosomal anomaly. Genitourinary tract anomalies are among the most common lesions and are present in 4–15% of patients with congenital heart disease. Major chromosomal anomalies with associated cardiac lesions of anesthetic significance are Down (trisomy 21), Turner, Noonan, and DiGeorge syndromes.

Prevention of Air Embolism

All patients with shunt lesions are at risk for air emboli to the systemic circulation irrespective of their usual shunting pattern. A left-to-right shunt may transiently reverse due to the earlier relaxation of the left ventricle compared with the right ventricle. Additionally, upon sudden obstruction to right ventricular output due to an air embolus, a left-to-right shunt will convert to a right-to-left shunt pattern. Therefore, the intravenous (IV) line should be meticulously debubbled and then rechecked after warming of the operating room, since this may have caused nitrogen to come out of solution in the IV fluid, forming additional hazardous bubbles. All IV lines should be connected while the IV fluid is flowing freely. In addition, all syringes should be cleared of air. Prior to injecting into an intravenous line, a small amount of fluid should be aspirated into the syringe to clear any air that may be in the needle or injection port. A recommended technique is to dilute any given medication such that 1 mL consists of a unit dose. With this technique, aspiration of IV fluid into the syringe will not significantly change the drug concentration. These precautions are important in any patient in whom a communication exists between the systemic and pulmonary circulations, regardless of the presence or absence of pulmonary outflow obstruction.

Endocarditis Prophylaxis

The majority of patients with congenital heart disease, pre- or post-correction or palliation, require antibiotic prophylaxis for the prevention of bacterial endocarditis prior to any surgical, diagnostic, or dental procedure that may result in bacteremia. Routine oral endotracheal intubation and flexible bronchoscopy do not require prophylaxis. However, manipulation of the genitourinary tract does. Current recommendations as published by the American Heart Association are listed in Table 69.2.

4. What should be included in the preoperative assessment?

A thorough history and physical examination are essential to assess the significance of the heart disease and how well it is managed. Most congenital cardiac anomalies are associated with a pathologic murmur.

The two major sequelae of significant congenital heart disease are congestive heart failure and cyanosis. Congestive heart failure should be controlled with digitalis, diuretics, and/or an afterload-reducing agent prior to any elective intervention. Drug therapy should be maintained perioperatively. Adequate serum potassium levels and avoidance of hypocarbia are important to avoid digitalis toxicity in the patient taking digitalis. Control of congestive heart failure will improve pulmonary function and reduce the possibility of perioperative hypoxemia or respiratory failure.

Cyanosis is a feature of cardiac lesions with right-to-left shunting, limited pulmonary blood flow, and/or venous admixture to the systemic circulation. Severe hypoxemia results in polycythemia with a concomitant increase in blood volume and viscosity, neovascularization, alveolar hyperventilation to maintain arterial normocarbia, and a poorly defined coagulopathy. Clubbing or osteoarthropathy of the distal phalanges of the fingers and toes is indicative of longstanding cyanotic heart disease. Increased blood viscosity increases cardiac work by increasing peripheral vascular resistance. Cerebral and/or renal thrombosis may occur with high hematocrits, particularly in the presence of dehydration. At hematocrits greater than 60–65%, oxygen transport is not improved and the frequency of serious thrombotic complications and coagulopathy increases. To improve organ perfusion and reduce cardiac workload, the hematocrit should be kept below these levels, if necessary by hemodilution. In most cases, increasing hematocrits are an indication for cardiac surgery to either improve pulmonary blood flow or correct the lesion. Because of the danger of hemoconcentration with prolonged fasting, preoperative fasting (NPO) times

TABLE 69.2	American Heart Association Recommendations for Endocarditis Prophylaxis

For low-risk procedures:
Amoxicillin or ampicillin 2 g or 50 mg/kg
One dose 30–60 minutes preoperatively

Or if penicillin-allergic:
Clindamycin 600 mg or 20 mg/kg 30 minutes
    preoperatively

For high-risk procedures:
Ampicillin and gentamicin:
Ampicillin 2 g or 50 mg/kg + gentamicin 1.5 mg/kg
    within 30 minutes of the procedure

And 6 hours later:
Ampicillin or amoxicillin 1 g or 25 mg/kg

Or if penicillin-allergic:
Vancomycin 1 g or 20 mg/kg + gentamicin 1.5 mg/kg
Complete infusion within 30 minutes of the
    start of the procedure

Prophylaxis not required:
ASD II° preoperatively
PDA, VSD, ASD
    6 months post-repair with no residual
Mitral valve prolapse without dysfunction
Kawasaki without valve dysfunction
Pacemakers, defibrillators, VA shunts

---

should be held to a minimum in cyanotic children or the patient should be hydrated intravenously.

5. What are the anesthetic implications of intracardiac lesions with left-to-right shunting?

Lesions with left-to-right shunting include all forms of atrial septal defect (ASD) and ventricular septal defect (VSD), patent ductus arteriosus (PDA), and other large aorto-pulmonary connections. The magnitude and direction of the shunt depends on the difference between the outflow resistances of the two connections and the size of the defect. The exceptions are communications between the left ventricle and right atrium where obligatory shunting of blood occurs due to the large pressure difference between these two cardiac chambers.

A left-to-right shunt only minimally influences uptake of inhalation anesthetic agents, unless cardiac output is depressed, in which case induction is accelerated. Induction with intravenous agents is delayed, since much of the injected drug is recirculated into the lung. Agents that cause myocardial depression are poorly tolerated in infants with limited cardiac reserve. Ketamine, opioid/relaxant techniques, or low-dose inhalation anesthesia with isoflurane or sevoflurane are usually well tolerated.

Infants with large left-to-right shunts have chronically congested lungs with decreased compliance, increased closing volume, and increased airway resistance. Therefore, they should have their airway secured and ventilation controlled during anesthesia. However, close attention

needs to be paid to maintenance of a relatively high pulmonary vascular resistance (PVR) to avoid excessive perfusion of the lungs. This can be accomplished by using the minimal oxygen concentration necessary to maintain adequate oxygen saturation and by maintaining normocarbia to mild hypercarbia.

Although mild afterload reduction leads to increased systemic output and a reduction in left-to-right shunting,

Left-To-Right Shunting

Pulmonary congestion
    Decreased compliance
    Increased closing volume
    Increased airway resistance
    Control ventilation under anesthesia

Maintain pulmonary vascular resistance
    Minimize delivered oxygen
    Normo- to mild hypercarbia

Risk for paradoxical emboli

Myocardial depression poorly tolerated

Intravenous induction delayed

excessive systemic vasodilatation can lead to right-to-left shunting and cyanosis if the PVR is high.

Endocarditis prophylaxis is required for nonrepaired VSD and PDA, the first 6 months following repair, or after 6 months if there is a residual lesion present.

Prevention of paradoxical air embolism from IV lines is mandatory.

6. What are the common intracardiac left-to-right shunting lesions?

ASD Secundum

The ASD is located in the area of the fossa ovalis and shunting occurs between two low-pressure circulations. Despite a large volume of shunting resulting in a marked increase in pulmonary blood flow, pulmonary artery pressure remains low over many years. These patients are generally asymptomatic throughout childhood and adolescence but may develop mild pulmonary hypertension in the third and fourth decades of life. In this lesion, the right ventricle is volume-overloaded. Treatment consists of elective closure of the defect during later childhood either surgically or with an intracardiac device. The main anesthetic concern in asymptomatic patients is prevention of systemic embolization from injection of air or debris from IV lines. Endocarditis prophylaxis is necessary only if it is within 6 months of repair or after 6 months if there is a residual lesion present.

Ventricular Septal Defect

Small VSDs restrict the amount of left-to-right shunting and thereby limit the hemodynamic consequences. With a large defect (approximating the size of the normal age-appropriate aortic orifice or larger), there is no restriction to flow and shunting depends largely on the relative ratio of the PVR to systemic vascular resistance (SVR). In the early neonatal period, the PVR is high and the patient may have no signs or symptoms related to the VSD. As PVR declines during the second to third weeks of life, the left-to-right shunting increases and may result in congestive heart failure due to the volume overload on the left ventricle. In this lesion, the pulmonary vascular bed is exposed to increased blood flow and systemic blood pressure.

An estimated 25–50% of small to moderate-sized VSDs close spontaneously, generally during the first year of life. Many become smaller throughout life and remain benign. Probably less than 5% of large VSDs undergo spontaneous closure. Surgery is indicated for primary closure of the defect during the first year of life in infants with congestive heart failure and failure to thrive despite medical therapy. Failure to close a large VSD will lead to progressive pulmonary vascular obstructive disease, particularly after the second year of life.

Before the development of pulmonary vascular disease, the volume of the shunt may be manipulated by changing PVR and/or SVR. High oxygen concentrations, hyperventilation, and alkalosis lead to pulmonary vasodilation and may cause massive increases in left-to-right shunting. With the limited cardiac output of the small infant, this can lead to severe systemic underperfusion and cardiovascular collapse. Increased afterload will lead to an increase in left-to-right shunting as long as PVR is less than SVR. Most patients with large shunts are, therefore, on anticongestive medications (digoxin and lasix) and an afterload-reducing agent (angiotensin converting enzyme inhibitor) prior to cardiac surgery or if only medically managed.

Large PDAs present clinically in a similar way to large VSDs and are managed surgically or with a device closure to protect the pulmonary vascular bed.

7. What are the anesthetic implications of right-to-left shunting lesions?

In older cyanotic patients with severe polycythemia, hemodilution to a hematocrit of 55–60% should be performed prior to elective surgery. This will improve cardiac output, peripheral perfusion, and oxygen transport. It may also improve the coagulation defects commonly found in polycythemic patients. However, hemodilution to normal levels may be detrimental because oxygen transport will be seriously limited. Maintenance of cardiac output is essential since the oxygen content of the blood is low. Therefore, bradycardia is poorly tolerated.

Patients with cyanosis have a blunted response to hypoxia, which may persist even after correction of the underlying lesion. In patients with reduced pulmonary blood flow, marked ventilation/perfusion inequalities exist. Positive pressure ventilation may worsen this problem, leading to an increase in dead space ventilation and raised arterial carbon dioxide tension ($PaCO_2$). However, to maintain normal $PaCO_2$ with severely reduced pulmonary blood flow, a moderate degree of hyperventilation is required. Capnography underestimates $PaCO_2$ in these patients, since only part of the cardiac output will reach the pulmonary circulation for gas exchange. The greater the right-to-left shunt, the higher the arterial to end-tidal CO_2 ($ETCO_2$) gradient. Thus, a markedly increased $PaCO_2$ may be present despite a normal $ETCO_2$.

In patients with systemic-to-pulmonary shunts, adequate systemic blood pressure is necessary to maintain pulmonary perfusion, besides reducing right-to-left shunting at the cardiac level.

The presence of a right-to-left shunt prolongs induction with poorly soluble inhalation anesthetics. This may be offset by the presence of a surgically created systemic-to-pulmonary shunt. Induction time with highly soluble agents may be nearly normal because these patients usually hyperventilate to maintain a normal $PaCO_2$. The onset of action of intravenous agents is accelerated since a significant proportion of the drug bypasses the lungs.

Right-To-Left Shunting

Polycythemia
    Hemodilute to hematocrit of 55–60%

Coagulation defects

Maintain cardiac output
    Bradycardia poorly tolerated

Cyanosis
    Blunted response to hypoxia
    Ventilation/perfusion abnormalities
    Increased arterial to end-tidal CO_2 gradient

Maintain adequate systemic blood pressure

Risk for systemic emboli

Induction of anesthesia
    Prolonged with poorly soluble inhalation
        anesthetics
    Accelerated with intravenous agents

All patients with right-to-left shunts are at an increased risk of systemic embolization of air or blood clots from IV lines.

8. What are the common right-to-left shunting lesions with reduced pulmonary blood flow?

Tetralogy of Fallot (TOF)

The combination of VSD, pulmonary valvular and/or right ventricular infundibular stenosis, right ventricular hypertrophy, and a large overriding aorta is known as TOF. It is the most common cyanotic defect seen after the first year of life, contributing to 10% of all congenital cardiac lesions. The degree of right ventricular outflow and/or pulmonic obstruction determines the onset and severity of cyanosis. With severe obstruction, cyanosis appears with closure of the ductus arteriosus in the neonatal period. Prostaglandin E_1 may be used to clinically stabilize the patient prior to surgical intervention. Many infants do not develop symptoms until 3–6 months of age and even then may not appear cyanotic at rest. However, episodes of severe cyanosis with hyperventilation and acidosis, known as hypercyanotic spells (or "tet" spells), may occur. These are caused by severe infundibular spasm, probably induced by changes in venous return and SVR. Reduction in SVR leads to decreased pulmonary blood flow, since blood tends to be shunted to the systemic circulation. Decreased venous return further decreases pulmonary blood flow. In older children, the squatting posture may improve symptoms through an increase in venous return from the lower extremities and by increasing SVR. The treatment of hypercyanotic spells is based on the goals of decreasing infundibular spasm by decreasing contractility and heart rate, and by increasing preload. Another goal (especially in fixed right ventricular outflow obstruction) is to increase SVR to decrease right-to-left shunting across the ventricular septal defect.

In TOF, both ventricles work at systemic pressure but volume overload does not occur and congestive heart failure is rare.

These patients should arrive in the operating room well sedated. Preoperative fluid restriction should be minimized and/or maintenance fluid given intravenously to prevent hemoconcentration and hypovolemia. A smooth induction is important to prevent increases in oxygen demand or hypercyanotic spells. The agents used should have minimal peripheral vasodilating effects. Thus, halothane is theoretically preferable to isoflurane or sevoflurane for this purpose. Mild myocardial depression may relieve infundibular obstruction and is, therefore, desirable. If intravenous agents are used, they should be carefully titrated to prevent relative overdose. Intravenous barbiturate requirements may be halved. Ketamine can be safely used, particularly in very sick patients, since it maintains SVR and does not cause "tet" spells.

Arterial oxygen saturation generally increases upon induction of anesthesia in cyanotic patients. The reasons for this are probably related to the reduction in oxygen consumption during anesthesia and the subsequent increase in venous saturation. Monitoring blood pressure may become problematic in patients with previous shunting procedures using the subclavian arteries. The contralateral arm should be used for invasive or noninvasive monitoring. For major surgery, intra-arterial and/or central venous pressures should be measured directly. This will also allow blood sampling for blood gas and acid–base measurements. Because the major myocardial stress rests on the right ventricle in these patients, central venous pressures can be used to assess cardiac performance.

Hypercyanotic spells may develop perioperatively because of the dynamic nature of the muscular infundibular obstruction present in TOF. Strategies to prevent and treat these complications are outlined in Table 69.3.

These patients require endocarditis prophylaxis for life.

Transposition of the Great Arteries (TGA) and Complex Lesions

These patients will have undergone repair or palliation prior to any elective noncardiac surgery and will be discussed below.

TABLE 69.3	Prevention and Treatment Measures for Hypercyanotic Spells

Prevention	Treatment
Preanesthetic sedation	Prevent and relieve airway obstruction
Continued β-blockade	100% oxygen
Maintain adequate anesthetic depth	Deepen anesthesia or provide sedation
Avoid hypovolemia	Give fluid bolus
Avoid afterload reduction	Increase SVR: phenylephrine 1–2 μg/kg IV
	Esmolol 100–200 μg/kg/min
	Aortic compression

9. How are congenital heart lesions repaired?

Repair or palliation of congenital heart disease attempts to establish normal physiology but cannot usually establish normal cardiovascular anatomy. Surgery may result in residual defects or in short- or long-term sequelae. True anatomic repair, in which further surgery is not anticipated, occurs in ligation of a PDA or suture closure of an ASD. Closure of a simple VSD, resection of a coarctation of the aorta with end-to-end anastomosis, or the arterial switch operation for correction of TGA also result in normal anatomy, but tend to result in late sequelae in some patients. Lesions in which anatomic repair is attempted but will result in residual lesions or requires use of prosthetic materials are repairs of TOF, atrioventricular canal defects, obstructive valvular lesions, any lesion requiring the insertion of a conduit between the ventricle and respective artery (usually the right ventricle and pulmonary artery), and any valve replacement.

In patients where anatomic repair is not feasible, surgical correction is aimed at trying to establish normal cardiovascular physiology. The initial repair of TGA by the Mustard or Senning operation results in redirection of blood flow at the atrial level (atrial switch). Pulmonary venous blood is directed to the aorta and systemic venous blood is directed to the pulmonary artery. This group of lesions also includes all patients whose cardiac malformation results in only one functional ventricle that supports the systemic circulation. This heterogeneous group of lesions requires several staged surgical interventions until the final Fontan operation, which results in separation of the two circulations without a pulmonary ventricle.

One of the most common sequelae following congenital heart surgery is rhythm abnormalities. Supraventricular dysrhythmias are the most common of these and can be life-threatening under certain conditions (e.g., atrial flutter in the post-Fontan patient). Supraventricular dysrhythmias are associated with a 2–8% incidence of sudden death. They are particularly common following repairs with extensive atrial suture lines and/or elevated atrial pressures. Atrial dysrhythmias may be tachycardias or bradycardias. They are often refractory to medical therapy and may require ablation or pacemaker insertion. Following the Senning or Mustard repair only 20–40% of patients are in sinus rhythm 5–10 years following surgery. Following Fontan repairs, performed with direct atrial to pulmonary anastomosis, there is at least a 30% incidence of atrial dysrhythmias. Newer surgical approaches, utilizing either a lateral tunnel or extracardiac conduits, diminish the incidence of late rhythm abnormalities. Atrial dysrhythmias are also seen in 5–10% of patients following repair of a secundum ASD, particularly when repair is carried out at an older age.

Ventricular dysrhythmias, although less common in the postoperative patient, are frequently more significant since they may indicate an underlying residual defect and may be the harbinger of sudden death. The etiologies for development of ventricular premature beats include right ventriculotomy and/or resection, elevated intracavitary pressure associated with valvular stenosis, and cardiomyopathies with decreased diastolic function. The latter occurs following surgery if there was suboptimal myocardial preservation during the procedure or when pressure and volume overload of the ventricle was present for a long time prior to corrective surgery, particularly if associated with a high hematocrit. On occasion, the stress of anesthesia and surgery may unmask an underlying rhythm disturbance. New ventricular extrasystoles observed during anesthesia in a patient with previous TOF repair should be brought to the cardiologist's attention so that appropriate follow-up can occur. TOF repair has the highest association of ventricular dysrhythmias and sudden death occurring long after surgical repair, particularly in patients operated later in life or in earlier series. These patients may require implantation of a cardioverting defibrillator (AICD) to prevent this complication.

10. Discuss the sequelae associated with the repair of specific cardiac lesions.

Atrial Septal Defect

Secundum ASD is associated with a 30% incidence of mitral valve prolapse. Patients need to be followed for the development of mitral regurgitation, which occurs in 5–10% of patients, or ventricular dysrhythmias. Early and late atrial dysrhythmias may occur, particularly if the patient was over the age of 20 years at the time of repair or if the dysrhythmias were present before surgery. Patients who develop paroxysmal or chronic atrial fibrillation will require anticoagulation to prevent systemic embolization. The risk of late development of atrial flutter or fibrillation 25–30 years following repair is 4% if the repair was done before age 10 years and 58% if it was carried out after age 40 years. The presence of a large left-to-right shunt prior to surgery is an additional risk factor for development of late atrial dysrhythmias. The most commonly observed dysrhythmias after repair of sinus venosus defects are sinus node dysfunction and sick sinus syndrome, which occur in at least 10% of patients.

Ventricular Septal Defect

The incidence of residual VSD following surgery is less than 5%. Patients with sub-arterial VSD may have aortic insufficiency, which is an indication to close even a small defect. In 3% of cases, the regurgitation is progressive. Many patients (30–50%) will exhibit a right bundle branch block on electrocardiogram (ECG). In older repairs, where a right ventriculotomy was commonly performed, serious ventricular dysrhythmias are seen in at least 34% of patients, with a 1–2% incidence of sudden death. Complete heart block is one of the risk factors of VSD closure, but with better surgical techniques the incidence is less than 2%. It is a late sequela in patients who exhibit bifascicular block following surgery (right bundle branch block and left anterior hemiblock). The majority of patients whose defects are closed before the age of 2 years have normal cardiovascular function; however, they have a higher risk for dysrhythmias than the normal population. Patients operated on later in life may have persistence of depressed myocardial reserve and progressive pulmonary hypertension.

Coarctation of the Aorta (CoA)

Fifty percent of patients with CoA have other associated cardiac lesions. Bicuspid aortic valve is seen in 85% of patients and 3–10% have berry aneurysms of the circle of Willis. Thirty-five percent of patients with Turner syndrome have CoA.

The technique of repair has changed over the years. Resection of the coarcted aorta and end-to-end anastomosis is the preferred surgical technique at this time. Older repairs included patch aortoplasty, subclavian flap aortoplasty, and interposition graft. Patch aortoplasty, which has a high incidence of aortic aneurysm formation that may rapidly expand and lead to aortic rupture and death, has been abandoned. Subclavian patch repair is still used occasionally. Blood pressure measurements in the left arm may be unreliable following this procedure. Bridging grafts are occasionally used in older patients with repeated coarctations. Repair in infancy is associated with a 15–20% incidence of recoarctation. Most of these patients can be managed effectively with balloon angioplasty. Balloon angioplasty of a primary coarctation in the newborn is not effective. A long-term sequela of balloon angioplasty is the development of an aortic aneurysm at the angioplasty site (2–14%).

Patients with repaired coarctation are at risk for development of late hypertension in the absence of recoarctation. Age at time of surgical repair is the strongest predictor for this complication. Repair after age 5 years has a 75% incidence of systolic hypertension at 25-year follow-up. Long-term survivors have an accelerated risk of coronary artery disease, myocardial infarction, and premature death. In addition, because of the high incidence of bicuspid aortic valve, 7–10% of patients develop aortic valvular disease requiring aortic valve replacement. In the perioperative period, patients who are normotensive at rest may develop significant hypertension with minimal stimulation. This may be due to underlying hypertensive disease or to unrecognized recoarctation.

Atrioventricular (AV) Septal Defects

AV septal defects are the most common cardiac defect associated with Down syndrome. The complete form results in severe congestive heart failure and pulmonary hypertension. The defect is usually repaired in infancy because of symptoms and to prevent development of obstructive pulmonary vascular disease. Primum atrial septal defects present similar to secundum ASD, unless associated with significant mitral regurgitation. Although the cleft mitral valve is competent in the majority of patients, 10–15% of patients have mitral valve regurgitation at the time of the initial surgery. Because of the abnormality of the mitral valve, long-term mitral insufficiency remains a serious problem after repair of primum defects and complete canals. More than 60% of patients followed long term after repair of partial AV septal defects have evidence of mitral regurgitation, which may eventually require mitral valve replacement. After repair of complete AV septal defects in infancy, the incidence of mitral regurgitation requiring re-intervention is quoted at about 7%. First-degree heart block is seen in 50% of patients after repair. Patients are at risk for development of malignant tachydysrhythmias as they age.

Tetralogy of Fallot

Older repairs of TOF have resulted in right ventricular dysfunction due to pulmonary insufficiency and a high incidence of dysrhythmias from extensive right ventriculotomies. Incomplete relief or right ventricular outflow obstruction, demonstrated by a RV:LV systolic pressure ratio of greater than 0.5, is an independent predictor of late mortality after repair. Repair at an older age is also associated with higher long-term mortality, as is the presence of a large outflow patch. The majority of patients are symptom-free following repair. There is, however, in the survivors of the earlier repairs a 6% incidence of sudden death and at least a 10% incidence of inducible ventricular tachycardia requiring AICD implantation. Nearly a third of patients at late follow-up have atrial tachycardias, which can also cause sudden death. Most patients have a right bundle branch block on the ECG. The presence of ventricular ectopy must be thoroughly evaluated preoperatively. Patients need to be evaluated for residual lesions, VSD, or right ventricular hypertension prior to a procedure. Sympathetic stress in the setting of right ventricular hypertension and an old ventriculotomy scar increases the propensity for ventricular dysrhythmias. Patients with significant pulmonary insufficiency may tolerate rapid fluid shifts poorly. Vascular access may be difficult in patients with multiple previous cardiovascular procedures. Patients with residual shunts are at risk for paradoxical emboli.

Transposition of the Great Arteries

TGA represents 5–7% of all congenital cardiac defects and is the most common cause of cyanotic congenital heart disease in the newborn. In this lesion, the aorta arises from the right ventricle and the pulmonary artery from the left, creating two parallel circulations. Unless some mixing between the circulations occurs, either through a patent ductus arteriosus, ASD, or VSD, survival past the neonatal period is not possible. Prior to surgical interventions 90% of patients with this lesion died within the first year of life. Surgical repair is aimed at either improving mixing, redirecting flow of systemic venous and pulmonary venous return to the pulmonary artery or aorta, or at anatomically correcting the problem. The initial physiologic repair for this condition was "switching" the blood return at the atrial level with the help of an intra-atrial baffle, the Mustard and Senning operations. This resulted in the right ventricle becoming the systemic ventricle and the creation of extensive suture lines in the atria. There is now more than 30-year follow-up for these patients. Twenty-year survival is 80% but late morbidity is common. Less than 20% of patients are in sinus rhythm and more than 10% of patients have developed right ventricular failure requiring either transplantation or conversion to an arterial switch. The intra-atrial baffle leads to systemic venous obstruction in 10–20% of patients, which may not be clinically apparent except for mild facial swelling. Monitoring of the central venous pressure may be quite misleading under these circumstances and may cause superior vena cava syndrome. Obstruction of the right pulmonary veins due to baffle shrinkage occurred in 5–10% of patients. Also the Senning procedure frequently required reoperation because of unilateral pulmonary venous hypertension. The most serious long-term complication, however, is the severe dysrhythmias which follow both operations. Sinus node dysfunction or atrial flutter can result in sudden death (25%). Late right ventricular dysfunction leads to ventricular tachycardia. Patients may be on multiple antiarrhythmic drugs and may require pacemaker implantation to prevent complications from this therapy. Patients with sick sinus syndrome require a pacemaker. Patients with tachydysrhythmias are presently treated with radiofrequency ablation, if possible, but may require an implantable anti-tachycardia device. After the Mustard procedure, 50% of patients required a pacemaker by age 30 years. Patients following the atrial switch procedure may have limited cardiac reserve. There may also be difficult central access problems and the course of central lines on the chest radiograph will appear quite abnormal, since the catheter will traverse from the superior vena cava along the baffle into the mitral valve, left ventricle, and then the pulmonary artery.

Because of the disappointing long-term results of the atrial switch procedures, anatomic correction at the arterial level has been the preferred approach since the mid-1980s. It involves transsection of both great vessels with relocation of the aorta above the pulmonary valve and the left ventricle, and the pulmonary artery above the aortic valve and the right ventricle. The coronary arteries are disconnected and relocated to the neo-aorta. Long-term follow-up is available for only 15 years, but already there is a significant reduction in dysrhythmias, better systemic ventricular function, and better exercise tolerance. In the initial series, supravalvular pulmonary stenosis occurred in more than 10% of patients requiring dilatation or reoperation. With modifications in the surgical technique this complication has become rare. Aortic insufficiency is now seen in long-term survivors, who may eventually require valve replacement. In addition, 1–3% of patients have asymptomatic occlusion of one coronary artery on follow-up coronary angiography. Patients following the arterial switch should be evaluated for supravalvular stenosis and may be at risk for development of myocardial ischemia due to coronary stenosis. They are otherwise similar to a person with a structurally normal heart.

Single Ventricle and the Fontan Operation

A multitude of complex congenital cardiac lesions have only one functional ventricle to support the systemic circulation or can only be repaired by converting them to single-ventricle physiology. Some of the more common lesions that are "repaired" in this way include tricuspid atresia, double inlet left or right ventricle, hypoplastic left heart syndrome, and pulmonary atresia with intact septum with hypoplastic right ventricle. In infancy, these patients undergo a procedure to balance pulmonary blood flow between the systemic circulation and the pulmonary circulation. This involves either the creation of an aortopulmonary shunt for pulmonary perfusion or banding of the pulmonary artery to restrict excessive flow. In hypoplastic left heart syndrome, the aorta is reconstructed in the same procedure (Norwood I). At about 6 months of age, in order to relieve the volume load on the single ventricle, the venous return from the upper extremity is diverted directly into the lung by anastomosis of the superior vena cava to the pulmonary artery (Bi-Glenn). The prior shunt or band is taken down at that time. All patients remain cyanotic following these procedures. The oxygen saturation in these patients is in the eighties when the cardiac output is normal because blood that equally perfuses the systemic and pulmonary circulation mixes in the single ventricle. The final stage consists of separating the two circulations (Fontan) by diverting inferior vena cava (IVC) blood to the pulmonary artery. There have been several modifications of this procedure over the years. At present, the IVC is channeled either through an intra-atrial lateral baffle or via an extracardiac conduit to the pulmonary artery.

Since pulmonary blood flow and hence cardiac output depend on a pressure gradient between the central venous pressure and the mean pulmonary or intrathoracic pressure, PVR has to be low and myocardial function relatively normal to avoid excessively high central venous pressure. Patients have limited potential to increase cardiac output because of limited flow across the venous channels. At present, a fenestration is created between the IVC channel and the right atrium (creating a right-to-left shunt) to allow decompression of high venous pressure, which would

Complications and Sequelae of the Repaired Heart

ASD secundum
- Mitral valve prolapse
- Mitral regurgitation
- Atrial dysrhythmias
- Ventricular dysrhythmias

VSD
- Residual defect
- Aortic insufficiency
- Right bundle branch block
- Ventricular dysrhythmias

Coarctation of the aorta
- Associated conditions
  - Bicuspid aortic valve
  - Berry aneurysm of the circle of Willis
  - Turner syndrome
- Recoarctation
- Aortic aneurysm at balloon angioplasty site
- Hypertension
  - Aortic valve disease

AV septal defects
- Mitral insufficiency
- First-degree heart block
- Malignant tachydysrhythmias

TOF
- Atrial tachycardias
- Right bundle branch block
- Ventricular ectopy/dysrhythmias
- Residual lesions
- Paradoxical emboli
- Difficult vascular access

TGA
- Mustard/Senning
  - Systemic venous obstruction
  - Right ventricular failure
  - Atrial/ventricular dysrhythmias
  - Right pulmonary vein obstruction
  - Pulmonary venous hypertension
  - Thrombosis
- Arterial switch
  - Supravalvular pulmonary stenosis
  - Aortic insufficiency
  - Coronary artery occlusion

Single ventricle and Fontan operation
- Elevated central venous pressure
- Protein-losing enteropathy
- Pleural effusion
- Atrial tachydysrhythmias
- Spontaneous thrombosis
- Paradoxical emboli

maintain cardiac output at the expense of full oxygenation. Survival after these procedures is 60–73% at 15 years.

Patients are at risk for several long-term problems. The persistently elevated central venous pressure leads to a protein-losing enteropathy in 5–13% of patients over 10 years, and to persistent pleural effusions. Atrial suture lines and atrial distention lead to a high incidence of atrial tachydysrhythmias. Atrial flutter occurs in 40–50% of patients 15 years following the procedure. In patients whose single ventricle is a right ventricle, ventricular function deteriorates progressively. Only half of Fontan patients have normal cardiac function 10 years after the repair. Patients also tend to develop spontaneous thrombosis and need to be on chronic low-dose anticoagulation. Afterload-reducing agents are prescribed to protect myocardial function and maintain low left atrial pressures. Maintenance of sinus rhythm is equally important to maintain cardiac output. All patients have reduced exercise tolerance.

Key considerations for anesthetic management are:

- Thorough preoperative cardiac evaluation including echocardiography is required to assess function of the atrioventricular valve and ventricle.
- Maintenance of adequate preload, sinus rhythm, and avoidance of cardiodepressant drugs is essential.
- Spontaneous ventilation should be maintained if at all possible to minimize any increase in intrathoracic pressure.

If controlled ventilation is necessary, positive intrathoracic pressure should be kept to a minimum.
- Central venous pressure lines should be used only when absolutely indicated because of the risk of thrombosis and obstruction to venous return.
- Regional anesthesia should be carefully titrated to allow for adjustment for acute preload and afterload reductions.
- Patients require endocarditis prophylaxis.
- Meticulous attention is necessary to prevent introducing air bubbles, since these patients are at risk for paradoxical emboli in the presence of a fenestration or baffle leak.

SUGGESTED READINGS

Hollinger I, Reich DL, Moskowitz D: Congenital heart disease. pp. 287–316. In Troyanos CA (ed): Anesthesia and the Cardiac Patient. Mosby, St. Louis, 2002

Laussen PV, Wessel DL: Anesthesia for congenital heart disease. pp. 467–539. In Gregory GA (ed): Pediatric Anesthesia. Churchill Livingstone, New York, 2002

Strafford MA: Management of the patient with repaired or palliated congenital heart disease. pp. 415–460. In Coté CJ, Todres ID, Goudsouzian NG, Ryan JR (eds): A Practice of Anesthesia for Infants and Children. WB Saunders, Philadelphia, 2001

70

PRETERM INFANT

Gregg Lobel, MD

A 10-week-old, former 29-week gestation infant is now ready for discharge home from the neonatal intensive care unit (NICU). Prior to discharge the infant presented for bilateral inguinal hernia repair.

QUESTIONS

1. What are the anatomic and physiologic differences between the infant and the adult?
2. What is the definition of prematurity?
3. Do the pharmacokinetics and pharmacodynamics of anesthetic drugs differ in this population as compared with adults?
4. What are the nil per os (NPO) guidelines for this case?
5. What anesthetic options are available and what are the concerns regarding each option?
6. If a general anesthetic is planned, what are the induction options?
7. What are the appropriate monitors for this case?
8. What are the options for postoperative pain control?
9. When can this infant be discharged home? Could this procedure have been done as an outpatient after discharge?

1. What are the anatomic and physiologic differences between the infant and the adult?

The anatomic and physiologic differences that exist between the infant and the adult clearly affect the anesthetic management.

Anatomic

There are multiple airway anatomic differences which affect anesthesia management.

Large Occiput Infants' upper airways are much more susceptible to collapse, especially with flexion of the neck. Flexion occurs naturally in the infant when lying supine because of their relatively large occiput. Hence, appropriate head position is important for maintenance of a patent upper airway. This may necessitate placement of a shoulder roll to extend the neck.

Relatively Large Tongue Infants have large tongues relative to the total size of their mouth, which can lead to airway obstruction and make mask ventilation difficult.

Cephalad Larynx The infant's larynx is situated more cephalad (C3–4) than the adult's (C4–5), making it appear "anterior." This results in a greater angle between the tongue and the glottic opening, making visualization of the larynx difficult with a curved laryngoscope blade. For this reason, a straight laryngoscope blade is usually used for intubation.

Narrow Epiglottis   The adult epiglottis is broad and parallel to the axis of the trachea whereas the infant's epiglottis is narrow (omega-shaped) and angled away from the axis of the trachea making it appear "floppy." Therefore, a straight laryngoscope blade is used to lift the epiglottis during intubation.

Cricoid Cartilage Narrowest Portion of the Airway   The narrowest portion of the infant's airway is at the cricoid cartilage. Therefore, an endotracheal tube (ETT) that passes easily through the vocal cords may not pass through the cricoid cartilage. In addition, an ETT that fits too tightly at the cricoid ring may cause subglottic edema and airway obstruction after extubation. Therefore, after placement of an ETT, the leak around the tube should be determined and the ETT changed if the leak is >30 cm H_2O.

Vocal Cords Are Slanted   The vocal cords in the infant are slanted, with the anterior commissure being more caudad than the posterior commissure. In the adult, the vocal cords are perpendicular to the axis of the trachea. Because of the slanting, ETTs are more likely to hit the anterior commissure, causing difficulty in passing the ETT and trauma to the vocal cords.

Pulmonary

Pulmonary compliance in the pediatric patient is less than in the adult patient due to differences in alveolar architecture, surfactant, and elastin. These differences are especially evident in the neonate and infant. Since Poiseuille's law (resistance = $8Ln/\pi r^4$) states that airway resistance is inversely proportional to the fourth power of the radius, airway resistance is greater in infants than in adults. In the child, and especially the neonate, the chest wall is very compliant, primarily because of the cartilaginous nature of their ribs. Minute ventilation is higher in the infant compared with the adult. This is mainly due to the increased respiratory rate. Tidal volume, on a cc/kg basis, is the same in the infant and the adult. Closing volume, the lung volume at which small airways begin to collapse, is higher in the infant than in the adult. This results in collapse of the small airways during normal tidal volume breathing. In addition, the infant has a higher alveolar ventilation to functional residual capacity ratio (V_A/FRC). In the infant this ratio is 5:1 whereas in the adult it is 1.5:1. These factors, along with the neonate's higher oxygen consumption (7–9 mL/kg/min), are responsible for the rapid desaturation seen in neonates. Also, the diaphragm of an infant has a much lower proportion of type I muscle fibers, which are fatigue resistant. This contributes to the main respiratory muscles being more susceptible to fatigue.

Because this case involves an ex-premature infant, there may be other significant issues involving the pulmonary system. Infants born prematurely are at risk for hyaline membrane disease (HMD), which may progress to chronic lung disease. Bronchopulmonary dysplasia (BPD) is diagnosed if supplemental oxygen is needed and abnormal chest radiograph findings are present at 36 weeks postconceptual age. The presence of apnea of prematurity must be evaluated and the factors that may affect it such as anemia, hypoglycemia, hypothermia, sepsis, or hypoxemia need to be evaluated as well.

Cardiac

The newborn myocardium has decreased compliance that limits its ability to increase stroke volume. Ultimately, this results in the cardiac output being dependent on heart rate. There is very little reserve in the neonatal heart since it routinely operates at close to its maximal level. Cardiac output in the infant is greater than in adults. In addition, the sympathetic nervous system is immature in the neonate and therefore cannot provide the usual support during periods of stress. This also results in the neonate being vagotonic and responding to most insults (e.g., hypoxia) with bradycardia rather than tachycardia, as most adults would. Also, one must always consider congenital heart disease and the effect of changes in preload, afterload, and contractility in that situation.

Renal

In term infants, the glomerular filtration rate (GFR) is about 40% of that of the adult and is even lower in preterm infants. GFR is proportional to the gestational age. The decreased GFR impairs the newborn's ability to concentrate or dilute urine, especially during the first week of life. The renal blood flow is low at birth and increases during the first year of life, especially during the first week. The neonatal kidneys cannot completely reabsorb sodium, and they excrete sodium even in the presence of a sodium deficit.

Hematologic

Full-term neonates have a higher hematocrit than older children or adults, but this begins to decline in the first week of life. At about 2–3 months of life, the physiologic nadir usually occurs. The same process occurs in premature infants, but it is more exaggerated with the physiologic nadir occurring even earlier. Also, fetal hemoglobin has a higher affinity for oxygen. Therefore, even with the same hemoglobin as an adult, less oxygen may be delivered to the tissues. The infant compensates for this with a higher blood volume per kilogram (90 mL) and a higher cardiac output per kilogram than adults.

Pharmacologic

The pharmacokinetics and pharmacodynamics of medications used in the pediatric population differ from those in the adult. This is particularly true in the neonate and premature infant. These differences are:

- Decreased protein binding results in a larger unbound fraction.
- Volume of distribution is larger. Total body water (TBW) is composed of intracellular fluid (ICF) and extracellular fluid (ECF). ECF consists of interstitial volume and plasma volume. These compartment sizes change dramatically as a neonate grows. For example, TBW is 80% in a preterm neonate and about 55% in an adult, while ECF is about 40% of TBW in a neonate and about 20% in a 1-year-old. These differences in body water composition effect drug dosages and distribution.
- Smaller proportion of body weight as fat and muscle mass. This proportion changes as the neonate grows. Medications that redistribute to fat and muscle may have higher initial and sustained peak blood levels.
- Hepatic metabolism is reduced resulting in prolonged half-lives of medications excreted by the liver.
- Renal function is decreased resulting in prolonged half-lives of medications excreted primarily through the kidneys.

Anatomic and Physiologic Differences Between the Infant and the Adult

Anatomic
   Relatively large tongue
   Large occiput
   Narrow epiglottis
   Cricoid cartilage narrowest portion of the
      airway
   Slanted vocal cords

Pulmonary
   Decreased pulmonary compliance
   Increased airway resistance
   Increased chest wall compliance
   Increased minute ventilation
   Increased closing volume
   Increased V_A/FRC
   Increased oxygen consumption
   Decreased Type I diaphragm muscle fibers

Cardiac
   Decreased myocardial compliance
   Increased cardiac output
   Cardiac output heart-rate-dependent
   Immature sympathetic system (vagotonic)
   Bradycardic response to insults (e.g., hypoxia)

Renal
   Decreased GFR
   Decreased renal blood flow
   Inability to concentrate urine
   Sodium wasters

Hematologic
   Increased hematocrit
   Fetal hemoglobin

---

2. What is the definition of prematurity?

Prematurity is defined as a gestational age less than 37 weeks from the last menstrual period at the time of birth. Prematurity may be subdivided into borderline prematurity (36–37 weeks' gestation), moderate prematurity (31–36 weeks' gestation), and severe prematurity (24–30 weeks' gestation.) Severely premature neonates have the most significant physiologic disturbances affecting multiple organ systems. A thorough review of the ex-premature infant's neonatal course is critical in providing the appropriate anesthetic care. This review should include discussions with the neonatologist as well as the nurses who were involved in the patient's care.

3. Do the pharmacokinetics and pharmacodynamics of anesthetic drugs differ in this population as compared with adults?

Pharmacokinetics refers to the changes in drug concentration in blood over time. In children, especially neonates and infants, pharmacokinetics is very different from that in adults. These differences are due to many factors including differences in the size of the fluid compartments, smaller muscle mass and fat stores, and the immature or absent hepatic enzyme systems necessary for metabolism of certain drugs. These hepatic enzyme systems mature at different rates; therefore the pharmacokinetics of all drugs do not progress toward the adult model at the same pace. The kidney is where most drugs or their metabolites are eliminated. The renal clearance of many drugs is altered because of the decreased GFR and other immature aspects of renal function in the neonate, such as secretion and resorption.

Neonates and infants have a faster uptake of inhaled anesthetics, which results in a more rapid induction of general anesthesia. There are several factors that contribute to this: the increased V_A/FRC ratio and the greater percentage of cardiac output that goes to the brain, which is part of the vessel-rich group. The minimum alveolar concentration (MAC) for the inhaled agents in a full-term infant is the same as for an adult. It is decreased in the preterm infant and increases until about 6 months of age. After 6 months, the MAC begins to decrease toward the adult level.

The respiratory and cardiovascular effects of inhaled agents are similar in adults and children. Respiratory and myocardial depression occur in a dose-dependent fashion. However, the blood pressure tends to decrease more in neonates than in adults. This may be due to the immature baroreceptors that prevent an appropriate compensatory response. Any anesthetic that decreases heart rate or cardiac contractility will cause hemodynamic instability until the child's cardiac output is no longer rate-dependent.

In conclusion, the pharmacology of anesthetic agents changes as a neonate becomes an infant, an infant becomes a child, and a child becomes an adult. As a result, drug dosages must be individualized to take into account the changes that occur in the many pharmacokinetic parameters as the neonate grows.

4. What are the nil per os (NPO) guidelines for this case?

There is a lot of variation among institutions regarding NPO policies for clears, formula, breast milk, and solids. Even among pediatric anesthesiologists, there is disagreement. The American Academy of Pediatrics and American Society of Anesthesiologists formed a task force, which made the following recommendations regarding NPO for various liquids and food:

- 2 hours for clear liquids
- 4 hours for breast milk
- 6 hours for non-human milk or a light meal
- 8 hours for fatty solid meals

The task force describes a light meal as tea and toast. The recommendation of 6 hours for non-human milk comes with the caveat that the amount of milk the patient drank may affect the amount of time necessary for complete emptying of the stomach. In other words, a longer time than 6 hours may be necessary to assure complete emptying of the stomach.

These recommendations apply to patients not considered "full stomachs." One must still use appropriate judgment in patients who have certain underlying medical conditions (gastroesophageal reflux) or who are presenting for emergency surgery. Pharmacologic agents used to increase gastric emptying and reduce gastric acidity should be considered in certain cases.

In general, NPO policies have been liberalized recently because longer fasting times were found to be unnecessary. Patients were becoming unnecessarily dehydrated. In the pediatric population, this also led to irritability, and in the very young neonate, possibly hypoglycemia. Prolonged fasting times also caused unnecessary distress to the child and the parents. Whatever policy you choose, it should be clearly communicated to the parents and the operating room staff to prevent unnecessary prolonged fasting times.

5. What anesthetic options are available and what are the concerns regarding each option?

Approximately 30% of preterm neonates have inguinal hernias and 20% of those have them bilaterally. These neonates are at increased risk for incarceration of the hernia and a decision on the timing of the surgical repair needs to be made. This decision may be affected by the experience of the surgeon and the anesthesiologist. The anesthetic options include general anesthesia and regional anesthesia. Since many ex-premature infants may have chronic medical problems, each case must be individually reviewed prior to determining the risks and benefits of each type of anesthesia.

A detailed history of the neonatal course is critical in preparing this patient for anesthesia and avoiding complications. The preoperative evaluation should include a discussion with the neonatologists and nurses who have been caring for the patient as well as a chart review. Specific areas of focus include severity of lung disease and current therapy, presence or absence of tracheal intubation, history of tracheal intubation (including size of ETT and duration of intubation), current oxygen requirements, frequency of apnea episodes, and use of respiratory stimulants. A history of intraventricular hemorrhage (IVH) should be sought. IVH is graded 1–4 with grades 3 and 4 being associated with hydrocephalus. Other medical problems include cerebral palsy, retinopathy of prematurity, and gastroesophageal reflux. Any history of prior anesthesia should be obtained and reviewed for any adverse events. Current medications, allergies, family history of anesthetic-related problems, current weight, and NPO status should be obtained in addition to performing a physical and airway examination.

There are several concerns if general anesthesia is chosen. First, maintaining normal body temperature is more difficult in the neonate due to the larger body surface area/volume ratio, which results in the loss of large amounts of heat through the skin. A warmed operating room and the use of a forced-air warming blanket help maintain normal body temperature. A lowered body temperature could contribute to postoperative apnea.

Secondly, the infant may require postoperative ventilation and may be at risk for postoperative apnea. There appears to be a direct correlation between the incidence of postoperative apnea and general anesthesia in specific ex-premature infants. Post-conceptual age, gestational age, and the presence of anemia are factors that compound this matter. Most institutions will require apnea monitoring in the postoperative period if the post-conceptual age is less than 60 weeks. Post-conceptual age is calculated in the following manner:

$$\text{Gestational age} + \text{Chronological age} = \text{Post-conceptual age}$$

Another concern associated with general anesthesia is retinopathy of prematurity (ROP). ROP is most likely a result of several factors, of which oxygen is a major one. This risk probably exists until the neonate is 44 weeks post-conceptual age. For this reason, it is important to limit the amount of oxygen delivered. A common goal is to maintain the oxygen saturation by pulse oximetry (SpO_2) in the mid-nineties. Preductal oxygen saturations should be measured if the ductus arteriosus is still patent.

The two regional anesthetics most commonly used are a spinal and continuous caudal. One major advantage of these techniques is the reduced incidence of postoperative apnea when compared with general anesthesia. This only appears to be true when no additional depressant drugs such as fentanyl, morphine, midazolam, or ketamine are administered at the same time. However, this does not preclude the need for postoperative apnea monitoring in infants identified to be at risk.

Spinal anesthesia has some limitations, most notably the shorter duration of action, even when 1 mg/kg of hyperbaric tetracaine is used. The maximum duration of surgical anesthesia is 60–90 minutes before supplementation would be necessary. Since there is no hemodynamic instability following spinal blockade in neonates (secondary to the immature sympathetic system), intravenous (IV) access may be placed after establishment of the spinal anesthetic in an area where there is sensory loss.

Continuous caudal anesthesia is accomplished by placing a catheter in the caudal space. Since caudal anesthesia requires higher doses of local anesthetics compared with spinal anesthesia, toxicity becomes a concern, especially if repeat dosing is necessary. In this scenario, 2% 2-chloroprocaine is preferable because it has a short serum half-life and a low systemic toxicity.

6. If a general anesthetic is planned, what are the induction options?

Either an inhalation or intravenous induction is appropriate. There are several factors to consider when making this decision. Does the patient have an intravenous catheter in place? Is there an increased risk of pulmonary aspiration? Are there any underlying medical conditions that make one technique preferable over another? IV access may be difficult to achieve in the patient with a long and complicated neonatal course. If there is no increased risk of pulmonary aspiration, IV access may be easier to achieve after an inhalation induction. However, be prepared for a rapid induction and the possibility of myocardial depression

and bradycardia. Some anesthesiologists may opt to premedicate these patients with intramuscular atropine prior to an inhalation induction. Obviously, if IV access is already present, an IV induction would be appropriate.

The airway may be secured either with an ETT or laryngeal mask airway (LMA). Common practice is to secure the airway with an ETT. Normally, the ETT size is based on age. But if there is a history of prolonged intubation, there may be subglottic narrowing and the need for a smaller ETT. Attention to the "fit" of the ETT, by checking for an adequate air leak (<30 cm H_2O), is key to the prevention of postoperative edema and airway obstruction. An LMA may be used if there are no contraindications, such as gastroesophageal reflux. LMA size #1 is appropriate for patients weighing <5 kg. Assisted ventilation is required when using an LMA.

7. What are the appropriate monitors for this case?

A precordial or esophageal stethoscope is the most important monitor. With the stethoscope, the anesthesiologist can listen for the presence of breath sounds, as well as to the quality and rate of heart sounds. Changes in these sounds are often the first sign of change in the patient's condition, occurring before any change in the other monitors. Monitoring should include pulse oximetry, electrocardiogram, noninvasive blood pressure, capnometry (if using general anesthesia), and temperature.

8. What are the options for postoperative pain control?

There are several options available for postoperative pain control. Regional anesthetic techniques are the preferable choice for these patients because excellent analgesia can be obtained without the use of opioids, which would increase the risk for postoperative apnea. These techniques include caudal block, ilioinguinal, and iliohypogastric nerve blocks, and local anesthetic infiltration of the wound

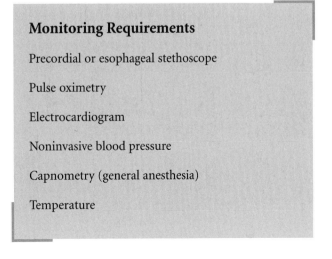

Monitoring Requirements

Precordial or esophageal stethoscope

Pulse oximetry

Electrocardiogram

Noninvasive blood pressure

Capnometry (general anesthesia)

Temperature

by the surgeon. It is important to keep track of the amount of local anesthetic injected to prevent toxic levels in these typically very low weight neonates. Acetaminophen administered orally or rectally is another option for pain control, especially as the regional block subsides. Finally, IV opioids may be administered but the patient must be closely observed for apnea.

9. When can this infant be discharged home? Could this procedure have been done as an outpatient after discharge?

Due to the risk of incarceration of the hernia, many of these procedures are scheduled just prior to discharge home from the NICU. After the procedure, the infant is monitored in the NICU for postoperative apnea for 24 hours and if there are no apneic events they are discharged home.

Recently, there has been increasing pressure to reduce length of stay. Many of these patients are now discharged home and brought back as outpatients for their hernia repairs. Current recommendations for postoperative admission vary depending on the gestational age at birth. In the full-term infant, the current recommendation is to monitor for postoperative apnea if they are less than 44 weeks post-conceptual age. In the preterm infant, these recommendations can vary from 50 to 60 weeks post-conceptual age and are institution-specific. The risk for incarceration of the hernia while waiting beyond this timeframe must be weighed against the risk of postoperative apnea and the need for overnight admission to the hospital. These risks vary and depend on other variables, including post-conceptual age, gestational age, hemoglobin concentration, and home apnea monitoring. Each case is unique and must be reviewed on a case-by-case basis to determine the proper treatment course.

SUGGESTED READINGS

Berry FA, Castro BA: Neonatal anesthesia. pp. 1171–1194. In Barash PG, Cullen BF, Stoelting RK (eds): Clinical Anesthesia, 4th edition. Lippincott Williams and Wilkins, Philadelphia, 2001

Bikhazi GB, Davis PJ: Anesthesia for neonates and premature infants. pp. 445–474. In Motoyama EK, Davis PJ (eds): Smith's Anesthesia for Infants and Children, 6th edition. Mosby-Year Book, St. Louis, 1996

Gregory GA: Pharmacology. pp. 19–51. In Gregory GA (ed): Pediatric Anesthesia, 4th edition. Churchill Livingstone, Philadelphia, 2002

Siedman L: Anesthesia for the expremature infant. pp. 369–379. In Gregory GA (ed): Pediatric Anesthesia, 4th edition. Churchill Livingstone, Philadelphia, 2002

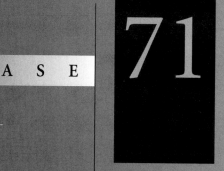

Cheryl K. Gooden, MD

A 4-year-old boy with Down syndrome (trisomy 21) presents for MRI of the brain for evaluation of an intracranial mass. Past medical history is also significant for a seizure disorder. Surgical history is significant for tonsillectomy and adenoidectomy under general anesthesia at age 2 years without complications.

QUESTIONS

1. What is magnetic resonance imaging (MRI)?
2. What are the magnetic field problems associated with MRI?
3. What are the specific problems encountered with physiologic monitors and equipment in the MRI suite?
4. What are possible patient problems encountered in the MRI scanner?
5. What are the clinical manifestations of Down syndrome?
6. Describe the pre-anesthetic evaluation of the child with Down syndrome.
7. What anesthetic alternatives are available for the child with Down syndrome undergoing MRI?
8. Describe the postanesthetic concerns in the child with Down syndrome after MRI.

1. What is magnetic resonance imaging (MRI)?

MRI incorporates the use of static and gradient magnetic fields with radiofrequency (RF) pulses to produce images of the body. Magnetic field strengths range from 0.15 to 3.0 tesla (T). The tesla is a measure of the strength of a magnetic field (1 T = 10,000 gauss). The quality of the image depends on the strength of the magnetic field.

Hydrogen is the element most commonly used in MRI. The reasons for this are that hydrogen is the most abundant element in human tissue and it can be magnetized. Atoms, such as hydrogen, with an unpaired number of protons and/or neutrons respond to, and align themselves within, the magnetic field of the MRI scanner.

Following placement of the patient within the cylindrical bore of the magnet, a steady state is established in which hydrogen atoms are in alignment. RF pulses are introduced and deflect the orientation of the atoms. When the RF pulses are eliminated, the hydrogen atoms return to their original position of alignment. As these atoms establish a resting state, the energy emitted is used to produce the resulting image.

2. What are the magnetic field problems associated with MRI?

The attractive force of the magnet exerts a substantial pull on objects that are ferromagnetic. The major concern is that these propelled ferromagnetic objects can lead to injury or lethal outcome to patients or personnel.

Devices/Objects Considered Unsafe for MRI

Pacemakers
Implantable defibrillators
Tissue expanders with metallic ports
Implantable infusion pumps
Cochlear implants
Intracranial aneurysm clips (certain types)

Care must be taken to avoid the use of, or to have in one's possession, objects such as pens, scissors, clamps, stethoscopes, non-lithium batteries, ferromagnetic compressed gas cylinders, and other objects that are ferromagnetic.

Patients with implanted ferromagnetic devices or objects which include pacemakers, tissue expanders with metallic ports, implantable defibrillators/cardioverters, implantable infusion pumps, cochlear implants, and certain types of intracranial aneurysm clips are generally excluded from MRI studies. The magnetic fields of the MRI scanner can potentially affect the function and safety of these devices. The newer aneurysm clips contain non-ferrous material and are not considered to be a problem. However, a thorough investigation of the type of aneurysm clip is required before proceeding with the MRI study. Metallic-based substances such as eye make-up or tattoos can produce local skin irritation during MRI scanning.

Metals that are known to be safe include stainless steel, titanium, alloys, and nickel. Equipment that is made of plastic is better for use in the proximity of the MRI magnet.

3. What are the specific problems encountered with physiologic monitors and equipment in the MRI suite?

The use of a conventional electrocardiogram (ECG) monitor in the MRI suite can cause distortion of the image as a result of the wire leads acting as antennas. In addition, the ECG monitor may not be able to distinguish the ECG from the background static magnetic field and RF pulses. Voltage induced in the wire leads can cause electrical shock hazards and burns to the patient.

The magnetic fields produced by the MRI scanner can cause interference and possible inactivation of the conventional operating room pulse oximeter. Either a nonferrous or fiberoptically cabled pulse oximeter should be used. The pulse oximeter probe should be placed on a distal extremity as far from the site to be scanned as possible, to prevent interference and possible scan artifact.

The oscillometric method is optimal for noninvasive blood pressure monitoring in the MRI suite because it is not affected by magnetic fields. Fiberoptic systems in conjunction with invasive blood pressure monitoring have been used successfully. In addition, central venous pressure can be monitored if necessary. There are several transducers that lack ferrous components and can be used in the MRI suite.

The use of side-stream capnography with a long sampling line allows for monitoring of patient ventilation, anesthetic gas concentrations, and circuit disconnection during the MRI scan. However, the long sampling line may create a greater lag time between the actual event and the time of its detection.

There are several MRI-compatible anesthesia machines available commercially. *Only oxygen, air, and nitrous oxide cylinders made of aluminum can be used in the MRI suite.* Ferromagnetic compressed gas cylinders are pulled by the attractive force of the magnet, and have resulted in either injury or death to patients or personnel.

Infusion pumps should be checked for MRI compatibility as well.

4. What are possible patient problems encountered in the MRI scanner?

The MRI environment creates an unavoidable distance between the patient and the anesthesiologist. The patient's inaccessibility following placement in the MRI scanner can be problematical when immediate access is required. Patient visibility is limited once the patient is placed within the gantry of the scanner. Some MRI systems are equipped with a closed-circuit camera which allows for continuous visualization of the patient.

Noise is produced by the MRI scanner as a result of the vibration of wire loops producing gradient current in the presence of RF pulses. This can at times be loud and may average approximately 95 decibels. Auditory protection, such as earplugs, should be provided to all patients undergoing a scan.

The risk of burns during MRI is another possible patient problem. The monitoring systems that may be associated with burns in the MRI scanner have been discussed above.

Patient-Related Considerations for MRI

Patient inaccessibility
Lack of patient visibility
Noise
Burns
Contrast agent reactions
Anxiety, claustrophobia (may be encountered in the awake patient)

Gadopentetate dimeglumine (gadolinium) is a commonly used MRI contrast agent. It is a low-osmolar ionic medium, with a slower clearance in neonates and infants compared with adults. Reported adverse effects include thrombophlebitis, hypotension, headache, nausea, and vomiting.

Anxiety and claustrophobia are possible problems encountered by the awake patient.

5. What are the clinical manifestations of Down syndrome?

Down syndrome (trisomy 21) is the most common autosomal chromosomal abnormality causing mental retardation. It occurs in approximately 1 in 800 live births. Children with Down syndrome can have associated congenital defects as well as other medical problems requiring surgical intervention. The anesthetic management of these patients can present many challenges.

The clinical manifestations of Down syndrome that are of particular concern to the anesthesiologist include macroglossia, micrognathia, obstructive sleep apnea, small subglottic area, and recurrent pulmonary infections. Other considerations for the anesthesiologist include hypotonia, atlantoaxial instability, seizure disorders, high arched palate, and varying degrees of mental retardation. The cardiovascular system presents other concerns. Congenital heart defects occur in 30–50% of children with Down syndrome. These lesions include endocardial cushion defects, ventricular septal defect, atrial septal defect, patent ductus arteriosus, and tetralogy of Fallot. Pulmonary hypertension may also be present. A review of systems specific to the patient with Down syndrome appears in Table 71.1.

6. Describe the pre-anesthetic evaluation of the child with Down syndrome.

The pre-anesthetic evaluation of the child with Down syndrome should include a complete history and physical examination. The anesthetic assessment should focus particularly on the organ systems most commonly involved in Down syndrome. A detailed systematic approach is necessary to prepare for potential intraoperative events. Further evaluation of these patients will depend on the extent of organ system involvement.

Atlantoaxial instability is present in 10–20% of children with Down syndrome and is a major source of concern in the perianesthetic period. Several neurologic deficits may be associated with atlantoaxial instability (Table 71.2).

Screening for atlantoaxial instability includes lateral cervical spine radiographs in the flexed, extended, and neutral positions. The atlas–dens interval is often used to quantify the movement of the atlantoaxial joint. This is measured from the posterior margin of the anterior arch of the first cervical spine to the anterior margin of the dens.

TABLE 71.1	Review of Systems: The Child with Down Syndrome

System	Clinical Features
Airway	Macroglossia
	Small mouth
	High arched palate
	Small nasopharynx
	Micrognathia
	Small glottic area
	Short and broad neck
	Tonsillar and adenoid hypertrophy
Cardiac	Endocardial cushion defect
	Patent ductus arteriosus
	Ventricular septal defect
	Atrial septal defect
	Tetralogy of Fallot
Pulmonary	Recurrent respiratory tract infections
	Pulmonary hypertension (associated with CHD)
	Obstructive sleep apnea
	Increased risk for postoperative pulmonary complications
Musculoskeletal	Hypotonia
	Temporomandibular joint laxity (and laxity of other joints)
	Atlantoaxial instability
Neurologic	Seizure disorder
	Mental retardation
Gastrointestinal	Duodenal atresia
	Increased incidence of Hirschsprung's disease
Immune/ Hematologic	Altered immune response
	Increased incidence of lymphocytic and myeloid leukemias
	Frequent infections (particularly respiratory)
	Polycythemia (neonates)

TABLE 71.2	Neurologic Deficits Associated with Atlantoaxial Instability

Gait abnormalities
Neck pain
Torticollis
Mild extremity weakness
Hyperreflexia
Spasticity

The normal atlas–dens interval for children is 4.5 mm or less.

The current recommendation is that screening for atlantoaxial instability should be done at 3–5 years of age. Follow-up cervical radiographs at 3 year intervals are no longer recommended. Obtaining a good history and neurologic assessment are key factors. When the child with Down syndrome presents for a general anesthetic, all precautions must be taken to maintain the cervical spine in a neutral position.

7. What anesthetic alternatives are available for the child with Down syndrome undergoing MRI?

Premedication for this child may be necessary to facilitate the induction of anesthesia. Oral midazolam may be considered for premedication. Intramuscular ketamine can be used quite successfully for premedication in the child with Down syndrome. However, the use of ketamine would not be considered an option in this particular patient, on account of his seizure disorder. Parental presence during the induction of anesthesia has been proven to be quite helpful. However, parental presence should not be viewed as a substitute for premedication.

If the airway examination appears normal, then either an inhalation or intravenous induction can be performed. General anesthesia with an endotracheal tube or laryngeal mask airway (LMA) are good options for this patient. Sedation with a propofol infusion may also be considered. The choice of anesthetic technique for the child with Down syndrome will involve similar decision-making as with any patient.

8. Describe the postanesthetic concerns in the child with Down syndrome after MRI.

Postanesthetic concerns after MRI are the same as following an anesthetic in the operating room. This child should be observed in either a postanesthesia care unit (PACU) or a recovery area at the MRI location equipped with monitors and nursing personnel. The child can be discharged as soon as criteria defined by the facility have been met. Since many MRI examinations are performed on an outpatient basis, a parent should be informed as to what to expect and observe in their child following discharge from the facility. In addition, instructions must be given to the parent to contact the facility immediately if they observe any untoward reaction in their child.

SUGGESTED READINGS

Coté C: Anesthesia outside the operating room. p. 571. In Coté C, Todres I, Goudsouzian N, Ryan J (eds): A Practice of Anesthesia for Infants and Children, 3rd edition. WB Saunders, Philadelphia, 2001

Gooden C, Dilos B: Anesthesia for magnetic resonance imaging. Int Anesthesiol Clin 41:29, 2003

Menon D, Peden C, Hall A, Sargentoni J, et al.: Magnetic resonance for the anaesthetist. Part I. Physical principles, applications and safety aspects. Anaesthesia 47:240, 1992

Mitchell V, Howard R, Facer E: Down's syndrome and anesthesia. Paediatr Anaesth 5:379, 1995

Patteson S, Chesney J: Anesthetic management for magnetic resonance imaging: problems and solutions. Anesth Analg 74:121, 1992

Peden C, Menon D, Hall A, Sargentoni J, et al.: Magnetic resonance for the anaesthetist. Part II. Anaesthesia and monitoring in MR units. Anaesthesia 47:508, 1992

Williams J, Somerville G, Miner M, Reilly D: Atlanto-axial subluxation and trisomy 21: another perioperative complication. Anesthesiology 67:253, 1987

Joel M. Kreitzer, MD

Gordon Freedman, MD

A 63-year-old man is scheduled to undergo an exploratory laparotomy and possible colon resection for colon carcinoma. A few years ago, he underwent a right total hip replacement. In the postoperative period, he received meperidine 75 mg intramuscularly every 4 hours on an as-needed basis for pain, with very poor pain control. He is scheduled to undergo a left total hip replacement in the future. He has no other significant medical problems. For the past 2 months, he has been taking sustained-release morphine, as well as oxycodone and acetaminophen (Percocet), for relief of his left hip pain. For the past 3 weeks, since being diagnosed with colon cancer, he has been taking diazepam to diminish anxiety.

QUESTIONS

1. Why has postoperative pain been undertreated in the past?
2. Which factors in this patient's history may impact on postoperative pain management?
3. Which organ systems are affected by postoperative pain?
4. Outline the major afferent pain pathways.
5. What are the primary chemical mediators of pain?
6. What are the advantages and disadvantages of intramuscular opioid therapy?

7. List alternative postoperative analgesic modalities for this patient.
8. What is patient-controlled analgesia (PCA)?
9. What are typical dosage schedules for intravenous PCA-administered opioids?
10. Compare the advantages and disadvantages of PCA opioids with those of intramuscular opioids.
11. Describe the regional analgesic techniques available for postoperative pain relief. Which are applicable to this patient?
12. By what mechanism does neuraxial (epidural and subarachnoid) opioid administration produce analgesia?
13. Outline the potential side-effects of neuraxial opioids and their treatment.
14. Describe the advantages and disadvantages of subarachnoid and epidural opioids.
15. Which opioids and adjuvants are commonly used in the subarachnoid and epidural spaces?
16. What is preemptive analgesia? Can it reliably be performed in this patient?

1. Why has postoperative pain been undertreated in the past?

Despite tremendous advances in medications, techniques, knowledge, and education about pain, both acute and chronic pain are still tremendously undertreated throughout the world. Because of undertreatment of both acute and chronic pain in the hospitalized patient in the United States, Joint Commission on the Accreditation of Hospital Organizations (JCAHO) has mandated that the patient's pain be assessed and treated, and both patients and hospital staff be educated about the modalities of pain therapies available.

Postoperative pain, in particular, has been undertreated in both the ambulatory and inpatient settings. Misconceptions about the pharmacokinetics and pharmacodynamics of analgesic medications, fear of opioid side-effects, and the historical use of unpredictable intramuscular administration of opioids have all led to undertreatment of pain in the postoperative setting. Other barriers which need to be broken include the misconception of a "standard" dose of an analgesic to control pain in all patients. Current theory states that individual titration is the best way to safely and effectively promote analgesia. It must also be recognized that one cannot judge another person's level of pain; the patient must be integrated into the process and rate his or her own pain.

2. Which factors in this patient's history may impact on postoperative pain management?

A patient's preoperative emotional and psychiatric state can greatly influence his or her response to pain in the postoperative period. Fear, uncertainty, and helplessness are factors which may influence a patient's anxiety level. In addition, psychiatric states, such as depression, can increase a patient's postoperative pain. This patient's past experience with improperly treated postoperative pain, as well as his knowledge of his recent diagnosis of cancer, may heighten his anxiety, and thus make his postoperative pain more difficult to control. In addition, his use of an opioid analgesic (oxycodone) for a few months prior to surgery may make him mildly tolerant to the effects of the opioids administered in the postoperative period. Tolerance means that a higher dose of medication will be needed to obtain the desired clinical effect.

In this patient, it would be wise to continue the use of a benzodiazepine in the postoperative period to avoid withdrawal symptoms. In addition, it would be prudent to give him the equivalent dose of his long-acting morphine throughout the postoperative period, as well as a higher dose of systemic opioids, thus taking into consideration the tolerance which he has developed. If possible, the use of epidural opioids and local anesthetics, in addition to non-opioid analgesics, such as ketorolac, a parenteral nonsteroidal anti-inflammatory drug (NSAID), may provide better analgesia.

3. Which organ systems are affected by postoperative pain?

Multiple organ systems are affected by improperly treated postoperative pain. After thoracic or upper abdominal procedures, postoperative pain is associated with a decrease in the ability to breathe deeply and cough, and with reduced lung volumes. These effects predispose patients to atelectasis and impaired pulmonary toilet, possibly leading to postoperative fevers. Involuntary splinting of thoracic and abdominal muscles, reflex muscle spasm, and premature airway closure cause ventilation-perfusion mismatch, leading to postoperative hypoxemia.

Pain causes stimulation of the sympathetic nervous system, resulting in release of catecholamines, such as norepinephrine and epinephrine. These circulating amines can result in tachycardia and peripheral vasoconstriction, increasing the workload on the heart. An increased incidence of ischemia, dysrhythmias, and hypertension has been shown to occur in patients whose pain is not adequately controlled.

The sympathetic discharge noted above has an adverse effect on the gastrointestinal (GI) system, causing an ileus and decreased GI motility. This effect must be considered with the use of systemic opioids, which can decrease the peristaltic activity of the GI tract even further.

Pain increases urinary bladder sphincter tone, with the potential for urinary retention.

The neuroendocrine stress response has been a topic of recent research. Postoperative pain has been demonstrated to be associated with a state of increased catabolism and decreased anabolism, leading to an overall catabolic state with negative nitrogen balance. This is associated with an increase in oxygen use and metabolism. This stress response has been associated with decreased wound healing. In addition, activation of the stress response may be associated with maintenance of a hypercoagulable state, predisposing the patient to thromboses and embolic events.

Poor postoperative pain control can result in states of helplessness, depression, and increased anxiety.

4. Outline the major afferent pain pathways.

Somatic pain is produced by activation of pain receptors in the periphery. There are two principal cutaneous nociceptors: high-threshold mechanoreceptors (HTMs) and polymodal nociceptors (PMNs). The HTMs respond to mechanical stimuli and have a receptive field of 1 cm^2. PMNs respond to mechanical, thermal, and chemical irritants. HTM axons conduct via myelinated A delta fibers at a rate of 5–25 m/sec and transmit sharp pain with a rapid onset. PMN axons conduct via unmyelinated C fibers at a rate of less than 2 m/sec and convey dull aching pain with a slow onset (Figure 72.1). Pain from visceral origins is carried away from the organs by myelinated visceral B fibers.

These nerves enter the dorsal horn of the spinal cord and terminate in different laminae, which were designated histologically by Rexed. A delta and C fibers synapse with wide dynamic range neurons (activated by tactile or noxious stimuli) in lamina V and nociceptive-specific

Physiologic Effects of Postoperative Pain

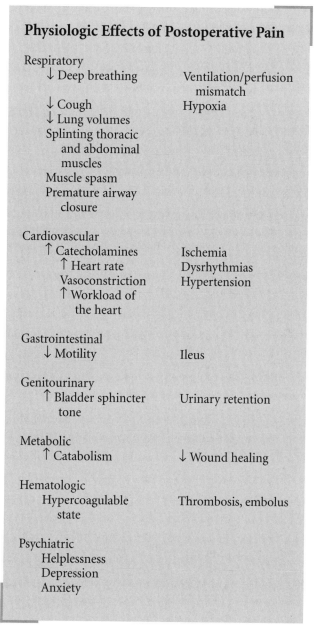

Respiratory
  ↓ Deep breathing   Ventilation/perfusion
                              mismatch
  ↓ Cough   Hypoxia
  ↓ Lung volumes
  Splinting thoracic
    and abdominal
    muscles
  Muscle spasm
  Premature airway
    closure

Cardiovascular
  ↑ Catecholamines   Ischemia
    ↑ Heart rate   Dysrhythmias
    Vasoconstriction   Hypertension
    ↑ Workload of
      the heart

Gastrointestinal
  ↓ Motility   Ileus

Genitourinary
  ↑ Bladder sphincter   Urinary retention
    tone

Metabolic
  ↑ Catabolism   ↓ Wound healing

Hematologic
  Hypercoagulable   Thrombosis, embolus
    state

Psychiatric
  Helplessness
  Depression
  Anxiety

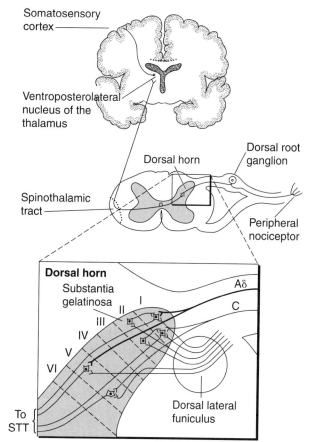

FIGURE 72.1 A schematic afferent nociceptive pathway. Inset, dorsal horn neural interrelationships. Abbreviations: STT, spinothalamic tract; Aδ, A delta fibers entering dorsal horn; C, C fibers entering dorsal horn.

somatosensory cortex. These neurons are associated with discrimination (location, duration, and intensity) of pain. Other axons project to the medial thalamic nuclei as well as the medulla, pons, midbrain, and hypothalamus (paleospinothalamic tract) and are associated with emotional aspects of pain.

5. What are the primary chemical mediators of pain?

At the peripheral pain receptor, mediators of inflammation such as serotonin, histamine, bradykinins, and prostaglandins decrease nociceptor thresholds, thus sensitizing the receptor to pain. Blocking production of these substances, such as with the use of NSAIDs which decrease prostaglandin production, decreases pain by this peripheral mechanism.

Centrally, substance P, an 11 amino acid peptide, is released in the dorsal horn of the spinal cord, activating the spinothalamic and other ascending pain tracts.

neurons in lamina I. Both types of fibers send branches into the substantia gelatinosa (laminae II and III), whose inhibitor interneurons modulate perceived nociception.

The axons of the neurons originating in laminae V and I cross over to the opposite ventrolateral funiculus of the spinal cord and ascend as the lateral spinothalamic tract. Some axons terminate in the ventroposterolateral nucleus of the thalamus (neospinothalamic tract), where they synapse with neurons that project to the

Peripherally, substance-P-releasing axons dilate blood vessels, degranulate mast cells, and stimulate sweat glands, mediating many of the secondary changes associated with pain.

Other physiologic mediators act to inhibit perceived pain stimulation. Endogenous analgesic peptides, such as enkephalins and endorphins, are found throughout the central nervous system and stimulate opioid receptors, inhibiting the release of substance P. These substances are found in the brain, as well as in the descending inhibitory tracks in the dorsal horn of the spinal cord. Neurotransmitters such as serotonin and norepinephrine are also involved in the activation of descending inhibitory tracts.

Amino acids, such as gamma-aminobutyric acid (GABA) and glycine, are known to inhibit synaptic transmission. These neurotransmitters may serve as inhibitory mediators in the substantia gelatinosa.

6. What are the advantages and disadvantages of intramuscular opioid therapy?

For years, intramuscular (IM) opioids were the mainstay of postoperative pain management. An order such as "meperidine 75 mg IM q4H prn pain" was the gold standard by which other analgesic regimens were judged.

Advantages of the use of IM opioids include ease of administration, familiarity with the technique, and low cost. Disadvantages include long delays from a patient's complaint of pain to actual time of drug administration, long onset of action, as well as variable and unreliable absorption. When IM opioids are administered every 3–4 hours, bolus doses lead to alternating periods of analgesic-induced over-sedation and painful under-medication. During IM administration, only during one third to one half of the time is the patient's blood opioid concentration in the "analgesic therapeutic window", where they are comfortable but not having side-effects. Standard IM opioid orders do not take into account the variability seen between patients with regard to dosing of opioids to achieve analgesia. Individual variability may account for up to a sevenfold difference in the plasma opioid concentration required to achieve analgesia. Each patient possesses particular plasma opioid concentration at which analgesia becomes adequate and only by individual titration can this be achieved.

7. List alternative postoperative analgesic modalities for this patient.

Alternative analgesic modalities include patient-controlled analgesia (PCA), neuraxial opioids (spinal or epidural), and local anesthetics. Infiltration of the surgical wound with local anesthetics may decrease pain in the immediate postoperative period. The use of non-opioid analgesics, such as parenteral NSAIDs, may have an opioid sparing effect, allowing pain relief to be achieved with less opioid use and with a better side-effect profile.

8. What is patient-controlled analgesia (PCA)?

PCA is a method by which patients self-administer opioids, by either the intravenous, epidural, or subcutaneous route. PCA devices consist of an infusion pump connected to a timing device (Figure 72.2). By pressing a button, the patient receives a predetermined bolus dose of medication. Another dose can only be obtained after a preset time interval (lock-out period) has passed. PCA devices also provide the option of administering a continuous infusion, called the basal infusion. Although patients determine when they will give themselves medication, the physicians prescribe the dose, as well as the frequency of administration. With demand dosing, a negative closed loop enhances the system's safety: excessive plasma opioid levels may induce a somnolent state, during which time the button is not depressed, and additional bolus doses are not administered until the plasma levels fall.

Features of PCA devices vary, but most include alarms noting occlusion in the line, low battery levels, and when the medication has run out or is low. The systems have a read-out, by which the prescription, as well as information regarding patient's opioid utilization can be obtained. To prevent unauthorized tampering, the prescription can only be changed by the use of a key and by keying a numerical code into the machine. In addition, access to the opioid in the machine is only with the use of a key or combination.

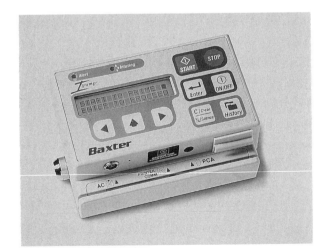

FIGURE 72.2   PCA pump. Not shown is the patient call button, which is attached to the pump and allows the patient to request medications. (Reproduced with permission from Baxter Healthcare, Round Lake, Illinois.)

9. What are typical dosage schedules for intravenous PCA-administered opioids?

Sample adult dosage schedules for commonly used opioid analgesics are noted in Table 72.1. Such schedules are only guidelines and require individual titration from patient to patient. In the elderly, or the patient with severe pulmonary or renal disease, basal rates may need to be eliminated, bolus doses may need to be decreased, and/or lock-out intervals may need to be lengthened. Conversely, in young, healthy patients, or in those tolerant to opioids, the bolus dose and basal rate might need to be increased or the lock-out interval may need to be shortened.

The choice of opioid used depends on many factors including the practitioner's familiarity with the drug, cost, and availability. Certain clinical situations may dictate the use of one opioid over another. For example, morphine, due to its propensity to release histamine, may not be the first-line drug of choice in the asthmatic patient. Meperidine should not be used routinely in the postoperative period because of its ability to cause tachycardia and because its primary metabolite, normeperidine, lowers the seizure threshold.

Debate exists over the benefits of using a constant, basal rate infusion with PCA. Opponents of its use note the fact that the use of a basal rate defeats the idea behind PCA, that patients only request medication when they need it, while proponents of its use believe that it improves analgesia. In a study involving post-cesarean section patients (Sinatra et al., 1989) the use of a basal rate improved analgesia, but also increased the incidence of nausea. Another study in gynecologic patients (Parker et al., 1992) failed to show any advantage to the use of basal rates. Although it may seem counter-intuitive, the use of a basal infusion has never shown to increase a patient's ability to sleep in the postoperative period.

10. Compare the advantages and disadvantages of PCA opioids with those of intramuscular opioids.

The idea behind PCA is to allow a patient to achieve a plasma opioid concentration in their "therapeutic window", which is the plasma level where they are comfortable but not suffering from side-effects. This "therapeutic window" is highly variable between patients. By titrating to their own level of analgesia, patients using PCA can achieve individual plasma opioid concentrations that provide pain control without the peak and trough levels seen with intramuscular opioids. This avoids periods of both profound sedation and inadequate pain control. PCA also provides the psychological advantage of allowing patients to influence an aspect of their care without blind dependency on medical personnel.

PCA provides a convenient method of increased dosing immediately prior to painful events, such as coughing and mobilizing. During the immediate postoperative period, patients utilizing PCA use smaller amounts of opioids than patients receiving intramuscular injections, and benefit from the absence of painful intramuscular injections. By reducing the total amount of opioids and by avoiding large intramuscular doses, opioid side-effects such as sedation, nausea, vomiting, and respiratory depression are reduced. Nursing time devoted to responding to a patient's call for analgesics, assessing the need for medication, checking the orders, signing out, and administering the opioid is decreased, thereby improving nursing efficiency.

There are disadvantages to the use of PCA. The pumps and disposable tubing are expensive. Patients must be instructed in the proper use of PCA prior to the use of the device. PCA is an excellent way to maintain analgesia; however, the patient needs to be bolused to comfort with opioids prior to the start of PCA therapy. Improper programming or pump malfunction can cause overdosing or underdosing. Opioid side-effects such as nausea, vomiting, sedation, and respiratory depression can occur, although with a decreased incidence when compared with intramuscular opioid administration. Potential for overuse and abuse still exists.

11. Describe the regional analgesic techniques available for postoperative pain relief. Which are applicable to this patient?

Regional analgesic techniques with local anesthetics are invaluable, underutilized techniques for the treatment of

TABLE 72.1	Sample Routine Adult PCA Dosing Schedules		
Drug	**Basal rate (mg/hr)**	**Bolus dose (mg)**	**Lock-out (minutes)**
Morphine	1	0.7–1.5	6–10
Hydromorphone	0.2	0.2–0.4	6–10
Fentanyl	0.01–0.015	0.01–0.02	6–10
Meperidine	10	10–15	6–10

postoperative pain. The simple infiltration of a wound with a long-acting local anesthetic can greatly decrease pain in the postoperative period. Blockage of peripheral nerves to the hands and arms (brachial plexus analgesia), legs (femoral or popliteal blocks), and chest and upper abdomen (intercostal blocks) can reliably provide up to 12 hours of analgesia postoperatively, as can blockade of the ilioinguinal and iliohypogastric nerves after inguinal hernia surgery. The recent resurgence of the use of indwelling catheters for peripheral nerve anesthesia and analgesia has greatly expanded the utility of these procedures. Analgesia obtained by these methods is free from the sympathectomy and its attendant hypotension seen with local anesthetic blockade of the neuraxis.

Interpleural catheters were utilized in the 1990s for unilateral thoracic or upper abdominal surgery. Local anesthetics may be administered into the interpleural space by placing a catheter between the parietal and visceral pleura of the lung. In this location, local anesthetics bathe the intercostal nerves and, to a lesser extent, the thoracic sympathetic nerves. Analgesia is obtained in the distribution of these nerves. Their use fell into disfavor for many reasons including difficulty of placement, risk of pneumothorax, high local anesthetic blood levels, and the inability to use them effectively with a chest tube in place.

Neuraxial opioids, by the spinal or epidural route, can provide profound analgesia, with a lower incidence of side-effects compared with the use of parenteral opioids, including those administered via PCA. Adding a dilute concentration of a local anesthetic (i.e., bupivacaine 0.1%) can enhance the analgesia, allow the use of lower doses of opioids (with a lower incidence of side-effects), and still avoid the motor blockade and hypotension seen with higher concentrations of epidural local anesthetics.

Appropriate choices for this patient include wound infiltration and the use of neuraxial opioids. Although intercostal blocks could be performed, the need to perform bilateral blocks at multiple levels makes this an impractical option.

12. By what mechanism does neuraxial (epidural and subarachnoid) opioid administration produce analgesia?

Neuraxial opioids were first used in humans in 1979. Since that time, they have been widely used for the treatment of postoperative and chronic cancer pain. Neuraxial opioids interact with the opiate receptors in the substantia gelatinosa of the spinal cord's dorsal horn, causing inhibitory modulation of afferent pain messages entering the cord, prior to their reaching the cerebral cortex. Thus, analgesia occurs in the absence of motor loss or autonomic blockade and resultant hypotension seen with neuraxially administered local anesthetics. Excellent analgesia can be obtained with small doses of neuraxial morphine, resulting

in serum concentrations far below those required for analgesia.

Epidural-administered lipid-soluble opioids, such as fentanyl, achieve higher serum opioid concentrations than similarly administered water-soluble opioids, such as morphine. Multiple studies have shown continuous intravenous and continuous epidural fentanyl infusions to yield similar plasma fentanyl concentrations after 18–24 hours of use. Thus, some researchers have questioned whether the analgesia obtained from epidural fentanyl is secondary to a spinal effect or whether it is due to high plasma fentanyl levels producing analgesia at a supraspinal level. A study (Salomaki et al., 1991) in patients undergoing thoracotomy showed a definite advantage to epidural fentanyl compared with intravenous administration. Similar analgesia was obtained with the use of smaller amounts of opioids, reduced plasma fentanyl levels, and a lower incidence of side-effects. However, this question is still being debated. To use epidural fentanyl appropriately, it is imperative to place the catheter tip as close to the middle of the surgical field as possible. It is the belief of these authors that when used in an appropriate manner, lipid-soluble epidural opioids produce an effect at the spinal cord level. Appropriate use means that the epidural catheter is in the middle of the surgical field, a low concentration of fentanyl (i.e., 5 µg/ml) is utilized in conjunction with a low concentration of local anesthetic (bupivacaine 0.1%), and careful titration is achieved. However, with prolonged use plasma levels will rise. This point is still being debated.

13. Outline the potential side-effects of neuraxial opioids and their treatment.

Side-effects of neuraxial opioids include respiratory depression, nausea, vomiting, pruritus, and urinary retention. Respiratory depression is the most serious of these. When severe, it requires aggressive treatment with an intravenous opioid antagonist (i.e., naloxone) and ventilatory support. However, with the use of proper dosing, respiratory depression should not be seen clinically. A recent study (Liu et al., 1999) looking at 1,030 patients being treated with epidural fentanyl and bupivacaine for postoperative analgesia, placed the incidence of respiratory depression at 0.3%.

After the initial administration of neuraxial opioids, minimally appropriate monitoring calls for respiratory/sedation checks every 2–4 hours. Respiratory depression can occur within the first 2 hours (early) or up to 24 hours (late) after opioid administration. Early respiratory depression is primarily associated with the lipid-soluble opioids and is secondary to vascular uptake. Late respiratory depression occurs mostly with hydrophilic opioids and results from migration of the opioid within the cerebrospinal fluid (CSF), up to the respiratory centers in the brain.

Other side-effects respond to symptomatic treatments. Antiemetics, such as metoclopramide and ondansetron, are generally useful for treating nausea. However, patients after abdominal surgery must be evaluated prior to administration of antiemetics to rule out any intra-abdominal pathology. Pruritus usually responds to diphenhydramine. Failing these measures, low-dose naloxone infusions (1–2 μg/kg/hr) will reduce the side-effects, while retaining analgesia.

Side-effects seem to occur more commonly with subarachnoid administration than with epidural administration. Lipid-soluble opioids may be associated with a decreased incidence of side-effects compared with hydrophilic opioids.

Low doses of epidural local anesthetics are often used to potentiate the analgesia obtained with neuraxial opioids. Although rare, motor blockade, hypotension, and urinary retention may occur. Motor strength in the lower extremities needs to be checked prior to a patient getting out of bed for the first time while utilizing this therapy.

14. Describe the advantages and disadvantages of subarachnoid and epidural opioids.

The advantages of subarachnoid opioids include simplicity of administration and small dose requirement. Although they can be administered through a subarachnoid catheter, it is more common to inject subarachnoid opioids as a bolus dose through a needle. Thus the ability to titrate small amounts of a medication to the desired effect is lost. In addition, the one-shot dosing provides analgesia of only a specified duration, with morphine lasting from 8 to 24 hours. The incidence of side-effects is greater with subarachnoid opioids compared with epidural opioids.

Epidural opioid via a continuous infusion is the preferred way to administer neuraxial opioids in the postoperative period. Because access to the epidural space is often provided through an indwelling catheter, multiple small doses or continuous infusions may be administered. If placed in a sterile fashion, the catheter can be kept in place for many days, allowing for a long duration of analgesia. The use of PCA via the epidural route adds the ability for a patient to self-administer additional boluses when pain increases, such as prior to mobilization. Combinations of opioid and local anesthetic can be used to enhance analgesia.

Disadvantages of epidural opioids include larger dose requirements, predisposing patients to higher plasma narcotic concentrations with lipid-soluble opioids. Indwelling catheters may migrate into the CSF or a blood vessel, placing patients at risk for complications. Any indwelling catheter can become a source of infection. If a patient is to receive an anticoagulant in the postoperative period, the catheter must be removed prior to institution of the medication, or, if appropriate, within the safe window of the drug's administration. If a patient develops a coagulopathy in the postoperative period, it must be decided on a risk–benefit basis whether or not to remove the catheter, for fear of dislodging a clot and causing an epidural hematoma. In addition, it is imperative to use tubing without ports or other access, to prevent inappropriate injections into the epidural space. Also, the epidural catheter may be difficult to place in some patients, such as the obese or those with a curvature of the spine.

15. Which opioids and adjuvants are commonly used in the subarachnoid and epidural spaces?

Morphine and fentanyl are the opioids most commonly used for neuraxial epidural analgesia. Because of its longer duration of action, morphine is the drug of choice when subarachnoid analgesia is desired. Although both epidural morphine and fentanyl can be used with a bolus dosing technique, a continuous infusion of either is desirable to provide continuous, titratable analgesia. Fentanyl has gained tremendous popularity for epidural use because of its quick onset of action and shorter duration, once administration is terminated. Neuraxial hydromorphone has been used by some practices, as an opioid with properties in between those of morphine and fentanyl in terms of duration of action.

Current practice is to use the lowest dose possible to obtain the best analgesia with the lowest incidence of side effects. Table 72.2 outlines dosage guidelines.

For enhanced analgesia, 0.0625–0.1% bupivacaine is often added to continuous epidural fentanyl infusions. Even with such low concentrations, partial sensory, autonomic, and motor dysfunction may occur, recovery from which must be documented before allowing the patient to ambulate.

Comparison of the Advantages and Disadvantages of Neuraxial Analgesia

Subarachnoid	Epidural
Advantages:	Advantages:
Simple to administer	Infinite duration
Smaller dose	Patient control (PCA)
Disadvantages:	Disadvantages:
Cannot titrate	Larger dose needed
Finite duration	Migration of catheter
Greater side-effects	Infection
	Difficult placement

TABLE 72.2	Sample Routine Adult Neuraxial Narcotic Schedules		
Route and drug	**Dose (mg)**	**Onset (min)**	**Duration (hours)**
Subarachnoid			
Morphine	0.1–0.7	30	8–24
Epidural			
Morphine	4–10	30–60	6–24
Continuous infusion	0.1–0.5 mg/hr		
Fentanyl	0.05	5–10	3–6
Continuous infusion	0.02–0.08 mg/hr		

Epidural clonidine has been investigated for the use in the treatment of postoperative pain. Although it is an effective analgesic, its widespread use has been limited because of associated hypotension.

16. What is preemptive analgesia? Can it reliably be performed in this patient?

Preemptive analgesia is a technique via which an analgesic modality is introduced prior to the painful procedure so that the patient will have less pain in the postoperative period. This idea is based on the theory of "central nervous system wind-up", whereby if the spinal cord receives a constant barrage of painful stimuli it becomes hyperexcitable and thus more prone to evoke a pain response, even to less painful stimuli. Different modalities have been investigated, such as the use of preoperative NSAIDs to provide peripheral analgesia, the use of local anesthetic peripheral nerve or neuraxial block to prevent transmission of painful impulses into the spinal cord, as well as the use of high doses of systemic narcotics, to blunt cortical perception.

Unfortunately, a reliable way to achieve preemptive analgesia in association with major abdominal surgery has not been achieved. A few small studies have shown efficacy with the use of neuraxial opioids, but no large study has been able to confirm this. In a recent study (Aida et al., 1999) epidural catheters were placed preoperatively in their respective areas (cervical placement for upper limb surgery, low thoracic placement for abdominal surgery, lumbar placement for lower limb surgery, etc.) and an appropriate anesthetic level with local anesthetics was achieved pre-incision. A preemptive analgesic effect was noted in the limb and mastectomy patients but not in the laparotomy patients. The authors concluded that to perform preemptive analgesia properly, one must completely block all afferent input into the spinal cord, and that as some input is provided via the vagus nerve which was not blocked with the epidural, preemptive analgesia could not be reliably achieved.

Many questions remain to be answered with respect to preemptive analgesia. The first and foremost is, does it clinically exist, and if so, by what modality can it be achieved? Perhaps a single procedure, such as the administration of a properly placed epidural with local anesthetic prior to the surgical stimulation, can provide pre-emptive analgesia. Most likely, we will discover that both central and peripheral modalities will need to be utilized. Another question is whether a single procedure prior to the initial stimulus will be sufficient for preemptive analgesia, or whether it will be necessary to continue this technique during the entire procedure, as well as into the postoperative period.

SUGGESTED READINGS

Aida S, Baba H, et al.: The effectiveness of preemptive analgesia varies according to the type of surgery: a randomized, double-blind study. Anesth Analg 89:711, 1999

Beattie WS, Badner NH, Choi P: Epidural analgesia reduces postoperative myocardial infarction: a meta-analysis. Anesth Analg 93:853, 2001

Crews JC: Acute pain syndromes. p. 169. In Raj PR (ed): Practical Management of Pain, 3rd edition. Mosby, St. Louis, 2000

Ellis DJ, Millar WL, Reisner LS: A randomized double-blind comparison of epidural versus intravenous fentanyl infusion for analgesia after cesarean section. Anesthesiology 72:981, 1990

Liu SS, Allen HW, Olsson GL: Patient-controlled epidural analgesia with bupivacaine and fentanyl on hospital wards. Anesthesiology 88:688, 1998

Luper KA, Ready LB, Downey M, et al.: Epidural and intravenous fentanyl infusions are clinically equivalent after knee surgery. Anesth Analg 70:72, 1990

Miaskowski C, Crews J, et al.: Anesthesia-based pain services improve the quality of postoperative pain management. Pain 80:23, 1999

Norris EJ, Beattie C: Double-masked randomized trial comparing alternative combinations of intraoperative anesthesia and postoperative analgesia in abdominal aortic surgery. Anesthesiology 95:1054, 2001

Owen H, McMillan V, Rogowski D: Postoperative pain therapy: a survey of patients' expectations and their experience. Pain 41:303, 1990

Parker RK, Holtman B, White PF: Effects of a nighttime opioid infusion with PCA therapy on patient comfort and analgesic requirements after abdominal hysterectomy. Anesthesiology 76:362, 1992

Rawal N: Ten years of acute pain services: achievements and challenges. Reg Anesth Pain Med 24:68, 1999

Ready LB: Acute pain: lessons learned from 25,000 patients. Reg Anesth Pain Med 24:499, 1999

Salomaki TE, Laitinen JO, Nuutinen LS: A randomized double-blind comparison of epidural versus intravenous fentanyl infusion for analgesia after thoracotomy. Anesthesiology 75:790, 1991

Sinatra R, Chung KS, Silverman DG, et al.: An evaluation of morphine and oxymorphone administered via patient-controlled analgesia (PCA) or PCA plus basal infusion in post-cesarean-delivery patients. Anesthesiology 71:502, 1989

Thomas T, Robinson C, et al.: Prediction and assessment of the severity of post-operative pain and of satisfaction with management. Pain 75:177, 1998

Woolf CJ, Chong M: Preemptive analgesia: treating postoperative pain by preventing the establishment of central sensitization. Anesth Analg 77:362, 1993

Gordon Freedman, MD

Joel M. Kreitzer, MD

A 42-year-old man presents to the Pain Management office with low back pain. The pain began after moving furniture and radiates down the lateral aspect of his right leg, through the knee, and into the foot. It is relieved somewhat with nonsteroidal anti-inflammatory drugs and bed rest. A computed tomography scan shows a herniated disk at L_4–L_5. He is otherwise in good general health.

QUESTIONS

1. What is the incidence of low back pain?
2. List the differential diagnosis of low back pain.
3. Describe the classic presentation of a patient with a herniated nucleus pulposus.
4. Differentiate the clinical presentation of a herniated nucleus pulposus from spinal stenosis.
5. Describe the pathogenesis and treatment of myofascial syndrome (trigger points).
6. What are the signs and symptoms of sacroiliac disease and how is it treated?
7. What are the facet joints and how does pathology in them manifest?
8. What is the mechanism of action by which epidural steroid injections work?
9. What are the pathogenesis, diagnosis, and treatment of internal disc disruption (IDD)?

10. What oral medications are prescribed for low back pain?
11. What is failed back syndrome (FBS) and how is it managed?

1. What is the incidence of low back pain?

Low back pain is one of the most common disabilities of modern life. It is the second most common reason for visiting a medical doctor and accounts for 3% of all hospital discharges. It has been estimated that at any one time, 17% of Americans suffer from low back pain and that 85% will complain of low back pain at some point in their lives.

2. List the differential diagnosis of low back pain.

Low back pain can be caused by a multitude of disease processes. The most common cause is muscular in origin, often presenting as myofascial syndrome, with trigger points noted on physical examination. Common skeletal causes include degenerative disease of the vertebral column (osteoarthritis), disc disease (herniated nucleus pulposus), and joint involvement (facet syndrome and sacroiliitis). Rheumatoid and other types of inflammatory arthritis can also cause low back pain. Less frequent skeletal causes include metabolic (osteoporosis), neoplastic, infectious (osteomyelitis), traumatic (fractures), or congenital (scoliosis). Back pain of neurologic origin may originate from irritation of nerves by herniated discs, osteophytes, tumors,

Differential Diagnosis for Low Back Pain

Muscular
      Myofascial syndrome

Skeletal
      Degenerative disease of the vertebral column
         (osteoarthritis)
      Disc disease (herniated nucleus pulposus)
      Joint involvement (facet syndrome,
         sacroiliitis)
      Rheumatoid or other inflammatory
         arthritis
      Metabolic (osteoporosis)
      Neoplastic
      Infectious (osteomyelitis)
      Traumatic (fractures)
      Congenital (scoliosis)

Neurologic
      Herniated disc
      Osteophytes
      Inflammation (herpes zoster)
      Neoplasms (intradural or epidural tumors)

Intrathoracic/intra-abdominal
      Aortic aneurysms
      Pancreatic cancer/inflammation
      Lower lobe pneumonia
      Sarcoma
      Lymphoma
      Visceral process involving the genitourinary or
         gastrointestinal systems

or disease of the neuraxis such as inflammation (herpes zoster) or neoplasms (intradural or epidural tumors). Low back pain may also be referred from intra-abdominal/thoracic diseases such as aortic aneurysms, pancreatic cancer/inflammation, lower lobe pneumonias, sarcomas, lymphomas, or visceral processes involving the genitourinary or gastrointestinal tracts. Because of the large differential diagnosis, a thorough investigation and evaluation is necessary to determine the cause of the lower back pain.

3. Describe the classic presentation of a patient with a herniated nucleus pulposus.

The average age of patients presenting with herniated discs is 30–50 years. The pain is primarily in the back and posterior aspects of the legs and typically occurs after lifting heavy objects. It is caused by either mechanical compression of nerve roots or chemical injury from substances released by degenerating intervertebral discs (e.g., phospholipase A). The nerve roots affected determine the distribution of the pain. The pain is aggravated by bending, coughing, or sneezing and is improved with resting and lying down. Motor or sensory deficits depend on the level and extent of nerve involvement. Rarely, bowel or bladder dysfunction can occur. Computed tomography (CT) or magnetic resonance imaging (MRI) scans are invaluable in confirming the diagnosis. However, imaging must be correlated with clinical symptoms because positive findings on scans may not necessarily be related to symptoms.

Physical examination demonstrates increased pain when tension is applied to the lumbosacral plexus. Thus, tests such as the bowstring sign (radicular pain elicited by popliteal pressure), Gower's sign (radicular pain secondary to foot dorsiflexion), and radicular pain with straight leg raising are indicative of nerve irritation.

4. Differentiate the clinical presentation of a herniated nucleus pulposus from spinal stenosis.

Spinal stenosis, which is primarily seen in older patients, is caused by a combination of enlarging posterior facet joints, osteophytes from osteoarthritis, hypertrophy of the ligamentum flavum, and bulging of a disc annulus. All these structures may impinge on nerve roots or the cauda equina and produce typical radicular low back pain. Patients with spinal stenosis experience neurogenic claudication, leg pain when walking. Sitting and resting relieve the pain. Neurogenic claudication differs from vascular claudication in that the sitting position relieves the pain in the former and cessation of walking relieves the pain in the latter.

The pain of spinal stenosis differs from that of disc disease in that sitting with flexion of the lumbar spine relieves spinal stenosis pain. Disc disease pain is typically relieved by reclining and may be increased with flexion of the lumbar spine. Another difference between spinal stenosis and disc disease is that pain and neurologic deficits can extend over several dermatomes with spinal stenosis because of the diffuse nature of the disease. A herniated nucleus pulposus manifests as a localized disease of specific dermatomal distribution. Spinal stenosis is characterized by chronic mild discomfort that progresses over time. Conversely, the hallmark of disc disease is the acute and severe onset of radicular pain.

A CT scan or MRI examination ultimately makes the definitive diagnosis. It is important that the findings on these scans are correlated with the clinical symptoms.

5. Describe the pathogenesis and treatment of myofascial syndrome (trigger points).

Trigger points can be found in more than 50% of the population. Acute muscle strain or chronic repetitive

Herniated Nucleus Pulposus Disease Versus Spinal Stenosis

Herniated Nucleus Pulposus Disease	Spinal Stenosis
Younger patient population	Older patient population
Acute onset of pain	Chronic onset of pain
Dermatomal distribution of pain	Multilevel distribution of pain
Pain relieved by supine position	Pain relieved by sitting position
Pain increases with flexion of the lumbar spine	Pain is relieved with flexion of the lumbar spine

motions lead to tissue damage and the release of calcium from the sarcoplasmic reticulum. This causes a localized sustained contracture of the muscle fibers. Myofascial syndrome manifests as discrete, well-localized, point pain and tenderness. A taut muscular band is often palpated causing a painful reaction (jump sign).

Treatment modalities consist of the spray and stretch technique (with ethyl chloride), trigger point injections with local anesthetic under pressure, massage therapy, transcutaneous electrical nerve stimulation (TENS), and acupuncture.

6. What are the signs and symptoms of sacroiliac disease and how is it treated?

The sacroiliac joint is a synovial joint bordered by strong ligaments. Strain and degeneration cause pain and restricted motion. Tenderness to palpation can be elicited over the joint. Immobility of the joint may be noted with leg lifting. Maneuvers causing joint movement such as the Gaenslen's test (extension) or the Faber Patrick test (external rotation) can produce pain.

Sacroiliac disease is treated by local anesthetic injections into and around the joint with or without steroids. Physiotherapy may help the restrictive motion component.

7. What are the facet joints and how does pathology in them manifest?

The facet joints are the paired posterior articulations of the vertebrae and are typical synovial joints. Synovitis and articular degeneration causes local tenderness over the involved joint with referred pain to the buttock and posterolateral leg.

Pain from facet disease, sacroiliitis, and lumbar sacral radiculopathy can often mimic each other. The diagnosis of facet joint disease can only be made by performing a complete physical examination and correlating the findings with radiographic information.

Treatment involves injecting local anesthetic and steroids directly into the facet joint. For longer-lasting effect,

neurolysis of the medial branch nerve that innervates the joint with radiofrequency lesioning can be done.

8. What is the mechanism of action by which epidural steroid injections work?

Radicular pain is caused by nerve inflammation from direct impingement or chemical irritation. Steroids injected into the epidural space produce anti-inflammatory effects on the nerve roots. A series of up to three injections is traditionally performed every 2 weeks as needed. A steroid such as methylprednisolone 80 mg, with or without local anesthetic, is diluted to a volume of 10 mL and injected into the epidural space. Success rates of greater than 80% have been reported in the treatment of radicular lower back pain of less than 6 months duration.

Large series have supported the relative safety of this procedure. Recognized complications include dural puncture, salt and water retention, congestive heart failure, hyperglycemia, epidural abscess, and hemorrhage.

If the radicular pain is in a specific dermatomal distribution, selective nerve root blocks of individual nerves, with local anesthetic and steroids, can be performed under fluoroscopic guidance.

9. What are the pathogenesis, diagnosis, and treatment of internal disc disruption (IDD)?

IDD may begin as a vertebral endplate fracture caused by chronic repetitive or acute strain leading to annular tears of varying degrees. Nerve endings may grow into the inner annulus and become sensitized by chemicals leaking from the nucleus pulposus via the tears. Clinically, there is a band-like axial back pain. MRI may be helpful in diagnosis but a provocative discogram correlating radiologic and clinical findings may be more specific and sensitive.

Treatment modalities include intra-discal electrothermocoagulation (IDET) and spinal fusion, if there is instability. Several theories have been proposed as to the mechanism of action of IDET. It may denervate the nerve supply to the disc, denature the chemical mediators of sensitization, or possibly coagulate the collagen in the disc to close the tear.

10. Which oral medications are prescribed for low back pain?

Nonsteroidal anti-inflammatory drugs (NSAIDs) are frequently taken to relieve low back pain. They serve a dual purpose, acting as both an anti-inflammatory agent and an analgesic. Prostaglandins sensitize nociceptors to painful stimuli and potentiate the algesic effect of bradykinins. By inhibiting the enzyme cyclo-oxygenase (COX), NSAIDs inhibit prostaglandin synthesis and analgesia occurs.

Side-effects of NSAIDs include gastric irritation, renal dysfunction, platelet inhibition, hepatic dysfunction, and tinnitus. New COX-2 specific inhibitors have been developed which maintain the analgesic, anti-inflammatory and beneficial effects on the stomach of COX-1 (i.e., increased gastric blood flow, increased protective gastric mucus secretion, decreased gastric acid secretion) while decreasing the detrimental side-effects of gastric ulceration and bleeding.

Tricyclic antidepressant drugs (TCAs) can be used as adjuncts to analgesic therapies. They decrease the reuptake of serotonin and norepinephrine, which are neurotransmitters in the descending inhibitory spinal cord pain neuropathways. Thus, TCAs have analgesic properties of their own. Other effects of TCAs that can be used in pain management include sedation (fostering a good night's sleep), potentiation of opioid analgesics, and mood elevation. If there is a strong neuropathic component to the pain, anticonvulsant agents may be beneficial.

11. What is failed back syndrome (FBS) and how is it managed?

FBS is the failure to return to normal activities and/or lose pain complaints after lumbar surgery. The incidence is between 15% and 30%. The etiology of FBS includes complications (scarring) from the surgery or diagnostic procedures, incorrect diagnoses, inadequate surgery, and new pathology.

Treatment modalities focus on decreasing inflammation around the nerve roots and/or decreasing scar tissue that may be causing irritation of the nerve roots. Pain management techniques that have been utilized for FBS include:

- Selective nerve root blocks with local anesthetic and steroid.
- Caudal/epidural steroid injections below or above the surgical scar.
- Epidurolysis, which lyses adhesions in the epidural space. This can be accomplished either mechanically with a spring-tipped catheter or chemically with large volumes of steroids, hyaluronidase, local anesthetic, and possibly hypertonic saline, which have a local anesthetic as well as anti-inflammatory effect.
- Epiduroscopy, which allows for lysis of adhesions and specific steroid injections under direct visualization.
- Spinal cord stimulation has also been used for FBS with varying success. In properly chosen patients, one can expect that 50% of the patients will have a 50% decrease in pain after insertion of the stimulator.
- Chronic analgesic regimens are frequently prescribed for patients with FBS in conjunction with the more definitive invasive techniques.

SUGGESTED READINGS

Abram SE: Treatment of lumbosacral radiculopathy with epidural steroids. Anesthesiology 91:1937–1941, 1999

Benzon HT: Epidural steroid injections for low back pain and lumbosacral radiculopathy. Pain 24:277–295, 1986

Czerniecki JM, Goldstein B: General considerations of pain in the low back, hips and lower extremities. pp. 1475–1507. In Loeser JD (ed): Bonica's Management of Pain, 3rd edition. Lippincott Williams and Wilkins, Philadelphia, 2001

Dipalma JR, Digregorio J: Management of low back pain by analgesics and adjuvant drugs. Mt Sinai J Med 58:101–108, 1991

Haldeman S: Differential diagnosis of low back pain. pp. 227–248. In Kirkaldy-Willis WH, Bernard TN Jr. (eds): Managing Low Back Pain, 4th edition. Churchill Livingstone, New York, 1999

Loeser JD, et al.: Low back pain. pp.1508–1564. In Loeser JD (ed): Bonica's Management of Pain, 3rd edition. Lippincott Williams and Wilkins, Philadelphia, 2001

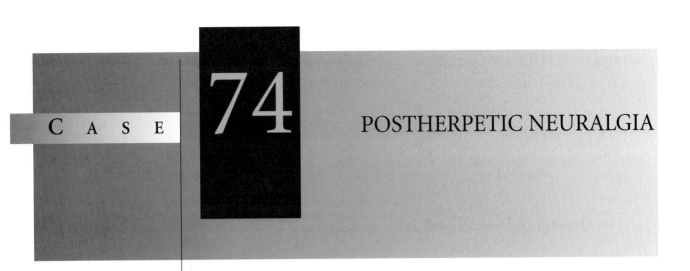

Joel M. Kreitzer, MD

Gordon Freedman, MD

A 73-year-old woman with a history of lymphoma suffered an acute herpes zoster infection, involving the left-sided T_9–T_{10} dermatomes. This process was manifested by vesicles and pustules, which over 2 weeks crusted over and healed. Three weeks after the lesions healed, she noted severe, burning pain in the area.

QUESTIONS

1. What is the pathogenesis of an acute herpes zoster infection?
2. How does an acute herpes zoster infection manifest itself?
3. What is postherpetic neuralgia (PHN)?
4. Which patients are at risk for the development of PHN?
5. How does PHN present?
6. What medications can be used for treatment of PHN? What is the mechanism of action of these medications?
7. What invasive procedures can be used for the treatment of PHN?
8. Can PHN be prevented?

1. What is the pathogenesis of an acute herpes zoster infection?

Acute herpes zoster (shingles) is an infection caused by the varicella zoster virus. This virus, the smallest of the double-stranded DNA herpes viruses, usually enters the body in childhood via the respiratory route and causes a varicella, or chickenpox, infection. When contracted as a child, this infection is usually a brief, benign illness; however, it can be a serious illness if contracted as an adult. Chickenpox presents as a systemic viremia, followed by a rash on the face, thorax, arms, and legs. During this infection, the virus gains access to the dorsal root ganglion, where it lays dormant. Later in life, the virus can become reactivated. Reactivation has been associated with aging, stress, malignancy, immunodeficiency, and steroid use, although in most cases of acute herpes zoster, no precise cause of reactivation can be noted. The reactivated virus replicates in the dorsal root ganglion, and spreads to the skin via the sensory nerves, causing acute herpes zoster, or shingles, infection.

2. How does an acute herpes zoster infection manifest itself?

The typical acute herpes zoster infection starts with pain in the affected area, which is usually described as burning or stabbing. During this time, the patient may have 'flu-like symptoms, such as fever or malaise. A few days later, lesions erupt. The lesions most commonly develop along one or more thoracic dermatomes, always unilateral and never crossing over the midline. Lesions may appear in the ophthalmic division of the trigeminal nerve, the cervical dermatomes, or rarely the lumbar or sacral dermatomes. These lesions are described as erythematous vesicles and pustules. Over the course of about 4 weeks, the lesions crust over and heal, sometimes causing scarring in the area. The lesions are accompanied by severe pain, usually of a burning nature, although some patients also complain of achy, itchy pain. The pain is worse when the area is touched.

3. What is postherpetic neuralgia (PHN)?

PHN is the development of severe pain in the area where an acute herpes zoster infection occurred. There is much debate about the precise definition of PHN, specifically at what point the disease changes from acute herpes zoster to PHN. Some state that pain which remains 4 weeks after the onset of lesions is PHN, while others state that pain in the area after the lesions have healed is PHN.

4. Which patients are at risk for the development of PHN?

Overall, the incidence of PHN is 5–10% in patients who develop an acute herpes zoster infection. The older the patient is when they develop acute herpes zoster, the greater the chance that they develop PHN. There is a greater than a 70% chance of developing PHN if the acute herpes infection begins at age 70 years. In addition, increasing age at the onset of infection is also correlated with a longer duration of the PHN. It has been proposed that patients who have a longer, more painful episode of acute herpes zoster have an increased chance of developing PHN, and thus aggressive treatment, including pain management, of the acute herpes infection is recommended (see question 8).

5. How does PHN present?

PHN presents as pain in the area where an acute herpes zoster infection was present. Although the rash and vesicles of the acute herpes zoster infection have healed, scarring in

the area may still be present. The area of pain is unilateral, never crossing over the midline, and usually mimics the distribution of the acute herpes zoster pain. The thoracic and ophthalmic division of the trigeminal nerve is most commonly involved, followed by the lumbar and sacral areas. However, the pain is sometimes in small, discrete locations, and may sometimes spread to areas outside the initial acute herpes zoster infection (see below). The patient's pain complaints are varied and numerous, ranging from mild, aching pain, to severe, burning, lancinating pain. The pain may be constant or intermittent, and may be provoked by touch, activity, or stress. The patient may complain of extreme hyperesthesia (increased sensitivity), hyperpathia (increased pain to a painful sensation), or allodynia (pain to a nonpainful stimulus) in the area, and may also present with pain over an area of numbness. The pain of PHN may be so severe as to push the patient to suicide and is a known cause of suicide in the elderly population.

The fact that there are so many different types of pain means that there are most likely multiple mechanistic reasons why patients develop pain, including sensitization and/or loss of peripheral nerve endings, damage to peripheral axons and the dorsal horn, ectopic firing of peripheral afferent nerves, infiltration of peripheral nerves with chronic inflammatory cells, and damage to the central nervous system. In addition, some investigators believe that central "wind-up" occurs, causing spreading of the painful area, as well as hyperesthesia.

6. What medications can be used for treatment of PHN? What is the mechanism of action of these medications?

Because of the various possible etiologies of PHN pain, multiple types of medications have been tried, all with variable degrees of success. Overall, medication management for PHN is not standardized and the treating physician must try different combinations of medications to see which will work for any individual patient. At present, the only medication approved by the US Food and Drug Administration for PHN pain is 5% lidocaine patch (Lidoderm™, Endo Pharmaceuticals, Chadds Ford, Pennsylvania). This patch is placed over the painful area for 12 hour periods, and then left off for 12 hours. Up to three patches may be placed to cover the painful area. Although the exact mechanism of action is unknown, it is believed to be secondary to decreasing the ectopic firing of peripheral nerve endings.

The most commonly used medications for the treatment of PHN pain include the tricyclic antidepressant agents (TCAs) and the antiepileptic drugs. Multiple studies looking at the TCAs, especially amitriptyline, have shown a benefit to their use. The mechanism of action relates to their ability to block reuptake of serotonin and norepinephrine in the central nervous system, thus enhancing the action of the central nervous system's descending inhibitory pathways. These medications are started at a low dose, usually in the evening, and titrated to effect or side-effects, which may include sedation, dry mouth, or urinary retention. As patients with PHN oftentimes have trouble in sleeping, a nighttime dose of a TCA, with its sedative properties, is often a useful medication.

The antiepileptic drugs are often used for pain for PHN. This is a varied class of drugs, encompassing multiple medications with various mechanisms of action. Gabapentin is a commonly used antiepileptic drug for PHN pain. This drug, a γ-aminobutyric acid (GABA) analog, has an unknown mechanism of action, which may be related to the increased metabolism of glutamate, an excitatory neurotransmitter. Overall, this medication is very well tolerated, the most common side-effect being sedation, which is usually seen in the elderly. Older antiepileptic drugs such as phenytoin and carbamazepine are prescribed for neuropathic pain; however, their use is decreasing because of their poor side-effect profile and multiple drug–drug interactions. Some of the newer antiepileptic medications (lamotrigine, oxcarbazepine) have been used for PHN pain, but there are no large studies to document their efficacy.

Nonsteroidal anti-inflammatory drugs (NSAIDs) and opiates are often prescribed for the pain of PHN. The NSAIDs work by decreasing prostaglandin production at the peripheral nerve receptors, thus desensitizing them, and the opiates work by binding to the opiate receptors in the brain and spinal cord, stimulating the descending inhibitory pathway. The use of opiates for PHN pain is slowly becoming accepted, as the literature increasingly shows that these drugs, when given appropriately, are safe and effective. A recent study showed the efficacy of long-acting oxycodone for treatment of PHN pain. NSAIDs may be given to prevent the pain from a peripheral mechanism, but there is little literature to support their use.

Other medications that have been described include capsaicin cream, baclofen, intravenous lidocaine, and mexiletine. Again, there is little in the literature to support the use of any one of these medications, and different combinations need to be tried until the patient is comfortable.

7. What invasive procedures can be used for the treatment of PHN?

Over time, various invasive measures have been employed for PHN pain; however, none has proven to be beneficial. When one looks at the literature, the lack of randomized, controlled studies does not enable one to recommend one invasive procedure over another. Sympathetic blocks have been used for the treatment of pain from PHN; however, their efficacy has not been proven in large-scale studies. Simple infiltration of the painful area with local anesthetics and steroids has been employed by some practitioners as a way to provide immediate pain relief, and

with the hope of benefiting the patient by the steroid's peripheral action on nerve endings. Somatic nerve blocks, while providing transient pain relief, have never shown any long-lasting benefit. A recent study from Japan showed excellent, sustained pain relief with the use of intrathecal methylprednisolone and lidocaine; however, the results have been questioned and this therapy has not gained widespread acceptance. Other modalities such as spinal cord stimulation and dorsal root rhizotomies have also been described with varying results.

8. Can PHN be prevented?

As mentioned earlier, the longer and more painful the patient's acute herpes zoster infection, the greater the chance that they will develop PHN. Thus, it makes sense that aggressive control of the pain and symptoms of acute herpes zoster will decrease the intensity of the PHN. However, as is the case with most topics related to PHN, this has not been proven in large-scale studies. Based on small studies, it makes sense to treat the patient early in the acute herpes zoster period with oral analgesics, as well as oral antiviral agents such as valacyclovir. The use of oral steroids during the acute herpes zoster infection has never been shown to decrease the intensity and frequency of PHN pain.

Another controversial topic is the use of sympathetic blocks during the acute herpes zoster episode. It has been debated that this technique can decrease the severity and intensity of PHN pain; however, this too has not been generally accepted as the truth. One may argue that because of the low risk factor in properly performing such a procedure and the potential debilitating consequences of PHN pain, these techniques should be employed early on during an acute herpes zoster infection.

SUGGESTED READINGS

Ali NM: Does sympathetic ganglionic block prevent postherpetic neuralgia? Reg Anesth Pain Med 20:227–233, 1995

Galer BS, Argoff CE: Zoster and postherpetic neuralgia: pain mechanisms and current management. p. 115. In Aronoff GM (ed): Evaluation and Treatment of Chronic Pain, 3rd edition. Lippincott Williams and Wilkins, Philadelphia, 1998

Kotani N, Kushikata T, Hashimoto H, et al: Intrathecal methylprednisolone for intractable postherpetic neuralgia. N Engl J Med 343:1514–1519, 2000

Rowbotham MC, Peterson KL: Zoster-associated pain and neural dysfunction. Pain 93:1–5, 2001

Watson CP, Babul N: Efficacy of oxycodone in neuropathic pain: a randomized trial in postherpetic neuralgia. Neurology 50:1837–1841, 1998

COMPLEX REGIONAL PAIN SYNDROME

Gordon Freedman, MD

Joel M. Kreitzer, MD

A 39-year-old secretary was healthy until 1 year ago when she tripped and fell onto her right arm while at work. Ten days later the patient awoke with severe burning pain from the palm to the mid-forearm. The arm began to swell and intermittently turned pale and red. The arm is exquisitely tender to touch and the patient is unable to wear long-sleeved shirts. The patient is unable to functionally use the arm and has become depressed.

QUESTIONS

1. Define complex regional pain syndrome (CRPS) type 1 and type 2.
2. What are the pathophysiologic theories leading to CRPS?
3. Delineate the different stages of CRPS.
4. What are the signs and symptoms of CRPS?
5. How is the diagnosis of CRPS made?
6. What different nerve blocks can be used for the diagnosis and treatment of CRPS?
7. What other modalities can be used to treat CRPS?

1. Define complex regional pain syndrome (CRPS) type 1 and type 2.

CRPS is a disease process consisting of continuous pain, often burning in nature, usually consequent to an injury or a noxious stimulus. CRPS usually presents with variable degrees of autonomic and trophic changes along with sensory and motor dysfunction.

CRPS type 1 was previously known as reflex sympathetic dystrophy (RSD) and CRPS type 2 was previously known as causalgia. The nomenclature has been changed to dispel some of the old theories as to the possible etiologies for these diseases.

CRPS types 1 and 2 have similar signs and symptoms. In CRPS type 2 a history is commonly elicited describing a gross nerve injury, whereas with CRPS type 1 the inciting event may never be determined.

2. What are the pathophysiologic theories leading to CRPS?

Multiple theories have been proposed regarding the etiology of CRPS. Current accepted theories focus on both the peripheral nerves and the central nervous system. Peripheral etiologies for CRPS describe the existence of ephapses, or neurologic short-circuits between the somatic and sympathetic nervous systems, possibly caused by trauma. It is unclear whether these connections are actual structural connections or "chemical" connections caused by release of neurotransmitters. These ephapses could explain the clinical findings. Stimuli that are usually mediated by the autonomic nervous system, such as responses to emotion, temperature, and weather, are rerouted through the somatic nervous system and cause pain. Stimuli that are usually mediated via the somatic nervous system, such as light touch, are rerouted through the autonomic nervous system and cause an uncoordinated sympathetic response.

Central theories that try to explain the etiology of CRPS look at the wide dynamic range neurons in the dorsal horn of the spinal cord. These are neurons that normally receive input from multiple types of nerve fibers and could serve as the anatomic correlate for the short-circuit connections between the somatic and sympathetic nervous systems.

3. Delineate the different stages of CRPS.

CRPS is usually described in three different stages.

- *Stage 1: acute or hyperemic stage.* This stage occurs within days to weeks of the initial injury and is significant for a predominance of severe burning or lancinating pain. It is notable for signs of sympathetic blockade; thus the area affected is red, warm, and dry. Hyperesthesia, an exaggerated response to stimuli, and allodynia, a painful response to non-painful stimuli, are prominent symptoms of this stage. Treatments instituted during stage 1 have the best prognosis for a cure.
- *Stage 2: dystrophic stage.* This stage occurs weeks to months after the initial insult. The signs and symptoms of this stage are consistent with sympathetic hyperexcitability. The area involved is pale or cyanotic and cool. Burning pain associated with hyperesthesia and allodynia is again very common. Although treatments in this stage can be successful, the longer the duration of the symptoms the poorer the prognosis.
- *Stage 3: atrophic stage.* This stage occurs months to years after the initial injury. Atrophy of the tissues in the involved area occurs because of prolonged vasoconstriction caused by increased sympathetic discharge over time. Burning and hyperesthesia become less prominent and trophic changes predominate. The skin in the area becomes smooth and glassy and the hair begins to fall out. The nails become brittle and the muscles atrophic. The bones in the area show a classic patchy demineralization on radiography known as Sudeck's atrophy of the bone. The prognosis for pain relief and functionality is very poor at this point.

It is common for a patient not to experience all three stages of the syndrome. Stages may be skipped or the progression may be halted with appropriate therapy.

4. What are the signs and symptoms of CRPS?

CRPS type 1 usually presents with a history of a very minor trauma or may even present with the patient having no recollection of an injury at all. In contrast, the initial history for CRPS type 2 will consist of a major injury with gross nerve damage. Rarely, cerebrovascular accidents or myocardial infarctions may be complicated by CRPS. The most common symptom of CRPS is burning pain. Although CRPS usually occurs in an extremity, it can occur anywhere in the body, including the face or major joints, such as the knee or shoulder. Because this syndrome demonstrates an abnormality involving sympathetic nerves, the affected areas can encompass unusual nondermatomal distributions. Neurologic abnormalities such as allodynia and hyperesthesia are common with CRPS but can occur with somatic neuropathies as well. Depending on the stage of the disease varying degrees of color, temperature, sweating, and trophic changes may be present. Motor and sensory dysfunctions are less common manifestations.

5. How is the diagnosis of CRPS made?

The diagnosis of CRPS is a clinical one, made by the history and physical examination. There is no one test that can make the diagnosis definitively.

The most commonly used diagnostic test involves blocking the sympathetic innervation to the affected area and noting any improvement in the clinical symptoms. Another modality that has been described is a continuous intravenous phentolamine infusion.

Indirect measures of sympathetic function that can be used to diagnose CRPS include skin probes and infrared thermography to measure temperature changes to the area affected, peripheral somatosensory mapping for allodynia/hyperesthesia, triple-phase bone scans, and sweat testing.

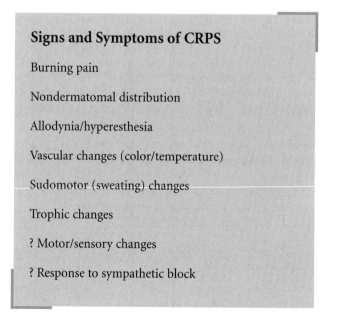

Signs and Symptoms of CRPS

Burning pain

Nondermatomal distribution

Allodynia/hyperesthesia

Vascular changes (color/temperature)

Sudomotor (sweating) changes

Trophic changes

? Motor/sensory changes

? Response to sympathetic block

6. What different nerve blocks can be used for diagnosis and treatment of CRPS?

The two most common sympathetic nerve blocks utilized for both diagnosis and treatment of CRPS are stellate ganglion and lumbar sympathetic blocks. The stellate ganglion is a sympathetic ganglion made up of the fusion of the inferior cervical and first thoracic sympathetic ganglia. Anatomically, it is located near the transverse processes of C_7 or T_1 and has axons that arise from sympathetic cell bodies from the T_1–T_5 spinal cord levels. Axons that pass through the stellate ganglion supply sympathetic innervation to the head, neck, and upper extremities. Stellate ganglion blocks can also be used to treat upper extremity peripheral vascular disease.

Traditionally, a stellate ganglion block is performed at the level of the transverse process of C_6, at Chaissagnac's tubercle. Some practitioners perform the procedure under fluoroscopic guidance at the C_7 level. A good indication of a successful sympathetic block to the head and neck region is Horner's sign (ptosis, miosis, and anhydrosis). A good indicator of a successful sympathetic block to the upper extremity is either vasodilatation or increased temperature in the arm.

Complications of a stellate ganglion block include hoarseness, intravascular (vertebral artery) injection causing seizures, pneumothorax, bradycardia, diaphragmatic paralysis, intrathecal/epidural injection, arm weakness, bleeding, and infection.

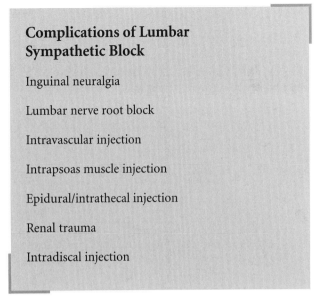

Complications of Lumbar Sympathetic Block

Inguinal neuralgia

Lumbar nerve root block

Intravascular injection

Intrapsoas muscle injection

Epidural/intrathecal injection

Renal trauma

Intradiscal injection

Lumbar sympathetic blocks are indicated for CRPS involving the lower extremities, as well as for peripheral vascular disease. These blocks should be done under fluoroscopic guidance with contrast dye confirmation of proper needle placement. The needle is placed anterolateral to the body of the lumbar vertebra at the L_2, L_3, and/or L_4 levels.

Complications that can occur include inguinal neuralgia, a selective nerve root block, intravascular injection, spinal/epidural anesthesia, renal trauma, and intradiscal injection.

7. What other modalities can be used to treat CRPS?

Intravenous regional bretylium Bier blocks can be performed along with or in lieu of sympathetic nerve blocks. Bretylium is a sympatholytic agent that decreases catecholamine release from nerve endings. Mixed somatic/sympathetic blocks such as epidurals or spinals can be used but will lack diagnostic specificity. Oral sympatholytics such as β-blockers will decrease sympathetic discharge but can cause systemic side-effects especially related to the cardiovascular system. Anticonvulsant agents, tricyclic antidepressants, oral steroids, and antiarrhythmic agents have also been described as therapies for CRPS. Spinal cord stimulation has recently shown very encouraging results for the treatment of refractory CRPS.

Physical therapy to prevent the trophic changes associated with CRPS is of the utmost importance in conjunction with other treatment modalities. The key to successful therapy seems pre-eminently dependent on treating the syndrome as early as possible. Psychotherapy is sometimes a productive adjunct.

Complications of Stellate Ganglion Block

Hoarseness

Intravascular (vertebral artery) injection/seizures

Pneumothorax

Epidural/intrathecal injection

Diaphragmatic paralysis (phrenic nerve block)

Arm weakness (brachial plexus block)

Bradycardia

Hematoma

Infection

SUGGESTED READINGS

Breivik H, Cousins MJ, Lofstrom JB: Sympathetic neural blockade of upper and lower extremity. pp. 411–443. In Cousins MJ, et al. (eds): Neural Blockade in Clinical Anesthesia and Management of Pain, 3rd edition. Lippincott-Raven, Philadelphia, 1998

Stanton-Hicks M, Hassenbusch S, Haddox JD, et al.: Reflex sympathetic dystrophy: changing concepts and taxonomy. Pain 63:127–133, 1995

Veldman PHJM, Reynen HM, Arntz IE, et al.: Signs and symptoms of reflex sympathetic dystrophy: prospective study of 829 patients. Lancet 342:1012–1016, 1993

Walker SM, Cousins MJ: Complex regional pain syndrome: including "reflex sympathetic dystrophy" and "causalgia". Anaesth Intensive Care 25:113–125, 1997

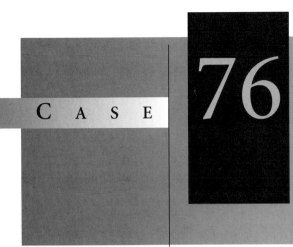

CANCER PAIN MANAGEMENT

Gordon Freedman, MD

Joel M. Kreitzer, MD

A 57-year-old man comes to your Pain Management office complaining of epigastric pain radiating to the back. His scleras are mildly icteric. A magnetic resonance imaging (MRI) study shows a mass at the head of the pancreas.

QUESTIONS

1. What is the prevalence of cancer pain?
2. What is the prevalence of cancer pain by organ system?
3. What are the different causes of pain in a cancer patient?
4. What is the WHO ladder?
5. What guidelines can be followed in devising a chronic analgesic regimen for treating cancer pain?
6. What are the advantages of set-dose-extended duration opioid management?
7. Describe the anatomy of the celiac plexus.
8. What are the indications for performing a celiac plexus block?
9. How is a celiac plexus block performed and what complications can occur?
10. What are the differences between alcohol and phenol neurolysis?
11. When would one use intrathecal versus epidural analgesia for cancer pain management?

1. What is the prevalence of cancer pain?

The number of cases of cancer in the United States is over 2 million per year. Of these, approximately 50% of patients with intermediate-stage cancers and approximately 75% of patients with advanced-stage cancers have pain. This leads to a prevalence of over 1 million cases of cancer pain per year.

2. What is the prevalence of cancer pain by organ system?

Different organ systems are variously associated with cancer pain. Pancreatic cancer is the most common type of cancer associated with pain, with bone cancer being the second most common. Both cancers cause pain in over 80% of cases. Breast, lung, and colon cancers are associated with pain in greater than 70% of cases, and with lymphomas and leukemias, nearly 60% of patients experience pain.

3. What are the different causes of pain in a cancer patient?

There are multiple causes of cancer pain. Approximately 65% of cases are caused by the cancer itself, either by direct invasion, involvement of nerves or the neuroaxis, obstruction of a viscus, or metastasis to a distant tissue. Anticancer treatments are responsible for 25% of cancer pain. These include surgery, diagnostic procedures, chemotherapy side-effects, and radiation complications. Syndromes unrelated to the cancer cause the remaining 10% of pain in the cancer patient. It is important to remember that patients with cancer may also have common noncancer-related pain syndromes such as lower back pain and headaches.

4. What is the WHO ladder?

The World Health Organization (WHO) has devised a protocol for treating pain utilizing a tiered approach. This protocol allows for the use of less potent medications initially (first tier), increasingly more potent medications (next tiers) being added in a stepwise approach until the patient is comfortable. The WHO states that about 85% of cancer patients can be kept comfortable using this protocol.

First-tier medications include non-opioid analgesics such as nonsteroidal anti-inflammatory drugs (NSAIDs), tricyclic antidepressants (TCAs), and anticonvulsants. Second-tier medications include "weak opioids," which have ceiling dosages due to their combination with acetaminophen or NSAIDs. Third-tier analgesics in the WHO ladder include all sole opioid preparations, both short-acting and extended release. Despite the addition of large doses of opioids in the third tier, the non-opioid medications from tier 1 should be continued. A good knowledge of opioid equipotency conversions is necessary to be able to change from one opioid to another.

The WHO ladder can be further extrapolated clinically to include invasive techniques. Thus, oral analgesics are tried first, followed by intravenous opioids, analgesia via tunneled epidural catheters, implantable analgesic devices, and finally neuroablative procedures.

Sequence For Management of Cancer Pain

WHO ladder
   Tier 1: non-opioid analgesics
   Tier 2: "weak opioids" (in combination with
      acetaminophen or NSAIDs)
   Tier 3: pure opioids

Tunneled epidural catheters

Implantable analgesic devices

Neuroablative procedures

---

5. What guidelines can be followed in devising a chronic analgesic regimen for treating cancer pain?

Guidelines frequently followed when treating cancer pain use a combination of different classes of analgesics to minimize the side-effects of any one medication. The combination should utilize drugs that work on the pain pathways at different levels, so that the analgesics can have additive/synergistic effects.

A typical cancer pain regimen includes:

- Opioids with a set dose and extended-release mechanism (Table 76.1): act on opioid receptors in the brain and the spinal cord.
- NSAIDs: act by primarily inhibiting prostaglandin synthesis causing desensitization of peripheral pain receptors.
- TCAs: act by inhibiting the reuptake of serotonin and norepinephrine, which results in stimulation of the descending inhibitory pain tracts in the spinal cord.
- Anticonvulsants (optional): act on the neuropathic components of pain.
- Fast-onset, short-duration analgesics: given on a "prn" basis for episodic, breakthrough pain.

6. What are the advantages of set-dose extended-duration opioid management?

Set-dose extended-release opioids maintain analgesic blood concentrations within the therapeutic window more consistently over time. The therapeutic window is the range of blood levels at which the desired clinical effect—in this case analgesia—is achieved. With blood levels above the therapeutic window, the patient begins to experience side-effects. Drug blood levels below the therapeutic window would be ineffective and result in the patient experiencing pain. In contrast, "prn" dosing of medications maintain analgesic blood concentrations within the therapeutic window for approximately one-third of the time. Therefore, set-dose extended-release medications provide better analgesia with less overall side-effects.

7. Describe the anatomy of the celiac plexus.

The celiac plexus is part of the sympathetic nervous system and is made up of the celiac, superior mesenteric, and aortico-renal ganglia. Nerve fibers that traverse the celiac plexus arise from cell bodies from T_5–T_{12} and leave the spinal cord without synapsing in the paravertebral ganglia. These sympathetic fibers form the greater, lesser, and least splanchnic nerves and coalesce around the celiac artery at approximately the L_1 level. Here they synapse with postganglionic fibers that supply the intra-abdominal organs below the diaphragm up to the splenic flexure of the large intestine. These include the stomach, small and large intestine, pancreas, hepatobiliary system, kidneys, adrenals, spleen,

TABLE 76.1	Common Extended-Duration Opioids	
Extended-Duration Opioid	**Dosing Interval (hours)**	**Equipotent Dose (morphine 10 mg iv)**
Methadone	6	20 mg po/10 mg iv
Continuous-release fentanyl patch (Duragesic, Janssen Pharmaceutica)	72	300 μg[a]
Extended-release oral oxycodone (Oxycontin, Purdue Pharma)	12	30 mg
Extended-release oral morphine (MS Contin, Purdue Pharma)	12	30 mg
Extended-release oral morphine (Kadian, Faulding Laboratories)	24	30 mg
Levorphanol	6–8	4 mg po/2 mg IV

[a]Fentanyl patch 100 μg/hr = iv morphine 3 mg/hr.

and omentum. The celiac plexus contains visceral afferent and efferent fibers, as well as, some parasympathetic fibers.

8. What are the indications for performing a celiac plexus block?

There are three main indications for blockade of the celiac plexus:

- Pain from upper gastrointestinal (GI) malignancies, as well as nonmalignant pain. This is the most common reason.
- To increase blood flow to the splanchnic vessels for cases such as abdominal angina.
- Dysmotility syndromes, such as with diabetes mellitus or scleroderma, to increase peristalsis in the GI tract.

9. How is a celiac plexus block performed and what complications can occur?

Celiac plexus blocks are performed under either fluoroscopic or computerized tomography (CT) scan guidance. The patient is placed in the prone position unless they cannot tolerate it because of ascites or other intra-abdominal processes. The plexus lies anterior to the aorta and posterior to the vena cava. A needle is placed from each side to lie anterior to the body of L_1. Dye injection confirms needle placement in the retroperitoneum. A maximum of 40 mL of either local anesthetic or neurolytic agent is injected. Complications that can occur with celiac plexus blockade include hypotension, injury to adjacent viscera (e.g., kidneys, pancreas, pleura, lung, aorta, and intestines), lower extremity dysesthesias or motor dysfunction, intravascular injections, retroperitoneal hematomas, and intrathecal, epidural, intrapsoas, or intraosseous injections. As is the

case with any invasive procedure, sterile technique is imperative to avoid infection, especially in the cancer patient who may be immunosuppressed.

10. What are the differences between alcohol and phenol neurolysis?

Neurolysis can be accomplished with either alcohol or phenol. Alcohol for neurolysis is usually used in concentrations of 50–70%. It causes neurolysis by extracting cholesterol, phospholipids, and cerebrosides and causing precipitation of lipoproteins and mucoproteins. This results in damage to both the Schwann cell and the axon. Clinically, alcohol is painful on injection and is hypobaric

Complications of Celiac Plexus Block

Hypotension

Trauma to the kidneys, pancreas, pleura, lung, aorta, intestines

Lower extremity dysesthesias/motor dysfunction

Intravascular injection

Retroperitoneal hematoma

Epidural/intrathecal/intradiscal/intraosseous/intrapsoas injection

Differences Between Alcohol and Phenol for Neurolytic Blocks

Alcohol	Phenol
Extraction of neuronal cholesterol, phospholipids, and cerebrosides; precipitation of lipoproteins and mucoproteins	Coagulation of neuronal proteins
Painful on injection	?Local anesthetic effect
Hypobaric (subarachnoid)	Hyperbaric (subarachnoid)
?More potent/longer acting	?Less potent/shorter acting
Safe for perivascular injection	?Can cause blood vessel wall necrosis

if used for intrathecal neurolysis. Relative to phenol, alcohol may be more potent with a longer duration of action.

Phenol's primary neurolytic effect is by coagulation of proteins. It also causes nonselective damage to neural tissue. Secondarily, phenol might have a local anesthetic effect. Intrathecally, phenol is hyperbaric. Phenol has a great affinity for vascular tissue and injury to adjacent blood vessels must be considered when it is used. For this reason, many pain specialists prefer alcohol to phenol for celiac plexus blocks. Radiofrequency lesioning, cryoablation, and glycerol are other modalities used for neurolysis.

11. When would one use intrathecal versus epidural analgesia for cancer pain management?

Both epidural and intrathecal analgesia systems allow the pain specialist to deliver a wide variety of opioids, local anesthetics, and adjuvants (e.g., clonidine, baclofen) directly into the central nervous system. This allows for smaller dosing and potentially less side-effects. In particular, the use of local anesthetics enables denser analgesia and a possible opioid sparing effect.

Permanent intrathecal analgesia reservoirs are more expensive to place than externalized epidural infusion systems but are less expensive to maintain in the long term. If the prognosis for life expectancy is greater than approximately 3–4 months, the intrathecal analgesia system with an internal pump is financially preferable.

SUGGESTED READINGS

Caraceni A, Portenoy RK: An international survey of cancer pain characteristics and syndromes. Pain 82:263–274, 1999

Eisenberg E, Carr DB, Chalmers TC: Neurolytic celiac plexus block for treatment of cancer pain: a meta-analysis. Anesth Analg 80:290–295, 1995

Mercadante S, Nicosia F: Celiac plexus block: a reappraisal. Reg Anesth Pain Med 23:37–48, 1998

Patt RB (ed): Cancer Pain. Philadelphia, Lippincott-Raven, 1993

Zech DFJ, Grond S, Lynch J, et al.: Validation of World Health Organization guidelines for cancer pain relief. A 10-year prospective study. Pain 63:65–76, 1995

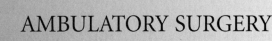

CASE 77 AMBULATORY SURGERY

Laurence M. Hausman, MD

James N. Koppel, MD

A 38-year-old woman is scheduled for an ambulatory diagnostic pelvic laparoscopy at 3 o'clock in the afternoon. She arrives 1 hour before scheduled surgery with her 11-year-old son and appears to be extremely apprehensive. Prior medical history is significant for asymptomatic esophageal reflux, long-standing stable asthma that has been successfully treated with inhaled sympathomimetics and steroids, and juvenile-onset diabetes mellitus, currently controlled with 25 U neutral protamine Hagedorn (NPH) and 6 U regular insulin every morning and 10 U NPH and 3 U regular insulin every night.

QUESTIONS

1. Are there advantages to performing surgery on an ambulatory basis?
2. Which patients are considered acceptable candidates for ambulatory surgery?
3. Are there any patients who should never have surgery on an ambulatory basis?
4. Are diabetic patients suitable candidates for ambulatory surgery?
5. What types of surgical procedures are appropriate for ambulatory surgery?
6. What is the appropriate fasting time before ambulatory surgery that necessitates an anesthetic?
7. Should drugs be administered to empty the stomach or change gastric acidity or volume before the administration of an anesthetic?
8. How can patients be appropriately screened for anesthesia when ambulatory surgery is planned?
9. What preoperative laboratory studies should be obtained before surgery?
10. Should an internist evaluate each patient before ambulatory surgery?
11. Is anxiolytic premedication advisable before ambulatory surgery, and what agents are appropriate?
12. What are the reasons for last-minute cancellation or postponement of surgery?
13. What is the ideal anesthetic for ambulatory surgery?
14. Are there relative or absolute contraindications to the administration of a general anesthetic in the ambulatory setting?
15. What are the advantages and disadvantages to performing a conduction anesthetic in the ambulatory patient?
16. What are the advantages and disadvantages of selecting a nerve block technique for the ambulatory patient?
17. Describe the intravenous regional anesthetic technique (Bier block) for surgery on the extremities.

18. What sedatives can be administered to supplement a regional anesthetic?
19. What complications of nerve block anesthesia are of special concern to the ambulatory patient?
20. Should patients having ambulatory surgery be tracheally intubated?
21. What is the role of propofol in ambulatory surgery?
22. What is total intravenous anesthesia (TIVA), and what are its advantages and disadvantages?
23. What is moderate sedation, when is it employed, and what advantages does it offer?
24. When tracheal intubation is required for a short procedure, can one avoid the myalgias associated with succinylcholine?
25. Can a relative overdose of benzodiazepines be safely antagonized?
26. Do the newer volatile agents offer advantages over enflurane and isoflurane?
27. What are the etiologies of nausea and vomiting, and what measures can be taken to decrease their incidence and severity?
28. How is pain best controlled in the ambulatory patient in the postanesthesia care unit (PACU)?
29. What discharge criteria must be met before a patient may leave the ambulatory surgery center?
30. What are the causes of unexpected hospitalization following ambulatory surgery?
31. When may patients operate a motor vehicle after receiving a general anesthetic?
32. What is the role of aftercare centers for the ambulatory surgery patient?
33. Are quality assurance and continuous quality improvement possible for ambulatory surgery?

1. Are there advantages to performing surgery on an ambulatory basis?

There are multiple advantages to performing surgery on an ambulatory basis. Most obviously, the patient returns much more quickly to the familiar home environment. This is especially important for both pediatric and geriatric surgical patients. Formerly, patients might have remained hospitalized for days, rather than a few hours. A reduction in the acquisition of nosocomial infections has also been noted. This is an extremely important consideration when dealing with immunocompromised patients such as organ transplant recipients or patients who are receiving chemotherapeutic agents. Furthermore, in the ambulatory model, the incidence of medication errors related to either faulty prescribing or dispensing of drugs has decreased. In addition, overall costs are usually significantly reduced. This cost saving is due in part to a decrease in the number of laboratory tests requested and medical consultations obtained, as well as pharmaceuticals dispensed. Of course, the significant expense of both the inpatient

hospitalization as well as the hospital facility fee is avoided. Other less tangible advantages include ease of scheduling procedures, without having to consider variables such as operating room block time, and an improved sense of patient privacy. This occurs because most offices are staffed by a small consistent group of personnel.

As a group, ambulatory patients tend to be more aware of the effects of the anesthetic they receive than the inpatient population. Because ambulatory patients usually undergo less intrusive surgical procedures and are less ill postoperatively, an attempt is made to resume usual preoperative activities at an earlier time. Therefore, nausea, vomiting, myalgias, headache, as well as disordered sensorium and vertigo may appear to be more significant to this group of patients. Unpleasant symptoms are spontaneously reported with greater frequency than in the inpatient group, and patients may tend to focus their attention on them. These discomforting symptoms, if present postoperatively, may be recalled in a vivid fashion if an additional surgical procedure is required. The negative recall may predispose the patient to extreme anxiety.

Only a small subgroup of patients may actually prefer hospitalization to ambulatory surgery.

2. Which patients are considered acceptable candidates for ambulatory surgery?

For patients to be considered acceptable candidates for ambulatory surgery, generally they should have a relatively stable medical condition. However, many centers now routinely accept American Society of Anesthesiologists (ASA) physical status III and IV patients for selected, relatively noninvasive surgical procedures or diagnostic studies. Generally, less invasive surgery is performed on patients who are less healthy, while more invasive surgery is performed only on ASA physical status I or II patients. Patients with cardiovascular disease have an increased risk of perioperative complications. Those with severe physical or mental handicaps are often excluded from consideration as candidates for ambulatory surgery. The ability to comprehend and comply with postoperative instructions is mandatory to the success of ambulatory surgery.

Ambulatory surgery is well suited for the pediatric patient population. Generally, ambulatory surgical procedures commonly performed on children are shorter in duration, less extensive, and less invasive than the majority of procedures performed on adults. Additional benefits to the pediatric group include less disruption of the child's normal feeding schedule and decreased separation time from parents. Exposure to the unfamiliar and frightening hospital milieu can be reduced to the bare minimum. Additionally, because recovery times are short for procedures such as myringotomy and tubes, circumcision, and inguinal herniorrhaphy, early discharge from the facility is feasible.

Preoperative communication and collaboration between anesthesiologists and their surgical colleagues are essential in the case of the questionable or problem patient. The surgeon who is to perform the procedure, the patient, and the family must be agreeable to the concept of ambulatory surgery. However, reimbursement schedules created by insurance carriers will often convince the occasional skeptic, because costs associated with hospitalization for procedures that can be readily performed on an ambulatory basis will usually not be covered. Overwhelming and incontrovertible evidence of medical necessity for inpatient care must be presented to obtain authorization for postoperative hospitalization.

3. Are there any patients who should never have surgery on an ambulatory basis?

An exception to the list of acceptable candidates is ex-preterm infants who are less than 55–60 weeks postconceptual age. These patients may have life-threatening episodes of postoperative apnea and bradycardia as many as 12 hours and up to 48 hours after receiving a general anesthetic. Therefore, in-hospital monitoring of these patients is recommended. For similar reasons, term infants less than 44 weeks postconceptual age should also have surgery performed only on an inpatient basis. Postoperative respiratory monitoring is mandatory for at least 12–18 hours. If at all possible, any required surgery or diagnostic procedures requiring the administration of either a sedative or a general anesthetic should be postponed until the child passes this period.

4. Are diabetic patients suitable candidates for ambulatory surgery?

Diabetic patients may present a major challenge for the anesthesiologist when scheduled for ambulatory surgery. Because of the critical nature of glucose homeostasis, it may be advisable to handle exceptionally brittle diabetics on an inpatient basis. Preoperatively, diabetic patients must be carefully assessed for the presence of end-organ damage. Cardiovascular disease, autonomic and renal insufficiency, and gastroparesis may lead to potential problems in the perioperative period.

It is preferable to schedule surgery on the insulin-dependent diabetic as the first or second case of the day. The major concerns, of course, are to avoid the extremes of plasma glucose, both hypoglycemia and hyperglycemia, as well as acidosis. Delays in insulin administration may lead to ketoacidosis despite the fasting state. For this reason, it is recommended that patients receive insulin along with a continuous infusion of dextrose on arrival at the ambulatory surgery facility. Insulin may be administered by either the subcutaneous or intravenous route. The relative advantage, if any, of administering a continuous infusion of regular insulin versus one third to one half of the usual long-acting insulin dose subcutaneously has not been demonstrated. Another option for early-morning surgical procedures is to administer the usual long-acting insulin dose subcutaneously immediately following surgery and shift the time of all meals and future insulin injections by the same offset.

Non-insulin-dependent diabetics who are controlled by one of the available oral hypoglycemic agents must also be carefully monitored in the perioperative period by periodic fingerstick or blood glucose determinations. The half-life of some of the oral agents may be as long as 60 hours (chlorpropamide). Fortunately, patients with adult-onset, non-insulin-dependent diabetes mellitus (NIDDM) rarely develop ketoacidosis. However, this group may develop hyperosmolar, nonketotic coma when significant hyperglycemia and dehydration occur.

Before discharge, it is critical that diabetic patients be capable of eating and be relatively free of significant nausea that might lead to emesis and inability to maintain adequate caloric intake.

5. What types of surgical procedures are appropriate for ambulatory surgery?

Initially, it was believed that procedures should be limited to those that could be easily accomplished within $1–1\frac{1}{2}$ hours. This was based on the premise that recovery time would be significantly prolonged after the administration of a lengthy general anesthetic and would perhaps prevent discharge. However, it has been well demonstrated that patients may be discharged safely and on a timely basis even after long operations performed with general anesthesia.

The types of surgical procedures that may be performed on an ambulatory basis will depend on whether an ambulatory surgery facility is truly a freestanding unit (geographically detached from a hospital) or is located within a hospital, or directly contiguous to an inpatient facility. Hospital-based units often accept patients with a greater severity of baseline illness and may perform more complex surgical procedures for a number of reasons. In the event of an unexpected massive surgical hemorrhage, availability of immediate blood bank support is crucial. However, when the need for blood may be anticipated preoperatively, even freestanding ambulatory surgery centers can arrange for blood products to be available, and transfusions may be administered if the need arises. Patients may also be asked to donate one or more units of autologous blood, which may be kept available for either intraoperative or postoperative use. Procedures in which blood might be administered include extensive liposuction or reduction mammoplasty. Radiology services, as well as subspecialty consultative services and the relative ease of hospital transfer for overnight admission, allow performance of more involved and invasive procedures in hospital-based ambulatory surgical facilities.

Ideal procedures for ambulatory surgery result in relatively minor postoperative physiologic changes including fluid shifts and blood loss. Commonly performed surgeries include procedures from all surgical disciplines and subspecialties. A few examples include cataract extraction, minor breast surgery, plastic surgery, dilatation and curettage, hysteroscopy, termination of pregnancy, laparoscopy, arthroscopy, inguinal and umbilical herniorrhaphies. The common denominator of all the procedures is that they are associated with only mild-to-moderate degrees of postoperative pain, which may be readily controlled by oral analgesic agents.

In the early days of ambulatory surgery, tonsillectomy was an example of a procedure that was considered to require overnight in-hospital observation. Today, it is being performed on an ambulatory basis in many centers, although the period of postoperative observation is increased compared with that for other ambulatory surgeries. After tonsillectomy, nausea and vomiting are the most common complications causing morbidity. Early bleeding, if it occurs, usually becomes evident within the first 6 hours. Therefore, it is now considered safe to discharge individuals to home who are otherwise in good health and reside within a reasonable distance from the facility with responsible adults. It is especially important that adequate fluid repletion be accomplished before discharge because early attempts at fluid intake after tonsillectomy may be relatively unsuccessful as a result of marked pharyngeal pain.

6. What is the appropriate fasting time before ambulatory surgery that necessitates an anesthetic?

The prescribed preoperative fasting period for both fluids and solids for patients scheduled for ambulatory surgical procedures should be identical to that required for an inpatient who is scheduled to receive an anesthetic. The ASA have released guidelines that recommend 8 hours for solids, 6 hours for a light meal (toast and tea), 4 hours for breast milk, and 2 hours for clear liquids. Eight ounces of orange juice without pulp or coffee without milk has not been demonstrated to increase gastric volume. In fact, both resting gastric volume and acidity may be reduced, which may further decrease the incidence and potentially devastating sequelae of an intraoperative aspiration.

Other benefits result from decreasing the fasting time in preoperative patients. Patients allowed to drink clear fluids are more content while they impatiently wait for a surgical procedure that was either delayed or was scheduled for the latter hours of the day. Thirst is relieved, and hunger may be diminished. Furthermore, the ingestion of glucose-containing solutions may also prevent relative degrees of hypoglycemia noted in both healthy patients and those with limited reserves. It is important to emphasize that medications required for the maintenance of homeostasis such as blood pressure and cardiac drugs can be taken orally up to 1 hour before surgery with an ounce of water.

Fasting guidelines should not be made on a case-by-case basis but rather should be reflected in facility- or institution-wide guidelines.

7. Should drugs be administered to empty the stomach or change gastric acidity or volume before the administration of an anesthetic?

Studies regarding differences in the resting gastric volume between the inpatient and ambulatory population have yielded conflicting results. Whereas some anesthesiologists administer liquid antacids before the induction of anesthesia, no evidence supports the notion that every patient must receive a soluble agent (0.3 molar sodium citrate, 30 ml). A soluble antacid is substituted for the conventional nonabsorbable antacid containing aluminum, magnesium, or calcium hydroxide to avoid the severe chemical pneumonitis that may result from aspiration of these particulate substances. Other pharmacologic agents include the H_2-receptor blockers (ranitidine or famotidine), which inhibit gastric acid production and decrease gastric volume. Mental confusion has been reported after intravenous administration of cimetidine in geriatric patients. Ranitidine is more potent and specific and has a longer duration of action than cimetidine. Metoclopramide increases the tone of the lower esophageal sphincter as well as facilitating gastric emptying. However, it does not guarantee a stomach free of gastric contents. It also possesses anti-emetic properties. Metoclopramide, in conjunction with an H_2-receptor blocker, may be more efficacious. However, the routine use of any of these drugs in patients without specific risk factors is not currently recommended.

Diabetes mellitus with evidence of autonomic dysfunction or gastric atony, documented hiatal hernia, a history of symptomatic gastroesophageal reflux, pregnancy, significant obesity, acute abdomen, or current opioid use or abuse are examples of diseases or conditions that appear to increase the incidence of aspiration during induction or emergence from general anesthesia or during heavy sedation. Therefore, prophylaxis in these situations is recommended. There is no advantage to administration of triple prophylaxis with H_2-receptor antagonists, soluble antacids, and metoclopramide. If prophylaxis with an H_2-blocker is employed, it should be given 1–2 hours preoperatively. Another effective regimen combines metoclopramide on the morning of surgery and a nonparticulate antacid immediately prior to surgery.

Despite the administration of pharmacologic agents and imposition of fasting, significant amounts of acidic gastric contents may still be present. Fortunately, aspiration of gastric material remains a relatively rare occurrence. If a patient is observed to aspirate and if symptoms of cough, wheeze, or hypoxemia while breathing room air do not develop within 2 hours, the development of significant respiratory sequelae is unlikely. Therefore, reliable and otherwise healthy ambulatory patients can probably be discharged after several hours of observation in the postanesthesia care area with the proviso that they immediately contact their physician at the onset of any symptoms.

8. How can patients be appropriately screened for anesthesia when ambulatory surgery is planned?

In the ideal situation, on the day before surgery a patient having an ambulatory procedure would have the opportunity to participate in a private conference with the anesthesiologist who will be caring for him or her. Rapport and trust could be established, and history and physical assessment could be conducted. Furthermore, appropriate laboratory tests could be ordered and additional consultations, if deemed necessary, could be requested. Finally, information from old medical records could be obtained.

To avoid an additional trip for the patient and family, some facilities may substitute a screening telephone interview for a personal interview, conducted by either a nurse or an anesthesiologist several days before surgery. Pertinent medical history can be elicited, general and specific instructions can be given, and reassurance offered to the patient. In this scenario, laboratory studies and additional components of the data base including an electrocardiogram (ECG) and radiographs, if necessary, are performed immediately before surgery. Previously established criteria will determine the tests that must be obtained. Of course, on the day of surgery the anesthesiologist must still review all information with the patient, conduct the appropriate examination, and obtain informed consent.

The surgeon who schedules surgery must assume a large degree of responsibility for the medical evaluation of the patient. The surgeon is often the only physician to see the patient until the day of surgery. Besides conducting a thorough history and physical examination, the surgeon may also request medical consultation when appropriate.

To aid in the screening process, surgeons may also selectively order laboratory and other examinations according to written guidelines established by the medical facility. However, a mechanism should be in place for free communication between the surgeon's office and the facility so that appropriate action may be taken when abnormal laboratory values or other reports are received.

The anesthesiologist's preoperative interview should be conducted in a relaxed, unhurried, and comprehensive manner both chronologically and geographically apart from the operating room. It is highly improper to conduct the preanesthesia interview and examination with the patient stripped of clothing and strapped to the operative room table. At this moment, the patient's anxiety level may be extraordinarily high. Therefore, the patient may neglect to communicate essential information that may have an impact on either general medical care or intraoperative anesthetic management. Under these circumstances, it is truly impossible to obtain informed consent for anesthesia, which is a moral as well as a legal necessity. Additionally, with the surgeon and nurses waiting and instrumentation prepared, the pressure on the anesthesiologist to proceed with anesthesia may be intense.

The anesthesiologist should not fail to question patients firmly regarding the use of illicit drugs. In one patient population, one quarter of the subjects were found to have positive urine findings for commonly abused substances. Depending on the drug involved, modifications in patient management including cancellation of surgery might be well advised. Additionally, users of illicit drugs may have diminished capability or interest in complying with postoperative instructions.

9. What preoperative laboratory studies should be obtained before surgery?

For an ambulatory surgery unit that is affiliated with or attached to a hospital, clinical laboratory testing guidelines should be identical to those required by the related institution. It has been well established that shotgun, nonselective screening batteries of both laboratory, radiographic, and other studies yield an extraordinarily low rate of abnormal findings, few of which may have a significant impact on patient management. Patients scheduled for surgery should have preoperative testing ordered with selectivity and based only on a screening including a careful history and physical examination. In fact, indiscriminate ordering of tests can have potentially serious and deleterious consequences. To explain abnormal results, additional series of tests may be obtained. Some invasive studies have inherent dangers. Often, abnormalities are simply ignored, creating a potential medicolegal liability. Indiscriminate screening often reveals abnormalities that fail to have any relevance to either the surgery or the choice of anesthetic agent or technique. Some centers use handheld computers to obtain the patient history. Branching lines of questioning dependent on previous answers allow extensive information to be gathered. At the conclusion of the interactive interview, the computer can provide a detailed printout of significant findings in the history and recommend the preoperative testing to be obtained. Many facilities do not require any preoperative testing for superficial surgical procedures on otherwise healthy men and women below the age of 40–50 years.

10. Should an internist evaluate each patient before ambulatory surgery?

The same rules and standards regarding a complete preoperative evaluation of patients apply to surgery scheduled on either an inpatient or an ambulatory basis. Accordingly, an internist or medical subspecialist should be consulted regarding the advisability of surgery at a particular moment in time whenever the stability of a patient's medical condition is questionable. Although it may be true that the resultant physiologic perturbations associated with some ambulatory surgery procedures may be characterized as minor, there is nothing minor about the administration of an anesthetic. A complete written history and physical examination are required as part of the medical record before the administration of anesthesia and commencement of surgery. For patients with no or stable co-existing medical conditions, the complete history and physical can be done by the surgeon. However, for patients with significant co-existing medical diseases and/or whose medical status may be questionable, there should be an evaluation completed by the internist or medical subspecialist.

11. Is anxiolytic premedication advisable before ambulatory surgery, and what agents are appropriate?

Because the goal of anesthesia for ambulatory surgery is to permit early discharge to home, there was concern that the administration of short-acting anxiolytic or analgesic premedication might delay recovery from anesthesia and thereby prolong time in the postanesthesia care unit (PACU) with a resultant delay in patient discharge. However, no significant differences in recovery times can be demonstrated after short-acting premedicants have been administered. The effects of more potent and longer-acting anesthetics and the surgical procedure itself contribute in a more significant fashion to the recovery time before a patient may be discharged. However, although time to discharge, a gross measurement, may remain unaffected, tasks that require fine coordination and speedy reaction times may still be deleteriously affected.

Many patients experience anxiety in the immediate preoperative period, and pharmacologic management is quite acceptable. The administration of either diazepam, 5–10 mg orally, 1–2 hours before surgery or midazolam, 1–2 mg intravenously, after an intravenous catheter is placed before surgery can ameliorate distress if deemed desirable. The amnestic effect of intravenous midazolam is powerful, and patients may not remember having seen their surgeon. Midazolam can also be given orally, although much larger doses are required because of first-pass hepatic degradation (0.5–1 mg/kg orally). Opioid premedication may contribute to the incidence of postoperative nausea and vomiting.

Preoperative oral doses of clonidine, a centrally acting α_2-adrenergic agonist have been used to provide sedation, reduce anesthetic requirements, and decrease episodes of hypertension and tachycardia during intubation and maintenance of anesthesia. Side-effects of this class of drugs may include dryness of the oral cavity, hypotension, as well as undesirable sedation extending into the postoperative period. Relaxation techniques have been taught preoperatively to patients and may aid in the reduction of anxiety level. Instruction of these techniques, however, is time-consuming and requires patient motivation, and is therefore usually reserved for selected patients with extreme phobias.

12. What are the reasons for last-minute cancellation or postponement of surgery?

The incidence of last-minute postponement or cancellation of ambulatory procedures exceeds the cancellation rate for the inpatient population. A multiplicity of factors can be operative. Repeat physical examination by the surgeon may reveal the disappearance of pathology. Patients may forget and ingest either solid food or liquids before arrival at the medical facility. Abnormal results on tests that were not available or not previously reviewed may be discovered. Communication between the surgeon and anesthesiologist regarding laboratory abnormalities will help to reduce the incidence of last-minute cancellation of surgery, the consequences of which distress both patient and surgeon and make for inefficient use of available operating room time. Additional questioning may reveal either new symptoms or significant history that was not previously elicited. Physical findings apparent on a last-minute assessment by the anesthesiologist may preclude the safe administration of an anesthetic. Examples include an acute upper respiratory tract infection or an exacerbation of bronchospastic pulmonary disease. Finally, patients may arrive late to the facility or without a responsible escort to accompany them home.

Because the escort's function in the postoperative period goes beyond merely ensuring a safe means of transportation home, in the absence of a designated appropriate escort, surgery should not proceed unless alternative care arrangements are made. If the patient speaks only a foreign language, the escort may serve as an interpreter throughout the perioperative period. After surgery, the escort will receive the postoperative instructions and serve as a companion to the patient during the first 24 hours following the completion of surgery. Assistance in the performance of activities of daily living will be rendered as required. Additionally, the escort will be available to summon medical assistance in the event of a medical, surgical, or anesthetic complication.

13. What is the ideal anesthetic for ambulatory surgery?

No single anesthetic is ideal for every procedure performed. However, the goal of the anesthetic is to allow for patient discharge shortly after the procedure's completion. An ideal general anesthetic agent would have a rapid onset, permit a rapid return to baseline levels of lucidity and equilibrium, and be free of deleterious cardiovascular and respiratory effects. It would provide intraoperative amnesia, analgesia, and muscle relaxation and would possess anti-nausea and anti-emetic properties. Unfortunately, such a marvelous single agent is not in existence at the present time. In an attempt to avoid some of the unpleasant side-effects associated with general anesthesia, regional anesthetic techniques including field blocks, intravenous regional block (Bier block), various approaches to the brachial plexus, ankle block, and spinal and epidural anesthesia have been offered to patients as an alternative to general anesthesia.

14. Are there relative or absolute contraindications to the administration of a general anesthetic in the ambulatory setting?

Sometimes the administration of a general anesthetic clearly should be avoided, if possible. Examples of such cases are a patient with severe, poorly controlled asthma or documented bullous emphysema. In these cases, lesser concern should be given to the possibility of a postdural puncture headache (PDPH) if more serious sequelae are likely to result during or after administration of a general anesthetic. This, however, is the exception rather than the rule, and in most instances the final choice of anesthesia should remain with the patient, guided, of course, by the anesthesiologist. Additionally, when a patient arrives for extremely minor surgery without an escort, a local anesthetic injection alone might suffice for anesthesia. This might allow the patient to return home unaccompanied. Unfortunately, it sometimes becomes necessary to supplement a local anesthetic with intravenous sedation, and under these circumstances an escort would then be mandatory.

15. What are the advantages and disadvantages to performing a conduction anesthetic in the ambulatory patient?

Employing regional anesthesia in the ambulatory surgery patient has a number of potential advantages. If little or no intraoperative sedation is required, little or none of the "hangover" effect will be present throughout the postoperative period. Patients who express fear about losing consciousness or the loss of control associated with a general anesthetic may prefer a regional technique. Some patients have a strong desire to remain awake to view arthroscopic surgery as it is being performed.

Spinal or epidural anesthesia, however, has potential disadvantages. There had been concern regarding the apparent increased incidence of PDPH in patients who ambulate postoperatively. However, experience has shown that the incidence of PDPH is equal among patients who are nonambulatory and ambulatory, but that the onset may be delayed in patients who remain recumbent for a longer period of time. If spinal anesthesia is chosen, the use of conventional smaller gauge needles as well as newer designs (Greene, Sprotte, Whitacre) that include modifications at the tip to be less traumatic appear to markedly reduce the incidence of PDPH. The theory behind the pencil-point Greene, the conical Sprotte, or side port Whitacre needles is that splitting rather than cutting of the dural fibers occurs, which may reduce the amount of cerebrospinal fluid (CSF) leak.

Reduction of the incidence of PDPH to approximately 1–2% or less would be an ideal goal. Technical failure rates of the various needles must also be figured into the overall equation.

Patients must always be informed regarding the potential for development of a PDPH because ambulatory patients usually expect to resume their normal activities shortly after surgery. Additional recommendations to reduce the incidence of headache include keeping the bevel edge of the conventional needle parallel to the longitudinal axis of the body and the dural fibers and avoiding multiple attempts at subarachnoid needle placement. Maintenance of adequate hydration intraoperatively and postoperatively and avoiding straining and lifting postoperatively are recommended.

Patients presenting with a persistent PDPH may require an epidural blood patch for relief. Therefore, it is especially important to follow up patients with a telephone call at 24–48 hours after surgery to inquire about the presence of any problems. Conservative treatment of a PDPH in the ambulatory patient includes traditional analgesics, fluids, and bed rest. Performance of an epidural blood patch should be considered early if the headache is perceived by the patient to be extraordinarily severe or incapacitating, or if the patient must return to work immediately, or care for children.

In an attempt to avoid the possibility of a PDPH in younger patients, an epidural anesthetic may be offered to patients if a regional technique is requested or medically indicated. Though an epidural requires greater technical expertise and may be slightly more time-consuming to perform when compared with a spinal, the insertion of a catheter allows additional incremental doses of anesthetic to be added if surgical time is unexpectedly lengthened. Additionally, the use of shorter-acting local anesthetics allows for timing the block to wear off shortly after the procedure is completed. However, the incidence of headache after unintended dural puncture with larger gauge epidural needles is significantly higher. It is interesting that the reported incidence of headache following a general anesthetic in ambulatory patients exceeds the incidence of headache after regional anesthesia, although it is usually much less incapacitating and is self-limiting. It is postulated that the cause of the headache is intraoperative and postoperative starvation and an element of dehydration.

Spinal anesthesia provided by tetracaine and bupivacaine has been associated with recovery room stays as long as 6–8 hours. This must be considered before performing a regional anesthetic, especially if the procedure is to be done later in the day. Another potential disadvantage of administering a spinal anesthetic in an ambulatory patient is the potential for persistence of autonomic blockade for 1–2 hours following restoration of motor function. This can result in the inability to urinate and the need for bladder catheterization. It appears that increasing duration of sympathetic blockade correlates with an increased incidence of urinary retention.

16. What are the advantages and disadvantages of selecting a nerve block technique for the ambulatory patient?

There are numerous advantages to selecting a nerve block technique when the type of surgery permits. The ability to continue profound analgesia into the postoperative period provides for patient comfort, which may allow early return home from the facility. However, rapid return to presurgical levels of mental alertness and acuity can be achieved only if judicious amounts of sedative drugs are administered during both performance of the block and surgery. Patients may have a decreased incidence of nausea in the early postoperative period if smaller amounts of intravenous opioids are required or can be avoided entirely. This may also allow earlier alimentation and a speedier return to normal functioning.

There are a few disadvantages to performing nerve blocks in the ambulatory surgical patient. Preparation and performance of a block anesthetic may require more time than the induction of a general anesthetic. In some instances, the actual performance of a regional block and establishment of surgical anesthesia may take longer than the proposed operation. Brachial plexus and other nerve blocks have a known failure rate, and incomplete or inadequate anesthesia will further delay the onset of surgery. Some patients will not tolerate any sensation whatsoever and may require inordinately large amounts of sedative drugs throughout the procedure. This might easily negate some of the advantages of selecting a regional approach.

Unfortunately, patients who have not been seen by an anesthesiologist before the actual day of surgery and arrive with the expectation of receiving a general anesthetic may be unprepared to accept another technique. The surgeon's preference will also influence the receptiveness of a patient to a regional technique. A surgeon who prefers the use of major conduction anesthesia or nerve blocks will often inform patients of the benefits and availability of these techniques during a preoperative discussion of the proposed surgery.

17. Describe the intravenous regional anesthetic technique (Bier block) for surgery on the extremities.

The intravenous regional anesthetic (Bier block) is an easily performed and extremely predictable method for providing anesthesia of the extremities. It is best reserved for procedures on the upper extremity below the elbow, although it can provide anesthesia for surgery on the distal lower extremity as well. The technique of intravenous regional block requires little technical skill other than the placement of an additional intravenous catheter in the hand or foot of the extremity to be anesthetized. The block has a rapid

onset, and the success rate approaches 100% in most hands. Only minor patient discomfort occurs during performance of the block. After the arm is exsanguinated, by wrapping it in an Esmarch bandage, the tourniquet is inflated to 100 mmHg over systolic pressure, and the elastic bandage is then removed. Fifty milliliters of 0.5% preservative-free lidocaine is then injected through the previously placed intravenous catheter. Surgical anesthesia is achieved within approximately 10 minutes.

Because a significant proportion of the infused medication may enter the systemic circulation, the anesthesiologist must remain vigilant at all times for the development of subtle central nervous system changes. Frank seizures may occur if the tourniquet fails shortly after the drug is injected.

Usually, little or no intraoperative sedation or adjunctive analgesia is required. On release of the tourniquet, anesthesia rapidly dissipates. Therefore, the Bier block is recommended where postoperative surgical pain is apt to be minimal. It is ideal for procedures such as ganglion excision, trigger finger repair, removal of foreign bodies, and carpal tunnel release.

18. What sedatives can be administered to supplement a regional anesthetic?

The best anxiolytic may be a solid relationship between the anesthesiologist and patient; however, excellent rapport may be difficult to establish within the confines of a fast-paced ambulatory surgery center. It has been shown that a preoperative visit with the anesthesiologist immediately before surgery may serve as a powerful anxiolytic itself.

In the pharmacologic realm, intravenous midazolam has proven to have excellent sedative and anxiolytic properties (Table 77.1). It is water-soluble, nonirritating to veins, painless on administration, provides superb amnesia with rapid onset, and it is therefore well accepted by patients. Diazepam can cause significant discomfort on intravenous infusion, and if patients are followed for a number of days after injection it has been shown to cause thrombophlebitis in a significant number of cases. Therefore, intravenous diazepam has been virtually eliminated from the practice of anesthesia. Compared with diazepam, midazolam's much shorter elimination half-life of 1–4 hours provides a significantly shorter time to recovery. Midazolam is best titrated every 2 minutes in 1- to 2-mg increments, because its onset is rapid and effects may be profound. Sedation after small-to-moderate intravenous doses usually lasts approximately 20–30 minutes. The profound amnestic properties may interfere with assimilating and following instructions, and patients may become unable to cooperate during surgery. Some patients who receive the drug may become completely disoriented, uncooperative, or even combative. This may necessitate either increasing the depth of sedation, pharmacologic reversal, or conversion to a general anesthetic.

TABLE 77.1   **Drugs Used During Ambulatory Surgery**

Drug	Class	Action	IV Dose Range	Potential Side-Effects
Midazolam	Benzodiazepine	Sedative/hypnotic	1–4 mg/70 kg	Apnea and potentiation of hypotension in combination with opioids
Propofol	Diisopropylphenol	Sedative/hypnotic induction agent	2.0–2.5 mg/kg, then 0.1–0.2 mg/kg/min infusion and 10–20 mg bolus prn	Pain on injection; hypotension; respiratory depression; apnea
Fentanyl	Opioid	Analgesia	1–3 µg/kg	Respiratory depression; apnea; nausea; vomiting; miosis; depression of cough; bradycardia; hypotension
Remifentanil	Opioid	Analgesia	Bolus 0.5–1.0 µg/kg, then infusion 0.1–0.3 µg/kg/min	Respiratory depression; apnea; nausea; vomiting; miosis; depression of cough; bradycardia; hypotension
Ranitidine	H_2-blocker	Histamine receptor antagonist	150 mg po or 50 mg IV preoperatively	Headache; fatigue; drowsiness; dizziness; nausea; vomiting; abdominal pain; diarrhea; constipation
Naloxone	Opioid antagonist	Competitive antagonist	20–40 µg bolus, titrate to effect	Precipitate withdrawal symptoms; hypertension; tachycardia; dysrhythmias
Flumazenil	Imidazobenzodiazepine	Specific benzodiazepine antagonist	0.2 mg every 1 min up to total dose of 1.0 mg May repeat every 20 min	Central nervous system excitation; seizures; nausea; vomiting; acute withdrawal
Metoclopramide	Benzamine	Anti-emetic Gastrokinetic	10–20 mg/70 kg 0.15–0.25 mg/kg	Dysphoria; extrapyramidal signs; dopamine antagonism; avoid with pheochromocytoma
Droperidol	Butyrophenone	Anti-emetic	10–20 µg/kg 0.625–1.25 mg/70 kg	Dysphoria; extrapyramidal signs; sedation; hypotension; la belle indifference; catatonia; torsades de pointes
Ondansetron	Serotonin receptor antagonist	Anti-emetic	4–8 mg/70 kg over 2.5 min	Pain on injection; rash; headache
Transdermal scopolamine	Anticholinergic	Anti-emetic Anti-motion sickness	0.5 mg slow-release patch	Dry mouth; dysphoria; sedation
Labetalol	α- and β-adrenergic blocker	Antihypertensive	5–20 mg increments every 5 min up to total dose of 80 mg	Bronchospasm; conduction delays; bradycardia
Esmolol	Relative β-1-selective adrenergic blocker	Antihypertensive	10 mg bolus, add increasing doses every 3 min prn up to 300 mg total; then may administer 50–200 µg/kg/min	Bradycardia; conduction delays; hypotension; bronchospasm; congestive heart failure

continued

TABLE 77.1		Drugs Used During Ambulatory Surgery—cont'd		
Drug	**Class**	**Action**	**IV Dose Range**	**Potential Side-Effects**
Mivacurium	Benzylisoquinoline	Nondepolarizing muscle relaxant	For tracheal intubation, 0.2–0.25 mg/kg in adults and 0.2–0.3 mg/kg in children. May also be administered via continuous infusion for maintenance	Cutaneous flushing; hypotension and wheezing via histamine release
Desflurane	Ether	General anesthesia	Minimum alveolar concentration = 6% Inhaled	Myocardial depression; respiratory depression; airway irritation

Remifentanil is an excellent addition for the patient who requires a short-acting opioid to provide analgesia either during the performance of a painful block or to provide adjunctive analgesia during an inadequate block. It can be administered by intravenous bolus or by continuous infusion. Bolus doses of 0.5 µg/kg may be administered with repeat doses titrated to desired effect. For a continuous infusion, the dose ranges from 0.02 to 0.3 µg/kg/min. Side-effects common to all drugs in the opioid class include nausea, vomiting, and the potential for significant respiratory depression. Alternatively, fentanyl administered in intravenous bolus doses of 25–50 µg can be employed to provide adjunctive analgesia. Instead of using a benzodiazepine to provide sedation, propofol can be administered by either bolus dose (10–20 mg) or continuous infusion (0.1–0.2 mg/kg/min) and titrated to the desired hypnotic effect. Inherent anti-nausea and anti-emetic properties of propofol provide a significant advantage in the ambulatory setting.

19. What complications of nerve block anesthesia are of special concern to the ambulatory patient?

The potential for pneumothorax must be considered when performing approaches to the brachial plexus other than the more commonly practiced and inherently safer axillary approach (supraclavicular, infraclavicular, and interscalene). This complication may necessitate placement of a chest tube or prolonged observation. The occurrence of central nervous system toxicity ranging from tinnitus to frank seizures secondary to an intravascular injection during an attempted block may delay the onset of surgery but should not prevent eventual discharge from the PACU on the day of surgery. General anesthesia, rather than a repeat block, should be induced after it has been determined that the patient has fully recovered neurologically and after this has been documented on the anesthesia record.

20. Should patients having ambulatory surgery be tracheally intubated?

Whether ambulatory patients have increased gastric volumes when compared with inpatients scheduled for surgery is now questionable. In view of the small incidence of documented aspiration with subsequent major pulmonary derangements in previously healthy patients presenting for elective surgery, routine tracheal intubation of every patient is not required. Tracheal intubation should be reserved for patients with any of the known risk factors that predispose patients to esophageal reflux or increased resting gastric volume. Of course, if the surgical procedure requires that the airway must be shared with the surgeon or where an airway cannot be easily or safely maintained using an oropharyngeal or nasopharyngeal airway, tracheal intubation should be performed.

The laryngeal mask airway (LMA), approved by the Food and Drug Administration (FDA) for use in 1991, has proven its value in both the inpatient and ambulatory surgery settings. It is presently manufactured in five sizes and is appropriate for the adult patient as well as the neonate. After induction of general anesthesia, the LMA is inserted blindly into the pharynx. Deep anesthesia is necessary for placement of the device. After inflation of the cuff, formation of a low-pressure seal allows both positive pressure as well as spontaneous ventilation. After recovery of normal reflexes, and when the patient is able to respond to commands and open the mouth, the device can be gently removed from the oral pharynx.

When properly placed, the LMA can free both hands of the anesthesiologist for other tasks including proper maintenance of the anesthetic record, adjustment of monitors, and other responsibilities. The incidence of sore throat following LMA use is less than that associated with tracheal intubation. Because muscle relaxants are not required for the insertion of the instrument, postoperative myalgias associated with the administration of succinylcholine can be avoided. Additionally, ocular and oral trauma associated with conventional facemasks and oral airways may be avoided. Edentulous patients, characteristically more difficult to ventilate by facemask, can be managed well with this device. Because the LMA does not interfere with the functioning of the larynx and glottic closure, an effective cough is possible with the airway in place.

Aspiration of gastric contents has been reported in conjunction with this device. It does not guarantee airway protection. However, in the event of a difficult airway where a patient cannot be intubated and facemask ventilation proves to be inadequate, the LMA may serve as a temporizing measure. Contraindications include oral pathology, pulmonary disease marked by low compliance, inability to open the mouth adequately, and conditions that may predispose the patient to gastric reflux.

21. What is the role of propofol in ambulatory surgery?

Propofol may be used to provide sedation during a regional anesthetic, to induce general anesthesia, and to maintain general anesthesia. It is a water-insoluble, highly protein bound, lipophilic compound that has unique pharmacokinetic characteristics that render it ideal for use with ambulatory surgery. It is rapidly redistributed, and hepatic and extrahepatic clearance (pulmonary) permit rapid recovery of cognitive function with less postoperative sedation and drowsiness compared with the traditionally employed ultra-short-acting barbiturates. Depressant effects on the central nervous system are dose-dependent and range from mild sedation to sleep and unconsciousness. Neither retrograde nor anterograde amnesia is associated with this drug. For the induction of anesthesia, propofol can be administered as a bolus dose (2–2.5 mg/kg slowly), and its effect can be maintained via a continuous intravenous infusion (0.1–0.2 mg/kg/min). Dosages are reduced for debilitated patients and for the geriatric population. For sedation during regional anesthesia, incremental doses of 10–20 mg (0.3 mg/kg) may be given, or an infusion begun. There is a known relationship between propofol (as well as other intravenous agents) serum drug levels and therapeutic effects. For propofol, the target concentration is between 3 and 6 μg/ml to provide surgical anesthesia.

When administered as the sole agent, propofol may not provide amnesia 100% of the time, and intraoperative awareness has been reported. Therefore, it is often used in conjunction with nitrous oxide, a volatile anesthetic, or midazolam. Propofol has no muscle relaxant or analgesic properties. For total intravenous anesthesia, a continuous infusion of a short-acting opioid, such as remifentanil, can be administered along with an infusion of propofol. Additional bolus doses of propofol can be infused to rapidly deepen the level of anesthesia. Another major advantage of propofol appears to be a significantly diminished

incidence of postoperative nausea and vomiting. Propofol's inherent anti-emetic properties allow earlier discharge of patients, even when emesis occurs in the PACU. When used for both induction and maintenance of anesthesia in cases lasting approximately 1 hour, faster recovery time is noted when compared with a thiopental induction followed by maintenance with isoflurane and nitrous oxide. Patients anesthetized with propofol appear to awaken with a positive mood, and they regain equilibrium including the ability to ambulate early. The requirement for pain medication in the postoperative period appears to be reduced, which may be related to an overall feeling of well-being.

Two disadvantages of propofol include the lack of analgesic properties and pain on injection. As for the former, the combination of propofol with an opioid, such as remifentanil or fentanyl, will provide required analgesia. The discomfort associated with administration can be avoided by infusion into large-bore veins as well as pretreatment with intravenous lidocaine. Injecting lidocaine, 10–25 mg intravenously, before giving propofol or drawing up the lidocaine into the syringe after first filling it with propofol will ameliorate or eliminate completely the discomfort in most patients.

Infectious hazards associated with propofol have been well documented because the base, which is composed of an emulsion of soybean oil and egg phosphatides, serves as an excellent culture medium for the growth of bacteria. It is important to draw up the drug in an aseptic fashion and shortly before it is to be administered. Additionally, it is imperative that the syringe be discarded after single patient use. Repeated use of the same syringe throughout the day for multiple patients has been associated with clusters of cases of bacterial septicemia.

22. What is total intravenous anesthesia (TIVA), and what are its advantages and disadvantages?

TIVA is a technique in which continuous or bolus doses of intravenous infusions of anesthetic drugs are administered for induction and maintenance of anesthesia (Table 77.2). The various components of a general anesthetic—hypnosis, amnesia, analgesia, as well as muscle relaxation—can be individually provided and controlled by varying the rates of infusion, thereby influencing serum concentrations. The depth of anesthesia can be controlled in a similar manner to dialing in desired concentrations on a vaporizer.

TIVA avoids the use of all gases with the exception of oxygen, compressed air, or helium. Therefore, contamination of the operating room suite that invariably occurs when using volatile agents, despite the use of scavenger systems, may be eliminated entirely. Intravenous drugs are used to provide unconsciousness, anesthesia, and muscle relaxation, if desired. Because nonflammable gases may be employed, the technique is ideal for laser surgery. For procedures on the upper airway, TIVA is perfect for use

TABLE 77.2	Administration of Total Intravenous Anesthesia (TIVA)

Infuse drugs into an intravenous line as close to the catheter as possible

No nitrous oxide or volatile anesthetic agents

Recommended continuous drug infusions

Propofol alone

Induction dose: 2.0–2.5 mg/kg

Maintenance dose: 0.5–2.0 mg/kg/min continuous infusion. In a 70-kg patient, the infusion rate is approximately the same as the percent isoflurane that would be used

As the sole agent does not provide reliable amnesia, and awareness is possible

Propofol plus adjuvants

Propofol plus tranquilizer (midazolam) plus opioid (either remifentanil or fentanyl)

If patient movement during surgery is undesirable, addition of a muscle relaxant is indicated

For signs of light anesthesia (hypertension, tachycardia, sweating, tearing, or movement), increase infusion rate of propofol, not opioid

or

Administer a propofol bolus dose of 10–40 mg

If blood pressure or heart rate are difficult to control within dosage guidelines, addition of a β-blocker (esmolol or labetalol) or vasodilator is recommended

Turn off opioid infusion 10–15 minutes before anticipated end of procedure

Turn off propofol about 5–8 minutes before anticipated end of procedure

---

with jet Venturi ventilation. Additionally, intravenous anesthesia does not depend on normal pulmonary function for either wash-in or washout of active agent.

The further refinement of computer-assisted infusion systems will allow the anesthesiologist to achieve therapeutic blood concentrations of various anesthetic and sedative drugs. Episodes of "light" anesthesia can be treated with bolus doses or increased rate of infusion. Additional benefits of the technique are the potential for attainment of rapid awakening at the conclusion of the surgical procedure and decreased nausea and vomiting in the postoperative period in patients who receive propofol.

Since few facilities have monitors that measure the blood concentration of the intravenous anesthetics, a potential disadvantage of the technique may include the risk of patient awareness during surgery. However, presently there are several monitors that use processed electroencephalography

(EEG) data to monitor the depth of sedation, and may in fact decrease the risk of awareness during a general anesthetic. Each monitor uses a proprietary algorithm to analyze EEG data to derive a linear score of 0–100. A score of 0 usually denotes complete EEG suppression while a score of 100 usually correlates with the awake unsedated state. Each monitor has its own range of numbers that correlate with general anesthesia. These monitors have proven to be very helpful intraoperatively in the decision-making tree of the anesthesiologist.

Traditionally, when a patient became hypertensive or tachycardic intraoperatively, the anesthesiologist would usually deepen the anesthetic. However, this change in vital signs can be attributed to several causes, and has been repeatedly shown to correlate very poorly with anesthetic depth. The most common of these causes are "light" anesthesia, pain, or intrinsic hypertension. If during this period of increased heart rate and blood pressure there is a concomitant rise in the score to above the general anesthesia level, the most likely cause is "light" anesthesia. Thus, the appropriate response would be to deepen the depth of anesthesia with a bolus of propofol. If, however, the score on the monitor of anesthetic depth remains within the range for general anesthesia, the response would be to give an opioid for pain. The choice of opioid would be either an ultra-short-acting opioid, such as remifentanil, for a short-lived painful stimulus (i.e., esophagoscopy) or a longer acting opioid, such as fentanyl, for a persistent painful stimulus (i.e., an incision). However, care must be taken to utilize the information gleaned from a depth of anesthesia monitor in conjunction with all clinical data, including the procedure being done, the medical condition of the patient, the patient's need for perfusion to the vital organs, as well as hemodynamic variables.

Monitors of anesthetic depth are particularly useful in the ambulatory setting since they have been associated with decreases in times to extubation, postoperative nausea and vomiting, and time to home readiness. Whether or not it is cost-effective to utilize this monitor on all patients has been heatedly debated in the anesthesia community.

23. What is moderate sedation, when is it employed, and what advantages does it offer?

Moderate sedation, previously known as conscious sedation, is a technique that strives to achieve a decreased level of consciousness during surgery whereby patients remain capable of independently maintaining the airway with reflexes intact, as well as responding appropriately to verbal instructions. When properly executed, moderate sedation provides anxiolysis, amnesia, and allows maximum patient comfort and safety. Moderate sedation should be considered to be a valuable accompaniment and adjunct to a properly placed local anesthetic or regional anesthetic. Because interference with short-term memory occurs, the patient experiences a markedly distorted perception of time. Therefore, the anesthesiologist can increase a patient's tolerance and acceptance of the discomforts associated with an ongoing procedure by providing encouragement and a sense of well-being and security. The goal is to allow the patient, anesthesiologist, and surgeon to communicate throughout the operative procedure.

Moderate sedation is achieved by careful titration of intravenous agents administered by either intermittent bolus injection or continuous infusion. Since moderate sedation is part of a continuum, it is possible for moderate sedation to progress to deep sedation or even general anesthesia. Propofol, midazolam, and remifentanil have ideal pharmacokinetic properties for the provision of moderate sedation. These characteristics include a rapid onset, easy titration, and a relatively short duration of action, which allow for an early recovery from their effects. It is useful to combine a benzodiazepine with an opioid. However, one must be vigilant for the insidious or sudden onset of respiratory depression including apnea. Hypoxemia or apneic episodes have been demonstrated to be more frequent when a combination of benzodiazepines and opioids is used, as compared with either drug used alone. Therefore, supplemental oxygen should be provided via mask or nasal cannula, and respiration should be carefully monitored.

Present standards of care require monitoring of heart rate, blood pressure, respirations and oxygen saturation, as well as the capability of measuring temperature and ECG. Nasal cannulae are now available with a separate tube that can be attached to the sampling probe from a capnograph, thereby allowing for end-tidal CO_2 monitoring. This is particularly useful during procedures where the anesthesiologist may be physically separated from the airway.

Though a patient may appear awake and fully recovered at the end of surgery using this technique, vigilance must be maintained throughout the postoperative period because delayed respiratory depression may occur. In the PACU, hypercarbia or even respiratory arrest may occur if the patient is left unstimulated.

24. When tracheal intubation is required for a short procedure, can one avoid the myalgias associated with succinylcholine?

Until the development of mivacurium, a short-acting nondepolarizing agent, patients who required tracheal intubation for surgical procedures less than 20 minutes in duration could be managed only by the administration of a bolus dose of succinylcholine to facilitate intubation followed by a continuous infusion for maintenance of neuromuscular blockade. Alternatively, after administering succinylcholine for intubation high concentrations of isoflurane could be administered to provide a satisfactory degree of muscle relaxation. Isoflurane could also be used to facilitate the action of small doses of a short-acting nondepolarizing

muscle relaxant. However, the use of high concentrations of a volatile anesthetic can result in delayed awakening, an undesirable consequence in the setting of ambulatory surgery.

Disadvantages of succinylcholine include postoperative myalgias and the potential triggering of malignant hyperthermia. At times, myalgias, which occur 5 times more commonly after ambulatory surgery than in the inpatient population, may far outlast the discomforts associated with the surgical procedure itself. These muscle pains may vary in intensity from mild to incapacitating in nature and often develop on the first postoperative day.

Mivacurium, like succinylcholine, is degraded by plasma cholinesterase. In the patient with atypical pseudocholinesterase, the effective duration of action is markedly prolonged. However, it may still be possible to antagonize the drug. Ordinarily, the majority of the mivacurium is rapidly hydrolyzed to inactive metabolites. The recommended intubating dose is 0.2–0.25 mg/kg in adults. When employing the 0.25 mg/kg dose, an initial dose of 0.15 mg/kg should be followed 30 seconds later by 0.10 mg/kg. In children, a dose of 0.2–0.3 mg/kg is often used. Satisfactory intubating conditions are usually achieved in approximately 1.5–2.5 minutes. The duration of neuromuscular blockade is 15–20 minutes in adults but only 9–11 minutes in children. Unfortunately, mivacurium is not free of side-effects. The drug may cause histamine release, which may cause cutaneous flushing and even bronchospasm and hypotension in some patients. Hypotension has not been a problem when dosage guidelines are not exceeded and the drug is administered slowly. Antagonism can be easily accomplished by conventional dosages of edrophonium or neostigmine administered in conjunction with the appropriate anticholinergic agent. Twenty minutes after a single bolus dose, it may be unnecessary to antagonize the block when the train-of-four has returned to normal and fade is not present to a tetanic stimulus.

25. Can a relative overdose of benzodiazepines be safely antagonized?

Flumazenil is an intravenously administered competitive benzodiazepine receptor antagonist at specific benzodiazepine binding sites in the central nervous system. It can be judiciously titrated to obtain the desired degree of benzodiazepine reversal as evidenced by patient arousal. Previously, two drugs were available for this purpose. Physostigmine, a nonspecific centrally acting arousal agent, appears to antagonize the central nervous system depressant effects of both volatile anesthetic agents and benzodiazepines with some success. Aminophylline also appears to be a nonspecific antagonist of benzodiazepine depression but itself has side-effects.

Within 1–2 minutes of an intravenous dose, flumazenil permits awakening of a patient who may have become oversedated by benzodiazepines. If necessary, restoration to baseline levels of lucidity and alertness may be possible. Anesthesiologists may find this new drug useful in three clinical situations. First, flumazenil may be useful in the intraoperative period when a patient becomes confused, uncooperative, or combative after benzodiazepine administration. Second, it may be infused at the conclusion of surgery, when the rapid return of consciousness was the desired objective but was not attained. Flumazenil might be useful either before or after extubation following upper airway surgery when bleeding or secretions might pose a significant problem in the patient who remains excessively somnolent. Third, either intraoperatively during moderate sedation or in the PACU, reversal of excessive midazolam sedation may allow a patient to safely tolerate the central nervous system depressant effects of other drugs that were administered concurrently.

The recommended dose of flumazenil is 0.2 mg given intravenously over 15 seconds. Its onset of action is 1–2 minutes, and its peak action is 6–10 minutes. Incremental doses may be administered every minute, up to a total of 1 mg. Some recommend administration of the full 1 mg dose as a single bolus. Because flumazenil is a specific reversal agent with selectivity for benzodiazepine-induced sedation, it does not interfere with the analgesic state afforded by previously administered opioids. Its duration of action is highly variable, ranging from 20 minutes to 3 hours. Resedation may occur, and close patient surveillance is important. Resedation might occur in someone who received excessive doses of benzodiazepines, especially those agents with longer half-lives such as diazepam or lorazepam. If recognized, resedation can be safely managed by repeat administration of flumazenil at 20 minute intervals as required. Although excessive sedation and tranquility may be antagonized, flumazenil may not sufficiently reverse all the psychomotor and cognitive impairments induced by benzodiazepines. Thus, a false sense of security may be engendered. Furthermore, flumazenil may not entirely reverse respiratory depression caused by benzodiazepines. Mild side-effects reported in association with flumazenil administration include pain at the site of injection, dizziness, headache, precipitation of nausea and vomiting, acute anxiety, and disorientation. Seizures have also been precipitated in patients who have chronically used excessive amounts of benzodiazepines for anxiety or seizure control.

Midazolam has varying effects at different dosages. With small doses, it is anxiolytic. Increasing the dose administered increases the amount of sedation encountered. With still additional midazolam, the hypnotic effects of the agent become manifest. Careful titration of flumazenil may allow partial antagonism of excessive benzodiazepine effect.

When contemplating the use of any reversal agent in the setting of ambulatory surgery, it is important to remember that the duration of action of flumazenil, as well as naloxone, is short-lived. Therefore, additional patient observation before discharge from the PACU is required whenever these agents have been administered.

26. Do the newer volatile agents offer advantages over older agents such as enflurane and isoflurane?

Two volatile anesthetic agents, desflurane and sevoflurane, both ethers, have been extensively tested. Desflurane is a clear nonflammable liquid that is extremely insoluble and requires a specially designed, heated vaporizer for administration. Unfortunately, the gas has a strong odor and is a powerful airway irritant. It can produce coughing, breath-holding, and laryngospasm; therefore its use as an inhalation induction agent is precluded. Its major advantage is low blood and tissue solubility, which allows for a fast emergence when compared with currently available volatile agents. Low solubility properties also allow rapid titration of anesthetic depth.

Although desflurane and isoflurane have similar muscle relaxing properties, higher levels of desflurane can be administered without concern about a delayed emergence. Studies to date have revealed that the times to ambulation and discharge with desflurane are similar to those seen with propofol, although patients anesthetized with desflurane appear to be less sedated in the early postoperative period. However, nausea and vomiting were less frequent with propofol.

Sevoflurane is nonpungent and odorless, and coughing and breath-holding are absent on rapid inhalation induction. Its solubility in blood approaches that of nitrous oxide. Fires have been reported when sevoflurane is used in the presence of desiccated soda lime. Both sevoflurane and desflurane can provide sufficient muscle relaxation to allow tracheal intubation. Both can trigger malignant hyperthermia.

27. What are the etiologies of nausea and vomiting, and what measures can be taken to decrease their incidence and severity?

Unfortunately, postoperative nausea and vomiting remain a significant problem in patients who receive either general anesthesia or intravenous sedation. They are among the most commonly reported complications associated with ambulatory surgery, and hospitalization following an ambulatory procedure is often attributable to them. Persistent and severe retching or vomiting can disrupt surgical repairs and cause increased bleeding; left untreated, they may lead to dehydration and electrolyte imbalance. From 10% to 40% of patients who have not received anti-emetic prophylaxis may be expected to experience some degree of nausea or frank vomiting. The incidence of nausea and vomiting depends on the type of surgical procedure performed, as well as the anesthetic administered. It has been demonstrated that patients undergoing laparoscopy

TABLE 77.3	Factors Associated with Postoperative Nausea and Vomiting

Associated conditions
  Obesity
  Pregnancy
  History of motion sickness
  History of previous postoperative vomiting
  Recent ingestion of food
  Anxiety
  Female gender
  Day 4–5 of the menstrual cycle
  Diabetes mellitus
  Age (uncommon less than 2 years of age)
Surgical procedure
  Strabismus correction
  Laparoscopy
  Dilatation and curettage
  Orchiopexy
  Varicocelectomy
  Ear surgery
Anesthesia-related
  Etomidate and ketamine more often than
    thiobarbiturates, which have a greater incidence
    than propofol
  Opioid/N_2O/relaxant more often than volatile
    anesthetic, which has a greater incidence than propofol
  Intraoperative and postoperative opioids
  Positive-pressure mask ventilation forcing air into
    the gastrointestinal tract
  Anticholinesterases
Miscellaneous
  Blood entering gastrointestinal tract during surgery
  Uncontrolled pain
  Rapid changes in positioning or during rapid transport
    on stretcher
  Early ambulation and oral intake
  Systemic hypotension
  Vasovagal episode

have a 35% incidence of nausea and vomiting. This may be due to manipulation of abdominal viscera, retained intraperitoneal carbon dioxide, and the use of electrocautery. Symptoms occur regardless of whether a general anesthetic or epidural technique is employed. Arthroscopic surgical procedures are associated with a much lower incidence of symptoms than laparoscopic surgeries or ovum retrievals.

The cause of postoperative nausea and vomiting is multifactorial (Table 77.3). Obesity, sudden movement or changes in patient position, a history of motion sickness, postoperative hypotension, female gender, days 4 and 5 of

the menstrual cycle, pain, opioid administration, the anesthetic technique used, and site of surgery may all contribute to the establishment and persistence of these symptoms. They are often disquieting and sometimes incapacitating. Physical measures as well as pharmacologic agents have been employed in an attempt to reduce the incidence of these distressing sequelae. Examples include the attempted removal of stomach contents by intraoperative gastric suctioning; avoidance of excessive positive pressure during mask ventilation, which may force gas into the stomach; and diminished use of opioid-based general anesthesia. These have proven to have variable effects in the reduction of nausea and vomiting, probably because the problem is strongly multifactorial in nature.

Nitrous oxide has been both implicated and exonerated in multiple studies. It is unlikely that this gas plays a major role in influencing the presence or absence of nausea in the postoperative period. However, the selection of induction agent does influence the incidence of postoperative symptomatology. Etomidate and ketamine are associated with a much higher incidence of these symptoms when compared with thiopental. General anesthesia induced and maintained with propofol is associated with the least number of episodes of nausea and emesis.

To help prevent symptoms, moving patients slowly from the operating room table to the stretcher, avoiding sudden turns during transport to the PACU, and allowing patients to wake up slowly have been applied with some measure of success. Warm blankets and repeated verbal reassurance may reduce overall anxiety by increasing feelings of well-being and a sense of security. A vigorous stir-up, sit-them-up regimen with early oral intake is likely to precipitate nausea and vomiting. The end result of significant symptomatology is an increased length of stay in the PACU. For the patient with unremitting symptoms, overnight admission for observation and further treatment with anti-emetics and intravenous fluids to prevent dehydration may be required.

Adequate hydration must be ensured during the operative period as well as maintained in the PACU. To avoid precipitating episodes of nausea or vomiting postoperatively, it is recommended to hydrate vigorously intraoperatively with at least 15–20 mL/kg of crystalloid solutions and to avoid pushing oral fluids and food. Intravenous fluid repletion allows oral fluids to be offered sparingly. Solids should be withheld until the patient expresses hunger. In addition, postponing early ambulation may help to reduce symptoms.

Prophylactic administration of dexamethasone (4–10 mg IV) at the beginning of the procedure, and metoclopramide (10 mg IV) have been advocated. Droperidol, a potent anti-emetic, has fallen into disfavor because of its association with QT prolongation and torsades de pointes. This led the FDA to issue a black-box warning regarding its use. The FDA's recommendations have been challenged because of droperidol's long history of efficacy and rare occurrence of adverse events. If one decides to administer droperidol, a baseline

TABLE 77.4	Prophylaxis and Treatment of Postoperative Nausea and Vomiting

Class and Drug	Dosage and Route of Administration
Benzamines metoclopramide	10–20 mg IV in adults 0.1–0.2 mg/kg IV in children
Phenothiazines prochlorperazine	5–10 mg/70 kg IV/IM
Steroid dexamethasone	4–10 mg IV in adults 0.5–1.0 mg/kg in children
Serotonin antagonists ondansetron	1–4 mg/40–80 kg IV in adults 0.1 mg/kg in children
Sympathomimetics ephedrine	10–25 mg/70 kg IV/IM
Anticholinergics scopolamine patch	Releases 0.5 mg over 3 days transdermally

ECG should be performed, and the QT interval should be measured. Furthermore, the ECG should be monitored during its administration (Table 77.4).

Unfortunately, clinically significant side-effects have been reported with these agents. These include prolonged sedation and delayed awakening, an increase in anxiety as well as restlessness, and extrapyramidal symptoms. Acute dystonic reactions including torticollis, tics, or an oculogyric crisis can be treated with diphenhydramine, 25–50 mg, or with benztropine, 1–2 mg, intravenously or intramuscularly.

Transdermal scopolamine, proven earlier to be efficacious in the prevention of motion sickness, has been studied for the prevention of postoperative nausea and vomiting. Although effective in reducing symptoms when applied 12 hours before surgery, significant side-effects including dry mouth as well as sedation, dysphoria, and urinary retention may occur. It is often reserved for preoperative use in patients who have a strong history of motion sickness. In the pediatric age group, the incidence of visual disturbances and hallucinations after application of the patch is increased. Some clinicians have placed the patch before discharge in patients whose nausea has not completely resolved. However, the patch should be avoided in the geriatric population, pregnant or lactating patients, and in patients with glaucoma.

Ephedrine has been used in the treatment of nausea and vomiting in the PACU. Hypotension or documented postural hypotension in the postoperative period is often due to an intravascular volume deficit and should be ruled out. Treatment consists of crystalloid infusion to correct hemodynamic instability. Ephedrine has been demonstrated to be useful in patients whose symptoms are causally related to assuming the upright position. Ephedrine, 0.5 mg/kg given intramuscularly, has been used in laparoscopy patients with some success. Patients who received ephedrine also had lower sedation scores, and no differences in mean arterial blood pressure were noted. It may be indicated in otherwise healthy patients who have a history of motion sickness or in those patients who experience dizziness, nausea, or vomiting when attempting to ambulate in the postoperative period.

A popular drug in the anesthesiologist's armamentarium against nausea and vomiting, ondansetron, is a serotonin receptor antagonist with possible central and peripheral sites of action. It does not appear to affect awakening from general anesthesia and has no extrapyramidal effects or sedative qualities. Ondansetron appears to offer improved control over both nausea and vomiting. The effective dose is 2–4 mg intravenously and has a duration of action of up to 24 hours. An oral formulation is also available. It has been demonstrated that a combination of agents, perhaps in conjunction with propofol, will prove to be most efficacious in the prophylaxis of nausea and vomiting.

Many surgical centers have abandoned the routine administration of prophylactic anti-emetics to every patient. However, anti-emetic regimens should be administered for specific surgical procedures, such as strabismus repair or laparoscopic surgery, that are associated with an extraordinarily high incidence of postoperative nausea and vomiting.

Sometimes simply relieving postoperative pain may alleviate nausea. The use of acupuncture has been reported in some studies to be effective, but its use is not widespread. A propofol-based anesthetic is associated with fewer emetic symptoms, earlier ability to tolerate oral alimentation, and shorter stays in the PACU when compared with induction with a thiobarbiturate and maintenance with isoflurane. Unfortunately, despite careful anesthetic management including propofol and even prophylactic medication, symptoms of nausea and vomiting in the postoperative period still remain a problem.

28. How is pain best controlled in the ambulatory patient in the PACU?

Management of postoperative pain in the PACU as well as after discharge is of major concern to the anesthesiologist. Adequate pain relief must be achieved before a patient may be discharged and patient comfort in the postoperative period is important. The prevention of postoperative pain appears much easier to accomplish than the treatment of pain that has been allowed to reach significant intensity. Unfortunately, the occasional inability to manage postoperative pain remains a cause of unexpected overnight hospitalization.

In procedures for which patients can be anticipated to experience significant postoperative discomfort, the addition of an opioid as part of the anesthetic is helpful. A propofol anesthetic will not provide postoperative analgesia. The intraoperative administration of long-acting local anesthetics such as bupivacaine, 0.25–0.5%, at the surgical site may provide hours of postoperative pain relief. This technique has proven to be most efficacious following inguinal and umbilical hernia repairs and minor breast surgery. The efficacy of intra-articular local anesthetics and opioids following arthroscopy of the knee joint has been shown to be of value. Other techniques such as performance of a penile block or the topical application of lidocaine jelly on the penis following circumcision have proven effective in reducing discomfort. The use of ilio-inguinal and iliohypogastric nerve blocks is efficacious in adults and children following herniorrhaphy. Repeating maxillary or mandibular nerve blocks at the conclusion of oral surgery is efficacious.

In the PACU, careful titration of small intravenous doses of opioids can safely provide satisfactory analgesia. The blood levels of opioids that are required to provide analgesia are less than those that usually result in significant respiratory depression or marked oversedation. Fentanyl is the narcotic of choice in the postoperative period for treating pain. Its duration of action is modest, and intravenous doses of 25–50 μg may be repeated every 5 minutes until satisfactory pain relief has been achieved. Medicating patients with oral opioid preparations before discharge will provide a patient with a more comfortable trip home because the intravenous drugs administered in the PACU have relatively short durations of action.

The home use of patient-controlled analgesia systems permits the discharge of patients who are expected to experience pain that may not be sufficiently controlled with oral agents. Experiments with patient-controlled analgesia in the home have found this modality of pain relief to be both safe and effective. Oxycodone and codeine are suitable for amelioration of mild-to-moderate pain but are not strong enough to prevent hospitalization in a patient who experiences severe pain.

Ketorolac, a nonsteroidal anti-inflammatory agent, has been administered orally, intramuscularly, and intravenously in an attempt to prevent and relieve pain and reduce opioid requirements. The drug itself is free of opioid-related side-effects including sedation and vomiting. Some are hesitant to employ this class of drugs because of their potential for causing bleeding. Further, when administered orally, gastric irritation may be encountered. COX-2 inhibitors minimize the potential for postoperative bleeding and the risk of gastrointestinal complications and thus are becoming popular as a non-opioid adjuvant for treating postoperative pain.

TABLE 77.5	Guidelines for Safe Discharge After Same-Day Surgery

Stable vital signs every 15 minutes × 4
Oriented to time, place, and person (or returned to preoperative status)
Capable of walking with minimal assistance (consider preoperative status)
Tolerable nausea and no active vomiting
Pain adequately controlled
Absence of surgical bleeding
Responsible adult present who will accompany the patient home and remain with patient
Able to tolerate oral fluids (optional)
Able to void (after gynecologic, genitourinary, groin and perineal procedures, and after epidural and spinal anesthetics)

29. What discharge criteria must be met before a patient may leave the ambulatory surgery center?

Most institutions divide postanesthesia care into two phases. The first phase begins when the patient first enters the recovery area. The second phase, or step-down phase, begins after stability of vital signs has been achieved and the major effects of anesthesia have dissipated. At this point, the patient can be comfortably transferred into a recliner chair, either in the same area or in another unit (Table 77.5).

Patients who have received a spinal or epidural anesthetic can only be discharged when full motor, sensory, and sympathetic function has returned. An inpatient who will remain at bed rest might be discharged from the PACU to the nursing unit while minimal residual neural blockade persists; in the case of the ambulatory patient, however, it is essential that the block has completely dissipated.

Following administration of an epidural or spinal anesthetic, the patient should demonstrate the ability to void. This provides evidence that residual sympathetic blockade has dissipated. Of course, before attempting to ambulate a patient, it is essential to ensure that all motor block has resolved.

Patients who have received an ankle block, brachial plexus block, or peripheral nerve block may be discharged despite the persistence of residual anesthesia or paresthesias. The arm or foot should be protected from harm with either a sling in the case of the arm or a bulky dressing in the case of the foot. The patient needs to be reminded that in time the block will dissipate and discomfort will appear. For this reason, instructions should be given to take the prescribed oral analgesic medication at the first sign of discomfort, because pain is most readily treated before it becomes excruciating.

Patients who have received general anesthesia may awaken either in the operating room or shortly after transfer to the PACU. Although the patient may appear to be lucid and oriented, numerous criteria must be satisfied before a patient may be considered to be ready for discharge from the facility. A restoration of vital signs within 15–20% of the preoperative baseline is ordinarily required. Patients should demonstrate an intact gag reflex and the ability to cough effectively and swallow liquids without difficulty. It is not necessary for patients to eat before discharge. Forcing patients to ingest unwanted food in the absence of hunger may simply serve to increase the incidence of postoperative nausea and vomiting. Ordinarily, the patient is asked to demonstrate the ability to tolerate a small amount of liquid. If a patient experiences mild nausea and has not been able to ingest more than a few sips without precipitating vomiting or increased nausea, it is foolish to persist. Discharge can still be considered, but written instructions must be provided regarding steps to be taken (contact facility or surgeon) if there is continued inability to tolerate fluids. It is important to ensure that a normal state of hydration has been achieved before discharge. This is especially important following surgery in the oral cavity, where postoperative pain may preclude early oral intake.

Unless the patient was previously unable to walk or the procedure performed precludes ambulation, patients should be able to walk with assistance and without experiencing dizziness. If crutches are required, it should not be assumed that the patient received preoperative instruction. Additional instruction should be offered. Hemostasis should be present at the surgical site, and control of pain should be satisfactory. The preoperative level of orientation should be achieved, although a mild degree of residual sedation is acceptable.

It is not essential for a patient to demonstrate the ability to urinate unless genitourinary, gynecologic, or other surgery has been performed in the inguinal or perineal region. The patient and the escort should be instructed of the need to contact either the ambulatory facility or the surgeon if the patient has not voided within 6 hours following discharge from the recovery area.

Postanesthesia discharge scoring systems have been proposed and developed for the purpose of assessing when home readiness is achieved in the postoperative period. Criteria such as mental status, pain intensity, ability to ambulate, and stability of vital signs are given numeric values. A total score above a particular number may indicate a high likelihood of readiness for discharge. To be practical, a scoring system must be readily understood, simple to employ, and objective. Sophisticated pen-and-paper and neuropsychological tests to assess recovery from anesthesia are reserved solely for research purposes. Actually, after stability in vital signs is achieved, the ability of a patient to walk and urinate may be the best measure of a patient's gross recovery from an anesthetic and signal readiness for discharge. These activities indicate return of motor strength,

central nervous system functioning, and restoration of sympathetic tone.

Each patient and escort should receive a set of detailed, written discharge instructions regarding activity, medications, care of dressings, and bathing restrictions. Instructions must be reviewed verbally with the patient and escort, and they must be signed by the patient or escort, if the patient is incapable. Both must be aware of the need to contact the facility in the event of untoward reactions or any difficulties that may arise such as bleeding, headache, severe pain, or unrelenting nausea or vomiting. The majority of postoperative complications occur after the patient has been discharged. Therefore, it is important to ensure comprehension of all information by the patient or designated escort (Table 77.6).

Most states have a mandatory requirement that patients who have received other than a local anesthetic be discharged in the company of a responsible adult. Current definitions of "responsible adult" vary and may be broadened to include emancipated minors or responsible older children. Theoretically, the companion should be willing and able to remain with the patient for at least the first 24 hours after surgery. This is especially important when dealing with the geriatric or debilitated patient. Problems may arise when an octogenarian patient is discharged in the company of an octogenarian spouse. Ideally, two adults should accompany pediatric patients from recovery room to home. After discharge, a child may suddenly experience nausea or vomiting, pain, fright, or disorientation. A parent who is driving a car cannot possibly attend to both responsibilities simultaneously.

A clear distinction is made between "home readiness" and "street fitness." Home readiness signals that the time has arrived to discharge the patient from the recovery area. On the other hand, "street fitness" is attained after approximately 24 hours have elapsed, when most of the more subtle and persistent central nervous system effects of general anesthesia have dissipated. Patients must be

TABLE 77.6	Functions of the Escort in Ambulatory Surgery

Provide translation when the patient speaks a foreign
   language
Receive and comprehend postoperative instructions
Accompany patient during transport home
Serve as companion to the patient during the first
   24 hours following completion of surgery and assist
   in the performance of activities of daily living
Remain available to summon medical assistance in the
   event of a medical, surgical, or anesthetic complication

advised not to resume normal activities immediately upon returning home.

Formal discharge criteria must be in place, and final evaluations should be conducted immediately before a patient's discharge from the unit. All perturbations from normal, including vital signs and unusual symptoms, must be addressed.

Every attempt must be made to avoid premature discharge of the patient from the PACU. The consequences of such faulty judgments may include the necessity for emergency care elsewhere and possible readmission to another health care facility. When any element of doubt exists as to the stability or suitability of a patient for discharge, the better part of valor is to arrange for hospital admission for overnight observation.

30. What are the causes of unexpected hospitalization following ambulatory surgery?

Although a patient may be scheduled to return home after surgery, admission may be required for a host of reasons. Approximately one quarter of the unexpected admissions following surgery are anesthesia-related. The remainder result from either medical or surgical complicating factors (Table 77.7)

TABLE 77.7	Reasons for Hospitalization Following Ambulatory Surgery

Surgical causes
   Improper designation as ambulatory surgery instead of
     day of admission surgery
   Surgery extended beyond anticipated procedure
   Surgical complication necessitating return to surgery
     or further observation
   Major intraoperative or postoperative hemorrhage
   Additional follow-up surgical or diagnostic procedure
     planned
Medical reasons
   Poorly controlled concomitant medical condition
   Requirement for intravenous antibiotic therapy
Anesthesia-related
   Unrelenting nausea or vomiting
   Aspiration pneumonitis
   Lethargy and lassitude
   Uncontrollable pain
Miscellaneous factors
   Patient refuses to leave for home
   Surgeon requests overnight observation or
     additional tests
   No escort or suitable person to care for the patient at
     home

Most ambulatory surgical facilities experience an unexpected hospital admission rate that ranges from less than 1% to approximately 4%. Unexpected hospitalization is greater with general anesthesia compared with local or regional anesthesia. As might be anticipated, the addition of intravenous sedation to a local anesthetic increases the complication rate. Nausea and vomiting, dizziness, bronchospasm, and delayed emergence from anesthesia are common causes of anesthesia-related hospital admission.

31. When may patients operate a motor vehicle after receiving a general anesthetic?

Current recommendations are to advise patients to refrain from operating heavy machinery including driving a car for approximately 24–48 hours after the administration of either a general anesthetic or intravenous sedation. While a patient may appear to himself or herself and to others to be completely recovered, subtle psychomotor disturbances and cognitive deficiencies may persist in the postoperative period. Important decision-making, as well as activities requiring fine motor coordination, should be postponed until after the first postoperative day. Despite admonitions to the contrary, postoperative patient surveys have revealed that some patients drive their automobiles within 24 hours after surgery, and some may even drive home from the facility.

As a result of central nervous system derangements or the surgery itself, patients may experience minor slips or even major falls after discharge. Some of these events may be related to confusion or subtle alterations in mental state. Others may be due to dizziness or pain. It is hoped that anesthetic agents of the future will be free of the prolonged and potentially hazardous central nervous system dysfunction seen with currently available drugs.

32. What is the role of aftercare centers for the ambulatory surgery patient?

Following some surgical procedures, patients may experience significant postoperative pain that cannot be readily controlled with oral opioids. Additionally, although they may require some skilled nursing observation or specialized care, these may be accomplished outside the setting of an acute care hospital both at lower cost and with greater comfort for the patient and family. With this in mind, the concept of a recovery care facility was born, thus creating a new category of inpatient postsurgical care. This healthcare model integrates ambulatory surgery with overnight or extended care outside of a hospital. Examples of procedures included in the present trial include hysterectomy, cholecystectomy via laparotomy, shoulder repairs, and mastectomies. If this type of facility is unavailable, appropriate use of home care services including newer modalities of pain control may still allow a patient to avoid inpatient postoperative care.

33. Are quality assurance and continuous quality improvement possible for ambulatory surgery?

To ensure quality as well as patient satisfaction, follow-up telephone calls by an anesthesiologist should be made to all patients on the first postoperative day. Some facilities make two additional calls, one on the evening of surgery and another 1 week following surgery. Postage-paid post-cards may be sent to patients requesting information on the overall experience as well as specific areas of care. Space may be allocated for the patient to note side-effects or adverse occurrences. Depending on surgeons to provide accurate feedback regarding complications is unreliable. Therefore, a mechanism for follow-up must be in place to uncover and identify patterns that may require remedial action.

SUGGESTED READINGS

Cameron D, Gan TJ: Management of postoperative nausea and vomiting in ambulatory surgery. Anesthesiol Clin North America 21:347, 2003

Gold BS, Kitz DS, Lecky JN et al: Unanticipated admission to the hospital following ambulatory surgery. JAMA 262:3008, 1989

Gupta A, Stierer T, Zuckerman R, et al: Comparison of recovery profile after ambulatory anesthesia with propofol, isoflurane, sevoflurane, and desflurane: a systematic review. Anesth Analg 98:632, 2004

Kallar SK, Everett LL: Potential risks and preventive measures for pulmonary aspiration: new concepts in preoperative fasting guidelines. Anesth Analg 77:171, 1993

Marshall SI, Chung F: Discharge criteria and complications after ambulatory surgery. Anesth Analg 88:508, 1999

Pennant JH, White PF: The laryngeal mask airway. Anesthesiology 79:144, 1993

Scarr M, Maltby JR, Jani J: Volume and acidity of residual gastric fluid after oral fluid ingestion before elective ambulatory surgery. Can Med Assoc J 141:1151, 1989

Warner MA, Warner ME, Weber JG: Clinical significance of pulmonary aspiration during the perioperative period. Anesthesiology 78:56, 1993

White PF: Studies of desflurane in outpatient anesthesia. Anesth Analg 75:S47, 1992

Merceditas M. Lagmay, MD

Laurence M. Hausman, MD

Yʏou arrive at the plastic surgeon's office where you have just started providing anesthesia care. A patient who was scheduled for liposuction that day has unexpectedly cancelled, but a new patient is willing to come in instead. The patient is a 54-year-old, American Society of Anesthesiologists (ASA) physical status 1 woman scheduled to undergo a rhytidectomy. During the preoperative evaluation you discover that her maternal grandmother had a complication with general anesthesia but she does not know the specifics. The patient states that she had a cup of black coffee prior to arriving at the office. You decide to go ahead with the case. The patient undergoes an uncomplicated total intravenous general anesthetic during which she receives midazolam, fentanyl, and a propofol infusion. However, during the recovery period she experiences nausea and vomiting.

QUESTIONS

1. Why have office-based procedures and anesthesia services grown so rapidly?
2. What do you need to consider before providing office-based anesthesia (OBA)?
3. What equipment is necessary to provide safe OBA? Is it the same as for the hospital setting?

4. Are there any differences in record keeping or documentation as compared with the hospital setting?
5. Does a history of malignant hyperthermia preclude OBA? How should you prepare for an untoward event?
6. Are there any limitations set for types of patients/procedures for office-based surgery?
7. What method/technique would you choose to provide anesthesia?
8. How will you treat postoperative nausea and vomiting (PONV)?
9. How will you determine when the patient is ready to be discharged?

1. Why have office-based procedures and anesthesia services grown so rapidly?

The number and types of surgical procedures performed in the office setting have risen dramatically over the last several years. This trend has been driven in part by the high facility fees charged by both hospitals and ambulatory surgery centers. These costs are usually not covered by third party payers for elective cosmetic procedures. Convenience for the patient, as well as the surgeon, also plays a major role in this changing trend. A surgical office is often a more comfortable setting for the patient, thus creating a more relaxing experience. Other advantages of an office-based procedure include a decreased risk of nosocomial infection, and improved patient privacy since the staff is usually a small consistent group of workers. It has been estimated that approximately 8 million procedures are done annually in offices. These procedures cross many medical specialties, including gastroenterology, urology, general surgery, dermatology, orthopedics, plastic surgery, podiatry, and dentistry.

2. What do you need to consider before providing office-based anesthesia (OBA)?

Before deciding to provide services for office-based procedures, there are a number of issues related to the procedure, the office, and the practitioners that need to be addressed. These are as follows:

Procedure:
- The patient is able to recover and be discharged from the facility in a timely fashion
- Patient selection

Office:
- Compliant with all federal, state and local regulations
- Monitoring and resuscitation equipment available
- Emergency and transfer protocols exist

Practitioners:
- Personnel qualifications to deliver appropriate level of clinical care
- Scope of practice within the capabilities of the practitioners and facility

3. What equipment is necessary to provide safe OBA? Is it the same as for the hospital setting?

An office-based anesthetic should be as safe as a traditional hospital-based anesthetic. A reliable source of oxygen with back-up, suction, resuscitation equipment, and emergency drugs should be available. Back-up electrical power should be available for lights, monitors, anesthesia machine, and surgical equipment in the event of an electrical outage. Monitoring must be consistent with the ASA "Standards for Basic Anesthetic Monitoring." This would include an electrocardiograph, end-tidal carbon dioxide monitor, pulse oximeter, noninvasive blood pressure device, and temperature monitor. Airway devices, such as oral and nasal airways, masks, laryngoscope handles, appropriate-sized blades, tracheal tubes, and laryngeal mask airways should also be readily available. There must also be a means of delivering positive-pressure ventilation. If the practice includes pediatrics, age appropriate equipment must be available. Proper maintenance, testing, and care of all equipment should be carried out in accordance with the manufacturer's recommendations and should be properly documented.

4. Are there any differences in record keeping or documentation as compared with the hospital setting?

Documentation in the office setting should be identical to that in a hospital. An appropriate preanesthesia evaluation and physical examination by an anesthesiologist is essential. If nonphysician personnel conducted the evaluation, it should be reviewed by the anesthesiologist and the information verified. Key elements of the evaluation should be documented. The anesthetic plan must be documented, as well as the discussion with and acceptance of the plan by the patient. An intraoperative and postoperative record must also be maintained. Confidentiality should be maintained.

5. Does the history of malignant hyperthermia preclude an office-based procedure and anesthesia? How should you prepare for an untoward event?

While the incidence of malignant hyperthermia is low, the occurrence of an episode of malignant hyperthermia in the office poses many problems unique to this setting. The resuscitation effort involved in malignant hyperthermia is quite complicated and labor-intensive and there may not be enough experienced personnel to run such an effort.

If triggering agents of malignant hyperthermia are to be used, the facility should have the resources necessary to begin the initial treatment of an event. This includes having at least enough dantrolene to treat a 70 kg patient for the initial intravenous dose (36 vials) while the patient is being transferred to a tertiary care facility. The emergency cart should contain sterile water, syringes, sodium bicarbonate, mannitol, lidocaine, procainamide, 50% dextrose, cold normal saline, and insulin.

6. Are there any limitations set for types of patients/procedures for office-based surgery?

According to the ASA "Guidelines for Ambulatory Surgery and Anesthesia," "patients who by reason of pre-existing medical or other conditions may be at undue risk for complications should be referred to an appropriate facility for performance of the procedure and administration of anesthesia." This leaves a very wide margin for interpretation. The anesthesiologist must determine on an individual basis the risk/benefit for each patient. Patients with a history of sleep apnea or obesity/morbid obesity present unique challenges in the office setting. Other conditions that may preclude an office-based anesthetic would include brittle diabetes, a history of substance abuse, moderate to severe chronic obstructive pulmonary disease, or risk of aspiration. Each case must be considered on its individual merits.

Over the past several years the procedures performed in offices have increased in complexity and become more invasive in nature. Some surgical procedures that may have required inpatient hospitalization 10 years ago can now safely be performed in an office. However, some procedures should still be avoided. These procedures would include those that are associated with significant blood loss, fluid shifts, or hypothermia. Procedures should not exceed 6 hours in duration and should be completed by 3:00 pm to insure adequate postoperative monitoring.

7. What method/technique would you choose to provide anesthesia?

All types of anesthesia ranging from monitored anesthesia care (MAC) through regional and general anesthesia have been safely performed in the office. Both general anesthesia and MAC have benefited from the introduction of newer faster-acting anesthetic agents, such as sevoflurane, desflurane, and remifentanil. These new agents provide rapid onset and offset that are perfect for the office setting.

Remifentanil is an ultra-short-acting opioid that can be easily titrated to various levels of surgical stimulation. It is a selective mu opioid agonist with potency similar to that of fentanyl. It is distinguished from fentanyl by its unique ester linkage. It has a rapid onset and offset making it ideal for use in the office setting. Remifentanil, 0.05–0.10 µg/kg/min, in combination with midazolam provides effective analgesia and sedation during MAC. Remifentanil can be titrated to provide deep levels of analgesia, if necessary; however, it does not provide long-term analgesia. Thus, it will be necessary to provide for postoperative analgesia for painful procedures.

Sevoflurane and desflurane are newer inhalation agents which have the distinction of rapid uptake and distribution, thereby allowing for a faster recovery from general anesthesia and short time to discharge.

Propofol, while not a new anesthetic agent, is widely used in office-based surgery because of its rapid onset and recovery times. A propofol infusion in combination with midazolam also provides good sedation during MAC, but does not provide analgesia.

Ketamine has recently gained popularity in the office-based arena. Ketamine is a phencyclidine derivative and provides intense analgesia without decreasing ventilation. In contrast to opioids, it is not associated with nausea and vomiting. However, ketamine is a dissociative anesthetic and has been linked to hallucinations. This effect can be attenuated or eliminated by the use of midazolam or propofol. Additionally, since ketamine can increase secretions, one should administer an antisialogogue, such as glycopyrrolate, when ketamine is used.

8. How will you treat postoperative nausea and vomiting (PONV)?

PONV continues to be a problem. In ambulatory anesthesia, where early discharge is an important issue, PONV can be a limiting factor in home readiness.

The first step in dealing with PONV is the identification of the high-risk patient. This particular patient is in the high-risk category because of gender (female), use of intraoperative opioids, and type of surgery. Other risk factors for PONV include being a non-smoker, history of PONV/motion sickness, use of volatile anesthetics, use of nitrous oxide, duration of surgery, and type of surgery (laparoscopy, ear-nose-throat, neurosurgery, breast, strabismus, laparotomy, and plastic surgery). Once the high-risk patient is identified, strategies to decrease the risk, such as use of regional anesthesia when appropriate, use of propofol for induction and maintenance of anesthesia, intraoperative supplemental oxygen, avoidance of volatile anesthetics and nitrous oxide, no to minimal use of opioids, and hydration should be employed.

Since the cause of PONV is considered to be multifactorial in nature, treatment and/or prophylaxis should be similarly directed. There are several drugs currently being used for PONV prophylaxis in adults. These include serotonin receptor antagonists, dexamethasone, and metoclopramide. Older anti-emetics such as promethazine, haloperidol, and perchlorperazine may be used as well. Combination therapy with drugs from different classes has been shown to be superior to treatment with a single drug. The serotonin receptor antagonists (5-HT$_3$), ondansetron, dolasetron, granisetron, and tropisetron, are most effective when given at the end of surgery. According to Gan et al. (2003) there is no difference amongst the various serotonin (5-HT$_3$) receptor antagonists in their efficacy and safety profiles.

Dexamethasone (2.5–5 mg intravenously) has also been shown to be effective as prophylactic treatment for PONV and is most effective when given before induction.

Low doses (0.625 mg) of droperidol are also effective as prophylactic therapy when given at the end of surgery. It is of note that the US Food and Drug Administration (FDA) issued a "black box" warning that droperidol may cause death or life-threatening events associated with QT prolongation and torsades de pointes. This warning is based on 10 reported cases. Gan et al. state that had it not been for the FDA warning, droperidol would have been their panel's first choice for PONV prophylaxis.

Treatment of patients with PONV in whom prophylaxis has failed includes the administration of small doses of serotonin receptor antagonists (ondansetron 1 mg, dolasetron 12.5 mg, granisetron 0.1 mg, or tropisetron 0.5 mg). In general, the rescue drug should be selected from a different class than was used for prophylaxis.

9. How will you determine when the patient is ready to be discharged?

Strong emphasis is placed on early discharge because there is usually limited space available. It is important to identify a set of criteria that helps to determine when a patient can be sent home to finish recovering.

TABLE 78.1	Aldrete Scoring System	

Category	Score
Activity	
Able to move all 4 extremities on command	2
Able to move 2 extremities on command	1
Unable to move	0
Respiratory	
Able to cough and breath deeply	2
Dyspnea or limited breathing	1
Apnea	0
Cardiovascular	
BP and HR +20% of pre-anesthetic level	2
BP and HR +20% to +50% of pre-anesthetic level	1
BP and HR −4% to −50% of pre-anesthetic level	0
Consciousness	
Fully awake (able to answer questions)	2
Arousable on calling (arousable only to calling)	1
Unresponsive	0
Oxygenation	
Able to maintain O_2 saturation > 92% on room air	2
Needs O_2 inhalation to maintain saturation > 90%	1
O_2 saturation < 90%, even with O_2 supplement	0

From Aldrete JA, Kroulik D: A postanesthetic recovery score. Anesth Analg 49:924?934, 1970.
BP, blood pressure; HR, heart rate.

Recovery itself can be divided into several phases that can overlap. Phase I, early recovery, generally begins at the end of an anesthetic and continues until the patient has recovered baseline activity, respiration, circulation, consciousness, and color. The Aldrete scoring system or a modification thereof is widely used in postanesthesia care units (Table 78.1). A score of 9 in the Aldrete system indicates that the patient is ready for phase II recovery. It is the physician's responsibility to determine when a patient is ready for discharge from the facility to complete their recovery at home (phase III). Home readiness criteria include such parameters as stable vital signs, ability to ambulate, control of surgical bleeding, pain control, and minimal nausea and vomiting. Marshall and Chung (1999) developed the Postanesthesia Discharge Scoring System (PADSS) (Table 78.2). When the score is 9 or greater the patient is ready for discharge.

TABLE 78.2	Postanesthesia Discharge Scoring System (PADSS)	

Category	Score
Vital signs	
Vital signs must be stable and consistent with age and preoperative baseline	
BP and pulse within 20% of preoperative baseline	2
BP and pulse within 20–40% of preoperative baseline	1
BP and pulse >40% from preoperative baseline	0
Activity level	
Patient must be able to ambulate at preoperative level	
Steady gait, no dizziness (or meets preoperative level)	2
Requires assistance	1
Unable to ambulate	0
Nausea and vomiting	
The patient should have minimal nausea and vomiting prior to discharge	
Minimal: successfully treated with oral medication	2
Moderate: successfully treated with intramuscular medication	1
Severe: continues after repeated treatment	0
Pain	
The patient should have minimal or no pain prior to discharge	
The level of pain that the patient has should be acceptable to the patient	
Pain should be controllable by oral analgesics	
The location, type, and intensity of pain should be consistent with the anticipated postoperative discomfort	
Acceptability: Yes	2
Acceptability: No	0
Bleeding	
Postoperative bleeding should be consistent with expected blood loss for the procedure	
Minimal: does not require dressing change	2
Moderate: up to two dressing changes required	1
Severe: more than three dressing changes required	0

From Marshall SI, Chung F: Discharge criteria and complications after ambulatory surgery. Anesth Analg 88:508–517, 1999.
BP, blood pressure.

In recent years, the idea of fast-tracking patients after general anesthesia has received much attention. Fast-tracking implies the bypassing of the high-care setting of the postanesthesia care unit and moving the patient directly to an ambulatory surgery unit (ASU). With the newer anesthetic agents and techniques it is possible to complete early recovery in the operating room and transfer a patient directly to an ASU. Proposed fast-track criteria include level of consciousness, physical activity, hemodynamic stability, respiratory stability, oxygen saturation status, postoperative pain assessment, and the absence of postoperative nausea and vomiting. These criteria presented by White incorporate pain and nausea assessment, which previous systems did not include. Much of the impetus is the cost-savings potential, which in a hospital setting or ambulatory surgery center can be significant. It may not be a factor in the office setting where the same personnel are responsible for both phase I and phase II recovery.

SUGGESTED READINGS

ASA Committee on Ambulatory Surgical Care and the ASA Task Force on Office-Based Anesthesia: Guidelines for Office-Based Anesthesia: Considerations for Anesthesiologists in Settting Up and Maintaining a Safe Office Anesthesia Environment. www.asahq.org

Dexter F, Macario A, Penning DH, Chung P: Development of an appropriate list of surgical procedures of a specified maximum anesthetic complexity to be performed at a new ambulatory surgery facility. Anesth Analg 95:78, 2002

Gan TJ, Meyer T, Apfel CC, et al: Consensus guidelines for managing postoperative nausea and vomiting. Anesth Analg 97:62, 2003

Guidelines for Ambulatory Anesthesia and Surgery. www.asahq.org

Hoefflin SM, Bornstein JB, Gordon M: General anesthesia in an office-based plastic surgical facility: a report on more than 23,000 consecutive office-based procedures under general anesthesia with no significant anesthetic complications. Plast Reconstr Surg 107:243, 2001

Iverson R, ASPS Task Force on Patient Safety in Office-Based Surgery Facilities: Patient safety in office-based facilities: I. Procedures in the office-based surgery setting. Plast Reconstr Surg 110:1337, 2002

Iverson R, Lynch DJ, ASPS Task Force on Patient Safety in Office-Based Surgery Facilities: Patient safety in office-based facilities: II. Patient selection. Plast Reconstr Surg 110:1785, 2002

Koch ME, Dayan S, Barinholtz D: Office-based anesthesia: an overview. Anesthesiol Clin North Am 21:417, 2003

Marshall SI, Chung F: Discharge criteria and complications after ambulatory surgery. Anesth Analg 88:508, 1999

Task Force on Postanesthetic Care: Practice Guidelines for Postanesthesia Care. Anesthesiology 96: 742-752, 2002

White PF, Song D: New criteria for fast-tracking after outpatient anesthesia: a comparison with the modified Aldrete's scoring system. Anesth Analg 88:1069, 1999

Levon M. Capan, MD

Navparkash S. Sandhu, MD

Sanford Miller, MD

A 46-year-old man is admitted to the trauma area of the Emergency Department approximately 30 minutes after being hit by a bus. The primary survey reveals no signs of upper airway obstruction, significant respiratory distress with chest wall splinting, blood pressure of 130/80 mmHg, heart rate of 120 beats per minute, Glasgow Coma Score of 15 with movement of all extremities, and no open wounds. The secondary survey reveals a left distal humerus fracture, left (5, 6, 7, 8, and 9) and right (6, 7, and 8) rib fractures, and abdominal guarding secondary to a grade 4 splenic injury, necessitating emergency laparotomy.

QUESTIONS

1. What are the consequences of thoracic trauma?
2. How are traumatic pneumothorax and/or hemothorax managed in a patient undergoing laparotomy for splenic injury?
3. What are the mechanisms of morbidity and mortality from flail chest?
4. What are the management options for flail chest and pulmonary contusion?
5. What are the perioperative management options for traumatic hemopericardium?
6. What are the clinical implications of blunt cardiac trauma?

7. When should traumatic thoracic aortic injury be suspected and how is the diagnosis made?
8. In blunt trauma patients with multiple injuries that include thoracic aortic injury, how is surgery prioritized?
9. What are the perioperative clinical and anesthetic pitfalls that can be encountered during management of patients with thoracic aortic injuries, and how should they be managed?
10. Describe the clinical management of transmediastinal gunshot wounds.

1. What are the consequences of thoracic trauma?

Of the 92,000 annual deaths caused by unintentional injuries, 41,000 result from motor-vehicle-related trauma, which carries a high risk of chest injury. Similarly, of the 52,000 deaths caused by intentional injuries, 21,000 are also highly likely to have injuries to the chest. It is estimated that 12–21% of all trauma deaths result primarily from blunt and penetrating chest injury. It has also been estimated that for each chest-trauma-related death, there are 100 nonfatal thoracic injuries. Not all intrathoracic organs are at equal risk of injury. The chest wall (50–71%) and lungs (21–26%) are the most commonly involved structures. The heart (7–9%), aorta and great vessels (4%), esophagus (7%) and diaphragm (0.5–7%) are less likely to be involved.

While cardiothoracic trauma is a major contributor to trauma mortality, in 80% of cases it coexists with other injuries which commonly require major surgery.

Some serious thoracic organ injuries may be clinically silent, thus active clinical suspicion and sophisticated diagnostic measures may be required to detect them. Physiologic derangements from chest injuries are multidimensional; some clinicians use the term "thoracic shock" to describe them. Pulmonary failure, hemorrhage, and cardiac failure, each of which may be caused by various injuries, are the main components of thoracic shock. Individually or in combination, each of these can interfere with oxygen delivery, consumption, and extraction, and potentially shift oxygen utilization from flow-independent to a flow-dependent state, with associated anaerobic tissue metabolism and lactic acidosis.

2. How are traumatic pneumothorax and/or hemothorax managed in a patient undergoing laparotomy for splenic injury?

Pneumothorax and/or hemothorax are the most frequent consequences of chest injury and require timely recognition and treatment. Concerns about exacerbating spine injuries or producing adverse hemodynamic changes preclude obtaining a chest radiograph in the sitting position, which is required for the diagnosis of a pneumothorax and recognition of the magnitude of a hemothorax. For these reasons, while supine chest radiographs are obtained routinely in all major trauma patients, additional measures may be necessary to diagnose pneumothorax and hemothorax when their presence is suspected. Computed tomography (CT) of the chest is highly specific for this purpose, and even a small amount of air in the pleural cavity can be recognized by this method. Unfortunately, in some instances a preoperatively undiagnosed pneumothorax may enlarge during surgery for associated injuries, and result in severe hemodynamic and oxygenation abnormalities and potentially death if not recognized in time.

The clinical signs and symptoms of pneumothorax in anesthetized patients receiving positive-pressure ventilation include elevation of peak airway pressure, decreased lung compliance, decreasing oxygen saturation, decreased breath sounds on the affected side and, in extremis, severe hypotension, and even cardiac arrest. A chest radiograph can provide the diagnosis even in the supine position if there is a large amount of intrapleural air; however it may be difficult or impossible to obtain during emergency surgery.

Without a radiologically confirmed diagnosis, placement of a 14G needle between the fourth and fifth ribs (the fourth intercostal space) in the midaxillary line, the thinnest region of the chest wall even in obese patients, may be indicated in unstable patients. Nevertheless, atelectasis, bronchial obstruction, or migration of intra-abdominal contents into the chest through a traumatic diaphragmatic defect can mimic the clinical findings of pneumothorax and lead to chest tube placement that is not indicated. Recently, the sonographic diagnosis of pneumothorax has gained some recognition.

Pneumothorax and Hemothorax

Pneumothorax
Diagnosis
  Chest radiograph in the sitting position
  Computed tomography
  Needle aspiration: 14G needle in the fourth intercostal space, midaxillary line
  Ultrasound: absence of lung movement and "comet-tail" artifact

Signs and symptoms under anesthesia
  Increased peak airway pressure
  Decreased lung compliance
  Decreasing oxygen saturation
  Decreased breath sounds on the affected side
  Severe hypotension
  Cardiac arrest

Differential diagnosis
  Atelectasis
  Bronchial obstruction
  Migration of intra-abdominal contents through a traumatic diaphragmatic defect

Hemothorax
Symptoms
  Hemorrhagic shock
  Mediastinal shift
  Airway management difficulties

Indications for thoracotomy
  Chest tube drainage
    >1200 mL upon placement of chest tube
    >200 mL/hr for 4 hours
    >100 mL/hr for 4 hours if >60 years old

Normally, when the lung is imaged by a 3.5–7.5 MHz ultrasound probe, it moves beneath the chest wall during each inspiration, and so-called comet-tail artifacts, multiple echodense spots at the surface of the lungs, appear in the image. In the presence of pneumothorax, neither lung movement (sliding) nor comet-tail artifacts can be observed in the ultrasound image.

Hemothorax may also cause hemorrhagic shock, mediastinal shift, and airway management difficulties. The volume and rate of blood drained via a chest tube determine the necessity of thoracotomy. Drainage of >1,200 mL of blood upon placement of a chest tube, and/or continuing drainage of >200 mL/hour for 4 hours, or >100 mL/hr for 4 hours in patients older than 60 years, are indications for thoracotomy. Other indications for emergency surgery include significant hypotension and/or tachycardia, persistence of "white lung" on the chest radiograph in the presence of a properly placed chest tube, difficulty of ventilation, pericardial tamponade, massive air leak from the chest tube, and cardiac or great vessel injury.

3. What are the mechanisms of morbidity and mortality from flail chest?

Flail chest is defined as fracture of several ribs at two or more sites, or disarticulation of ribs from their cartilaginous attachment to the sternum in addition to a fracture. The resulting respiratory impairment may lead to arterial hypoxemia and/or hypercarbia. Two mechanisms are involved: paradoxical ventilation and pulmonary contusion. Paradoxical chest wall motion—manifested by "caving" of the flail segment on inspiration and "bulging" on exhalation—is dyssynchronous with movement of the uninjured part of the chest wall and diaphragm. By itself, a flail segment may increase the work of breathing, but it usually is not the primary cause of acute respiratory failure, unless there is a pneumothorax from injury to the underlying pleura. The "Pendelluft" effect, a pendulum-like motion of gas from one lung to the other during respiration as a result of inequality of pressures between two hemithoraces, does not seem to be a significant cause of respiratory impairment either. It is currently believed that the primary cause of morbidity and mortality after blunt chest trauma is severe pulmonary contusion. An increase in elastic recoil from this cause makes it difficult to expand the lung during inspiration, which not only increases the work of breathing but also causes a decrease in functional residual capacity (FRC) and lung compliance that may not return to normal for several weeks. All these events result in exaggeration of paradoxical chest wall movement.

The pathology of lung contusion involves atelectasis, interstitial and intra-alveolar hemorrhage, and alveolar disruption. Although these changes begin within a few minutes after injury, they may take up to 3–4 hours to complete. Thus, chest radiographs and arterial blood gases will deteriorate gradually within the first few hours of injury. Generally, age >45 years, pre-existing diseases, a higher injury severity score, and the need for large volumes of fluids predict increased morbidity and mortality.

4. What are the management options for flail chest and pulmonary contusion?

Diagnosis

The presence of a flail segment obviously suggests an underlying pulmonary contusion, but if the patient is breathing rapidly and shallowly, this sign may not be evident. It should be emphasized, however, that neither the extent of the flail nor the number of ribs fractured accurately predicts respiratory failure. Chest wall bruising, rib cage deformities, and crepitus and/or pain during palpation of the thorax should suggest the presence of rib fractures or dislocation even in the presence of a normal chest radiograph. Cartilaginous injuries and fractures of poorly calcified ribs may not be detected by chest radiograph. The initial film often does not show an underlying lung injury since pulmonary edema appears late. If present, a focal infiltrate beneath an area of multiple rib fractures makes the diagnosis of pulmonary contusion. Clinical signs such as dyspnea, tachypnea, intercostal muscle retraction, and the use of accessory muscles of respiration should suggest underlying lung pathology. Monitoring with pulse oximetry in the initial stage is useful only if the patient is breathing room air; supplemental oxygen administration may mask inadequate ventilation, delaying the diagnosis and maneuvers that restore FRC and lung compliance toward normal. Likewise, arterial blood gases measured with the patient breathing room air may be useful. Of course, managing these patients without supplemental oxygen necessitates direct observation by a physician or qualified person. The usual pattern is a progressive decrease in arterial oxygen (PaO_2) and increase in carbon dioxide ($PaCO_2$) tensions resulting in a decrease in pH (respiratory acidosis). Although arterial hypoxemia may precede radiographic abnormalities, it may not reflect the size of the contusion because of restriction of blood flow to the injured lung by hypoxic pulmonary vasoconstriction. A PaO_2/F_IO_2 <300 after the initial resuscitation phase is considered a risk factor for the development of subsequent acute respiratory failure. Quantifying the contusion volume with a chest radiograph, and preferably with a CT scan, may have a prognostic value for identifying the patient who will develop acute respiratory distress syndrome (ARDS). Patients with contusion volumes greater than 20% of total lung volume are more likely to develop ARDS and pneumonia.

Treatment

Early treatment is of utmost importance. A delay of even a few hours may result in progression of underlying lung pathology, with increasing morbidity and mortality. The goal is to decrease elastic recoil and the work of breathing, and to improve arterial blood gases without adverse hemodynamic effects. In patients without acute respiratory failure or associated injuries requiring tracheal intubation this can best be accomplished by continuous positive airway pressure (CPAP) of 10–15 cm H_2O applied by face mask. The routine use of early tracheal intubation and mechanical ventilation with alveolar recruitment maneuvers, the usual practice before 1975, has fallen into disfavor because of an unacceptably high incidence of tracheobronchitis and pneumonia leading to sepsis, multiorgan failure, and death. At present, except in instances when tracheal intubation and mechanical ventilation are necessary (PaO$_2$ <60 mmHg in room air, or <80 mmHg with supplemental oxygen, and conditions other than thoracic injury), the vast majority of patients do well with CPAP. When impending respiratory failure indicates tracheal intubation, airway pressure release ventilation (APRV) may be a reasonable choice. With this mode of ventilation in the spontaneously breathing patient, CPAP is intermittently decreased for short periods with the device shown in Figure 79.1. In other words, spontaneous breathing is superimposed on mechanical ventilation. In addition to decreased work of breathing, the advantages of this technique over controlled mechanical ventilation are improved ventilation/perfusion ($\dot{V}/\dot{Q}$) matching, increased systemic blood flow, lower sedation requirement, greater oxygen delivery, and shorter periods of intubation.

In patients with severe life-threatening unilateral pulmonary contusion unresponsive to mechanical ventilation or APRV, differential lung ventilation via a double-lumen endobronchial tube should be considered. In bilateral severe contusions with life-threatening hypoxemia, high-frequency jet ventilation has been shown to improve systemic oxygenation effectively (Figure 79.2). This mode of ventilation may also improve depressed cardiac function caused by concomitant myocardial contusion or ischemia.

Irrespective of the mode of ventilation, effective removal of tracheobronchial secretions has a significant effect on outcome. Likewise, monitoring with pulse oximetry, an arterial line and, when indicated, a pulmonary artery catheter is important. The pulmonary artery catheter not only guides fluid management, which should be adjusted to the minimum consistent with adequate end-organ perfusion, but it also helps in ventilatory management, as it permits calculation of oxygen delivery and intrapulmonary shunt fraction and thus helps to adjust the optimal level of CPAP.

Supplemental oxygen should be administered judiciously in order to permit the acquisition of maximal information from the initial oxyhemoglobin saturation with pulse oximetry or arterial blood analysis, as well as to avoid its detrimental effects, such as absorption atelectasis, interference with hypoxic pulmonary vasoconstriction in damaged lung regions, decreased mucociliary clearance, free radical formation, and decreased surfactant production.

Overzealous fluid infusion may result in an increase in the size of the lung contusion and a decrease in PaO$_2$. Although it is possible to remove excess fluid with diuretics, their use is associated with electrolyte abnormalities, cardiac dysrhythmias, and hypovolemia. At least during

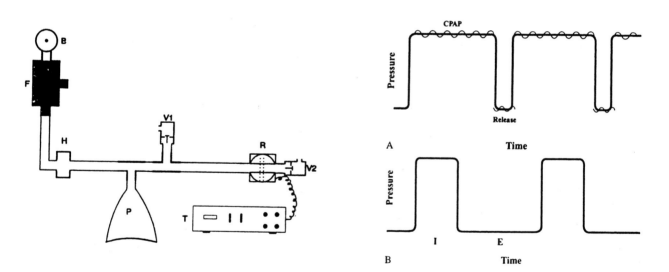

FIGURE 79.1   Left panel: Schematics of the airway pressure release ventilation (APRV) circuit. Right panel: Airway pressure pattern produced by APRV (A) compared with that produced by conventional mechanical ventilation (B). The circuit consists of a flow generator (F) that produces continuous positive airway pressure as it exits through a threshold resistor valve (V1). APRV breaths are produced by a timer (T) controlled release valve (R) in the expiratory limb of the circuit. This valve allows the circuit pressure to decrease intermittently below the continuous positive airway pressure; the level is determined by a second threshold resistor valve (V2). B, gas source; H, humidifier; P, patient. On the right panel note spontaneous breathing superimposed on CPAP, and the opposite inspiration/expiration (I/E) ratios of APRV and conventional ventilation. APRV can be described as a time-cycled, time-initiated, volume-variable device that limits peak airway pressure. (Adapted from Rasanen et al. Crit Care Med 19:1234–1241, 1991; and McCunn and Habashi, Int Anesthesiol Clin 40:89–102, 2002.)

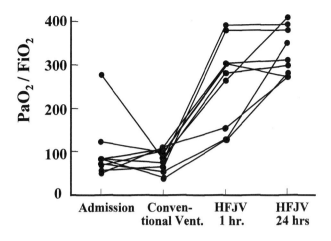

FIGURE 79.2 PaO_2/FiO_2 ratio in patients with severe bilateral lung contusion before and after high-frequency jet ventilation (HFJV). Each line represents an individual patient. (Adapted from Riou et al. Anesthesiology 94:927–932, 2001.)

initial resuscitation, the type of fluid used does not seem to affect outcome. Crystalloid solutions are favored because they are less expensive. In the presence of concomitant blunt cardiac injury, the complications of pulmonary contusion can easily confuse the clinical picture. In this situation, transesophageal echocardiography (TEE) or, if TEE is not available, pulmonary artery and wedge pressures are the best guides to fluid management.

Continuous epidural analgesia is the best pain management technique available for blunt chest trauma. It improves lung function and thus decreases overall morbidity. Other modalities, such as parenteral opioids, are not nearly as effective, while multiple intercostal blocks are labor-intensive and short-lasting, and thus must be repeated at least twice a day. Continuous thoracic paravertebral block has been described but awaits further clinical evaluation.

5. What are the perioperative management options for traumatic hemopericardium?

Traumatic hemopericardium can develop after both blunt and penetrating chest injuries. Unlike chronic effusions, in which as much as 600 mL of pericardial fluid may not cause hemodynamic depression, even small accumulations of blood following acute injury result in cardiac tamponade with significant hypotension and even cardiac arrest. Inflow occlusion of the atrioventricular valves, resulting from external compression by pericardial blood, leads to decreased ventricular filling, especially in the right heart. As a relatively small amount of acute fluid accumulation can cause major hemodynamic changes, evacuation of even a small amount of blood from the pericardium usually restores the blood pressure. Thus, hypotensive

Flail Chest and Pulmonary Contusion

Definition
> Flail chest: rib fractures at two or more sites, with or without disarticulation
> Pulmonary contusion: atelectasis, interstitial and intra-alveolar hemorrhage, alveolar disruption

Diagnosis
> Clinical symptoms
>> Dyspnea
>> Tachypnea
>> Intercostal muscle retractions
>> Use of accessory muscles of respiration
> Physical examination
>> Chest wall bruising
>> Rib cage deformities
>> Crepitus/pain on palpation
> Radiologic
>> Chest radiograph not always diagnostic
>>> Infiltrate seen in area of trauma
>> CT scan
> Laboratory
>> Progressive hypoxia
>> Progressive hypercarbia
>> Respiratory acidosis

Treatment
> CPAP 10–15 cm H_2O by facemask
> Tracheal intubation/mechanical ventilation
>> Airway pressure release ventilation
> Differential lung ventilation
> High-frequency jet ventilation
> Limit fluids
> Epidural analgesia

Monitoring
> Pulse oximeter
> Arterial line
> Pulmonary artery catheter
>> Calculate oxygen delivery and intrapulmonary shunt fraction to adjust optimal CPAP

patients who may have cardiac tamponade may benefit from pericardiocentesis. Transthoracic echocardiography (TTE) or, in intubated patients without suspected esophageal injury, TEE can aid in diagnosing as well as evacuating the pericardial blood. Diastolic collapse, defined as approximation of the left ventricular walls during diastole, is a sign of tamponade and is associated with a reduction in systemic blood pressure of 15–20% or more. During evacuation, simultaneous imaging of the needle and the pericardial sac prevents cardiac perforation. The clinical signs that are characteristic of chronic cases are virtually useless in acute traumatic tamponade. Beck's triad (cervical venous distention, hypotension, and muffled heart sounds) is seen in less than 50% of cases of traumatic tamponade. Agitation, combativeness, and cool vasoconstricted extremities are seen in patients with cardiac tamponade, but they are also present in patients with hypovolemic shock. Paradoxical inspiratory distention of the neck veins (Kussmaul's sign) is characteristic of cardiac tamponade, but it may be extremely difficult to demonstrate in the acutely traumatized patient.

Paradoxical pulse, although not specific for cardiac tamponade, is probably the most reliable clinical sign in these circumstances. It refers to a greater than 10 mmHg decline in the systolic arterial pressure during inspiration with the patient breathing spontaneously, and is simply an exaggeration of the normal 3–6 mmHg respirophasic variation. This sign lacks specificity, since it can also occur in patients with uncomplicated hypovolemia. Furthermore, its absence does not exclude cardiac tamponade. A concurrent septal defect, severe left ventricular failure, or aortic regurgitation may preclude a paradoxical pulse.

Two synergistic mechanisms during inspiratory reduction of intrathoracic pressure are responsible for the development of paradoxical pulse: (1) increase in transmural aortic pressure and thus in left ventricular afterload and (2) underfilling of the left ventricle because of leftward displacement of the interventricular septum. The increased venous pressure during inspiration in normovolemic patients makes the paradoxical pulse more obvious because it increases right ventricular filling and thus enhances the leftward septal shift. In hypovolemic trauma patients, however, right ventricular filling and thus the septal shift are limited, rendering pulsus paradoxus less perceptible. Equalization of elevated intrapericardial and right ventricular filling pressures is an inevitable phenomenon in compensated cardiac tamponade. With further accumulation of blood, these pressures rise toward the left ventricular diastolic pressure. With diastolic underfilling, cardiac output becomes rate dependent. A decrease in heart rate may result in catastrophic hypotension and cardiac arrest. Severe cardiac tamponade can also produce a reduction in coronary blood flow but myocardial ischemia and decreased contractility are unlikely, probably because of a proportional decrease in myocardial work resulting from decreased systemic blood pressure and stroke volume.

Associated injuries often overshadow the clinical manifestations of cardiac tamponade even when the classical signs of this entity are evident. Thus it is important to be familiar with the ancillary diagnostic findings of this readily treatable emergency. Radiographic findings are not helpful. Cardiomegaly is unlikely to be present in traumatic cardiac tamponade and is nonspecific. Electrocardiographic (ECG) findings are also not specific, although elevation of the ST segment and diminished QRS voltage may be observed if significant pericardial blood accumulates. Electrical alternans (the phasic alteration of R wave amplitude) may be more specific but can also occur in patients with tension pneumothorax. Total electrical alternans (phasic alteration of P and R wave amplitudes), although rare, is considered a pathognomonic sign. As mentioned, echocardiography is the most reliable diagnostic tool for this entity. Of the four sites examined during a focused abdominal sonographic study (FAST) the first involves exploration of the pericardium via a subxiphoid window. Transthoracic and transesophageal views can also be used. The ultrasound may demonstrate not only pericardial blood and its volume but also right ventricular diastolic collapse. Diastolic collapse may be absent in patients with a hypertrophic right ventricle or in those with high intraventricular pressures from tricuspid regurgitation.

Management priorities depend on pre-existing cardiac conditions, the type and extent of associated injuries, intravascular volume, the quantity of pericardial blood, and patient cooperation. If the severity of associated injuries permits, pericardiocentesis with echocardiographic guidance or surgical drainage and intravascular volume restoration should precede any anesthetic. Unlike pleural blood, pericardial blood clots easily. Thus it may be possible to drain only a fraction of the pericardial fluid, but even this amount will produce significant hemodynamic improvement.

Any drug that decreases myocardial contractility or produces peripheral vasodilation may precipitate hemodynamic depression. The classical anesthetic induction agent is ketamine, but even with this drug the blood pressure may deteriorate. Positive-pressure ventilation should be carefully maintained with low airway pressures and without positive end-expiratory pressure (PEEP). In most instances of major trauma with pericardial tamponade, invasive monitoring other than an arterial line may be difficult to place. But, if present, a pulmonary artery catheter can be helpful; equalization of cardiac chamber pressures, the cardiac output, and any response to therapeutic intervention can be observed. Bradycardia during direct laryngoscopy or surgical manipulation should be avoided at all cost.

6. What are the clinical implications of blunt cardiac trauma?

By definition, blunt cardiac trauma encompasses a wide variety of pathologic conditions, including varying degrees of myocardial damage; coronary artery injury; cardiac free wall, interatrial or interventricular septal or valvular ruptures; and, with impalement by a fractured sternum or rib, a penetrating injury from blunt trauma. The term blunt cardiac injury (BCI), formerly called myocardial contusion, refers to myocardial damage involving myofibrillar disintegration, edema, bleeding, or necrosis that, depending on its

Cardiac Tamponade

Diagnosis

Classic signs present < 50%
Cervical venous congestion
Hypotension
Muffled heart sounds
Paradoxical pulse – most reliable in acute trauma
ECG – nonspecific
Elevation of ST segment
Diminished QRS voltage
Electrical alternans
Echocardiography
Pericardial fluid
Right ventricular diastolic collapse

Treatment

Pre-induction of anesthesia
Pericardiocentesis with echocardiographic
guidance
Surgical drainage
Volume replacement
After anesthesia induction
Avoid cardiac depressants and bradycardia
Spontaneous ventilation
If positive-pressure ventilation necessary,
low airway pressure, no PEEP

severity, clinically presents as minor ECG or cardiac enzyme abnormalities, complex dysrhythmias, or cardiac pump failure. Some of these injuries may be caused by myocardial damage from direct mechanical injury or indirectly as a result of coronary occlusion or exacerbation of pre-existing coronary artery disease by the stress of trauma. Cardiac lesions, seen as ECG abnormalities and troponin release, may also be the result of increased catecholamine activity following severe central nervous system injury and hemorrhagic shock with little or no direct trauma to the heart.

In major trauma, multiple injuries frequently coexist with BCI. The perioperative physician must be able to:

- anticipate the possibility of cardiac-induced hemodynamic and rhythm abnormalities that may occur during the clinical course of a patient who may initially be stable;
- determine the contribution of cardiac trauma to the existing overall circulatory abnormality caused by hemorrhage, hypothermia, acid–base and electrolyte abnormalities, or various other causes; and
- implement the most appropriate management based on these findings.

The incidence of BCI in blunt thoracic trauma is approximately 20%, although it may be as high as 76% in severe injuries. Nevertheless, major cardiac complications requiring treatment are considerably less likely to occur; however, when they do occur they may be fatal.

Diagnosis

BCI may be associated with direct precordial impact, crush injury of the chest causing compression of the heart between the sternum and the spine, deceleration injuries, and blast injuries. Suggestive signs and symptoms include chest pain, angina responding to nitroglycerine, dyspnea, chest wall ecchymosis, and fractures of ribs and/or sternum. There is no gold standard for diagnosing blunt cardiac trauma. However, ECG, blood concentration of troponin I, and echocardiography are important. In addition, coronary angiography or ventriculography may very rarely be indicated to diagnose coronary lesions, cardiac rupture, or valve injuries.

A 12-lead ECG is the best screening test. Nonspecific changes such as tachycardia, bradycardia, or occasional atrial or ventricular premature contractions occur in 50–70% of patients, and usually do not require treatment. More serious alterations such as ST or T wave changes, conduction delays, and complex atrial and ventricular dysrhythmias occur less frequently (4–30%) but often need to be treated. Although sensitive, the ECG is not specific and a normal trace cannot rule out the diagnosis. Because of its anterior position, the right ventricle is injured more frequently than the left. However, standard leads, which are primarily useful to detect left-sided abnormalities, will miss some right heart events. Overall the sensitivity, specificity, and negative predictive value of ECG for predicting cardiac complications are 100%, 47%, and 90%, respectively. Although delayed (>24 hours) appearance of serious ECG abnormalities may very rarely occur, it has been demonstrated that a normal ECG on admission virtually eliminates the risk of complications of blunt cardiac trauma and the need for further evaluation, as long as the patient is hemodynamically stable, has no history of cardiac disease, is less than 55 years old, and does not have multiple injuries or significant chest wall trauma. If these compromising conditions exist, however, cardiac monitoring for at least 24 hours in a telemetry ward or intensive care unit is indicated. Of course, an abnormal ECG should be followed by continuous cardiac monitoring. Additionally, obtaining serum troponin I concentration 6 and 12 hours after the injury in hemodynamically stable patients, and echocardiography in hemodynamically unstable patients, should be considered.

Serum creatine kinase (CK) and creatine kinase MB (CK-MB) determinations, which were frequently used to diagnose myocardial contusion, are no longer performed because of their low specificity. Skeletal muscle, colon, lung, liver, and pancreatic tissue contain both CK and CK-MB. Thus in multiple trauma, a positive value may not indicate cardiac injury. Troponin I, on the other hand, is specific for cardiac muscle. However, negative levels of CK-MB or troponin I do not rule out clinically relevant BCI, because in many cardiac trauma patients muscle disintegration is not significant enough to release detectable enzyme levels. Yet even a small area of myocardial damage can cause dysrhythmias if it is in a critical location.

Echocardiography may be helpful in many ways in BCI. It provides information about myocardial function (wall motion abnormalities, increased end-diastolic wall thickness), cardiac structural abnormalities (echo-dense areas on the ventricular walls, valve malfunction, hemopericardium, intracardiac thrombi), cardiac preload (end-diastolic area), systolic cardiac function (fractional ventricular area change), and air embolism (air bubbles in the cardiac chambers, patent foramen ovale). Echocardiography can help not only with the diagnosis of BCI but also in hemodynamic management. TEE is a much more valuable monitor than TTE, whose usefulness is limited by mechanical ventilation, pleural effusion, pneumothorax, and difficulty in placing the patient in left lateral decubitus position. Furthermore, myocardial contusion, hemopericardium, valvular lesions, hemomediastinum, and aortic rupture are more likely to be recognized with TEE than with TTE. Nevertheless, it is important to eliminate esophageal injury before attempting TEE in chest trauma patients. However, dysrhythmias, unexplained hypotension, and/or heart failure are definite indications for TTE or TEE.

Perioperative Management

Depending on its type and extent, BCI can increase surgical risk. Although most patients with cardiac chamber perforation do not reach the hospital, some, especially those with atrial lesions, may reach the operating room. Thus preoperative information about the nature of injury is important. Some retrospective reports have documented an increased incidence of intraoperative dysrhythmias and hypotension in patients with preoperatively diagnosed myocardial contusion. It is not entirely clear whether these occurrences were due to the myocardial injury itself or to the complications of associated injuries. Nevertheless, the combination of atrial fibrillation, old age, and aortic rupture with myocardial contusion appears to increase perioperative mortality. The duration of complications is also a relevant issue for the anesthesiologist, since many trauma patients present days to months after injury. In the vast majority of patients, dysrhythmias last no more than a few days. Ventricular wall motion abnormalities may persist for up to a year, but any increased risk of perioperative complications appears to last for no more than 1 month. An intracardiac thrombus, a well-known complication of myocardial contusion, may be present more than 1 year after injury, further emphasizing the need for preoperative echocardiography even well after the accident.

The clinical presentation of patients with BCI varies; sometimes more than one compromising condition may be present in the same patient. Orliguet et al. (2001) proposed an algorithm describing the management principles for each of these scenarios (Figure 79.3). Dysrhythmias appear to respond readily to antiarrhythmic agents. Hypotension may be caused by hypovolemia, pump failure, or both. Fluid loading, with monitoring of heart function by echocardiography or right heart catheterization, will improve hypovolemia. Pump failure is usually caused by right ventricular dysfunction exacerbated by increased pulmonary vascular resistance due to pulmonary contusion, aspiration of gastric contents, or ARDS. An initial right ventricular free wall dilatation may be followed by leftward ventricular septal shift, which alters the geometry and compliance of the left ventricle increasing left ventricular filling pressure and decreasing cardiac output. This should by no means be a signal to decrease fluid loading. On the contrary, volume replacement should continue with concomitant use of inotropes and pulmonary vasodilators. Positive-pressure ventilation may also be adjusted to minimize intrathoracic pressure and thus right ventricular afterload. High-frequency jet ventilation with its relatively low mean airway pressure may be beneficial in these circumstances. As shown in the algorithm, hemopericardium is treated by drainage, either surgically or by placement of a large-bore catheter with echocardiographic guidance. Anticoagulants, if used, should be stopped. Myocardial infarction and valvular, septal, and coronary

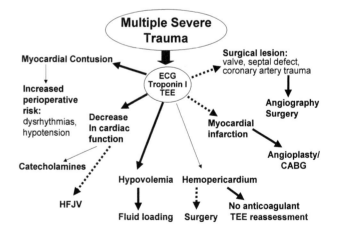

Figure 79.3 Algorithm for management of various clinical scenarios produced by severe blunt cardiac injury. Evaluation of multiple severe trauma-induced BCI is with ECG, troponin I and TEE. Arrows represent the frequency of occurrence of each scenario and the frequency of management measures. Thick arrows represent high-frequency occurrence, thin arrows low-frequency occurrences, and dotted arrows very rare occurrences. (Adapted from Orliguet et al. Anesthesiology 95:544–548, 2001.)

vascular injuries are treated in the same way as they would be in the absence of trauma. Of course, severe trauma may dictate surgery before angioplasty, coronary artery bypass, or repair of injured cardiac valves or a septal defect.

Very rarely pump failure may be unresponsive to pharmacologic measures and requires cardiac assistance. The ventricular balloon pump has been used in these rare cases of BCI. However, in most patients dysfunction originates from the right ventricle. Thus, if assistance is needed, biventricular assist devices would probably be preferable.

7. When should traumatic thoracic aortic injury be suspected and how is the diagnosis made?

Traumatic thoracic cardiovascular injury is a potentially lethal sequela of chest trauma carrying an almost 80% mortality in the first hour following the trauma. It should be suspected in every patient with blunt chest trauma. Although the majority of patients sustain the injury from sudden body deceleration after a motor vehicle accident or fall, other mechanisms such as sudden compression of the thoracic vessels between the spine and sternum or ribs can also produce this injury. In almost 90% of instances, the aorta is injured at the isthmus, the junction of its free and fixed portions. Injuries to the ascending portion and the aortic arch are much less frequent than isthmic injuries. A history of violent deceleration, ejection of an unrestrained passenger from the vehicle, death of anyone involved in the accident, a motor vehicle/pedestrian or bicyclist collision, or the presence of high-impact injuries such as diaphragmatic rupture or mesenteric tear should enhance the suspicion for this injury. Additionally, chest trauma patients who develop unexplained hypotension, external signs of direct chest injury, pulse deficits between right and left arms or between upper and lower extremities, requirement for mechanical ventilation, presence of retrosternal or interscapular pain, hoarseness, systolic precordial flow murmur, or lower extremity neurologic deficits may also have an aortic injury. All patients should have a chest radiograph following chest trauma. Only 20–30% of instances of mediastinal widening on chest films are associated with thoracic aortic injury. Other chest radiographic findings suggestive of aortic injury are blurred aortic contours, wide paraspinal interface, opacified pulmonary window, broad paratracheal stripe, displaced left mainstem bronchus, rightward deviation of the esophagus and trachea, and left hemothorax.

Aortography is the gold standard for the diagnosis of traumatic aortic injury. However, recent improvements in CT and ultrasound technologies permit reliable noninvasive diagnosis in the majority of patients. Contrast-enhanced spiral CT and multiplanar TEE are highly accurate and have substantially decreased the need for aortography. These two techniques are equally capable of diagnosing subadventitial aortic injuries which require surgical intervention. Lesions of the intima and media, which can be treated conservatively

---

Traumatic Thoracic Injury

Mechanism of injury
  Sudden body deceleration
  Compression of thoracic vessels between the spine and ribs/sternum

Site of injury
  Aortic isthmus 90%
  Ascending aorta
  Aortic arch

Suspicious of injury
  Unexplained hypotension
  Evidence of direct chest injury
  Pulse deficits between right and left upper extremities or upper and lower extremities
  Mechanical ventilation
  Retrosternal or interscapular pain
  Hoarseness
  Systolic precordial flow murmur
  Lower extremity neurologic deficits

---

but which may later result in a pseudoaneurysm, and concomitant BCI are much more likely to be detected by TEE than by CT. The high diagnostic accuracy of TEE is valuable for both patients and anesthesiologists. Most patients who are admitted do not have major aortic tears, thus their hemodynamic abnormality generally originates from other injuries, such as to the spleen or liver, which require immediate surgery without time for further evaluation of the chest. Intraoperative TEE in these instances eliminates the uncertainty about the presence of this injury that was common in the past, and permits appropriate intervention for nonaortic injuries while the diagnosis is made by the anesthesiologist. Aortic branch injuries, however, are difficult to be detected by TEE; angiography provides more accurate diagnosis for these injuries. TEE is also contraindicated in patients with suspected esophageal injuries. These patients frequently manifest bloody nasogastric tube drainage, severe facial trauma, unstable cervical spine injuries, and pneumoperitoneum. Although TEE is a useful technique in stable patients with mediastinal widening, flail chest, or pulmonary contusion, contrast-enhanced spiral CT appears to be the method of choice for definitive diagnosis.

The TEE findings of traumatic thoracic aortic injury include dilated aortic isthmus with abnormal contour, acute false aneurysm formation or an intraluminal medial flap associated with subadventitial disruption or both, a mobile image appended to the thoracic aortic wall consistent with an intimal tear or a mural thrombus, or a crescentic or circumferential thickening of the aortic wall suggesting the presence of intramural hematoma. In addition, a traumatic hemomediastinum should be considered if the distance between the esophageal probe and the anteromedial wall of the aortic isthmus is >3 mm or there is blood between the posterolateral aortic wall and the left visceral pleura. A left-sided hemothorax can be detected if there is blood between the left lung and the thoracic wall.

The CT findings of traumatic aortic injury include: polypoid or linear intraluminal areas of low attenuation suggesting clot or medial flap, false aneurysm, irregular aortic wall or contour, pseudo-coarctation, intramural hematoma, and aortic dissection.

8. In blunt trauma patients with multiple injuries that include thoracic aortic injury, how is surgery prioritized?

A patient with an injury that involves complete or a nearly complete circumferential transection of all three layers of the aortic wall is unlikely to arrive in the operating room. Those who make it to the surgery with this pathology generally have either a small perforation or a partial transection that is temporarily sealed with perivascular clot formation or a relatively large transection that bleeds at a relatively slow rate because of hypotension and possibly perivascular barriers such as adjacent tissues or clot covering the lesion. In our experience, patients who have up to 70% transection of the aortic circumference can survive until surgery. Most patients who arrive in the operating room have relatively small sealed subadventitial posterior wall injuries, which require surgical repair because of impending rupture. In addition, there are a significant number of patients who have intimal and/or medial layer injury, which can be managed conservatively or surgically, if necessary, on an elective basis. Undoubtedly, thoracic aortic injury represents a true surgical emergency but not all types of traumatic lesions carry the same degree of urgency. Thus, in hemodynamically stable patients with no intracranial pathology, assessment of the type of vascular injury with contrast-enhanced spiral CT provides important information for surgical prioritization.

Another important factor is the type and extent of associated injuries. Traumatic intracranial lesions and gross bleeding into body cavities are more emergent than stable aortic injuries seen on CT scan. In most instances, hypotension in these patients is caused by the associated injuries rather than the aortic injury itself, and at times these patients may have to be rushed to the operating room without any radiologic investigation. As mentioned, TEE in those circumstances helps immensely to determine the extent of aortic injury intraoperatively while the other injuries are being managed.

In summary, actively bleeding aortic injuries with hemodynamic instability have the highest surgical priority. If they occur concomitantly with unstable abdominal injuries or head injury, which is a relatively rare event,

---

Traumatic Thoracic Injury: Radiographic Findings

Chest radiograph
- Mediastinal widening
- Blurred aortic contours
- Wide paraspinal interface
- Opacified pulmonary window
- Broad paratracheal stripe
- Displaced left main stem bronchus
- Right deviation of esophagus and trachea
- Left hemothorax

Aortography – gold standard

CT scan
- Polypoid or linear intraluminal areas of low attenuation
- False aneurysm
- Irregular aortic wall or contour
- Pseudocoarctation
- Intraluminal hematoma
- Aortic dissection

TEE
- Dilated aortic isthmus with abnormal contour
- Acute false aneurysm formation
- Intraluminal medial flap
- Mobile image appended to thoracic aortic wall
- Crescentic or circumferential thickening of the aortic wall

---

simultaneous intervention should be considered. In the absence of an unstable associated injury, the aortic injury should be repaired as early as possible.

Surgical repair of the thoracic aorta requires clamping of the vessel. In the presence of intracranial pathology this maneuver may result in an uncontrollable rise in intracranial pressure. Thus, a significant intracranial hematoma must be evacuated with at least a burr hole. For small intracranial traumatic lesions, monitoring of the intracranial pressure during the aortic repair may suffice.

9. What are the perioperative clinical and anesthetic pitfalls that can be encountered during management of patients with thoracic aortic injuries, and how should they be managed?

Diagnostic Pitfalls

Coexisting more obvious injuries, lack of obtaining appropriate studies, and misinterpretation of radiographic findings result in diagnostic difficulties and at times missed diagnosis. For example, initially missed aortic injury may be recognized a few days after injury during an emergency sternotomy to relieve a cardiac tamponade and to control bleeding caused by cardiac free wall rupture.

Airway Management Pitfalls

Airway management difficulties may be encountered for several reasons. Bleeding from the aorta may reach the prevertebral space. A hematoma in this area may shift the larynx and trachea anteriorly creating difficulty during laryngoscopy and intubation. A prevertebral hematoma can easily be detected with a lateral neck film. Laryngoscopic visualization of the larynx may be difficult in the presence of a cervical collar placed for documented or suspected cervical spine injury, because neck extension is limited. Combined with a prevertebral hematoma this limitation may make conventional laryngoscopy impossible. However, neck extension should be avoided not only because of the possibility of cervical spine injury but also for preventing sudden hemorrhage from an aortic arch vessel injury; the perivascular hematoma that seals the injury may be distracted by extension of the neck.

Subadventitial and perivascular hematomas or pseudo-aneurysms may compress the left main stem bronchus and cause narrowing of its lumen. Double-lumen tubes have the advantage of preventing spillage of blood into the right bronchus from the left lung during dissection of the aorta. However, forcing a left-sided endobronchial tube blindly into the left main stem bronchus may result in a burst of peribronchial bleeding. Visualization of the left main stem bronchus with a fiberoptic bronchoscope before advancing the endobronchial tube can prevent this complication.

Central Line Placement Pitfalls

Bleeding into the left, and rarely into the right, hemithorax is a frequent complication of thoracic aortic rupture. At times a large quantity of blood may fill the pleural cavity, not only causing collapse of the lung and mediastinal shift but also giving false information when attempting to cannulate the internal jugular or subclavian vein. A free flow of blood may not necessarily indicate vascular puncture; it may be secondary to entry into the blood-filled interpleural space. If this situation is not recognized, rapid infusion of fluids into the pleural space may result in catastrophic complications.

Pitfalls Related to the Use of Anesthetic Drugs

The primary goal of anesthetic management in patients with vascular injuries is to prevent dislodgment of a perivascular clot to avoid bleeding. This can be accomplished by deep anesthesia and complete muscle relaxation. This can be achieved easily in hemodynamically stable patients. However, deep anesthesia may not be possible in unstable patients, who may only be able to tolerate oxygen, muscle relaxation, and possibly a minimal dose of intravenous anesthetic. Nevertheless, another important objective is to decrease viscous drag, which is the pulling force against the vascular wall by flowing blood. Viscous drag has the potential to displace the clot sealing the site of injury. It is proportional to the viscosity and blood flow, and inversely proportional to the third power of the radius. Thus, it is important to decrease the contractile force of the myocardium. In a young and healthy patient, the contractile force may increase to maximum levels to compensate for hypovolemia. Blunting this response with anesthetics may produce a catastrophic outcome. These conflicting objectives may be addressed by titration of the anesthetic while monitoring myocardial contractility with the TEE along with measuring the systemic blood pressure. Control of the blood pressure in the preoperative period and before clamping of the aorta during surgery is crucial to prevent rupture. Preoperative use of β-blocking or calcium channel blocking agents with or without sodium nitroprusside can usually maintain systolic blood pressure at 80–90 mmHg.

The surgical mortality from traumatic aortic injury averages 20% (5–35%). Mortality appears to correlate with patient age, presence of preoperative hypotension, delay in diagnosis and surgical treatment of the injury, and location of the lesion. Proximal aortic injuries have a greater mortality than isthmic injuries. Also injuries located less than 1 cm from the origin of the left subclavian artery are associated with a greater likelihood of technical difficulty, rupture, and mortality during surgical manipulation than those in other locations.

Pitfalls Related to Spinal Cord Ischemia

Spinal cord ischemia resulting in paraplegia or paraparesis is a well-known complication of thoracic aortic injury and its repair. A complete preoperative neurologic evaluation should be documented to avoid confusion regarding neurologic deficits after surgery. The blood supply to the spinal cord is from one anterior and two posterior spinal arteries, all of which originate from branches of the vertebral artery at the base of the skull and descend along the cord. The anterior spinal artery supplies the anterior two thirds and the posterior spinal arteries the posterior third of the cord. Anastomoses between the anterior and posterior blood supply within the cord are rather weak and there are areas with marginal blood supply within the spinal cord. The anterior spinal artery receives a few radicular branches that originate from the thoracic intercostals. The largest of those branches is the great radicular artery of Adamkiewicz (arterial radicularis magna).

The two most common mechanisms of spinal cord ischemia in traumatic aortic injury are occlusion of a subclavian artery, which supplies the vertebral and thus the spinal arteries, either by injury or by clamp placement during repair; and surgical interference with the intercostal vessels supplying the artery of Adamkiewicz. In 75% of patients, the blood supply to the artery of Adamkiewicz originates from the last four thoracic segments, in 15% from L_1 or L_2, and in 10% from the fifth to eighth intercostal arteries. The surgical technique is the likeliest cause of spinal cord injury in patients without a preoperative neurologic deficit or long periods of hypotension.

There are three techniques for repair of aortic injuries: clamp and sew; passive shunting between the proximal and distal aorta; and cardiopulmonary bypass. The latter may be achieved in several ways: partial femoral-femoral bypass, left heart bypass (left atrioaortic or atriofemoral), and right atrial to distal aortic bypass. The advantage of left or right atrial to distal aortic bypass techniques is that they can be used with minimal or no anticoagulation.

The clamp and sew technique is associated with the highest rate of spinal cord complications. However, the incidence of paraplegia is lower if the clamp time is less than 30 minutes. The use of passive shunt placement between the proximal and distal portions of the aorta does not significantly decrease the incidence of neurologic deficit. Partial bypass, e.g., femoral-femoral, decreases the rate of paraplegia, but the need for heparinization is a significant disadvantage of this technique. Left atriofemoral bypass is more frequently used than left atrioaortic or right atrioaortic techniques. If used with a centrifugal pump, these approaches result in the best spinal cord protection. Heparin-bound cannulae are used, which obviates the need for systemic heparinization. Left heart bypass also has two important additional advantages in that unloading the left heart may decrease cardiac complications, and possibly decreases ischemic reperfusion injury. The particular surgical technique will be dictated by surgeon preference and other associated injuries.

The recent development of endovascular stents promises not only to virtually eliminate spinal cord complications but also to decrease the overall morbidity and mortality compared to open repair. Although the routine clinical use of this technique awaits further convincing data, several of the advantages it offers (no need for thoracotomy, single-lung ventilation or aortic bypass, and decreased blood loss) make it an extremely desirable technique.

10. Describe the clinical management of transmediastinal gunshot wounds.

Injuries to internal organs caused by this type of trauma are unpredictable. Any organ, even outside of the thorax, may be injured depending on the path of the bullet. Penetrating trauma to the cardiac window, defined as a quadrangle bounded by the midclavicular lines laterally, the clavicles superiorly and 11th ribs inferiorly, is highly likely to damage the heart. Evaluation must include not only the heart but the other intrathoracic organs. Diagnostic algorithms for transmediastinal gunshot wounds suggest transferring unstable patients directly to the operating room. Stable patients may be evaluated by chest radiograph, pericardial ultrasound, and spiral CT. A patient with abnormal ultrasound findings should be transferred directly to the operating room. Patients with abnormal spiral CT findings may need further study with esophagram, angiogram, bronchoscopy, or esophagoscopy. Positive findings in any of these examinations requires surgery.

Patients with penetrating injury, and to a lesser extent with blunt injury, who require intubation and ventilation may develop systemic air embolism. This complication results from entry of higher-pressure alveolar air into injured lower-pressure pulmonary veins. Clinical signs and symptoms of this frequently fatal complication include sudden cyanosis, hypotension or cardiac arrest, loss of consciousness, and air bubbles in the radial, retinal, or coronary arteries. Although surgical measures such as emergency thoracotomy and clamping of the hilum of the lacerated lung have been recommended, the immediate measure to minimize further embolism is to ventilate the patients with the lowest peak inspiratory pressure. Placement of a double-lumen tube or a bronchial blocker to isolate the injured lung, thus avoiding ventilation to the injured lung, is another measure when time and equipment become available.

Anesthetic management of these patients is challenging. The massive requirement of fluid and blood necessitates insertion of large-bore intravenous lines. Abnormal coagulation requires factor and platelet replacement. Airway management may be difficult because of airway injury or mediastinal shift from hematoma, often necessitating fiberoptic-guided technique to facilitate intubation or to avoid entry into a false passage. Acid–base and electrolyte balance should be maintained. Cardiac injuries must be repaired immediately, possibly requiring the availability of cardiopulmonary bypass for safe repair of major coronary artery injuries.

SUGGESTED READINGS

Cardarelli MG: The management of traumatic aortic rupture. Adv Surg 37:123–137, 2003

Cardarelli MG, McLaughlin JS, Downing SW, Brown JM, Attar S, Griffith BP: Management of traumatic aortic rupture: a 30-year experience. Ann Surg 236:465–470, 2002

Jahromi AS, Kazemi K, Safar HA, Doobay B, Cina CS: Traumatic rupture of the thoracic aorta: cohort study and systematic review. J Vasc Surg 34:1029–1034, 2001

Karmakar MK, Ho AM-H: Acute pain management of patients with multiple fractured ribs. J Trauma 54:615–625, 2003

Orliaguet G, Ferjani M, Riou B: The heart in blunt trauma. Anesthesiology 95:544–548, 2001

Pretre R, Chilcott M: Blunt trauma to the heart and great vessels. N Engl J Med 336:626–632, 1997

Riou B, Zaier K, Kalfon P, Puybasset L, Coriat P, Rouby JJ: High-frequency jet ventilation in life-threatening bilateral pulmonary contusion. Anesthesiology 94:927–932, 2001

Schweiger JW: The pathophysiology, diagnosis and management strategies for flail chest injury and pulmonary contusion: a review. IARS Review Course Lectures Anesth Analg Suppl:86–93, 2001

80

ASTHMA

Andrew B. Leibowitz, MD

Arthur Atchabahian, MD

A 30-year-old woman presents for elective uterine myomectomy. She has a history of asthma dating back to childhood for which she is taking a slow-release aminophylline preparation and an unknown inhaler. Preoperatively, her chest is clear to auscultation.

QUESTIONS

1. What is asthma?
2. How is asthma classified?
3. How would you distinguish obstructive from restrictive lung disease, and asthma from chronic obstructive pulmonary disease (COPD), using preoperative pulmonary function tests?
4. Briefly describe the pharmacology of medications available to treat asthma. Which medications are used for long-term control, and which ones for acute attacks? Outline a treatment plan based on the degree of severity.
5. What are the indications for mechanical ventilation in severe asthma (status asthmaticus)? What are the specific concerns?
6. What preoperative evaluation and preparation would you order for this patient? Would you cancel the case if the patient said that she was just recovering from a "bad cold" and had a few scattered wheezes on auscultation? Would you continue the aminophylline during the perioperative period?
7. Would you choose general anesthesia (with endotracheal intubation, with a laryngeal mask airway) or a neuraxial block for this patient?
8. What are the signs and causes of perioperative bronchospasm?
9. The patient refused to have "a needle stuck in her back". Induction of general anesthesia and intubation were uneventful. During the procedure, the peak airway pressures suddenly rose, and wheezes are heard on auscultation. What would you do?

1. What is asthma?

Asthma is an obstructive lung disease, characterized by reversible constriction of the small airways, mucosal inflammation and edema, and increased mucous secretions. Attacks are characterized by episodes of shortness of breath or wheezing lasting minutes to hours. Between attacks there is an absence of symptoms. Exacerbations are periods of increased airway reactivity. Both attacks and exacerbations are often precipitated by allergic causes (pollen, dust) or by airway irritation (smoking, pollution, cold, respiratory infections). Local trigger factors (leukotrienes, prostaglandins) are released and contribute to inflammation, while vagal stimulation plays a role in bronchoconstriction.

TABLE 80.1		Classification of Asthma According to the National Heart, Lung and Blood Institute	
Stage	**Attacks**	**Nocturnal awakening**	**PEF or FEV_1 between attacks**
Mild intermittent	≤2 times/week	≤2 times/month	≥80% predicted
Mild persistent	< once a day	>2 times/month	≥80% predicted
Moderate persistent	Daily	> once a week	60–80%
Severe persistent	Continuously	Frequent	<60%

PEF, peak expiratory flow; FEV_1, forced expired volume in the first second.

2. How is asthma classified?

The National Heart, Lung and Blood Institute consensus classified asthma into four stages, with therapeutic implications. This classification is shown in Table 80.1.

3. How would you distinguish obstructive from restrictive lung disease, and asthma from chronic obstructive pulmonary disease (COPD), using preoperative pulmonary function tests?

Pulmonary function tests (PFT) are comprised of spirometry and flow-volume loops. An arterial blood gas and diffusion of carbon monoxide (DL_{CO}) can also be included. Typical values in obstructive and restrictive lung disease are shown in Table 80.2.

Asthmatic patients usually have normal PFT values between attacks and periods of exacerbation. Narrowing limited to the small airways can yield a normal FEV_1/FVC, but the FEF_{25-75} will be decreased. Bronchospasm may be triggered during PFT evaluation with methacholine or histamine to assess airway reactivity in patients suspected of asthma with normal baseline PFT values.

For patients with COPD, measurements are repeated after inhaled bronchodilators to evaluate the degree of reversibility or the spastic component, as opposed to the fixed component due to inflammation and airway destruction.

FEV_1/FVC is effort-dependent and requires patient cooperation for accurate measurement, while FEF_{25-75} is effort-independent. It is obtained by dividing the volume expired between 75% and 25% of the FVC by the time elapsed between these two points.

Flow-volume curves may also be helpful. A normal curve as well as typical curves from patients with obstructive and restrictive disease are shown in Figure 80.1. By convention, inspiration is below the baseline and expiration above. In restrictive disease, airway resistance is normal with no flow limitation, while lung volumes are reduced. In obstructive disease, the expiratory flow curve shows a characteristic flattening due to increased airway resistance. Curves from patients with fixed airway obstruction and variable extrathoracic and intrathoracic obstructions are shown in Figure 80.2. Fixed obstruction, such as is seen in tracheal stricture or compression by a tumor or a goiter, causes a decrease in inspiratory and expiratory flows. Variable extrathoracic obstruction (e.g., caused by vocal cord paralysis or marked pharyngeal muscle weakness) causes collapse of the airway during inspiration, as the transmural pressure gradient is negative. On the other hand, with variable intrathoracic obstruction (e.g., caused

TABLE 80.2	Results of Pulmonary Function Tests in Obstructive and Restrictive Lung Disease		
Value	**Obstructive**	**Restrictive**
FVC	Normal or decreased	Decreased
FEV_1/FVC	Decreased	Normal or increased
MMEFR (FEF_{25-75})	Decreased	Normal
MBC	Decreased	Normal
TLC	Normal or increased	Decreased
RV	Increased	Decreased
DL_{CO}	Decreased in COPD Normal in asthma	Decreased

FVC, forced vital capacity; FEV_1, forced expired volume in the first second; MMEFR, mid-maximal expiratory flow rate; FEF_{25-75}, forced expiratory flow between 25 and 75% of the FVC; MBC, maximum breathing capacity; TLC, total lung capacity; RV, residual volume; DL_{CO}, diffusion capacity of the lung for carbon monoxide; COPD, chronic obstructive pulmonary disease.

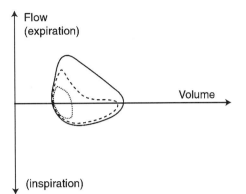

FIGURE 80.1 Flow-volume curves in a normal patient (continuous curve), in a patient with obstructive lung disease (dashed curve) and in a patient with restrictive lung disease (dotted curve).

by tracheal or endobronchial tumor) the airway narrowing increases during forced expiration.

Typically, the arterial blood gas (ABG) is normal in asthmatic patients between attacks. Depending on the severity of the attack, they will first show hypocapnia with normoxemia or mild hypoxemia. As the attack becomes more severe, normocapnia then hypercapnia will be seen, with worsening hypoxemia. The onset of hypercapnia is an ominous sign of impending respiratory failure. In patients with COPD, the ABG shows a variable degree of hypercapnia

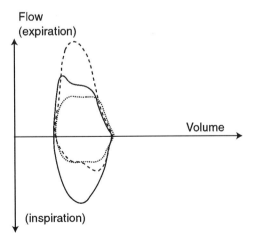

FIGURE 80.2 Flow-volume curves in a patient with fixed airway obstruction (dotted curve), in a patient with variable extrathoracic obstruction (dashed curve) and in a patient with variable intrathoracic obstruction (continuous curve).

and hypoxemia. Patients with restrictive disease can have a normal ABG at rest with hypercapnia and hypoxemia developing during exercise, or they can have baseline abnormalities.

4. Briefly describe the pharmacology of medications available to treat asthma. Which medications are used for long-term control, and which ones for acute attacks? Outline a treatment plan based on the degree of severity.

The medications used to treat asthma are detailed in Table 80.3.

Short-acting β_2-agonists and systemic steroids are used for the treatment of acute attacks. All other medications are used for the long-term control of asthma. Patients with severe disease occasionally need to be given oral steroids for long periods of time.

A detailed discussion of the long-term treatment of asthma is beyond the scope of this chapter, and recommendations vary among authors. Suggested regimens are as follows:

- *Mild intermittent asthma*: short-acting β_2 agonist used on an as-needed basis.
- *Mild persistent asthma*: low dose of inhaled steroid or a leukotriene antagonist as a long-term treatment, in addition to a short-acting β_2-agonist inhaler.
- *Moderate persistent asthma*: medium dose of inhaled steroid with or without a long-acting β_2-agonist.
- *Severe persistent asthma*: high dose of inhaled steroid and a long-acting bronchodilator. In addition, long-term oral steroids are often required. An extended-release theophylline can be used to decrease the frequency of attacks and nocturnal symptoms.

Acute attacks not responding to self-administered metered-dose inhaler (MDI) β_2-agonist are usually treated with β_2-agonist nebulizers and systemic steroids (e.g., methylprednisolone 125 mg IV) that will then be tapered over a few days. In case of failure after escalating doses of a β_2-agonist (15 mg of albuterol nebulized over 1 hour), subcutaneous epinephrine (0.3 mg q 20 min) can be used with electrocardiogram (ECG) monitoring. Magnesium has been used as a last-resort bronchodilator for refractory bronchospasm.

5. What are the indications for mechanical ventilation in severe asthma (status asthmaticus)? What are the specific concerns?

The indications for tracheal intubation and mechanical ventilation in severe asthma are the absence of response to treatment, worsening physiologic variables such as tachypnea,

TABLE 80.3   Pharmacology of the Medications Used to Treat Asthma

Drug	Action	Dose	Onset	Duration	Side-effects
Metaproterenol (Alupent)	Selective β_2-agonist	2–3 puffs q3–4h prn; 0.2–0.3 ml 5% sol nebulizer q4h	Seconds	4 hr	Cardiac arrest, tachycardia, hypokalemia
Terbutaline (Brethine)	Selective β_2-agonist	5 mg po q6h prn	Seconds	4 hr	Cardiac arrest, tachycardia, hypotension, hypokalemia
Albuterol (Proventil)	Selective β_2-agonist	1–2 puffs q4–6h prn; 2.5 mg nebulizer q4h	Seconds	4 hr	Ventricular dysrhythmias, tachycardia, hypokalemia
Salmeterol (Serevent)	Selective β_2-agonist (long-acting)	2 puffs q12h	20 min	12 hr	Ventricular dysrhythmias, tachycardia, hypokalemia, anaphylaxis, angioedema
Epinephrine	Nonselective β- and α-adrenergic agonist	0.1–0.5 mg SQ q 20 min	Seconds	<1 hr	Hypertension, ventricular dysrhythmias
Aminophylline	Antagonizes phosphodiesterase; increases intracellular cAMP	SR: 400–600 mg PO qd; : 0.5–0.8 mg/kg/hr; load if no prior use with 6 mg/kg	4 hr	SR: 24 hr; : 4–6 hr	Seizures, dysrhythmias, nausea, headache, insomnia, tachycardia
Systemic cortico-steroids	Block phospholipase A_2; block transcription of cyclooxygenase; suppress IL-1, IL-2, IL-6, and IF-gamma	Hydrocortisone 200–500 mg/methyl-prednisolone 60–125 mg IV; prednisone 40–60 mg po	6 hr	24 hr	Multiple (hypothalamo-adrenal axis suppression; water and salt retention; glucose intolerance; peptic ulcer; cataracts; glaucoma; osteoporosis, etc.)
Inhaled cortico-steroids (e.g., beclomethasone, Vanceril)		2 puffs q6h	3 days to 2 weeks	Days	Oral candidiasis
Cromolyn sodium (Aarane, Intal)	Prevents mastocyte degranulation	2–4 puffs q6h	Days	Days	Bronchospasm, anaphylaxis, nausea, headache
Ipratropium bromide (Atrovent)	Inhibits vagally mediated bronchoconstriction	2 puffs q6h 1 unit dose (500 μg) via nebulizer q4h	Seconds	4–6 hr	Cough, dry mouth, palpitations, blurred vision
Zafirlukast (Accolate)	Antagonizes leukotriene D4 and E4 receptors	20 mg po bid	Days	Days	Churg-Strauss syndrome, may inhibit metabolism of fentanyl; alfentanil, may increase INR when given with warfarin
Montelukast (Singulair)	Selectively binds to cysteinyl leukotriene receptors	10 mg po qhs	Days	Days	Churg-Strauss syndrome, angioedema, anaphylaxis

NB: Onset and duration refer to clinically significant effects.

hypoxemia, hypercapnia and obtundation, and physical exhaustion in face of maximal therapy.

The main concerns regarding the ventilation of asthmatic patients are increased airway resistance with high peak insufflation pressures and prolonged expiration with the risk of auto-PEEP and "stacking" of mechanical breaths. It is unclear, in these patients with high airway resistance, whether high peak pressures measured at the ventilator level actually correspond to high alveolar pressures. The mainstay of mechanical ventilation in patients with obstructive disease is to use, for a given minute ventilation, an elevated tidal volume (10–12 mL/kg or more), slow respiratory rates (6–8 breaths/minute), prolonged expiratory times, high inspiratory peak flows (80–100 L/ min), and a low I/E ratio (e.g., 1:4 to 1:6.) Most modern respirators allow auto-PEEP to be measured by triggering an expiratory pause (provided the patient is sedated enough to prevent spontaneous breathing). Occasionally, in patients with extreme bronchospasm, neuromuscular blockade might be used to increase chest wall compliance and make ventilation somewhat less difficult.

A strategy of permissive hypercapnia might reduce the risk of barotrauma, but is not supported by studies as it is in patients with acute respiratory distress syndrome.

A concern when ventilating a patient with bronchospasm in the operating room is the inability of most anesthesia ventilators to maintain flows at high impedance. Moreover, the high compliance of the anesthesia circuit may result in as much as 7–10 mL/cm H_2O of the delivered tidal volume lost in the circuit. This would ultimately result in decreasing the effectiveness of patient ventilation.

6. **What preoperative evaluation and preparation would you order for this patient? Would you cancel the case if the patient said that she was just recovering from a "bad cold" and had a few scattered wheezes on auscultation? Would you continue the aminophylline during the perioperative period?**

History and physical examination are the first step. Important information to elicit is the frequency and severity of attacks, the response to treatment, the need for emergency room visits, hospital admissions and mechanical ventilation, and the use of systemic steroids (dose, duration, last use). If the patient uses a peak expiratory flow (PEF) device, the best PEF and the current value should be obtained. There is probably no benefit in obtaining preoperative PFTs for a patient with asthma. Although the importance of the presence of wheezing on physical examination is often discussed, it should be noted that severe bronchospasm often manifests as almost absent breath sounds with little to no wheezing.

Patients with mild asthma do not need any special testing or preparation. Oral medications such as cromolyn,

leukotriene inhibitors, and steroids should be continued until the day of surgery. The patient should use their MDI β_2-agonist before entering the operating room because this has been shown to decrease the incidence of intraoperative bronchospasm. As appropriate, infection should be eradicated with antibiotics; chest physiotherapy should be used to improve bronchial drainage; and cessation of smoking should be maintained for at least 2 months to restore ciliary function and decrease mucus production. Cessation of smoking for 12–48 hours preoperatively decreases carboxyhemoglobin concentrations but has been shown to increase mucus production and possibly lead to an increased incidence of postoperative pulmonary complications.

The 1991 National Institutes of Health (NIH) expert panel recommended that asthmatics with an FEV_1 <80% of predicted receive a preoperative course of oral steroids. This has been shown to decrease perioperative pulmonary complications. Wound healing and infection is not affected by a short course of steroids. Treatment should be initiated 24–48 hours before surgery and can consist of 40–60 mg of prednisone per os once a day or 100 mg of hydrocortisone intravenously (IV) 8-hourly. This should be continued for 1 or 2 days after surgery and can usually be discontinued without tapering.

A history of recent airway viral infection increases airway reactivity in normal patients, and is one of the main triggers for exacerbations. In the adult patient with a clear chest auscultation, it is probably safe to proceed. Whether an elective case should be delayed in a symptomatic patient is controversial and no clear cut-off point can be given beyond which the risks justify the inconvenience. Response to treatment with inhaled β_2-agonists and steroids might help in determining the risk. A small child, on the other hand, would have more severe bronchospasm with the same trigger, because the airway diameter is smaller. Therefore, an elective case should be delayed for a few weeks. A recent study confirmed the increased incidence of adverse respiratory events in children with upper respiratory infections, but no long-term sequelae were noted.

If there are no signs of toxicity, such as tachycardia, tremulousness, nausea or vomiting, aminophylline should be continued during the perioperative period, with drug levels checked as indicated.

7. **Would you choose general anesthesia (with endotracheal intubation, with a laryngeal mask airway) or a neuraxial block for this patient?**

Regional anesthesia would be preferable since airway instrumentation can be avoided. However, a reduction in risk has been shown only for patients with ongoing bronchospasm. Groebel et al. (1994) reported that high thoracic epidural did not alter airway resistance and did attenuate the response to provocation tests in patients with bronchial hyperreactivity.

One concern with neuraxial block is the change in pulmonary function due to high block, but the reduction in expiratory reserve volume usually does not impair breathing. A theoretical concern is sympathetic blockade with unopposed vagal action and bronchospasm. However, no difference was found between parturients anesthetized with high epidurals $(T_2–T_4)$ and those receiving general anesthesia with ketamine and isoflurane.

The main issue with regional anesthesia is the risk for failed block and the need for emergent intubation. Preparations should be made for general anesthesia induction and intubation, and a difficult airway should be recognized in advance. All attempts should be made, if this situation arises, to obtain a deep plane of anesthesia before intubation to prevent bronchospasm.

Laryngeal mask airway (LMA) insertion has been shown to increase airway resistance less than endotracheal intubation and might be preferable. However, the LMA does not protect against aspiration of gastric contents, and administration of positive pressure ventilation through an LMA is controversial.

Propofol appears to have a bronchodilator effect and is currently the preferred agent for induction in asthmatics, provided they are not allergic to eggs or soy. Ketamine is also among the first choices for induction because of its sympathetic-stimulating action. Lidocaine 1.5 mg/kg IV administered 1–3 minutes before intubation prevents reflex bronchoconstriction. Intratracheal lidocaine may trigger bronchospasm and should be avoided. All volatile anesthetics are bronchodilators. A recent study suggests that halothane and sevoflurane are better bronchodilators than isoflurane at doses <1.7 MAC, but the clinical significance is unclear.

8. What are the signs and causes of perioperative bronchospasm?

Bronchospasm is recognized by expiratory wheezing, a high-pitched noise accompanied by a prolonged expiratory time. Tachypnea and dyspnea are usually present in the awake patient. Increased airway resistance manifests as high peak inspiratory pressures and an expiratory flow that does not return to zero at end-expiration, exposing the patient to barotrauma, auto-PEEP and stacking of mechanical breaths.

Not all perioperative bronchospasm is asthma! Important perioperative precipitants of wheezing are listed in Table 80.4.

9. The patient refused to have "a needle stuck in her back". Induction of general anesthesia and intubation were uneventful. During the procedure, the peak airway pressures suddenly rise, and wheezes are heard on auscultation. What would you do?

A. Rule out mechanical causes, such as an endotracheal tube positioned against the carina or endobronchially, kinked, or obstructed by secretions. Consider a pneumothorax, which while only rarely causing actual wheezing, can significantly increase insufflation pressures and confuse the diagnosis.

B. Deepen the plane of anesthesia (propofol, ketamine, sevoflurane) and obtain adequate neuromuscular blockade. Even if the blood pressure is dropping, deepening the plane of anesthesia might relieve the increased intrathoracic pressure, thus increasing venous return and decreasing pulmonary vascular resistance, which may result in improved hemodynamics.

C. Increase the percent oxygen delivered. Unless the arterial oxygen tension (PaO_2) drops significantly, nitrous oxide can be used.

D. Administer inhaled β_2-agonists. Two to four puffs are commonly given. However, Manthous et al. (1995) suggest that the optimal dose may be 15 puffs of

TABLE 80.4	**Etiologies of Perioperative Wheezing**

Congestive heart failure
Local irritation
  Cigarette smoke
  Pungent inhalation anesthetics (isoflurane, desflurane)
  Foreign body in the airway (ETT, suction catheter, oral or nasal airway, vomitus, blood)
Partial obstruction of ETT by secretions, blood, herniating cuff, carina
Histamine release
  Morphine
  Thiopental
  d-Tubocurarine, metocurine (atracurium, rapacuronium)
  Blood transfusion reaction
  Anaphylactic/anaphylactoid reaction
Surgical stimulation
Cholinesterase inhibitors
β-Blockers
Pulmonary embolus/edema

ETT, endotracheal tube.

albuterol with a spacer. These agents are very safe and can be administered in high doses with minimal side-effects. Do not use salmeterol, a long-acting β_2- agonist, because of its delayed onset of 20 minutes.

E. Administer steroids (e.g., hydrocortisone 200–500 mg IV or methylprednisolone 60–125 mg IV). Their effect might take up to 6 hours to manifest itself, but if the bronchospasm persists, it will be a good thing to have started steroids early.

F. Consider bringing in an intensive care unit ventilator. Higher inspiratory flows allow for shorter inspiratory time, longer expiratory time, and lower auto-PEEP. The only downside is the need to switch from inhaled to intravenous anesthetics.

SUGGESTED READINGS

Bremerich DH: Anästhesie bei Asthma bronchiale. Anaesthesiol Intensivmed Notfallmed Schmerzther 35:545–558, 2000 (Excellent review on asthma and anesthesia for those who can read German)

Brown RH, Wagner EM: Mechanism of bronchoprotection by anesthetic induction agents: propofol vs. ketamine. Anesthesiology 90:822–828, 1999

Groeben H, Schwalen A, Irsfeld S, et al.: High thoracic epidural anesthesia does not alter airway resistance and attenuates the response to an inhalational provocation test in patients with bronchial hyperreactivity. Anesthesiology 81:868–874, 1994

Kabalin CS, Yarnold PR, Grammer LC: Low complication rate of corticosteroid-treated asthmatics undergoing surgical procedures. Arch Intern Med 155:1379–1384, 1995

Kil HK, Rooke GA, Ryan-Dykes MA, et al.: Effect of prophylactic bronchodilator treatment on lung resistance after tracheal intubation. Anesthesiology 81:43–48, 1994

Manthous CA, Chatila W, Schmidt GA, et al.: Treatment of bronchospasm by metered-dose inhaler albuterol in mechanically ventilated patients. Chest 107:210–213, 1995

NHBLI: NIH Publication 97-4051, July 1997

Tait AR, Malviya S, Voepel-Lewis T, et al.: Risk factors for perioperative adverse respiratory events in children with upper respiratory tract infections. Anesthesiology 95:299–306, 2001

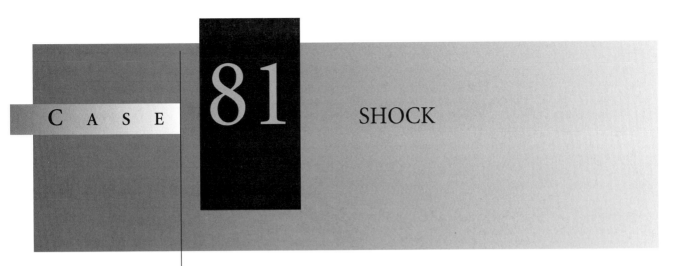

Andrew B. Leibowitz, MD

Arthur Atchabahian, MD

A 62-year-old man with a history of emphysema, coronary artery disease, and esophageal cancer underwent a prolonged esophagogastrectomy. Postoperatively, he remains intubated and ventilated. While in the postoperative care unit, he develops hypotension (blood pressure = 60/30 mmHg) and tachycardia (heart rate = 120 beats per minute).

QUESTIONS

1. What are the determinants of blood pressure?
2. How should postoperative hypotension be approached?
3. What is the definition of shock?
4. What are the different types of shock and the basics of treatment for each type? What would you do for this changed?
5. A pulmonary artery catheter (PAC) was inserted. For each etiology of shock described above, in which direction would the main hemodynamic parameters be changed?
6. What is the classification of hemorrhage according to the American College of Surgeons? Is it a good guide for deciding whether to transfuse a patient?
7. The heart rate suddenly goes up to 170 beats per minute with wide QRS complexes and the blood

pressure drops further. What are the diagnostic possibilities?
8. What are the treatment options for each of the discussed dysrhythmias? What would you do for this patient?

1. What are the determinants of blood pressure?

Mean arterial pressure (MAP) is determined by the cardiac output (CO) and the systemic vascular resistance (SVR) as follows:

$$MAP = \frac{CO \times SVR}{80}$$

CO is the product of the stroke volume (SV) and the heart rate (HR) and depends on preload (the end-diastolic myocardial fiber stretch), contractility (the forcefulness of the contraction), and afterload (the tension developed by the fibers during the contraction). A reduction in either cardiac output or systemic vascular resistance without a counteractive change in the other will tend to decrease the blood pressure.

2. How should postoperative hypotension be approached?

Keeping in mind the physiologic principles outlined above will standardize the approach to the diagnosis and management of hypotension.

- *Preload* can be decreased either by a decrease in the blood volume (hypovolemia due to inadequate fluid replacement, continued postoperative third-spacing or, most critical to diagnose, postoperative bleeding) or because of obstruction of venous return leading to decreased cardiac filling (cardiac tamponade, tension pneumothorax, positive pressure ventilation, positive end-expiratory pressure). Hypovolemia is the most frequent cause of postoperative hypotension and, therefore, the first steps are to assess fluid intake and output, and to examine the operative site, wound, and drains for signs of bleeding.

  A few facts regarding hypovolemia deserve special mention:
  - Acute hemorrhage will not cause a fall in hematocrit until there is intravascular absorption of interstitial water or intravenous volume administration; therefore, early failure of the hematocrit to fall is *not* strong evidence against acute hemorrhage.
  - Blood loss alone without hypovolemia usually does not cause hypotension.
  - In a patient with a nonfailing (i.e., preload-sensitive, afterload-insensitive) heart, decreased preload usually leads to a wide systolic variation of the blood pressure with the inspiratory cycle that can easily be detected on the arterial line tracing.
- A decrease in *contractility* may result from anesthetic administration, electrolyte imbalance (particularly hypocalcemia), ischemia, myocardial infarction, dysrhythmias, hypothermia, and any disease causing chronic cardiomyopathy. Therefore, the electrolytes and electrocardiogram should be checked in all hypotensive patients. On occasion, despite the lack of clear causative factors, postoperative echocardiography will reveal a major change in contractility. In patients with renal failure or mediastinal manipulation, suspicion should be maintained for the occurrence of pericardial effusions that cause tamponade and require rapid treatment with pericardiocentesis.
- A decrease in *afterload* may result from general or regional anesthesia, vasodilator administration, anaphylaxis, sepsis, and neurologic injury.
- *Rate* (extreme bradycardia or tachycardia) or *rhythm* alterations can also lead to decreases in blood pressure through a decrease in cardiac output.

If physical examination, review of the pertinent laboratory data, electrocardiogram, chest radiograph, and empiric fluid challenge do not lead to diagnosis and improvement, echocardiography or insertion of a pulmonary artery catheter (PAC) should be considered. A PAC will yield data on filling pressures, cardiac output, and systemic vascular resistance, as well as on oxygen delivery and consumption, that may help in further management. Data analysis by an experienced physician is needed if beneficial interventions are to result. Transthoracic or transesophageal echocardiography can provide helpful information as well, is less invasive than a PAC, but is more operator-dependent and does not allow for continuous monitoring.

In patients who develop hypotension when mechanically ventilated, consideration must be given to the diagnosis of pneumothorax.

3. What is the definition of shock?

Shock is the failure to meet tissue demand for oxygen. The notion that a certain blood pressure is equated with shock should be dispelled. Instead, signs and symptoms consistent with the failure to meet demand should be reviewed.

Decline in mental status, poor distal perfusion of the extremities, low urinary output, and lactic acidosis would

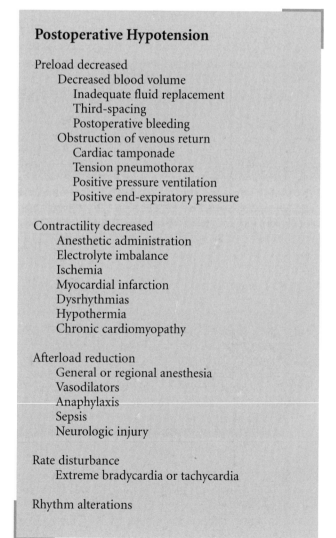

Postoperative Hypotension

Preload decreased
    Decreased blood volume
        Inadequate fluid replacement
        Third-spacing
        Postoperative bleeding
    Obstruction of venous return
        Cardiac tamponade
        Tension pneumothorax
        Positive pressure ventilation
        Positive end-expiratory pressure

Contractility decreased
    Anesthetic administration
    Electrolyte imbalance
    Ischemia
    Myocardial infarction
    Dysrhythmias
    Hypothermia
    Chronic cardiomyopathy

Afterload reduction
    General or regional anesthesia
    Vasodilators
    Anaphylaxis
    Sepsis
    Neurologic injury

Rate disturbance
    Extreme bradycardia or tachycardia

Rhythm alterations

be the most common manifestations of shock. One of these signs and symptoms without any of the others is rarely encountered in true shock. Some patients may experience a greater than 25% reduction in blood pressure, with a mean pressures in the fifties, and show none of these signs and symptoms. They should be classified as having a significant reduction in blood pressure that requires explanation, but not shock.

No single measurement can confirm the diagnosis of shock. In most types of circulatory shock, the mixed venous hemoglobin oxygen saturation will be decreased, as a reflection of the increased oxygen extraction by peripheral tissues. In septic shock, however, oxygen utilization by cells is impaired and the mixed venous saturation will be inappropriately high.

4. What are the different types of shock and the basics of treatment for each type? What would you do for this patient?

Many classifications of shock have been described. Schematically, shock can be divided into cardiogenic, obstructive, hypovolemic, and distributive.

- *Cardiogenic* shock is due to a primary pump failure with a decrease in cardiac output. It can be further classified as nonventricular (e.g., acute mitral regurgitation due to rupture of chordae) or ventricular (e.g., dilated or hypertrophic cardiomyopathy, myocardial ischemia). The treatment is to correct a nonventricular cause surgically, if amenable, after temporizing with medical treatment. In ventricular causes, treatment is aimed at correcting the decreased contractility, such as treating the ischemia or administering inotropes. Occasionally, an intra-aortic balloon pump (to improve myocardial perfusion and decrease afterload) or a ventricular assist device (usually as a bridge to transplantation) may be indicated.
- *Obstructive* shock results from impediment to blood return (tension pneumothorax, pericardial tamponade). In addition to fluid resuscitation, the cause needs to be treated, such as chest tube insertion or drainage of a pericardial effusion.
- *Hypovolemic* shock is due to absolute hypovolemia secondary to dehydration, third-spacing or hemorrhage. The treatment is fluid or blood administration, respectively.
- *Distributive* shock is due to relative hypovolemia secondary to loss of vascular tone. It can be secondary to sepsis or nonseptic systemic inflammatory response syndrome (SIRS), anaphylaxis, or neurogenic shock. Anaphylactic and neurogenic shock benefit from fluid resuscitation, but the primary treatment is restoration of vascular tone with vasopressors. Septic shock has a complex pathophysiology. The main characteristics are a hyperdynamic state with increased cardiac output (CO)

(in spite of depressed myocardial contractility) and decreased SVR. Besides the treatment of the septic focus with antibiotics and surgery if needed, therapy is mainly supportive. This would include adequate fluid resuscitation and pressors to maintain MAP within acceptable limits. Recent studies have shown the administration of human recombinant activated protein C (brand name XIGRIS), an inhibitor of coagulation, improves outcome from sepsis. A full discussion of sepsis is beyond the scope of this chapter.

For this patient, the first step should be an oriented physical examination, to gather elements suggesting one of the above diagnoses. The most likely causes of hypotension in this case are hypovolemia due to bleeding or third-spacing, sepsis, or myocardial ischemia. In the absence of a presentation suggesting cardiogenic shock, fluid and/or blood administration is appropriate. At the same time, more diagnostic data should be obtained from a 12-lead electrocardiogram (ECG), invasive hemodynamic monitoring, and possibly an echocardiogram. Vasopressors can be used with caution pending restoration of intravascular volume.

In spite of the result of meta-analyses suggesting that colloid administration might lead to poor outcomes, no broad consensus has emerged as to the best type of fluid to use for fluid resuscitation.

5. A pulmonary artery catheter (PAC) was inserted. For each etiology of shock described above, in which direction would the main hemodynamic parameters be changed?

The changes are summarized in Table 81.1. Cardiac tamponade typically presents with "equalization of pressures": the central venous pressure (CVP), right ventricular diastolic pressure, pulmonary artery diastolic pressure (PAP), and the pulmonary artery occlusion pressure (PAOP) are equal and usually approximately 20 mmHg.

6. What is the classification of hemorrhage according to the American College of Surgeons? Is it a good guide for deciding whether to transfuse a patient?

The American College of Surgeons' classification distinguishes four categories according to the importance of blood loss and the resulting clinical changes. It is presented in Table 81.2.

While this classification is helpful in estimating the severity of hypovolemia, its weakness lies in that it does not distinguish between intravascular volume loss and decrease in oxygen-carrying capacity. The need for transfusion should be based on clinical judgment and depends, among other things, on the patient's hematocrit before the blood loss occurred and after crystalloid or colloid

TABLE 81.1	Changes in Hemodynamic Parameters According to the Etiology of Shock					
Etiology of Shock	**CVP**	**PAP**	**PAOP**	**CO**	**SVR**	**SvO$_2$**
Hypovolemic	↓	↓	↓	↓	↑	↓
Cardiogenic						
Left ventricular	=/↑	=/↑	↑	↓	↑	↓
Right ventricular	↑	↓/↑[a]	=/↓	↓	↑	↓
Distributive						
Septic (hyperdynamic)	=/↓	=/↓	=/↓	↑	↓	=/↑
Anaphylactic	↓	↓	↓	=/↑	↓	↓
Neurogenic	↓	↓	↓	=	↓	↓
Obstructive						
Tamponade	↑	↑	↑	↓	↑	↓
Massive pulmonary embolism	↑	↑	=/↓	↓	↑	↓

↑, increased; ↓, decreased; =, unchanged.

[a]Depending on the etiology of RV failure: failure due to RV infarction will lead to low PAP, while failure due to pulmonary hypertension will present with high PAP.

administration, and on whether control of bleeding is achieved.

7. The heart rate suddenly goes up to 170 beats per minute with wide QRS complexes and the blood pressure drops further. What are the diagnostic possibilities?

Tachycardia may be supraventricular or ventricular in origin. Assuming p waves cannot be seen and the easy diagnosis of an atrial tachycardia therefore excluded, it is imperative to differentiate supraventricular dysrhythmias, which are usually easily treated and relatively benign, from ventricular dysrhythmias, which are life-threatening and require immediate intervention.

Any wide-complex dysrhythmia (QRS>0.12 second) should generally be assumed to be ventricular tachycardia until proven otherwise. Further criteria suggestive of ventricular tachycardia are the presence of atrioventricular dissociation, fusion beats, left axis deviation, right bundle branch pattern with a QRS>0.14 second, or a left bundle branch pattern with a QRS>0.16 second.

Supraventricular rhythm diagnosis rests on the determination of the rate, regularity, and the observation of p waves. Sinus tachycardia has identical-appearing p waves, a regular rate, and a fixed PR interval. The diagnosis of sinus tachycardia is less likely as the rate exceeds 150 beats per minute (bpm), especially in the elderly patient. Atrial fibrillation is an irregularly irregular rhythm without recognizable p waves, and the ventricular response often exceeds 150 bpm. Atrial flutter is more difficult to diagnose

than atrial fibrillation. It often presents with a rate of exactly 150 bpm and a sawtooth baseline on ECG. Multifocal atrial tachycardia is a common rhythm in patients with underlying pulmonary disease and presents with at least three different p wave morphologies preceding QRS complexes. Re-entry tachycardia has p waves hidden in the QRS complex and may often present with a rate of 150 bpm or greater. Administration of adenosine (6–12 mg intravenous push) will temporarily slow most supraventricular tachycardias. Although the dysrhythmia might quickly recur, diagnosis will be facilitated.

8. What are the treatment options for each of the discussed dysrhythmias? What would you do for this patient?

Complete discussion of all the treatment options for every dysrhythmia is beyond the scope of this discussion.

Sinus tachycardia should be treated by identification and correction of the underlying cause (e.g., hypovolemia, hypoxemia, anemia, pain, side-effect of medication). In the absence of a treatable cause in a patient at risk for developing ischemia from the tachycardia, a trial of β-blocker administration may be warranted. A short-acting agent such as esmolol should be used so that the therapy may be rapidly stopped if side-effects, such as hypotension, supervene.

In patients who develop new-onset atrial fibrillation or flutter complicated by significant hypotension, congestive heart failure, or ischemia, *synchronized* cardioversion starting at 100 joules (J) (50 for flutter) is the therapy of choice.

Supraventricular Dysrhythmias

Ventricular tachycardia
    QRS>0.12 second
    Atrioventricular dissociation
    Fusion beats
    Left axis deviation
    Right bundle branch block with
        QRS >0.14 second
    Left bundle branch block with
        QRS >0.16 second

Sinus tachycardia
    Identical p wave morphology
    Regular rate
    Fixed PR interval
    Less likely if heart rate >150 bpm

Atrial fibrillation
    Irregular rhythm
    Unrecognizable p waves
    Ventricular response >150 bpm

Atrial flutter
    Rate 150 bpm
    Sawtooth baseline on ECG

Multifocal atrial tachycardia
    Three different p wave morphologies

Re-entry tachycardia
    p wave in QRS complex
    Rate ≥150 bpm

In the absence of such life-threatening side-effects, chemical conversion to sinus rhythm may be accomplished with:

- β-*Blockers*: Metoprolol 5 mg intravenously (IV), repeat q5 min up to 25 mg.
- *Calcium-channel blockers:* Diltiazem, 5–10 mg IV q5 min up to 30 mg, is usually preferred over verapamil, 5 mg IV, because it is less of a negative inotrope.
- *Amiodarone:* load with 150 mg IV over 10 minutes, then 1 mg/min IV for 6 hours followed by 0.5 mg/min for 18 hours.
- *Digoxin:* 0.5 mg IV, then 0.25 mg IV q6h × 2; additional 0.25 mg doses can be given if the rate is not controlled. It is effective in controlling the rate, but equivalent to placebo for conversion to sinus rhythm. Digoxin will generally require a minimum of 30 minutes to have an effect but it is hemodynamically well tolerated. The other agents will act within minutes of administration but may cause hypotension.

Re-entry ("paroxysmal supraventricular") tachycardia is treated like atrial flutter but will more often convert to sinus rhythm when treated with intravenous diltiazem. Intravenous adenosine (6 mg IV push, then 12 mg up to 2 times) may also be used, but because of its very short half-life, the rhythm may quickly revert to the re-entry tachycardia.

Multifocal atrial tachycardia usually results from a primary respiratory problem such as decompensated chronic obstructive pulmonary disease. Treatment should be aimed at the underlying cause, most often hypoxemia and/or hypokalemia, although rate control can sometimes be achieved by administration of intravenous diltiazem or β-blockers.

TABLE 81.2   **Classification of Hemorrhage into Four Categories According to the American College of Surgeons**

	I	II	III	IV
Blood loss (mL)	≤750	750–1,500	1,500–2,000	≥2000
Blood loss (% blood volume)	≤15	15–30	30–40	≥40
Heart rate (beats/min)	<100	>100	>120	≥140
Blood pressure	Normal	Normal	Decreased	Decreased
Pulse pressure	Normal/increased	Decreased	Decreased	Decreased
Capillary refill	Normal	Delayed	Delayed	Delayed
Respiratory rate (breaths/min)	14–20	20–30	30–40	>35
Urine output (mL/hr)	≥30	20–30	5–10	Negligible
Mental status	Slightly anxious	Mildly anxious	Anxious, confused	Confused, lethargic
Fluid replacement	Crystalloid	Crystalloid	Crystalloid + blood	Crystalloid + blood

Reproduced with permission from American College of Surgeons' Committee on Trauma, Advanced Trauma life support® for Doctors, Student Course Manual, 6th Edition, Chicago American College of Surgeons, 1997, page 98.

Treatment Options for Supraventricular Tachycardias

Ventricular tachycardia
    Unstable: Cardioversion
    Stable: Amiodarone

Sinus tachycardia
    Treat underlying cause
    ? β-Blockers in the presence of myocardial
        ischemia

Atrial fibrillation/flutter (new onset)
    Unstable: Synchronized cardioversion
    Stable: β-Blockers
        Calcium-channel blockers
        Amiodarone
        Digoxin

Multifocal atrial tachycardia
    Treat underlying pulmonary disease
    Treat hypokalemia
    Diltiazem
    β-Blockers

Re-entry tachycardia
    Diltiazem
    Adenosine

Unstable patients with ventricular tachycardia should immediately be cardioverted (start with 100 Joules), whereas stable patients should be given intravenous amiodarone (150 mg IV infusion over 10 minutes). Wide complex dysrhythmias that cannot be clearly identified as aberrantly conducted supraventricular dysrhythmias should not be treated with calcium-channel blockers because these can lead to intractable cardiac arrest if given to patients with ventricular tachycardia. In this context, adenosine given for diagnostic purposes is no longer recommended. Untreated ventricular tachycardia will usually deteriorate into ventricular fibrillation, which should be immediately treated with DC defibrillation starting with 200 Joules. If a defibrillator is not immediately available, a precordial thump can be used in an attempt to restore sinus rhythm. If this fails, cardiopulmonary resuscitation (CPR) should be initiated until defibrillation is possible.

In this patient's case, the main diagnoses are ventricular tachycardia, aberrantly conducted atrial fibrillation with rapid ventricular response, or paroxysmal supraventricular tachycardia. Since the dysrhythmia is poorly tolerated, immediate *synchronized* cardioversion should be attempted, starting with 100 J and increasing to 200, 300, then 360 J if needed. Amiodarone is probably the drug of choice to prevent recurrence, since it will be effective both on ventricular tachycardia and on supraventricular dysrhythmias.

Most defibrillators automatically revert to the nonsynchronized mode after a synchronized shock is delivered, in order to permit immediate defibrillation should ventricular fibrillation result. One should not forget to select the synchronized mode again if the original dysrhythmia persists or recurs, in order to prevent "R on T" phenomenon leading to ventricular fibrillation.

Remember to avoid calcium-channel blockers (as well as adenosine) in patients with pre-excitation syndromes such as Wolff-Parkinson-White syndrome who develop atrial fibrillation, because of the risk of increased conduction through the accessory pathway causing ventricular fibrillation.

SUGGESTED READINGS

American College of Surgeons' Committee on Trauma. Life Support for Doctors, Student Course Manual, 6th Edition. American College of Surgeons, Chicago, 1997

Atlee JL: Perioperative cardiac dysrhythmias: diagnosis and management. Anesthesiology 86:1397–1424, 1997

Bunn F, Alderson P, Hawkins V: Colloid solutions for fluid resuscitation (Cochrane Review). Cochrane Database Syst Rev 2:CD001319, 2001

Carcillo JA, Cunnion RE: Septic shock. Crit Care Clin 13:553–574, 1997

Hasdai D, Topol EJ, Califf RM, et al.: Cardiogenic shock complicating acute coronary syndromes. Lancet 356:749–756, 2000

Jimenez EJ: Shock. pp. 359–387. In Civetta JM (ed): Critical Care, 3rd edition. Lippincott-Raven, Philadelphia, 1997

Wilkes MM, Navickis RJ: Patient survival after human albumin administration. A meta-analysis of randomized, controlled trials. Ann Intern Med 135:149–164, 2001

82

BRADYCARDIA AND HYPERTENSION

Andrew B. Leibowitz, MD

Arthur Atchabahian, MD

A 33-year-old man with a frontal meningioma underwent an uneventful resection. In the postanesthesia care unit he experiences a rise in blood pressure to 210/130 mmHg and a fall in heart rate to 35 beats per minute.

QUESTIONS

1. What is the differential diagnosis of bradycardia? What is the treatment for the different types of bradycardia?
2. What is the differential diagnosis of postoperative hypertension?
3. What intravenous agents may be administered to treat hypertension?

1. What is the differential diagnosis of bradycardia? What is the treatment for the different types of bradycardia?

Bradycardia is said to exist when the heart rate is less than 60 beats per minute. Bradydysrhythmias are usually noncardiogenic in etiology, reflecting stimuli such as increased vagal tone, drug side-effects, hypoxemia, and hypercarbia. The bradycardia may be either a sinus bradycardia, which is almost always benign, junctional rhythm, or second- and third-degree atrioventricular blocks,

which require a greater sophistication in diagnosis and management.

Sinus bradycardia is usually well tolerated in the absence of hypovolemia, systemic vasodilation and myocardial hypocontractility. The treatment for sinus bradycardia is directed at removing the cause. Surgical stimulation that results in increased vagal tone, such as the oculocardiac reflex or peritoneal traction, should be stopped. Medications that cause bradycardia, such as phenylephrine and fentanyl, should be replaced by alternative drugs or combined with a vagolytic drug (e.g., pancuronium). In the event that removing the stimulus cannot be accomplished or is ineffective and there is a direct hemodynamic consequence of the bradycardia, atropine 0.4–1.0 mg intravenously (IV) or glycopyrrolate in increments of 0.2 mg IV may be administered. Glycopyrrolate may be preferable because it is longer acting and is less likely to induce severe tachycardia. If necessary, a dopamine infusion of 5–10 μg/kg/min can be used to increase the heart rate. Isoproterenol is now rarely used because of the concomitant potent vasodilation that can lead to severe hypotension. As a last resort, transcutaneous or transvenous pacing may be required.

Junctional rhythms are due to decreased automaticity of or damage to the sinus node. Cells further down the pathway leading to the bundle of His take over but with a lower heart rate. The p waves on electrocardiogram (ECG) are morphologically different from those seen on an ECG recorded when the patient was in sinus rhythm. Depending on the level of escape focus, the PR interval can be shortened or the p waves can be seen within the QRS complex. Junctional rhythms are often seen with volatile anesthetics, especially halothane, and after cardiac surgery. They are usually benign and well tolerated, unless the loss of atrial "kick" leads to a significant decrease in cardiac output, as in patients with diastolic dysfunction and impaired ventricular filling. Atropine or dopamine can be used to restore sinus node activity. If this fails, atrial or atrioventricular (AV) pacing may be necessary.

Second-degree AV block may be further classified into two major groups. Mobitz I (Wenckenbach) block is characterized by a progressive increase in the PR interval resulting in a periodic failure to transmit the atrial impulse. The cause is usually an intrinsic heart disease involving the AV node or digitalis toxicity. Because the AV node is usually supplied by the right coronary artery, this dysrhythmia commonly complicates inferior wall myocardial infarctions. It is usually a benign and self-limited problem rarely requiring treatment. Mobitz II AV block originates below the AV node and is characterized by a failure of atrial depolarization to conduct. This failure to conduct may occur in an unpredictable manner or in a manner characterized by the "dropping" of every other or every third beat, respectively termed 2:1 and 3:1 block. Importantly, the PR interval for the conducted beats remains constant. Progression to complete heart block is frequent and pacemaker insertion is usually necessary.

Third-degree block is almost always pathologic and is characterized by a dissociation of the atrial depolarization and ventricular response. Blockage may occur within or below the AV node. Blockage within the node will present with narrow complex junctional rhythm usually at a rate of 40–60 beats per minute. Blockage below the node, so-called infranodal block, will present with a wide complex rhythm usually at a rate of 30–45 beats per minute. Treatment will entail transcutaneous or transvenous pacing when there is hemodynamic compromise. Blockage within the AV node may be transient and, with close observation, permanent pacemaker placement may not be necessary.

2. What is the differential diagnosis of postoperative hypertension?

Postoperative hypertension is an extremely common finding, even in patients with no previous history of hypertension. The most common cause is pain. The blood pressure should normalize as pain is controlled with analgesics. Other common causes include: (1) a full urinary bladder, which should be suspected after any prolonged procedure or administration of large amounts of intravenous fluids in a patient without a bladder catheter, (2) respiratory distress, especially when there is hypercapnia, (3) head and neck or carotid artery surgery, with carotid sinus denervation, and (4) cyclosporin or tacrolimus administration in patients undergoing transplantation. Of course, a previous history of hypertension should always be taken into account, especially if the patient did not take their antihypertensive medication(s) on the day of surgery.

The presence of a combined bradycardia and hypertension in a patient who had a craniotomy leads one to suspect a primary neurologic event causing what is known as the Cushing response or Cushing's triad. This consists of an increase in systemic blood pressure, a reflex bradycardia, and bradypnea, and occurs when there is an elevation in intracranial pressure. In this situation, hypertension should not be aggressively treated because it is a compensatory mechanism in an attempt to maintain cerebral perfusion pressure. Rather, measures should be taken to control intracranial pressure (head elevation, mannitol, hyperventilation, possibly cerebrospinal fluid drainage after neurosurgical consultation). Diagnostic imaging

---

Differential Diagnosis and Treatment of Bradycardia

Sinus bradycardia
    Stop the stimulus
    Anticholinergics: atropine or glycopyrrolate
    Dopamine
    Cardiac pacing

Junctional rhythm
    Atropine
    Dopamine
    Atrial or atrioventricular pacing

Heart block—second or third degree
    Cardiac pacing (Mobitz II)

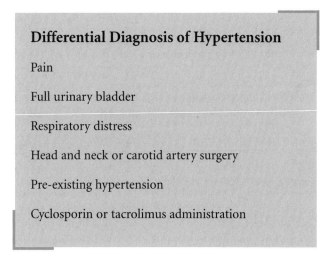

Differential Diagnosis of Hypertension

Pain

Full urinary bladder

Respiratory distress

Head and neck or carotid artery surgery

Pre-existing hypertension

Cyclosporin or tacrolimus administration

| TABLE 82.1 | The Most Common Intravenous Agents Used to Treat Hypertension | | |

Agent	Class	Dose	Comments
Propranolol (Inderal)	β-Adrenergic antagonist, nonselective	0.25–1.0 mg IVP	
Esmolol (Brevibloc)	β-Adrenergic antagonist, selective β_1	0.25–0.5 mg/kg IV load, then 50–200 µg/kg/min	The half-life of esmolol is 9 minutes. It is eliminated by red blood cell esterase
Labetalol (Trandate)	α- and β-adrenergic antagonist	Start with 5–10 mg IVP, up to 100 mg IVP 1–2 mg/min IV infusion	Ratio of β- to α-blockade of 7:1 when given IV and 3:1 when given PO
Phentolamine (Regitine)	α-Adrenergic antagonist	5 mg IVP	Used almost exclusively in patients with pheochromocytoma Treatment of extravasation of norepinephrine or dopamine: 5–10 mg diluted in 10 mL of normal saline infiltrated into the area of extravasation within 12 hours
Hydralazine (Apresoline)	Direct arterial vasodilator	Start with 5 mg IVP, repeat up to 20 mg	Peak effect may occur after 20 minutes Do not administer more frequently to avoid severe hypotension
Enalaprilat (Vasotec)	ACE inhibitor	Start with 1.25 mg IVP, up to 5 mg IVP q 6 hours	Enalaprilat is contraindicated during pregnancy ACE inhibitors may have no effect in certain patients
Nicardipine (Cardene)	Calcium-channel blocker	Start with 5 mg/hr IV infusion; increase as needed by 2.5 mg/hr every 15 minutes up to 15 mg/hr	Ongoing dose adjustment may be necessary since only 50% of the blood pressure decrease is achieved after 45 minutes
Nitroglycerin	Direct venous vasodilator	Start with 0.25–0.5 µg/kg/min IV infusion, up to 200 µg	The main effect is a decrease in preload. Very high doses, with which arterial dilation occurs, may be needed to control blood pressure
Sodium nitroprusside (Nipride)	Direct arterial and venous vasodilator	Start with 0.5–1.0 µg/kg/min IV infusion, up to 10 µg/kg/min	Sodium nitroprusside is contraindicated during pregnancy There is a potential for severe hypotension. Invasive blood pressure monitoring is necessary Risk of cyanide toxicity. Do not administer more than 1 mg/kg over a 2.5-hour period

should be obtained to delineate the need for neurosurgical intervention.

3. What intravenous agents may be administered to treat hypertension?

The most common intravenous medications used to acutely treat hypertension are compared in Table 82.1. As a general rule, vasodilators are best avoided in tachycardic patients, who might instead benefit from adrenergic blockade. Combining a β-blocker and a vasodilator can be very effective in lowering blood pressure.

SUGGESTED READINGS

Atlee JL: Perioperative cardiac dysrhythmias: diagnosis and management. Anesthesiology 86:1397–1424, 1997

Plets C: Arterial hypertension in neurosurgical emergencies. Am J Cardiol 63:40C–42C, 1989 (Good description of the Cushing response. The therapeutic recommendations, however, are outdated)

83

HYPOTHERMIA

Andrew B. Leibowitz, MD

Arthur Atchabahian, MD

A 69-year-old man underwent a cystectomy and ileal conduit complicated by hypothermia. He is brought to the recovery room with a temperature of 32°C.

QUESTIONS

1. How is hypothermia defined and graded?
2. What mechanisms lead to hypothermia in a patient under general anesthesia in the operating room?
3. What are the physiologic responses to hypothermia?
4. What are the physiologic consequences of hypothermia?
5. Are there any benefits to mild intraoperative hypothermia?
6. Where are the different sites at which temperature can be monitored?
7. What are the modalities to prevent and treat perioperative hypothermia?
8. Is prevention of hypothermia warranted in a patient who received a central neuraxial block?

1. How is hypothermia defined and graded?

Hypothermia is defined as a core body temperature less than 35°C. It is often further characterized as mild (32–35°C), moderate (28–32°C), or severe (less than 28°C).

2. What mechanisms lead to hypothermia in a patient under general anesthesia in the operating room?

In the first phase, the main mechanism is redistribution hypothermia. The core temperature decreases by 0.5–1.5°C during the first hour after induction of general anesthesia due to redistribution from the core to the periphery.

In the second phase, which lasts for 2–3 hours, heat loss exceeds metabolic heat production, which is decreased by about 20% after induction of general anesthesia.

Heat loss is multifactorial: 60% by radiation, 20% by evaporation (humidification of inspired gases and fluid loss from the surgical field, especially if the abdomen or thorax is opened), 5% by conduction (contact with the operating room table), and 15% by convection (warming of air flowing over the skin).

The core temperature will plateau after 3–4 hours because of peripheral vasoconstriction triggered by a core temperature of 33–35°C, while the peripheral temperature will continue to drop.

In other settings, hypothermia can be the result of loss of central thermoregulation (e.g., stroke, head trauma, or spinal cord injury), drug-related (e.g., alcohol or barbiturate overdose), or secondary to metabolic changes (e.g., hypoglycemia, hypothyroidism, sepsis, burns, or hepatic failure).

3. What are the physiologic responses to hypothermia?

Vasoconstriction

Vasoconstriction occurs secondary to sympathetic stimulation. Volatile agents reduce the threshold for vasoconstriction by 2–4°C. It is about 1°C lower in patients 60–80 years old than in patients 30–50 years old. Vasoconstriction is more or less an "on-off" response.

Shivering

The threshold for shivering is decreased by general anesthetics even more than that for vasoconstriction. Two types of shivering are described. One type is a tonic pattern, resembling normal shivering, with a 4–8 cycles per minute waxing-and-waning component. The second is a phasic, 5–7 Hz bursting pattern resembling clonus, which is specific to the postanesthesia care unit (PACU). This latter type of shivering is secondary to volatile anesthetics and probably results from anesthetic-induced disinhibition of normal descending control over spinal reflexes. Shivering can increase the oxygen consumption by 300–500%, thus leading to myocardial ischemia in susceptible patients. It can also increase the serum potassium level.

Nonshivering Thermogenesis

Nonshivering thermogenesis can double the metabolic heat production in infants but it plays an unimportant role in adults. It is inhibited by general anesthesia.

4. What are the physiologic consequences of hypothermia?

The physiologic consequences of hypothermia are summarized in Table 83.1.

Electrocardiogram (ECG) changes occur as well and include sinus bradycardia, widened PR interval, widened QRS, and prolonged QT. The Osborn wave is characteristic for hypothermia. This wave is a deflection at the J point (the junction between the QRS complex and the ST segment) in the same direction as that of the QRS complex, with a height proportional to the degree of hypothermia.

Deleterious clinical consequences have been documented:

- Impaired coagulation has been shown to lead to higher transfusion requirements in patients undergoing total hip replacement.
- The incidence of wound infection is increased because of a direct impairment of the immune function and a decrease in oxygen delivery to the tissues.
- The incidence of postoperative myocardial infarction and ventricular dysrhythmias is increased.

- Duration of hospitalization was increased in patients who developed hypothermia during surgery and anesthesia.

The current recommendation is to maintain the temperature at or above 36°C in order to avoid these adverse outcomes. Hypothermic patients, especially those with coronary artery disease, might benefit from maintaining anesthesia into the postoperative period until they have been rewarmed, rather than being awakened at the conclusion of surgery.

5. Are there any benefits to mild intraoperative hypothermia?

Mild intraoperative hypothermia seems to protect against cerebral hypoxia and ischemia, not only by a reduction in metabolic rate but maybe also by a decrease in excitatory neurotransmitters. While many neuroanesthesiologists would consider mild hypothermia during craniotomy as a standard of care, conclusive evidence is still lacking.

6. What are the different sites at which temperature can be monitored?

Temperature may be monitored via the oral, rectal, esophageal, nasopharyngeal, and tympanic membrane sites. It can also be monitored via a pulmonary artery catheter (PAC) or a urinary bladder catheter. With the exception of the oral route, all other methods provide a generally accurate and reproducible measurement of the core temperature in the general surgical patient. However, in the patient undergoing hypothermic cardiopulmonary bypass, significant gradients can exist between core, blood, and peripheral temperatures. Blood temperature, as measured by the PAC, reflects the temperature of the blood coming from the heart-lung machine, with core temperature (esophageal, nasopharyngeal, tympanic) lagging somewhat behind, and envelope temperature (rectal) taking even more time to equilibrate during both cooling and rewarming. Bladder catheter measurements should reflect peripheral temperature, but with high urine flows they are more likely to closely reflect blood temperature.

7. What are the modalities to prevent and treat perioperative hypothermia?

- *Redistribution* is best prevented by initiating skin warming before induction.
- *Radiation* heat loss is proportional to the fourth power of the difference between the absolute temperatures of the surfaces and can be limited by increasing the room temperature. Radiant warmers are only used for infants, facilitate keeping the patient warm while still visible, and preclude the need to increase the room temperature.

| **TABLE 83.1** | **Physiologic Consequences of Hypothermia** |

Factor	Effect	Comment
Oxygen and CO_2 solubility	Increased	pH increases by 0.015 per 1°C
Volatile anesthetic solubility	Increased	
MAC	Decreased	This can lead to delayed awakening and postoperative confusion
Cardiac output	Decreased	Blood flow is first decreased to muscle, then kidneys and gut, and eventually to brain and heart
Speed of induction	Unchanged	Since both MAC and cardiac output are decreased, speed of induction is unchanged
Oxygen consumption and CO_2 production	Decreased	Decreased by 7–9% per 1°C
$PaCO_2$	Decreased	Decreased by 1.5% by 1°C, i.e., the $PaCO_2$ equals the temperature in °C
Plasma catecholamines	Increased	This leads to hypertension, tachycardia, and hyperglycemia
Plasma insulin	Decreased	Glycogenolysis and neoglucogenesis are activated, leading to hyperglycemia
Affinity of hemoglobin for oxygen	Increased	Increased by 6% per 1°C
Hypoxic ventilatory drive	Depressed	Ventilation is essentially driven by hypercarbia
Bronchomotor tone	Decreased	Anatomic dead space is increased
Hypoxic pulmonary vasoconstriction	Decreased	Ventilation/perfusion mismatch is worsened
Threshold for ventricular fibrillation	Decreased	The risk of ventricular fibrillation becomes significant below 32°C
Systemic vascular resistance (SVR) and pulmonary vascular resistance (PVR)	Increased	However, coronary artery resistance seems to decrease
Hepatic blood flow	Decreased	The decrease is proportional to the decrease in cardiac output
Renal blood flow	Decreased	Renal blood flow decreases proportionately more than cardiac output
Diluting and concentrating capacity	Decreased	This "cold diuresis" can lead to hypovolemia and hemoconcentration
Tubular transport of sodium, chloride, water, and potassium		
Blood viscosity	Increased	Increased by 2–3% per 1°C
Coagulation	Impaired	Circulating factors are decreased and platelets are sequestered in the portal circulation
Platelet function	Impaired	Platelet dysfunction is related to local temperature (skin, surgical field) rather than core temperature
Urinary nitrogen excretion	Increased	Urinary nitrogen excretion remains high for several days postoperatively
Drug metabolism	Decreased	The effect of drugs such as vecuronium or propofol is prolonged

However, radiant warmers become less effective as the distance to the patient increases. In addition, they do not decrease convection heat loss.

- *Gas and fluid heating* have limited efficacy. Less than 10% of the heat loss is via respiration. Fluid warming should be used if a large volume of fluid is administered. One liter of crystalloid at room temperature or one unit (250 mL) of refrigerated blood will decrease the temperature by about 0.25°C.
- *Insulation* will decrease heat loss by only 30% with one layer of fabric (sheet or blanket), with little additional benefit from additional layers.

- Overall, *forced-air warming* (e.g., Bair Hugger blankets) is the most effective warming and rewarming method. It is more effective when patients are vasodilated. It is, therefore, better to maintain normothermia from the start of the procedure rather than to rewarm postoperatively. Rewarming a vasoconstricted patient can lead to hypotension secondary to vasodilation if the volume status is not maintained.
- *Circulating-water mattresses* placed on the operating room table have little efficacy, since 90% of the heat is lost from the surface of the body that is exposed and is not in contact with the table.

- *Never use hot-water bottles*! They are the leading cause of perioperative thermal injury according to the ASA Closed-Claims database.
- *Shivering* can be treated by skin-surface warming (core hypothermia is better tolerated before response mechanisms are activated when cutaneous warm inputs are increased) and/or pharmacologically, with either meperidine 12.5–25 mg intravenously or clonidine 75–150 µg intravenously. The mechanism of action of meperidine is unclear and may be due to kappa receptor activation. The mechanism of action of clonidine is a decrease in vasoconstriction and shivering thresholds.

8. Is prevention of hypothermia warranted in a patient who received a central neuraxial block?

Yes. In a patient with a neuraxial block, the area blocked is vasodilated and autoregulation is lost. Shivering is precluded if a motor block is present. Central control is impaired as well, owing to the incorrect perception by the central nervous system that the skin temperature is elevated in the blocked area. Significant hypothermia can occur, leading to discomfort and shivering, although the shivering threshold is lowered.

SUGGESTED READINGS

Bremmelgaard A, Raahave D, Beir-Holgersen R, et al.: Computer-aided surveillance of surgical infections and identification of risk factors. J Hosp Infect 13:1–18, 1989

Marion DW, Penrod LE, Kelsey SF, et al.: Treatment of traumatic brain injury with moderate hypothermia. N Engl J Med 336: 540–546, 1997

Michelson AD, MacGregor H, Barnard MR, et al.: Reversible inhibition of human platelet activation by hypothermia in vivo and in vitro. Thromb Haemost 71:633–640, 1994

Schmied H, Kurz A, Sessler DI, et al.: Mild intraoperative hypothermia increases blood loss and allogeneic transfusion requirements during total hip arthroplasty. Lancet 347:289–292, 1996

Sessler DI: Perioperative heat balance. Anesthesiology 92: 578–596, 2000

84

CASE

POSTANESTHESIA CARE
UNIT DISCHARGE
CRITERIA

Andrew B. Leibowitz, MD

Arthur Atchabahian, MD

A 32-year-old woman underwent an uneventful diagnostic laparoscopy under general anesthesia. In the postanesthesia care unit she is complaining of severe nausea and vomiting. She wants to be discharged home.

QUESTIONS

1. What is the cause of nausea and vomiting?
2. What are the risk factors for postoperative nausea and vomiting (PONV)?
3. What is the incidence and importance of nausea and vomiting after anesthesia and surgery?
4. What are the treatment options available for PONV?
5. What are the main complications occurring in the postanesthesia care unit (PACU)?
6. What are the discharge criteria for the PACU?

1. What is the cause of nausea and vomiting?

The vomiting center is located in the medulla and receives input from the chemoreceptor zone and the gastrointestinal tract. The vomiting center may be activated by a variety of stimuli including medications, body motion, stimulation of the posterior pharynx, odors, and visual images.

2. What are the risk factors for postoperative nausea and vomiting (PONV)?

Contributing factors to a higher incidence of PONV are young age, female gender, large body habitus, history of motion sickness or previous PONV, anxiety, and concomitant disease.

There is no evidence that any anesthetic technique or drug regimen results in a lower incidence of postoperative nausea and vomiting, except for propofol, which has intrinsic antiemetic properties. There is, however, little benefit if propofol is used only as an induction agent. Conflicting evidence exists regarding nitrous oxide. Similarly, claims of an increased incidence of PONV with higher opioid doses are questionable, and the incidence of PONV appears to be similar with different opioids.

The procedure performed has a major influence on the incidence of PONV, with the highest incidence in patients undergoing laparoscopic surgery or head and neck surgery involving the oropharynx, inner ear, or eyes (especially strabismus correction). A longer duration of the surgical procedure is also associated with a higher risk of PONV.

3. What is the incidence and importance of nausea and vomiting after anesthesia and surgery?

PONV is the most common postoperative complication and the leading reason for delayed discharge from the PACU. In one review of 8,995 pediatric outpatient cases,

26 patients required admission for persistent nausea and vomiting, accounting for 36% of all unanticipated hospital admissions.

4. What are the treatment options available for PONV?

There are several medications that are commonly admin-istered either prophylactically or as direct treatment. The following five drugs will be reviewed: droperidol, 5-HT3 antagonists, metoclopramide, scopolamine, and dexamethasone.

- *Droperidol* is a pharmacologic relative of the more widely used antipsychotic drug haloperidol. It is a potent α-adrenergic antagonist. Historically, it was combined with fentanyl and used in neuroleptic anesthesia. In smaller doses, ranging from 0.25 to 2.5 mg given intravenously, it significantly decreases the incidence of PONV. When given in higher doses, it may be associated with excessive sedation and delay in discharge from the PACU. A new controversial US Food and Drug Administration (FDA) "black box" warning notes that droperidol can cause QT prolongation, has been associated with precipitating lethal arrhythmias (e.g., torsades de pointe), and should not be administered in the presence of known QT prolongation. Further, in the absence of a prolonged QT interval, patients who receive droperidol should have electrocardiogram (ECG) monitoring for 3 hours afterwards.
- *Ondansetron, dolasetron,* and *granisetron* are the only 5-HT3 antagonists currently FDA-approved for PONV. There does not seem to be any significant difference in efficacy between these two drugs. These medications are devoid of the side-effects of the other medications, but their cost is much higher. The optimal dose of ondansetron is 4 mg intravenously, but the optimal timing of administration seems unclear, with the most recent manufacturer's recommendation being that it should be administered at the time of induction. The dose of dolasetron is 12.5 mg intravenously, with the time of administration reportedly not critical. Conflicting evidence has been published regarding the efficacy of 5-HT3 antagonists versus older agents, such as droperidol. In the best of cases, a minimal benefit is seen with 5-HT3 antagonists.
- *Metoclopramide* is a methoxychlorinated derivative of procainamide and is a dopamine antagonist. The antiemetic effect results from its ability to increase acid clearance, esophageal peristaltic amplitude, lower esophageal sphincter pressure, gastric emptying, and gastric contraction rate and amplitude. It may be administered orally, intramuscularly and intravenously in doses of 10–20 mg. The most problematic side-effects are extrapyramidal reactions. Metoclopramide should not be used in epileptics or in patients taking other medications likely to cause extrapyramidal reactions.

- *Scopolamine* is an anticholinergic drug that is usually administered as a premedicant. A transdermal preparation that has been widely used to prevent motion sickness has been shown in small studies to reduce PONV without significant side-effects. Scopolamine, when administered intramuscularly or intravenously, may cause central cholinergic syndrome, which consists of sedation, amnesia, and euphoria.
- *Dexamethasone* has been found to be as effective as ondansetron in the prevention of PONV in gynecologic surgery. Most corticosteroids have antiemetic properties through a poorly understood mechanism. A dose of 2.5 mg is sufficient and appears to be free of side-effects. Moreover, dexamethasone is inexpensive. However, its effectiveness in treating established PONV has not been studied.

Non-pharmacologic therapies that have been shown to be effective include:

- Administration of supplemental oxygen ($FiO_2 > 0.3$), even if limited to the intraoperative period. This may be the result of decreased nitrous oxide administration. There are studies suggesting that an intraoperative FiO_2 of 0.8 might be as effective as ondansetron in preventing PONV in patients undergoing laparoscopic gynecologic surgery.
- Aggressive intravenous rehydration.
- Transcutaneous acupoint electrical stimulation.

Combining available therapies in a "multimodal" management of PONV has been shown to be highly effective, with vomiting rates of 0, versus 7% with ondansetron alone and 22% with placebo.

There is little difference in outcome or patient satisfaction (97% vs. 93%) between patients receiving prophylaxis and those being treated as needed in the PACU, suggesting that prophylaxis might be warranted only in high-risk patients.

Although gastric suctioning prior to the completion of the procedure will empty the stomach and theoretically reduce the incidence of nausea and vomiting, no published evidence has documented its efficacy.

5. What are the main complications occurring in the postanesthesia care unit (PACU)?

The incidence of complications in the PACU is surprisingly high. A review of over 18,000 PACU admissions in a university hospital showed an overall complication rate of 26%, the most common being PONV (9.8%). Other complications are the need for airway support (6.9%), hypotension (2.7%), dysrhythmias (1.4%), hypertension (1.1%), altered mental status (0.6%), rule-out myocardial infarction (0.3%), and major cardiac events (0.3%). Another review of 120 incidents occurring in the PACU found that two-thirds were related to respiratory complications.

6. What are the discharge criteria for discharge from the PACU?

Discharge of patients to home after surgery and anesthesia is safest when predetermined discharge criteria are rigorously applied to all patients. Although criteria may vary somewhat from center to center, the following summarizes what is typically done on discharge.

Examination

1. Stable vital signs for at least 30 minutes and consistent with the patient's age and preanesthetic examination.
2. Ability to swallow and cough.
3. Ability to walk or return to preoperative status.
4. Minimal nausea, vomiting, and dizziness allowing for the ability to swallow and retain liquids and to ambulate.
5. Absence of any respiratory distress.
6. Alert and oriented.
7. No surgical contraindication to discharge (e.g., excessive pain, bleeding, etc.).

Instructions to the Patient

1. You may experience sleepiness or fatigue and should not drive, operate machinery, or make any complex decisions until tomorrow.
2. You may have a sore throat and should gargle with dilute salt water or take acetaminophen.
3. You may experience muscular soreness that may also be treated with acetaminophen (this is more likely if succinylcholine has been administered).
4. In case of any unforeseen emergent problem, call … [provide an emergency telephone number to contact].
5. An adult escort has to accompany you home. (Availability of an escort should be ascertained prior to starting surgery.)

Follow-up

1. A member of the anesthesia care team should call the patient the day after surgery and confirm that there are no complaints and that their recovery is as expected.

SUGGESTED READINGS

Gan TJ: Postoperative nausea and vomiting—can it be eliminated? JAMA 287:1233–1236, 2002

Goll V, Akca O, Greif R, et al.: Ondansetron is no more effective than supplemental intraoperative oxygen for prevention of postoperative nausea and vomiting. Anesth Analg 92:112–117, 2001

Greif R, Laciny S, Rapf B, et al.: Supplemental oxygen reduces the incidence of postoperative nausea and vomiting. Anesthesiology 91:1246–1252, 1999

Hines R, Barash PG, Watrous G, et al.: Complications occurring in the postanesthesia care unit: a survey. Anesth Analg 74:503–509, 1992

Scuderi PE, James RL, Harris L, et al.: Antiemetic prophylaxis does not improve outcome following outpatient surgery when compared to symptomatic treatment. Anesthesiology 90:360–371, 1999

Scuderi PE, James RL, Harris L, et al.: Multimodal antiemetic management prevents early postoperative vomiting after outpatient laparoscopy. Anesth Analg 91:1408–1414, 2000

Van der Walt JH, Webb RK, Osborne GA, et al.: The Australian incident monitoring study: recovery room incidents in the first 200 incident reports. Anaesth Intensive Care 21:650–652, 1993

Yogendran S, Asokumar B, Cheng DC, et al.: A prospective randomized double-blinded study of the effect of intravenous fluid therapy on adverse outcomes on outpatient surgery. Anesth Analg 80:682–686, 1995

85

RESPIRATORY FAILURE

Arthur Atchabahian, MD

Andrew B. Leibowitz, MD

A 59-year-old woman with a history of heavy smoking, chronic obstructive pulmonary disease (COPD), and type 2 diabetes mellitus has undergone resection of a thoraco-abdominal aortic aneurysm through a left thoracotomy and abdominal approach. At the end of the procedure, the double-lumen endotracheal tube was changed to a single-lumen tube, but airway visualization was difficult and the patient might have aspirated gastric contents. She is brought to the postanesthesia care unit (PACU) because of the lack of available space in the surgical intensive care unit (SICU).

QUESTIONS

1. How is postoperative respiratory failure defined? What are the two main types of acute respiratory failure?
2. The arterial blood gas (ABG) is pH 7.35, PCO_2 37 torr, and PO_2 54 torr on control-mode ventilation (CMV) with a rate of 12 breaths per minute, a tidal volume of 650 mL, an FiO_2 of 0.5, and a positive end-expiratory pressure (PEEP) of 5 cm H_2O. Peak inspiratory pressures (PIP) are 26 cm H_2O. What are the four primary causes of hypoxemia and how are they distinguished? Which is most likely in this patient, and how would you treat it?
3. If the ABG is pH 7.26, PCO_2 66 torr, PO_2 59 torr on the same ventilator settings, how would this ABG be interpreted? What treatment should be prescribed?

4. The next day, the patient is still in the PACU. The chest radiograph shows bilateral fluffy infiltrates, and the ABG is pH 7.32, PCO_2 54 torr, and PO_2 55 torr on CMV with a respiratory rate of 14 breaths per minute, a tidal volume of 550 mL, an FiO_2 of 0.8, and a PEEP of 5 cm H_2O. A pulmonary artery catheter is inserted, showing a pulmonary artery pressure (PAP) of 54/32 mmHg, pulmonary artery occlusion pressure (PAOP) of 13 mmHg, central venous pressure (CVP) of 12 mmHg, and a cardiac output (CO) of 5.4 L/min. How would you manage this patient?
5. Briefly describe the most common ventilatory modes.
6. After several days in the SICU, the patient's respiratory status has improved. What criteria are used to determine whether extubation will be successful?

1. How is postoperative respiratory failure defined? What are the two main types of acute respiratory failure?

Postoperative respiratory failure is defined as the need for continued mechanical ventilation beyond 48 hours after surgery, or the need for reintubation and mechanical ventilation after extubation.

There are two categories of respiratory failure: hypoxemic or type I (usually with a low or normal PCO_2) and hypercapnic or type II. Hypoxemia is discussed in detail in the next section. Hypercapnia is caused by either ineffective minute ventilation or, much less commonly, excessive carbon dioxide (CO_2) production (e.g., malignant hyperthermia or overzealous carbohydrate feeding). Ineffective ventilation may result from a low respiratory rate (e.g., opioid effect), a low tidal volume (e.g., neuromuscular weakness or splinting from pain), or an increase in physiologic dead-space (e.g., COPD, pulmonary embolus, acute respiratory distress syndrome, or shock).

2. **The arterial blood gas (ABG) is pH 7.35, PCO_2 37 torr, and PO_2 54 torr on control-mode ventilation (CMV) with a rate of 12 breaths per minute, a tidal volume of 650 mL, an FiO_2 of 0.5, and a positive end-expiratory pressure (PEEP) of 5 cm H_2O. Peak inspiratory pressures (PIP) are 26 cm H_2O. What are the four primary causes of hypoxemia and how are they distinguished? Which is most likely in this patient, and how would you treat it?**

The four primary causes of hypoxemia are hypoventilation, shunt, ventilation/perfusion ($\dot{V}/\dot{Q}$) mismatch, and diffusion impairment.

Hypoventilation

Hypoventilation means that there is a reduction in fresh gas flow to the alveoli such as is seen in a circuit disconnect. The hallmark feature is an increased arterial PCO_2. Two basic equations relate to this condition:

$$PCO_2 = \frac{\dot{V}CO_2}{V_A} \times k \tag{1}$$

where $\dot{V}CO_2$ is the CO_2 produced, V_A is the alveolar ventilation, and k is a constant equal to 0.863. This means that if the alveolar ventilation is halved, the PCO_2 doubles and vice versa.

$$PAO_2 = \left(FiO_2 \times \left[P_{atm} - P_{H_2O}\right]\right) - \frac{PaCO_2}{RQ}$$
(alveolar gas equation) (2)

where PAO_2 is the alveolar partial pressure of oxygen, P_{atm} is the atmospheric pressure, usually 760 mmHg at sea level (but in the low 600s in Denver, Colorado), P_{H_2O} is the saturated pressure of water at 37°C (47 mmHg), and RQ is the respiratory quotient, between 0.7 and 1.0 depending on the carbohydrate/lipid ratio in the diet (usually a value of 0.8 is used). This equation predicts that even severe hypoventilation may be overcome by administration of high FiO_2. Thus, postoperative patients with respiratory depression receiving supplemental oxygen by mask are more likely to suffer the effects of respiratory acidosis than hypoxemia.

Shunt

A shunt exists when blood passes from the venous circulation to the arterial circulation without exposure to ventilated areas of the lung. The primary feature of a significant shunt is the failure of the PO_2 to rise to normal values with the administration of oxygen. The PCO_2 is not raised because the central chemoreceptor sensitivity to a rise in the PCO_2 and hypoxemia will both act as a stimulus for greater ventilation. The degree of shunting is calculated by the shunt equation:

$$\frac{\dot{Q}_S}{\dot{Q}_T} = \frac{\left(C_c - C_a\right)}{\left(C_c - C_{\bar{v}}\right)} \tag{3}$$

where $\dot{Q}_S$ and $\dot{Q}_T$ refer to the shunt and total pulmonary blood flows, respectively, and C_c, C_a, and C_v refer to the oxygen content of pulmonary end-capillary, arterial and mixed venous blood, respectively. Blood oxygen content is calculated as follows:

$$CO_2 = \left(Hb \times SaO_2 \times 1.39\right) + \left(PO_2 \times 0.031\right) \tag{4}$$

Where Hb is the hemoglobin concentration in mg/dL, SaO_2 the oxygen saturation of hemoglobin, and PO_2 the partial pressure of oxygen. Hemoglobin concentration and oxygen saturation are thus the main determinants of blood oxygen content, with the partial pressure of oxygen playing a comparatively small role, except in special situations such as severe anemia or hyperbaric oxygen therapy.

Ventilation/perfusion mismatch

Ventilation/perfusion mismatch is the most common cause of hypoxemia and refers to the inefficient and incomplete transfer of gas because of mismatching of blood flow to ventilation. In practice, ventilation/perfusion mismatching is said to occur when hypoventilation, shunt, and diffusion defect (to be discussed next) are excluded from the differential diagnosis by studying the PCO_2 to rule out hypoventilation, the response to oxygen administration to rule out shunt, and a lack of history and radiographic findings to suggest diffusion impairment.

Diffusion impairment

Diffusion impairment implies that there is an incomplete equilibrium between the gas in the alveolus and the capillary blood because of an abnormality in the normally thin-walled and easily crossed alveolar–capillary barrier. This may occur in a variety of chronic lung diseases such as interstitial fibrosis, asbestosis, and sarcoidosis. Although diffusion capacity may be measured in a pulmonary function laboratory setting using carbon monoxide, bedside quantification of diffusion-limited hypoxemia using standard laboratory tests is impossible.

In the case of this patient, the alveolar to arterial (A–a) gradient is 256, while the PaO_2/FiO_2 ratio is 108. The most likely cause of hypoxemia is $\dot{V}/\dot{Q}$ mismatch. The PCO_2 is normal, virtually excluding hypoventilation. Shunt can be excluded if an increase in PO_2 is seen after increasing the FiO_2. Several etiologies could account for the $\dot{V}/\dot{Q}$ mismatch: pre-existing lung disease, fluid overload after an operation with major fluid shifts, aspiration pneumonitis, and atelectasis after general anesthesia with neuromuscular blockade and one-lung ventilation. Increasing the FiO_2 will help raise the PO_2, but an FiO_2 greater than 0.6 for prolonged periods of time should be avoided, if possible, because of the risk of oxygen toxicity. Increasing the PEEP, as hemodynamically tolerated, can recruit additional alveoli, reduce the shunt component, and redistribute lung water to areas that do not participate in gas exchange. Diuresis is indicated if fluid overload is clinically suspected or confirmed by invasive monitoring.

3. If the ABG is pH 7.26, PCO_2 66 torr, PO_2 59 torr on the same ventilator settings, how would this ABG be interpreted? What treatment should be prescribed?

This patient has acidemia by definition because the pH is <7.35. To determine the origin of the acidosis, especially in a patient with COPD who may have an elevated PCO_2 at baseline, it is necessary to measure the blood bicarbonate content. Caution should be exercised as the bicarbonate is usually calculated on ABG results but measured on the electrolyte panel. When the serum bicarbonate concentration is 24 mEq/L, elevation of the arterial PCO_2 by 10 mmHg results in a fall in the pH of 0.08 pH units. Normal or high bicarbonate is suggestive of respiratory acidosis with the pH decrease being caused by the increased PCO_2. In the case of this patient, an acute increase in PCO_2 by 20 mmHg (e.g., from 46 to 66) would change the pH from 7.42 to 7.26. Decreased serum bicarbonate suggests that there is a metabolic acidosis due to organic acids, such as lactic acid. However, mixed syndromes are common. Calculating the anion gap ($Na^+ - [Cl^- + HCO_3^-]$, normal 12 ± 4) can help differentiate the causes of metabolic acidosis.

Increasing the minute ventilation can treat the respiratory acidosis, keeping in mind Equation (1). In this case, both the tidal volume (since the PIP is only 26 cm H_2O) and respiratory rate can be increased. Experience with permissive hypercapnia shows that, even when the pH is allowed to decrease to values as low as 7.15, few adverse effects are seen except for obtundation (probably secondary to intracellular acidosis). Therefore, the risk of barotrauma should be carefully weighed before increasing mechanical ventilation parameters.

Metabolic acidosis requires treatment of the cause. The most common cause for metabolic acidosis in postoperative patients is lactic acidosis due to hypoperfusion. Fluid resuscitation and optimization of hemodynamics usually results in spontaneous resolution of the acidosis. Intravenous sodium bicarbonate should be used only in cases of extreme acidosis (pH <7.10) with hemodynamic instability.

4. The next day, the patient is still in the PACU. The chest radiograph shows bilateral fluffy infiltrates, and the ABG is pH 7.32, PCO_2 54 torr, and PO_2 55 torr on CMV with a respiratory rate of 14 breaths per minute, a tidal volume of 550 mL, an FiO_2 of 0.8 and a PEEP of 5 cm H_2O. A pulmonary artery catheter is inserted, showing a pulmonary artery pressure (PAP) of 54/32 mmHg, pulmonary artery occlusion pressure (PAOP) of 13 mmHg, central venous pressure (CVP) of 12 mmHg, and a cardiac output (CO) of 5.4 L/min. How would you manage this patient?

This patient presents with adult respiratory distress syndrome (ARDS). The criteria of the American-European Consensus Conference are:

- Acute onset ≤48 hours.
- Bilateral infiltrates on chest radiograph.
- PaO_2/FiO_2 ratio <200. [If the ratio is between 200 and 300, the syndrome is termed acute lung injury (ALI).]
- No cardiogenic pulmonary edema defined as a PAOP ("wedge") <18 mmHg.

ARDS is remarkable for heterogeneous lung lesions, with normal alveoli, obliterated alveoli, and "recruitable" areas. Mortality remains >50%, but only 20% is due to respiratory failure. The main cause of death is multiple organ failure.

Obviously, in spite of the definition, a patient can have ARDS and fluid overload. In those cases, the treatment for ARDS should be administered concurrently with that of fluid overload.

The current trend in treating ARDS is based on the following:

- *PEEP* improves oxygenation by recruiting alveoli (increases functional residual capacity (FRC) and redistributing lung water. Its side-effects are hemodynamic (decrease in venous return) and volutrauma. "Best PEEP" can be determined by plotting a static pressure–volume curve, and is usually greater than 12.5 cm H_2O. The "open lung" strategy aims at avoiding the repetitive opening and closing of recruitable alveoli.
- *Low tidal volumes*, 6 mL/kg of ideal body weight, is the only modality shown in a randomized trial to decrease mortality. Whether volume-controlled or pressure-controlled ventilation is used is unimportant. The aim is to limit the hyperinflation of normal alveoli. Plateau pressure is more important than peak pressure, the goal being to keep plateau pressure (including PEEP) below 30–35 cm H_2O. Lowering the tidal volumes, even with an increased respiratory rate, often leads to an increase in the PCO_2. The strategy of permissive hypercapnia consists

in tolerating a higher PCO_2 in order to prevent ventilator-induced lung injury. Keeping the pH >7.2 is recommended with sodium bicarbonate administration as needed.

- *Prone positioning* may lead to an improvement in oxygenation in up to 70% of patients that can persist even after return to the supine position. This strategy has not been shown to decrease mortality and is fraught with practical difficulties.
- *Steroids* are ineffective and even deleterious during the acute phase, but may be beneficial during the proliferative phase (7–10 days), presumably by limiting fibrosis.
- *Fluid management,* is directed at keeping the patient as dry as tolerated from the hemodynamic and renal points of view, in attempt to decrease the extent of pulmonary edema. However, there is no evidence to support this approach.

5. Briefly describe the most common ventilatory modes.

The most commonly used ventilatory modes are detailed in Table 85.1. "Trigger" refers to the event that initiates a breath. The set trigger can be time, in which case the set rate determines how often a breath will be delivered, or patient, in which case the ventilator will detect an inspiratory effort by the patient. The inspiratory effort can be detected either by the generation of negative pressure or inspiratory flow. "Target" refers to the set point for the ventilator during the breath. The target can be flow, in which case a set number of liters per minute will be delivered, or pressure, in which case a set pressure is attained. "Cycle" designates the event that terminates the breath. It can be volume, i.e., the set tidal volume has been delivered, patient, for spontaneous breaths, flow, in which case the breath is terminated when the inspiratory flow reaches 25% of the peak flow, or time.

CMV is also called volume-controlled (VC) ventilation. The respiratory rate and tidal volume are set on the ventilator, and the patient cannot take any spontaneous breaths.

It is only appropriate for a patient under deep sedation, neuromuscular blockade, or general anesthesia.

Assist-control ventilation (ACV) allows a patient to receive a preset number of machine breaths per minute. The ventilator will detect additional inspiratory efforts by the patient and deliver a machine breath with the set tidal volume.

Intermittent mandatory ventilation (IMV) is remarkable in that it combines machine breaths at a set rate (breaths will be synchronized with inspiratory efforts in synchronized intermittent mandatory ventilation, SIMV) and spontaneous breaths, either without assistance, or, almost exclusively nowadays, in combination with pressure support. It is used to permit a patient to take additional breaths, or as a weaning mode by progressively decreasing the rate of machine breaths.

Continuous positive airway pressure (CPAP) was initially devised as a mode to deliver PEEP to a spontaneously breathing patient. Quite often, however, it is informally used to designate spontaneous breathing on a ventilator, regardless of whether the pressure is positive at end-expiration.

Pressure support (PS) is used to assist spontaneous breaths. The ventilator detects an inspiratory effort and maintains a preset pressure until the inspiratory flow drops to 25% of the peak flow. A pressure support of 5–10 cm H_2O should be equivalent to breathing spontaneously without an endotracheal tube. It compensates for the resistance of the endotracheal tube, the ventilator tubing, and valves. A higher value provides additional support. This mode is mainly used for weaning from the ventilator. The controversy as to the best weaning mode—SIMV with PS versus PS alone—is far from resolved.

Pressure control (PC) was devised to limit hyperinsufflation, especially in patients with ARDS. It can be delivered as either CMV or ACV. Tidal volume is not set. Instead, a target pressure and an inspiratory time are programmed. Thus, the tidal volume received by the patient will depend on lung and chest wall compliance. This has not been shown to improve outcome.

TABLE 85.1   **The Most Common Ventilatory Modes**

Mode	Trigger	Target	Cycle	Type of breaths delivered
Controlled mechanical ventilation (CMV)	Time	Flow	Volume	Machine
Assist-control ventilation (ACV)	Patient	Flow	Volume	Machine
Synchronized intermittent mandatory ventilation (SIMV)	Patient	Flow	Volume	Machine/Spontaneous
Continuous positive airway pressure (CPAP)	Patient	Flow	Patient	Spontaneous
Pressure support (PS)	Patient	Pressure	Flow	Assisted
Pressure control (PC)	Time/Patient	Pressure	Time	Machine

6. After several days in the SICU, the patient's respiratory status has improved. What criteria are used to determine whether extubation will be successful?

Several criteria should be met to consider extubation:

- The patient should be alert and cooperative on no sedation.
- Muscular strength should be adequate, with a negative inspiratory force (NIF) ≤ -25 cm H_2O and/or a forced vital capacity (FVC) ≥ 15 mL/kg.
- The hemodynamics should be stable, with no or minimal vasoactive infusions.
- The PaO_2 should be ≥ 60 mmHg on a FiO_2 ≤ 0.5 and PEEP ≤ 5 cm H_2O.
- The $PaCO_2$ should be ≤ 50 torr, or near the patient's baseline.
- The patient should tolerate a trial of spontaneous ventilation, either on the respirator with a PS of 5–10 cm H_2O or on a T-piece. No tachypnea, dyspnea, tachycardia, hypertension, dysrhythmias, signs of myocardial ischemia, or desaturation should be observed. Obtaining an ABG after 30 minutes of such a trial does not add any further information to the clinical examination and the pulse oximeter data.

Protocols driven by non-physician staff, such as nurses or respiratory therapists, have been shown to lead to significantly earlier discontinuation of mechanical ventilation and should probably be the rule.

Numerous criteria have been proposed to predict successful extubation, but the most helpful may be the "rapid shallow breathing index" or RSBI, calculated in a patient breathing spontaneously with a low PS.

$$RSBI = \frac{RR}{V_T} \qquad (5)$$

RR is the respiratory rate in breaths per minute and V_T is the tidal volume in liters. A value below 105 suggests that extubation will be successful.

SUGGESTED READINGS

Ely EW, Meade MO, Haponik EF, et al.: Mechanical ventilator weaning protocols driven by nonphysician health-care professionals: evidence-based clinical practice guidelines. Chest 120:454S–463S, 2001

Meade M, Guyatt G, Cook D, et al.: Predicting success in weaning from mechanical ventilation. Chest 120:400S–424S, 2001

Schmidt GA, Hall JB, Wood LDH: Ventilatory failure. pp. 2443–2470. In Murray JF, Nadel JA (eds): Textbook of Respiratory Medicine, 3rd edition. WB Saunders, Philadelphia, 2000

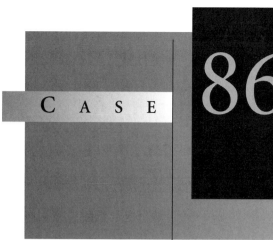

CASE 86

DELAYED EMERGENCE, COMA, AND BRAIN DEATH

Arthur Atchabahian, MD
Andrew B. Leibowitz, MD

A 56-year-old man has undergone craniotomy for clipping of a saccular aneurysm of the right middle cerebral artery. The aneurysm was discovered during the investigation of persistent headache and did not appear to have bled. At the conclusion of a seemingly uneventful procedure, the patient does not wake up.

QUESTIONS

1. What are the possible causes, investigation, and treatment for delayed emergence from anesthesia?
2. The CT scan shows a large left thalamic hemorrhage with intraventricular blood and a mild midline shift. The patient remains comatose. How would you manage this patient in the intensive care unit?
3. On the following day, the patient responds only to noxious stimuli by posturing in extension. The pupils are 4 mm, fixed, and nonreactive to light. The family asks whether the patient is brain dead. What is your response? What are the criteria for brain death?

1. What are the possible causes, investigation, and treatment for delayed emergence from anesthesia?

Anesthetic or preoperative medication overdose, or prolonged effect

The effect of hypnotic agents or inhalation anesthetics can last longer than expected. The amount of the medications administered should be reviewed. The effect of hypnotics and volatile agents should clear rapidly (i.e., within 90 minutes), provided that a gross overdose was not administered. Analysis of expired gases can rule out the persistence of volatile agents, especially after prolonged administration of high concentrations. Benzodiazepines can be reversed by titrating flumazenil up to 1.0 mg intravenously (IV). Physostigmine can reverse the effect of some sedatives, especially the central effects of anticholinergic agents such as scopolamine.

The prolonged effect of opioids should be considered. The patient will typically present with pinpoint pupils and apnea, or a slow respiratory rate with normal to high tidal volumes. Diagnosis and treatment can be made by carefully titrating naloxone IV in 40 μg increments, up to 400 μg, or more if the suspicion is high, until the patient is somnolent but arousable. Complete opioid reversal is not desirable since it might lead to severe pain or withdrawal symptoms, with tachycardia, dysrhythmias, hypertension, an increase in intracranial pressure (ICP), myocardial ischemia, and pulmonary edema.

Prolonged neuromuscular blockade is another cause of delayed emergence. Measuring the response to train-of-four stimulation can easily assess residual blockade. Care must be taken not to stimulate nerves in an area where upper motor neuron disease is present (e.g., hemiplegia) because the response can be brisk while the patient is effectively paralyzed in all other areas. The typical behavior of a patient with residual neuromuscular blockade is rapid, shallow breathing, and "flapping" of the limbs, described as "a fish out of water", as the weakness predominates proximally. Additional cholinesterase inhibitors can be given for reversal, or more time can be allowed to elapse. If that is the option chosen, the patient should be adequately sedated in order to avoid an awake but paralyzed patient. Inadequate reversal of neuromuscular blockade (despite administration of an adequate reversal dose of neostigmine or edrophonium) may result from several circumstances including: (1) a block that was too dense to overcome, (2) severe acidosis, (3) hypothermia, and (4) administration of antibiotics (e.g., aminoglycosides) or other medications that potentiate neuromuscular blockade.

Alcohol or recreational drugs present prior to the start of the anesthetic can be the cause of delayed emergence. This is most frequently seen in the trauma patient when a complete investigation could not be performed preoperatively. Blood, urine, and possibly gastric contents should be analyzed for these substances.

Metabolic disorders

The blood glucose should be measured to rule out profound hypoglycemia or marked hyperglycemia and hyperosmolar coma. Hypoglycemia is treated with the IV administration of glucose. If the suspicion is high that the patient may be hypoglycemic, treatment with 50% dextrose intravenously should be initiated without waiting for the laboratory results.

Blood analysis for electrolytes and an arterial blood gas (ABG) should be performed, and any significant abnormality (especially hypoxemia, hypercapnia, and hypo- or hypernatremia) should be corrected.

In patients whose immediate preoperative neurologic status is unknown or questionable, other etiologies such as hypothyroidism or adrenal insufficiency should be considered.

Neurosurgical disorders

A neurologic examination for focal deficits should be performed. If the cause of delayed awakening remains unclear, especially after a craniotomy, a computed tomography (CT) scan of the head should be performed to rule out a cerebral vascular accident (CVA), hemorrhagic or ischemic. It should be noted that ischemic CVAs are not apparent on CT scan before 48–72 hours have elapsed. Less commonly, CT scan may diagnose tension pneumocephalus, caused by nitrous oxide or global cerebral hypoxic damage.

2. **The computed tomography (CT) scan shows a large left thalamic hemorrhage with intraventricular blood and a mild midline shift. The patient remains comatose. How would you manage this patient in the intensive care unit?**

- Maintain cardiorespiratory function
  - Fluid resuscitation.
  - Vasopressors or inotropes as needed.
  - Mechanical ventilation.
- Decrease ICP
  - Elevate the head 30°.

Differential Diagnosis of Delayed Emergence

Medication
  Hypnotic agents, opioids, or inhalation
    anesthetics – prolonged effect
    Flumazenil – reverse benzodiazepines
    Naloxone – reverse opioids
  Neuromuscular blocking agents
    Inadequate reversal
      Block too dense at time of reversal
      Severe acidosis
      Hypothermia
      Concomitant administration of
        medications that potentiate the
        neuromuscular blockade
  Alcohol or recreational drugs

Metabolic disorders
  Hypoxemia
  Hypercapnia
  Hyponatremia
  Hypernatremia
  Hypoglycemia
  Hypothyroidism
  Adrenal insufficiency

Neurologic
  CVA
  Tension pneumocephalus

- Avoid positive end-expiratory pressure (PEEP), which may increase central venous pressure (CVP) and decrease blood return from the brain.
- Administer mannitol (0.5–1 g/kg IV) for acute intracranial hypertension to raise the serum osmotic pressure.
- Hyperventilation used to be routine practice. However, it has been shown to increase the risk of brain ischemia, therefore, ventilator settings should aim at normocapnia. Hyperventilation to a $PaCO_2$ of 25–30 mmHg can be used if there is an acute deterioration.
- Consider insertion of an ICP monitor (e.g., a ventriculostomy), which also permits withdrawal of cerebrospinal fluid in case of acute intracranial hypertension.
- In extreme cases, a salvage craniectomy can be performed to remove part of the skull vault to control the ICP.
- Avoid rebleeding
  - Control of the systolic blood pressure (SBP). Avoid SBP >160 mmHg.
  - Cerebral perfusion pressure (CPP) should be maintained >70 mmHg. CPP is calculated by subtracting the CVP or ICP (whichever is the higher value) from the mean arterial pressure. Although data are available only for closed head injury, the potential for further ischemic damage in areas where autoregulation is abolished exists with most intracranial lesions.
  - Correct any coagulopathy.
  - Do not use anticoagulants.
- Prevent seizures
  - Administer fosphenytoin 1500 mg IV (equivalent to 1000 mg of phenytoin) over 30 minutes, then phenytoin 100 mg IV every 8 hours, adjusted based on plasma levels.
- Prevent hyperthermia
  - While the cerebral protective effect of hypothermia is still controversial, the deleterious effect of hyperthermia on the injured brain is well established.
  - Administer antipyretics and active cooling as needed.
- Prevent gastrointestinal bleeding
  - Administer anti-H_2 agents (e.g., famotidine 20 mg IV every 12 hours).
- Prevent deep venous thrombosis
  - Sequential compression stockings.

3. On the following day, the patient responds only to noxious stimuli by posturing in extension. The pupils are 4 mm, fixed, and nonreactive to light. The family asks whether the patient is brain dead. What is your response? What are the criteria for brain death?

The patient is not brain dead, but if he survives, the likelihood of a persistent vegetative state is very high. If the patient does not have a living will stating his wishes, the discussion with the family should first provide information regarding the current status and prognosis in a way that nonmedical people can comprehend. The discussion should then center on attempting to elicit the wishes of the patient. If no wishes were clearly stated, the patient's values should be explored to reach a decision regarding pursuit or withdrawal of treatment.

The criteria for brain death are the irreversible absence of brain function, including cortex and brainstem, and the absence of hypothermia, or toxic, or metabolic disorder. Precise protocols for determining brain death vary among institutions. If the cause of the coma is unknown, a period of observation of at least 24 hours without neurologic change is necessary.

Several criteria have to be met to affirm the diagnosis of brain death.

- Absence of hypothermia (temperature <32°C).
- Absence of hypotension (SBP <90 mmHg).
- Absence of a significant metabolic disorder (hypoglycemia, hypo- or hypernatremia, acidosis or alkalosis, uremia, adrenal insufficiency, hypothyroidism, etc.).
- Absence of toxic substances that can cause depressed brain function. Blood and urine analysis for toxins may be performed.
- Coma with absence of purposeful movements. Spontaneous movements of spinal origin are possible and do not contravene the diagnosis of brain death.
- Absence of brainstem function as evidenced by the absence of all of the following:
  - Corneal reflex—no blinking when the corneas are gently touched with a clean sponge.
  - Oropharyngeal (gag) reflex and coughing during deep tracheal suctioning.
  - Oculocephalic (doll's eyes) reflex—no movement of the eyes when the patient's head is turned from side to side.
  - Oculovestibular reflex—no movement of the eyes when iced water is injected into each ear.
  - Pupillary response to light—dilated pupils if cervical sympathetic pathways are intact.
  - Respiratory reflex—assessed by performing an apnea test. To perform this test, the patient is ventilated with 100% oxygen for 10 minutes (or more if there is underlying lung disease). The ventilator is then disconnected and a catheter providing 6 L/min of oxygen is inserted into the endotracheal tube. ABGs are drawn before initiating the test and 5 and 10 minutes later. The $PaCO_2$ should reach 60 mmHg or rise by >20 mmHg if the baseline $PaCO_2$ was >40 mmHg. This appears to be adequate for spontaneous ventilation to resume if the medullary respiratory centers are functional. The test is interrupted if the patient develops dysrhythmias, or becomes hypotensive, or hypoxemic. An ABG should be drawn at that time to determine whether the $PaCO_2$ had increased sufficiently for the test to be conclusive.

- Confirmatory tests, such as a cerebral angiogram or a radionuclide scan, demonstrating the absence of blood flow to the brain, are sufficient to affirm brain death. A transcranial Doppler ultrasound examination showing small systolic peaks with no diastolic flow has similar value. The absence of signal on both electroencephalogram (EEG) and brainstem evoked potentials is also sufficient. Some of these tests are required by policy in some institutions; however, brain death can be affirmed based purely on clinical criteria.

All evidence should be adequately documented in the chart, and two concurring physicians should confirm the diagnosis of brain death. The family can then be approached for solid organ and tissue donation.

In children, these criteria are slightly different in two respects:

- No interval between the two determinations is mandated in adults, i.e., patients over 18 years of age. From term to 2 months old the determinations should be separated by at least 48 hours, between the ages of 2 months and 1 year by 24 hours, and by 12 hours between the ages of 1 and 18 years.
- Confirmatory tests are optional beyond the age of 1 year. Two confirmatory tests are needed between term and 2 months of age, while only one confirmatory test is required between 2 months and a year.

SUGGESTED READINGS

Quality Standards Subcommittee of the American Academy of Neurology: Practice parameters for determining brain death in adults: report of the Quality Standards Subcommittee of the American Academy of Neurology. Neurology 45:1012, 1995

Wijdicks EFM: The diagnosis of brain death. N Engl J Med 344:1215–1221, 2001

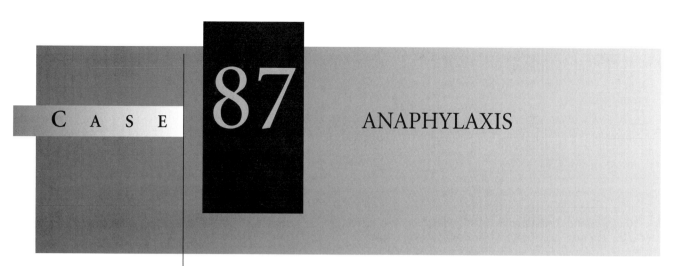

CASE 87

ANAPHYLAXIS

Arthur Atchabahian, MD
Andrew B. Leibowitz, MD

A 23-year-old man is scheduled to undergo an open reduction and internal fixation of a carpal scaphoid fracture, using a bone graft to be harvested from the iliac crest. Induction of general anesthesia and intubation were uneventful. When cefazolin 1 g is administered intravenously a rash appears over the face and chest. The heart rate is 135 beats per minute and the blood pressure drops to 70/40 mmHg.

QUESTIONS

1. What is the mechanism of anaphylaxis? What is the difference between anaphylactic and anaphylactoid reactions?
2. What treatment should be administered to this patient? What else should be checked on physical examination?
3. What are the medications most often implicated in anaphylaxis? In anaphylactoid reactions?
4. What is the percentage of patients allergic to penicillin who will have a reaction when challenged with a cephalosporin? What antibiotic would you use for "clean" orthopedic surgery in a patient reporting a penicillin allergy or a reaction to cephalosporins?
5. Once the blood pressure and heart rate returned to normal, the rash was subsiding and the chest auscultation was clear. Should surgery be allowed to proceed or should the case be cancelled? What will you tell the patient postoperatively?

1. What is the mechanism of anaphylaxis? What is the difference between anaphylactic and anaphylactoid reactions?

Anaphylaxis is an IgE-mediated allergic reaction. Antigens crosslinking two molecules of IgE bound on a mast cell or a basophil trigger degranulation of the cell with release of factors such as histamine, platelet-activating factor (PAF), eosinophil and neutrophil chemotactic factors, vasodilating prostaglandins and leukotrienes, adenosine, and serotonin. These factors in turn activate the complement and coagulation cascades. They also have direct effects, the most relevant being systemic arteriolar vasodilation, with an acute increase in vascular permeability and bronchoconstriction.

Anaphylactoid reactions are clinically indistinguishable from anaphylaxis. However, the mechanism of action differs in that IgE is not involved. Anaphylactoid reactions are a result of direct degranulation of mast cells and basophils with release of the same mediators as in anaphylactic reactions.

2. What treatment should be administered to this patient? What else should be checked on physical examination?

The A and B of the ABCs are already addressed in this case, since the patient is intubated and mechanically ventilated. Epinephrine 50–100 μg (0.5–1 mL of a 1:10,000 solution found in pre-filled syringes, or 0.05–0.1 mL of the more commonly used 1:1,000 solution), or 0.01 mg/kg in children, should be administered subcutaneously if the patient is merely hypotensive, and may be repeated as needed. Higher doses and the intravenous route should be used if the reaction is severe, or if cardiac arrest supervenes. High doses of epinephrine are more efficacious but cases of myocardial ischemia or even infarction after epinephrine administration have been reported. A review of 164 cases of fatal anaphylaxis in the United Kingdom showed that epinephrine overdose caused at least three of these fatalities. An intravenous infusion of epinephrine (1 mg in 250 mL at a rate of 0.05–2 μg/min) should be considered if repeat doses are necessary.

Epinephrine acts by two mechanisms: it reverses vasodilation by its α-agonist effects, and it blocks further degranulation of mast cells or basophils through its β-agonist effects. It may also improve cerebral perfusion independent of its effect on blood pressure by $β_2$-mediated vasodilation, and it is very effective in the treatment of bronchospasm.

Other measures to be taken are:

- Ventilation with 100% oxygen.
- Fluid resuscitation with crystalloids or colloids. Increased vascular permeability can transfer 50% of intravascular fluid into the extravascular space within 10 minutes. The amount of fluid administered should be based on hemodynamic parameters.
- Intravenous steroids (e.g., methylprednisolone 1–2 mg/kg intravenously (IV); repeat q4–6 hourly as needed). Steroids may have no effect for 4–6 hours, but may prevent persistent or biphasic anaphylaxis.
- Anti-H_1 medications (e.g., diphenhydramine 25–100 mg IV).
- Anti-H_2 medications (e.g., ranitidine 1 mg/kg IV).
- Glucagon (1–5 mg IV) in severe reactions. Glucagon directly activates adenyl cyclase and bypasses the β-adrenergic receptor. It may reverse refractory hypotension and bronchospasm. Glucagon or atropine should be used in β-blocked patients to increase an inappropriately slow heart rate.
- In case of refractory hypotension, military antishock trousers (MAST) may significantly improve hemodynamics.

If cardiac arrest supervenes, advanced cardiac life support (ACLS) protocols should be followed, including epinephrine, atropine, and transcutaneous pacing in case of pulseless electrical activity. In addition, rapid volume expansion is mandatory. Prolonged resuscitative efforts are encouraged, since recovery is more likely to be successful in anaphylaxis, in which the subject is often a young individual with a healthy cardiovascular system.

Therapeutic options for anaphylaxis are presented in Table 87.1.

The chest should be auscultated since bronchospasm is often triggered by anaphylactic or anaphylactoid reactions. If bronchospasm does not respond to the treatment administered for anaphylaxis, inhaled $β_2$-agonists and possibly aminophylline should be added to the regimen. Volatile anesthetics can also be used (if that is not already the case, and if the blood pressure allows) for their bronchodilating properties.

3. What are the medications most often implicated in anaphylaxis? In anaphylactoid reactions?

Anaphylaxis is commonly caused by antibiotics (predominantly the β-lactam antibiotics, which account for about 75% of anaphylaxis in the United States), radiology contrast dye, and protamine. The rate of anaphylactic reactions with iodinated contrast has significantly decreased because sensitive individuals are being pretreated with steroids and antihistamines, and non-ionic contrast with less potential to cause allergic reactions is being used. Latex has emerged as a cause of anaphylactic reaction (as well as other allergic reactions), probably because of the increasing use of latex gloves and barriers. Patients with spina bifida, patients who have undergone multiple surgeries, and healthcare workers are especially at risk.

Anaphylactoid reactions are commonly caused by morphine, d-tubocurarine, certain antibiotics (e.g., vancomycin, ciprofloxacin), aspirin (possibly through inhibition of cyclooxygenase), and succinylcholine. While not causing histamine release per se, β-blockers have been found to increase the incidence of anaphylactoid reactions.

4. What is the percentage of patients allergic to penicillin who will have a reaction when challenged with a cephalosporin? What antibiotic would you use for "clean" orthopedic surgery in a patient reporting a penicillin allergy or a reaction to cephalosporins?

True allergic reaction is defined as hives, edema, or anaphylaxis. A morbilliform rash (i.e., resembling measles), consisting of macular lesions that are red and are usually 2–10 mm in diameter but may be confluent in places, is a benign reaction that does not qualify as "allergic". In patients with true allergy to penicillin, a 3–7% rate of allergic reaction to cephalosporin is expected, versus 1–2% in patients with no history of penicillin allergy. History is the most important element here. In a patient who had a morbilliform rash, cephalosporins can be given safely. If true

TABLE 87.1	Treatment of Anaphylaxis

I. Immediate measures
   a. Assess airway, breathing, circulation, and adequacy of mentation (if applicable)
   b. Administer epinephrine SQ 50–100 μg or 0.01 mg/kg in children; repeat as needed
II. General measures
   a. Expedite surgery; position the patient supine; elevate lower extremities
   b. Establish and maintain the airway, possibly with an endotracheal tube or cricothyrotomy
   c. Administer 100% oxygen
   d. Administer normal saline or colloids if there is severe hypotension
III. Specific measures
   a. Epinephrine 1 mg in 250 mL of normal saline or D5W (4 μg/mL) at a rate of 0.5–2 μg/min
   b. H_1 antagonists: diphenhydramine 25–100 mg IV
   c. Glucocorticoids: methylprednisolone 1–2 mg/kg IV; repeat q 4–6 hourly as needed
   d. H_2 antagonists: ranitidine 1 mg/kg IV
   e. Glucagon: 1–5 mg IV
   f. Nebulized β_2-agonists: 0.5 mL or 2.5 mg of a 5% solution diluted in 3–5 mL of NS
   g. Aminophylline: 5 mg/kg IV over 30 min, then 0.9 mg/kg/hr IV; follow serum levels (therapeutic range 8–15 μg/mL)
   h. Military antishock trousers (MAST)
IV. Supervening cardiac arrest, in addition to ACLS protocol
   a. Rapid volume expansion
   b. Prolonged resuscitative efforts

(Adapted with permission from Kemp SF: Current concepts in pathophysiology, diagnosis and management of anaphylaxis. Immunol Allergy Clin Am 21:611–634, 2001.)

allergy to penicillin or cephalosporins is reported, it is prudent to use clindamycin 600 mg intravenously. Vancomycin 1,000 mg intravenously administered over 30–60 minutes can be used as well. However, widespread use of vancomycin seems to lead to a rise in the prevalence of vancomycin-resistant enterococci, and possibly of vancomycin-resistant staphylococci, and is best avoided. Rapid vancomycin administration may cause the "red man syndrome" secondary to a non-immune-mediated release of histamine, i.e., an anaphylactoid reaction.

5. Once blood pressure and heart rate returned to normal, the rash was subsiding and the chest auscultation was clear. Should surgery be allowed to proceed or should the case be cancelled? What will you tell the patient postoperatively?

The case can probably be allowed to proceed after rapid resolution of the event. Upper airway edema should be excluded prior to extubation. The presence of a leak around the endotracheal tube should be determined by deflating the endotracheal tube cuff and occluding the tube manually. However, anaphylaxis may respond poorly to treatment and acute respiratory distress syndrome (ARDS) and myocardial ischemia or infarction can ensue.

The patient should be told that the administration of any β-lactam antibiotic might be fatal. He should be given

a letter detailing the reaction and specifically naming the medication involved, and he should be instructed to wear a bracelet indicating his allergy. Allergy specialists sometimes perform skin tests to identify the causative drug, but the tests themselves are not without risk. In case of severe infection necessitating the administration of β-lactam antibiotics, an allergist can attempt desensitization. These techniques are not always successful and may be fatal.

SUGGESTED READINGS

Erffmeyer JE: Reactions to antibiotics. Immunol Allergy Clin North Am 12:633–648, 1992

Kelkar PS, Li JTC: Cephalosporin allergy. N Engl J Med 345:804–809, 2001

Kemp SF: Current concepts in pathophysiology, diagnosis and management of anaphylaxis. Immunol Allergy Clin North Am 21:611–634, 2001

Lang D, Alpern M, Visintainer P, et al.: Increased risk of anaphylactoid reaction from contrast media in patients receiving beta-adrenergic blockers or with asthma. Ann Intern Med 115:270–276, 1991

Sussman GL, Beezhold DH: Allergy to latex rubber. Ann Intern Med 122:43–46, 1995

INDEX

A

Abdominal aortic aneurysm (AAA), 195–199
  anesthetic techniques for surgery, 196
  hemodynamic consequences of aortic cross-clamping, 197–198
  monitoring devices for surgery, 196–197
    pulmonary artery catheters, 197
    transesophageal echocardiography (TEE), 197
  natural history, 195
  postoperative analgesia options, 198–199
    epidural anesthesia/analgesia, 198–199
    intravenous narcotics, 198
  preoperative evaluation, 195–196
Abruptio placenta, 364, 369
  anesthesia for emergency cesarean section, 369
  comparison with placenta previa, 370
  diagnosis, 364
  labor analgesia concerns, 369
  obstetric management, 364
  risk factors, 364
  signs and symptoms, 364
Accelerography, 134
Acetaminophen
  for pain control in preterm infants, 423
  toxicity, 190–191
Acetazolamide, in IOP reduction, 236, 238
Acetylcholine receptor antibodies, in myasthenia gravis diagnosis, 138
Acidemia, definition, 523
Acidosis, 523
Acquired inhibitors, 282, 283–284
Acquired platelet dysfunction, 283
Acromegaly, 113–116
  airway management, 115
  anesthetic considerations, 114
  postoperative concerns, 115–116
  structures within transsphenoidal surgical field, 115
  symptoms, 113–114
    airway changes, 114
    peripheral effects of excess growth hormone, 114
  treatment, 114
ACTH. *See* Adrenocorticotropic hormone

Activated protein C, in severe sepsis treatment, 283, 285–286, 505
Acute herpes zoster
  pathogenesis, 443–444
  presentation, 444
  treatment, 445
Acute isovolemic hemodilution (AIHD), 289–290
  advantages, 289, 295
  indications and contraindications, 290
  means of accomplishment, 289–290
  physiologic response to, 289
ACV. *See* Assist-control ventilation
Addisonian "crisis," 166
Addison's disease, 166
Adenoidectomy, without tonsillectomy, 261
Adenosine, in supraventricular tachycardia treatment, 5, 6
Adenotonsillectomy, 261–264
  ambulatory, suitable candidates for, 263–264
  anesthetic alternatives, 263
  anesthetic management of post-tonsillectomy hemorrhage, 264
  indications and contraindications, 261–262
  postanesthesia care unit problems, 263
  premedication, 262–263
  preoperative evaluation, 262
Adrenal reserve, evaluation, 167
Adrenocorticotropic hormone, 165
  stimulation test, 167, 168
Adult respiratory distress syndrome, 177, 523–524
  criteria for, 523
  mortality, 523
  treatment, 523–524
Advanced Cardiac Life Support (ACLS) protocol, 2
Afferent pain pathways, 430–431
Aftercare centers, 473
AICD. *See* Automatic implantable cardioverter-defibrillator
AIHD. *See* Acute isovolemic hemodilution
Airway pressure release ventilation (APRV), 484

Albumin
  levels as indicator of hepatic dysfunction, 188
  synthesis, 182–183
Alcoholic cardiomyopathy, 21–22
Aldosterone, 165, 166
Aldrete scoring system, 478
Alfentanil, central nervous system effects, 91, 92
Allergic reaction, definition, 532
Allowable blood loss (ABL), 397
α-Adrenergic agonists, contraindication during pregnancy, 376
Ambulatory surgery, 455–474
  acceptable candidates for, 456–457
  advantages, 456
  aftercare center role, 473
  anxiolytic premedication, 460
  benzodiazepine overdose reversal, 467–468
  choice of anesthetic, 460–461
  conduction anesthetic advantages and disadvantages, 461
  contraindications to general anesthetic, 461
  on diabetic patients, 457
  discharge criteria, 471–473
    "home readiness," 472
    "street fitness," 472
  drug administration prior to anesthesia, 458–459
  drugs used during, 463–464
  escort functions, 472
  hospitalization following, 473
  last-minute postponement reasons, 460
  moderate sedation in, 466–467
  motor vehicle operation after general anesthetic, 473
  nerve block anesthesia
    advantages and disadvantages, 462
    complications, 464
  newer vs. older volatile agents, 468
  patients not acceptable for, 457
  postoperative myalgias, 467
  postoperative nausea and vomiting, 468–470
  postoperative pain control, 470–471
  preoperative fasting period, 458
  preoperative internist evaluation, 459–460

Ambulatory surgery (Continued)
  preoperative laboratory studies, 459
  quality assurance, 473–474
  role of propofol, 465
  screening for anesthesia, 459
  sedatives to supplement regional
    anesthetic, 462–464
  surgical procedure types
    appropriate, 457–458
  total intravenous anesthesia
    in, 465–466
  tracheal intubation of
    patients, 464–465, 467
Aminophylline, 467
Amiodarone
  in congestive heart failure patients, 25
  in supraventricular dysrhythmias
    treatment, 507
Ammonia detoxification, 184, 185
Amyotrophic lateral sclerosis, and spinal
  anesthesia, 330
Anaphylactoid reactions
  distinguished from anaphylaxis, 531
  medications implicated, 532
Anaphylaxis, 531–533
  allergy to penicillin and cephalosporins,
    532–533
  distinguished from anaphylactoid
    reactions, 531
  mechanism, 531
  medications implicated, 532
  postoperative information to
    patient, 533
  surgery resumption after rapid
    resolution, 533
  treatment, 532, 533
Androgens, 165
Angiotensin converting enzyme (ACE)
  in hydrolysis of bradykinin, 275
  hypotensive reactions in patients on ACE
    inhibitors, 274–275
Angiotensinogen, 182
  effects of decreased
    production, 182
Anterior ischemic optic neuropathy
  (AION), 112
Anterior larynx, 249
Anticonvulsants, in cancer pain
  treatment, 452
Antidysrhythmics, 5, 6–7
Antiepileptic drugs, in PHN pain
  treatment, 445
Antithrombin III (ATIII), in DIC
  treatment, 283
Aortic stenosis, 27–30
  anesthetic strategy in patients
    with, 29–30
  aortic valve area calculation, 28
  etiology, 28
  hemodynamic goals in, 29

Aortic stenosis (Continued)
  importance of sinus rhythm
    maintenance, 28
  long-term prognosis, 27
  perioperative monitoring of patients
    with, 29
  symptoms, 27–28
  treatment of dysrhythmias in patients
    with, 28, 29
  treatment of hypotension in patients
    with, 28–29
APAP. See Acetaminophen
Apgar score, 391
Apnea, 212
APRV. See Airway pressure release ventilation
Aqueous humor, 236
ARDS. See Adult respiratory distress syndrome
Arndt blocker, 86
Arterial carbon dioxide tension. See $PaCO_2$
Arterial oxygen content. See CaO_2
Arterial oxygen tension. See PaO_2
Aspiration
  course, treatment and
    prognosis, 176–177
  mechanisms for protection
    against, 176
  pharmacologic interventions for
    prophylaxis, 177, 178
  problems associated, 176
  risk factors, 176
    when can occur during perioperative
      period, 176
Aspiration pneumonia, 351–352
Assist-control ventilation (ACV), 524
Asthma, 495–501
  aminophylline use in perioperative
    period, 499
  classification, 496
  etiologies of perioperative
    bronchospasm, 500
  general anesthesia vs. neuraxial block in
    patients with, 499–500
  indications for mechanical
    ventilation, 497–499
  management of peak airway pressure rise
    during general anesthesia, 500–501
  obstructive vs. restrictive lung disease,
    496–497
  pharmacology of medications to treat,
    497, 498
  preoperative evaluation and preparation
    in patients with, 499
  treatment plans, 499
  vs. chronic obstructive pulmonary
    disease, on pulmonary function tests,
    496–497
Asymmetric septal hypertrophy. See
  Hypertrophic obstructive
  cardiomyopathy
Atenolol, in cardiac risk patients, 13

Atlantoaxial instability, 427–428
Atracurium, central nervous system
  effects, 91, 92
Atrial fibrillation, 506
  treatment options, 506–507
Atrial flutter, 506
  treatment options, 506–507
Atropine
  in anaphylaxis treatment, 532
  in bradycardia treatment, 509
Automatic implantable cardioverter-
  defibrillator (AICD), 53–54
  deactivation, 55
  Guidant, 55
  perioperative management of patient
    with, 45
  in treatment of dilated cardiomyopathies,
    53–54
Axilla, anatomic landmarks, 336
Azathioprine, 61, 62

B

Baclofen, 327
BaCon study, 275
BACTHEM study, 275
Barbiturates, central nervous system
  effects, 91, 92
Bariatric surgery
  anesthetic plan for, 213–214
  equipment to anesthetize for, 213
Barrier pressure, 175
BCI. See Blunt cardiac injury
Beck's triad, 48, 486
Beckwith-Wiedemann syndrome, 394
Bellscope, 254
Benzocaine, toxic effects, 319
Benzodiazepines
  as Category D drugs, 374
  central nervous system effects, 91, 92
β-Blockers
  in hypertrophic obstructive
    cardiomyopathy treatment, 40
  in pheochromocytoma
    treatment, 172
  in supraventricular dysrhythmias
    treatment, 506, 507
Bezold-Jarisch reflex, 337
  treatment, 337
Bi-coherence, 111
Bier block, 316, 462
Bi-Glenn procedure, 417
Biguanides, 151
Bile salts, synthesis, 183
Bilirubin, overload, 191
Bioavailability, 185
Bispectral index state (BIS), 111
Blood oxygen content, calculation, 522
Blood pressure, determinants, 503
Blood product irradiation, 277

Blood replacement, 287–295. *See also* Acute isovolemic hemodilution; Cell salvage; Preoperative autologous blood donation
blood loss compensatory mechanisms, 288
oxygen transport, 287–288
sources of autologous blood, 289
comparison, 294–295
Blood substitutes, 301–302
Blood transfusions
Jehovah's Witnesses and, 298–299
in minor patient, 299
strategies for avoidance, 289, 300
Blunt cardiac injury (BCI), 486–489
diagnosis, 487–488
incidence in blunt thoracic trauma, 487
perioperative management, 488–489
Blunt cardiac trauma, 486
Body mass index (BMI), 211
Brachial plexus
anatomic course, 335
approaches to blocking, 336–337
axillary, 336, 337
infraclavicular, 336, 337
interscalene, 336, 336–337
supraclavicular, 336, 337
complications from upper extremity blocks, 337, 338
contraindications to interscalene block, 338
chronic obstructive pulmonary disease (COPD), 338
innervation of nerves of, 336
local anesthetics for blocks and doses, 337–338
amides, 338
esters, 338
Bradycardia
differential diagnosis and treatment, 509–510
junctional rhythm, 509–510
management strategies, 5
second-degree atrioventricular block, 510
sinus bradycardia, 509
third-degree atrioventricular block, 510
Bradydysrhythmias, treatment, in patients with aortic stenosis, 28, 29
Bradykinin, metabolism of, 275
Brain death
confirmatory tests, 530
criteria for, 529
in children, 530
Brainstem function, absence of, 529
Bretylium, 318, 320, 449
Bromocriptine, in acromegaly treatment, 114

Bronchopulmonary dysplasia (BPD), 420
Bullard laryngoscope, 254
Bupivacaine
for brachial plexus anesthesia, 338
in dental procedures, 319
for epidural anesthesia, 316, 317
with sodium bicarbonate, 316
for spinal anesthesia, 316–317, 326–327, 333, 461
toxic effects, 318, 319

C

Calcitonin, 162
Calcitriol, in hypocalcemia treatment, 164
Calcium homeostasis, 182
Calcium metabolism, 161–164. *See also* Hypercalcemia; Hypocalcemia
anesthetic considerations for parathyroid resection, 164
location of calcium in body, 161–162
postoperative concerns after parathyroid resection, 164
regulation of calcium, 162
role of calcium in body, 161
Calcium-channel blockers, in supraventricular dysrhythmias treatment, 507
Cancer pain management, 451–454
advantages of set-dose extended-duration opioid management, 452
causes of cancer pain, 451–452
celiac plexus block
complications, 453
indications, 453
differences between alcohol and phenol neurolysis, 453–454
guidelines for chronic analgesic regimen, 452
intrathecal versus epidural analgesia, 454
prevalence of cancer pain, 451
by organ system, 451
WHO ladder, 452
CaO_2, 287–288
Capnography, 74–75
end-tidal value, 74
inspiratory value, 74
Carbicarb, 4
Carcinoid syndrome, 225–229
anesthetic concerns in patients with, 227–228
bronchospasm, 227–228
hypertension, 227, 228
hypotension, 227–228
carcinoid tumors, 225–226
locations occurring, 227
chemoembolization treatment usage, 229

Carcinoid syndrome *(Continued)*
clinical manifestations, 226, 227
mechanism of action of somatostatin, 228
precautions for anesthetizing patients with, 228–229
Cardiac failure, definition, 52
Cardiac output (CO), 287, 503
Cardiac pacemakers. *See* Pacemakers
Cardiac tamponade, 47–49, 485–486, 487
clinical signs and symptoms, 48
diagnosis, 486, 487
implications for conduct of general anesthesia, 49
initial management, 48–49
intraoperative monitoring techniques, 49
pathophysiology, 47–48
treatment, 486, 487
Cardiac transplantation
immunosuppressive medications used following, 61–62
mechanisms of action, 61–62
side-effects, 61–62
non-cardiac surgery after, 62–64
anesthetic techniques applicable, 63
anticholinergic agent use when muscle relaxants reversed, 63–64
emergency drugs, 63, 64
intraoperative monitors, 63
pre-anesthetic concerns, 62–63
physiology of transplanted hearts, 59–60
cardiac denervation results, 59–60
intrinsic myocardial mechanisms, 60
post-transplant electrocardiogram, 61
reinnervation of transplanted heart, 60–61
as treatment for cardiomyopathy, 53–54
Cardiac window, 492
Cardiomyopathy, 51–56
definition, 52
dilated (DCM). *See* Dilated cardiomyopathy
etiologies, 52
hypertrophic (HCM), 39, 52, 53. *See also* Hypertrophic obstructive cardiomyopathy
ischemic (ICM), 52–53
management with LVAD. *See* left ventricular assist device
pathophysiology, 52
restrictive (RCM), 52, 53
Cardiopulmonary bypass (CPB), 65–67. *See also* Coronary artery disease
effects on hemostasis, 67
effects on major organs, 67
intraoperative monitoring, 66–67

Cardiopulmonary resuscitation (CPR), 1–9
    antidysrhythmic therapy in VF/pulseless
        VT, 5
    complications, 4
    indications
        for calcium salt administration, 5
        for magnesium therapy, 8
        for open cardiac massage, 8
        for pacemaker, 8
        for sodium bicarbonate
            administration, 4–5
        for vasopressin, 4
    initial response to cardiac arrest, 1–2
    management strategies in bradycardias, 5
    management strategy for pulseless
        electrical activity, 8–9
    optimal dose of epinephrine, 4
    recommended rates of compression, 2
    recommended rates of
        ventilation, 2–4
    serum glucose monitoring, 8
    "thoracic pump" theory, 2
    treatment of supraventricular
        tachydysrhythmias, 5–8
    treatments used, 6–7
Carotid artery angioplasty, 101
Carotid endarterectomy, 101–103
    alternatives, 101
    choice of anesthetic agent, 103
    indications, 101
    interventions reducing risk of neurologic
        injury, 103
    neurologic status monitoring, 102
        with general anesthesia, 102
        with regional anesthesia, 102
    perioperative complications, 101–102
Cauda equina syndrome, 319, 329,
    330, 333
Causalgia, 447
CBF. See Cerebral blood flow
CDH. See Congenital diaphragmatic hernia
CEA. See Carotid endarterectomy
Celiac plexus, anatomy, 452–453
Cell salvage
    characteristics of blood obtained
        by, 290
    intraoperative, 290–291
        advantages and disadvantages, 295
        controversies and contraindications,
            291–292
        indications, 291
    postoperative, 294
Central nervous system wind-up, 436
Central vein cannulation, during aortic
    surgery, 197
Central venous pressures (CVPs), 197
Cephalosporins
    allergic reaction to, 532–533
    in bariatric surgery, 214
Cerebral autoregulation, 89–90

Cerebral blood flow (CBF)
    effects of anesthetic agents and vasoactive
        drugs, 90–93
    major determinants of, 89–90
Cerebral edema, with ESLD, 186
Cerebral perfusion, decreased,
    treatment, 103
Cerebral perfusion pressure (CPP), 89
Cerebral vascular accident (CVA), 528
Cerebral vasospasm, 98
    treatment, 98–99
Cerebrospinal fluid (CSF), 90
    specific gravity, 325
    in spinal anesthesia, 324, 328, 330
Cesarean section. See also Labor and
        delivery
    in patient with abruptio placenta, 369
    in patient with placenta previa, 370
    in patient with preeclampsia, 361
Channel blockade, 120
CHF. See Congestive heart failure
Chickenpox, 443
Child-Turcotte-Pugh scoring
        system, 188–189
Child's classification, 188
Chloroprocaine, toxic effects, 330
Cholecystectomy, laparoscopic, 165, 166
Cholinergic crisis, 141
Chronic obstructive pulmonary disease
        (COPD)
    as contraindication to interscalene
        block, 338
    vs. asthma, on pulmonary function tests,
        496–497
Chvostek's sign, 163
Cimetidine, 177, 178, 458
Cisatracurium, central nervous system
    effects, 92
Citrate intermediate metabolism, 184
Clindamycin, 533
    effect on neuromuscular
        blockade, 126–127
Clonidine
    preoperative administration, 460
    in shivering treatment, 516
    in subarachnoid space, 327, 328
CMV. See Controlled mechanical
        ventilation; Cytomegalovirus
CO (cardiac output), 287, 503
Coagulation. See also Disseminated
        intravascular coagulation
    primary hemostasis, 380
    role of platelets, 380
    secondary hemostasis, 380
Cobb method, 298
Cocaine, toxic effects, 318–319
Codeine, 471
Cohen blocker, 86
Coma, management in intensive
        care unit, 528–529

Complex regional pain syndrome
        (CRPS), 447–449
    diagnosis, 448
    pathophysiologic theories, 447–448
    signs and symptoms, 448
    stages, 448
        stage 1 (acute/hyperemic), 448
        stage 2 (dystrophic), 448
        stage 3 (atrophic), 448
    treatment, 449
        intravenous regional bretylium Bier
            block, 449
        lumbar sympathetic block, 449
        modalities other than blocks, 449
        stellate ganglion block, 449
    type 1, 447, 448
    type 2, 447, 448
Congenital diaphragmatic hernia
        (CDH), 399–402
    anesthetic considerations for neonate
        with, 401
    clinical features, 400
    diagnosis, 400
    embryology and pathophysiology,
        399–400
        irreversible physiologic changes, 400
        reversible physiologic changes, 400
    incidence, 399
    intraoperative problems, 401–402
    permissive hypercapnia, 401
    postoperative problems, 401–402
    preoperative management, 400–401
    techniques for fetal surgery, 402
Congenital heart disease, 409–418
    differentiation between innocent and
        pathologic systolic murmurs, 409
    general anesthetic considerations for
        common cardiac lesions, 410
        endocarditis prophylaxis, 410, 411
        extracardiac defects, 410
        prevention of air embolism, 410
    incidence, 409–410
        frequency of most common congenital
            cardiac lesions, 410
    intracardiac lesions with left-to-right
            shunting anesthetic implications,
            411–412
        atrial septal defect (ASD)
            secundum, 412
        patent ductus arteriosus (PDA), 412
        ventricular septal defect (VSD), 412
    intracardiac lesions with right-to-left
            shunting
        anesthetic implications, 412–413
        tetralogy of Fallot (TOF), 413
        transposition of the great arteries
            (TGA), 413–414
    preoperative assessment, 410–411
    repair of congenital heart
            lesions, 414

Congenital heart disease (Continued)
  sequelae associated with repair of cardiac
    lesions, 415–418
    atrial septal defect (ASD)
      secundum, 415, 417
    atrioventricular (AV) septal defects,
      415, 417
    coarctation of the aorta (CoA),
      415, 417
    single ventricle, 416–417, 417
    tetralogy of Fallot (TOF), 416, 417
    transposition of the great arteries
      (TGA), 416, 417
    ventricular septal defect (VSD),
      415, 417
Congestive heart failure (CHF), 21–25
  anesthetic management, 23–25
  control, 410
  etiologies for dilated cardiomyopathy,
    21–22
  hemodynamic goals in, 24
  pathophysiology of dilated
    cardiomyopathy, 22–23
    "backward" failure, 23
    "forward" failure, 23
  perioperative monitoring, 23
  as predictor of perioperative cardiac
    events, 16
  prognosis, 16
Conscious sedation, 466–467
Continuous positive airway pressure
    (CPAP), 524
  for hypoxemia during one-lung
    ventilation, 86
Controlled mechanical ventilation
    (CMV), 524
COPD. See Chronic obstructive pulmonary
    disease
Cori cycle, 183
Corneal reflex, 529
Coronary artery bypass grafting. See
    Cardiopulmonary bypass
Coronary artery disease, 11–14. See also
    Myocardial infarction
  coronary steal, 13
  determinants of myocardial oxygen
    demand, 11–12, 65
  determinants of myocardial oxygen
    supply, 11, 65
  intraoperative monitoring of patients
    with, 13–14, 67
  medications used to treat, 65–66
  perioperative β-adrenergic blockade in
    patients with, 13
  pharmacologic alternatives for
    treating myocardial
    ischemia, 12–13
  pre-anesthetic concerns in patient
    with, 66
Coronary perfusion pressure (CPP), 28

Corticosteroids
  and adrenal suppression, 167
  clinical scenarios requiring
    administration, 167
  following cardiac transplantation, 61
  mechanism of action, 61
  in myasthenia gravis treatment, 138
  normal cortisol production, 166
  physiologic effects, 165
  relative potencies, 166
  in rheumatoid arthritis
    treatment, 307–308
  in septic shock treatment, 167–168
  side-effects, 61
Cortisol, 165
  normal production, 166
Cosyntropin, 167, 168
Coumadin, 281
Couvelaire uterus, 364
COX-2 inhibitors, in adenotonsillectomy,
    262, 263
CPAP. See Continuous positive airway
    pressure
CPP. See Cerebral perfusion pressure
CPR. See Cardiopulmonary resuscitation
Cricoid pressure, 177–178
Cricothyroid puncture, 257–259
CRPS. See Complex regional pain
    syndrome
Cryoprecipitate, 285, 305
  discovery, 304
CSF. See Cerebrospinal fluid
Curare
  central nervous system effects, 91
  poisoning, 138
Cushing disease, 166
Cushing response, 510–512
Cushing syndrome, 166
CVPs. See Central venous pressures
Cyanosis, 410–411, 413
Cyclophosphamide, effect on neuromuscular
    blockade, 127
Cyclosporine
  effect on neuromuscular
    blockade, 127
  side-effects, 61
CYP. See Cytochrome P450 (CYP) system
Cytal, 208
Cytochrome P450 (CYP) system, 185–186
  CYP2A6, 191
  CYP2E1, 185, 191
  CYP3A, 185
  CYP3A4, 191
Cytomegalovirus, 278

D

Dantrolene
  contraindication in pregnant patient, 145
  effect on neuromuscular blockade, 127

Dantrolene (Continued)
  in malignant hyperthermia treatment,
    144, 145
  pharmacology, 144
DCM. See Dilated cardiomyopathy
DDAVP. See Desmopressin
Defibrillators, 45, 508. See also Automatic
    implantable cardioverter-defibrillator
Delayed emergence from anesthesia
  causes, investigation and
    treatment, 527–528
    medication overdose or prolonged
      effect, 527–528
    metabolic disorders, 528
    neurosurgical disorders, 528
Delivery. See Labor and delivery
Depolarizing neuromuscular blockade,
    117–123. See also Succinylcholine
  effects of other drugs on, 127–128
  extrajunctional receptors, 118–119
  normal neuromuscular transmission,
    117–118
Desflurane, 468
  central nervous system effects, 91, 92
  in office setting, 477
Desmopressin (DDAVP)
  in diabetes insipidus treatment, 115
  in hemophilia A treatment, 304, 305
Destination therapy, 54
Dexamethasone
  following adenotonsillectomy, 263
  in postoperative nausea and vomiting
    treatment, 469, 477, 518
  relative potency, 166
Diabetes insipidus (DI), 115
Diabetes mellitus (DM), 149–154
  acute complications, 153–154
  ambulatory surgery on patients with, 457
  effects on perioperative morbidity and
    mortality, 152
  gestational (GDM), 150
  hypoglycemia causes and
    symptoms, 152–153
  insulin-dependent (IDDM/Type I),
    149–150, 151, 153–154, 457
    type IA, 149
    type IB, 149
  major types, 149–150
  malnutrition-related, 150
  maturity onset-type diabetes of the young
    (MODY), 150
  non-insulin-dependent (NIDDM/Type
    II), 149–150, 151, 153, 154, 457
  perioperative management, 153
  physiologic effects of insulin, 150
  and renal transplantation, 231
  risk of neuropathy in, 66
  treatment
    insulin preparations, 151
    oral hypoglycemic agents, 150–151

Diabetic ketoacidosis (DKA), 150, 153–154
    treatment, 154
Diastolic collapse, 485–486
Diazepam
    in ambulatory surgery, 462
    as Category D drug, 374
    preoperative administration, 460
    in seizure control, 319
Dibucaine, 327
DIC. See Disseminated intravascular
    coagulation
Difficult airway, 247–259
    approach to anticipated difficult
        intubation, 252–253
    Difficult Airway Algorithm, 256
    management options for difficult
        intubation after anesthesia
        induction, 253–255
    maneuvers if mask ventilation and
        intubation impossible after
        anesthesia induction, 255–259
    postoperative extubation following
        difficult intubation, 259
    predictors of difficult mask ventilation,
        247–248, 251
    probability of difficult intubation for
        combinations of risk factors, 253
    risk factors for difficult intubation,
        248–251
        dentition, 249
        mouth opening, 248–249
        reliability as predictors of difficult
            intubation, 251–252
        sniffing position, 248
        tongue, 249–251
    verification of tracheal intubation, 259
Diffusion constants, 353
Digitalis, in congestive heart failure
    control, 410
Digoxin, in supraventricular dysrhythmias
    treatment, 507
Dilated cardiomyopathy (DCM)
    etiologies, 52
    idiopathic, 52
    pathophysiology, 51–52
    treatment options, 53–54
        devices, 53–54
        medications, 53
        preventative measures, 53
        surgery, 53, 53–54
Disease-modifying anti-rheumatic drugs
    (DMARDs), 307
    and interstitial lung disease, 308
    and renal problems, 308
Disseminated intravascular coagulation
    (DIC), 283
    clinical presentation, 364–365
    as complication of cardiopulmonary
        bypass, 67
    as complication of TURP, 207

Disseminated intravascular coagulation
    (DIC) (Continued)
    diagnosis, 364–365
    etiology, 282, 283
    laboratory tests, 282, 283, 365
    treatment, 282, 283, 365
DMARDs. See Disease-modifying
    anti-rheumatic drugs
Do-not-resuscitate (DNR) orders, 69–70
    discussion with patient prior to surgery,
        69–70
    options available, 70
    re-evaluation for perioperative
    period, 70
    temporary and reversible adverse clinical
        events, 70
    temporary revocation in operating room, 69
DO_2, 287
Dolasetron, in postoperative nausea and
    vomiting treatment, 243, 477, 518
L-Dopa, in acromegaly treatment, 114
Dopamine
    in aortic surgery, 198
    in bradycardia treatment, 509
    in cardiac transplantation patient, 63
    metabolism, 170
Dopants, 265
Double-burst stimulation, 135
Down syndrome
    anesthetic considerations for MRI
        examination of child with, 428
    and atrioventricular septal defects, 415
    clinical manifestations, 427
    pre-anesthetic evaluation of child
        with, 427–428
    and predisposition to airway
        obstruction, 262
    review of systems specific to patient
        with, 427
Down-lung syndrome, 79
Doxazosin, in pheochromocytoma
    treatment, 171
Droperidol, in postoperative nausea and
    vomiting treatment, 469, 477, 518
Drugs, classification by extraction ratio, 186
Dual-chamber pacemaker. See Pacemakers,
    dual-chamber
Dysrhythmias
    following thoracotomy, 87
    following VAT, 87
    treatment in patients with aortic stenosis,
        28, 29

E

EA. See Esophageal atresia
ECG. See Electrocardiogram
Echothiophate, effect on neuromuscular
    blockade, 127
ECT. See Electroconvulsive therapy

Edrophonium, 129–130
    test for myasthenia gravis, 138
EEG. See Electroencephalogram
Eisenmenger syndrome, 35–38
    anesthetic considerations for patient
        with, 35–36
    antibiotic prophylactic regimens
        for dental, oral, respiratory tract, or
            esophageal procedures, 36, 37
        for genitourinary and gastrointestinal
            procedures, 37, 38
    association between bacterial
        endocarditis and structural heart
        disease, 36
    endocarditis prophylaxis
        recommendations, 37
    pathogens involved, 37–38
Electrocardiogram (ECG)
    in blunt cardiac injury diagnosis, 487
    in myocardial ischemia detection,
        13–14, 67
Electroconvulsive therapy (ECT), 105–108
    anesthesia for patient with
        gastroesophageal reflux
        disease, 107–108
    anesthetic agents for, 105–106
    anesthetic implications of psychotropic
        agents, 106–107
    contraindications, 108
    physiologic effects, 105, 106
    pre-anesthetic evaluation, 106
Electroencephalogram (EEG), for
    neurologic function monitoring, 102
Electromyograph (EMG), 133–134
    in myasthenia gravis diagnosis, 138
Embolization, during surgery,
    treatment, 103
EMG. See Electromyograph
Enalaprilat, in hypertension treatment, 511
Endotracheal tubes (ETT), 395
    in infants and young children, 395
    placement in patient with TEF, 407
    in preterm infants, 423
Endovascular aortic repair, 201–204
    anesthetic techniques, 202–203
    incidence of spinal cord ischemia
        after, 203–204
    perioperative surgical complications
        associated, 202
    "post-implantation syndrome," 204
    problems anticipated during proximal
        graft deployment, 203
    role of transesophageal echocardiography
        in, 203
    thoracic, outcomes following, 202
End-stage liver disease (ESLD)
    extrahepatic problems associated,
        186–188
    cardiac, 187
    hematologic, 187–188

End-stage liver disease (ESLD) *(Continued)*
    metabolic, 188
    neurologic, 186
    pulmonary problems, 186–187
    renal, 187
    hepatorenal syndrome in, 182, 187
    hypoglycemia with, 183, 186
End-stage renal disease (ESRD), 231
End-tidal CO_2. *See* $ETCO_2$
Enflurane
    central nervous system effects, 91
    hepatic injury following exposure to, 191
Enoxaparin, 384
Ephedrine
    in Bezold-Jarisch reflex treatment, 337
    in cardiac transplantation patient, 63
    in hypotension treatment, 328
    in postoperative nausea and vomiting
        treatment, 470
Epidural anesthesia
    addition of vasoconstrictors, 315–316
    in ambulatory patient, 461
    choice of local anesthetic, 317
    comparison with spinal anesthesia,
        331, 332
Epidural steroid injections, 441
Epinephrine
    actions, 532
    addition to local anesthetics,
        315–316, 327–328
    in allergic reaction treatment, 320
    in anaphylaxis treatment, 532
    in Bezold-Jarisch reflex treatment, 337
    in cardiac transplantation patient, 63
    in cardiopulmonary resuscitation, 4, 6
        optimal dose, 4
    in dental procedures, 319, 320
    in femoral and sciatic nerve
        blocks, 344
    metabolism, 170
    in neonatal resuscitation, 390
Erythropoietin, 292
ESLD. *See* End-stage liver disease
Esmolol
    in hypertension treatment, 511
    in pheochromocytoma treatment, 172
Esophageal atresia (EA)
    incidence, 405, 406
    types, 406
Esophageal surgery, with VAT, 85
Esophageal-tracheal combitube
    (ETC), 255, 257
Esophagectomy, Ivor Lewis, 85
Esophagomyotomy, 85
ESRD. *See* End-stage renal disease
Estimated blood volume (EBV), according
    to age, 397
$ETCO_2$, 94, 218, 221, 222
Ethanol, 185–186
Etidocaine, 316, 318

Etomidate
    central nervous system effects, 91, 92
    in congestive heart failure patients, 23
    in electroconvulsive therapy, 106
    and nausea and vomiting, 469
    in open-eye injury treatment, 237
ETT. *See* Endotracheal tubes
Extracellular fluid (ECF), 421
    in infants, 421
Extraction ratio, definition, 186
Extrajunctional receptors, 118–119
Extubation criteria, 132, 141

F

Faber Patrick test, 441
Facet joints, 441
    disease pathology, 441
Factor VIII
    deficiency in hemophilia A, 303
    recombinant, 304
Failed back syndrome (FBS), 442
Famotidine, 458
Fast-tracking, after general anesthesia, 479
Fat embolus syndrome (FES), 310–311
    causes, 310
    diagnostic criteria, 310
    management, 310–311
Fatty acid metabolism, 183
FBS. *See* Failed back syndrome
Femoral nerve block, 343
    choice of local anesthetic, 344
    sedation for, 344
Fentanyl
    in ambulatory surgery, 463, 464, 471
    central nervous system effects, 91
    crossing placenta by, 353
    in motor evoked potential
        monitoring, 111
    in subarachnoid space, 327
FES. *See* Fat embolus syndrome
Fetal circulation, 387, 388
Fetal distress, diagnosis, 365–366
Fetal heart rate (FHR)
    baseline features, 365
    monitoring during nonobstetric
        surgery, 376
    periodic features, 365–368
        early decelerations, 365, 367
        late decelerations, 365, 367, 368
        variable decelerations, 366, 367, 368
    reactive tracings, 365, 366
    tracings with poor variability, 365, 367
Fibrinolysis, 282, 283
Fick's equation, 352
Flail chest, 483–485
    diagnosis, 483, 485
    mechanisms of morbidity and mortality
        from, 483
    treatment, 483–485

Flexible fiberoptic laryngoscope (FFL),
    254–255
Flumazenil
    in benzodiazepine reversal, 467–468, 527
    side-effects, 468
Fluoxetine, effects, 107
Fogarty embolectomy catheter, 86
Fontan operation, 414, 417, 418
FRC. *See* Functional residual capacity
Full stomach, 175–179. *See also* Aspiration;
    Regurgitation
    anesthetic plan for patient with, 178–179
Functional residual capacity (FRC)
    decrease after pulmonary
        contusion, 483
    effect of morbid obesity, 212
Furosemide, in brain edema treatment, 93

G

Gabapentin, 445
Gaenslen's test, 441
Gastro-esophageal reflux, 175–176
    mechanisms for protection against,
        175–176
Gastroschisis and omphalocele, 393–397
    anesthetic plan, 396
    blood loss replacement, 397
    differences between gastroschisis and
        omphalocele, 393, 394
    fluid deficit replacement, 396–397
    intraoperative concerns, 396
    maintenance fluid management, 396
    operating room equipment for anesthesia,
        394–395
        airway, 395
        drugs, 395
        intravenous, 395
        machine, 394–395
        monitors, 395
        suction, 395
    postoperative concerns, 396
    preoperative management of
        neonate, 393–394
    third-space loss replacement, 397
Gilbert syndrome, 191
Glomerular filtration rate, in infants, 420
Glucagon, in anaphylaxis treatment, 532
Glucocorticosteroids, 165. *See also*
    Corticosteroids
    normal production, 166
Glucose homeostasis, 182, 184
α-Glucosidase inhibitors, 151
Glycerol, in IOP reduction, 236
Glycine
    as irrigating fluid, 208
    toxicities associated, 208
Glycogenesis, 182
Glycopyrrolate, 177, 178
    in bradycardia treatment, 509

Goiters, 158, 160
Gorlin formula, 28
Granisetron, in postoperative nausea and
    vomiting treatment, 243, 477, 518
Graves' disease, 157
Growth hormone (GH), excess, peripheral
    effects, 114
Gunshot wounds, transmediastinal, 492

H

H_2-receptor blockers, 177, 178, 458
Halothane
    in carotid endarectomy patients, 103
    central nervous system effects, 91
    effect on hepatic blood flow, 189
    in hypertrophic obstructive
        cardiomyopathy treatment, 41, 42
    toxicity, 191
Hashimoto's thyroiditis, 157
"Hassan" mini-laparotomy technique, 218
HCM. See Hypertrophic cardiomyopathy
HCV. See Hepatitis C virus
Heart failure, stages, 53
Heart transplantation. See Cardiac
    transplantation
Heartmate LVAS, 54, 55
HELLP, 357
Hemoglobin solutions, 301–302
Hemolysis, elevated liver function tests
    and low platelet count
        (HELLP) syndrome, 357
Hemophilia A, 303–305
    clinical presentation, 303–304
    compared with von Willebrand
        disease, 305
    laboratory findings, 304
    primary deficiency, 303
    treatment options, 280
        gene therapy, 304
Hemorrhage, classification, 505, 506
Hemostasis, role of liver in, 182
Hemothorax
    symptoms, 482
    treatment, 482–483
Heparin, 67, 311, 383. See also
    Low-molecular-weight heparin
Hepatic encephalopathy, 186
Hepatic functions
    basic, 181–185
    detoxifying, 184, 185–186
    effects of anesthesia, 189–190
    effects of surgery, 189
    endocrine, 182, 184–185
    metabolic, 183–184
        first-pass, 185–186
    synthetic (anabolic), 182–183, 185
Hepatitis, 190
    viral, 190
        concerns associated, 190

Hepatitis A virus, 190
Hepatitis B virus (HBV), 190
    tests for, 277
Hepatitis C virus (HCV), 190
    tests for, 277–278
Hepatopulmonary syndrome, 187
Hepatorenal syndrome, in end-stage liver
    disease, 182, 187
High frequency jet ventilation (HFJV),
    484, 485
High-threshold mechanoreceptors
    (HTMs), 430
Hip arthroplasty, 307, 309–312
    agitation management, 309–310
    anesthesia induction options, 309
    fat embolus syndrome during, 310–311
    postoperative pain control, 311–312
    thromboembolism prophylaxis and
        neuraxial anesthesia, 311
Histamine-releasing drugs, 227–228
HIV. See Human immunodeficiency virus
HOCM. See Hypertrophic obstructive
    cardiomyopathy
Homovanillic acid (HVA), 170
HPV. See Hypoxic pulmonary
    vasoconstriction
HTLV. See Human T-cell lymphotrophic
    virus
HTMs. See High-threshold
    mechanoreceptors
Human immunodeficiency virus (HIV)
    risk of transmission, 330, 331
    tests for, 277–278
Human T-cell lymphotrophic virus (HTLV),
    tests for, 277
Hunt–Hess Clinical Grade classification, 98
Hyaline membrane disease (HMD), 420
Hydralazine
    central nervous system
        effects, 91, 93
    in hypertension treatment, 359, 511
Hydrocortisone
    in allergic reaction treatment, 320
    relative potency, 166
    in septic shock treatment, 168
Hydroxyapatite, 161
β-Hydroxybutyrate, 183
5-Hydroxyindoleactic acid (5-HIAA),
    levels as carcinoid syndrome
        monitor, 225
5-Hydroxytryptamine (5-HT) antagonists,
    in prevention/treatment of
        postoperative nausea and
        vomiting, 243, 477, 518
Hyperammonemia, 208
Hypercalcemia
    correction prior to parathyroid
        resection, 164
    symptoms, 162–163
    treatment, 162, 163

Hypercapnia, 218
    causes, 521
    differential diagnosis, 144, 218
    maternal, effects on fetus, 376
Hypercarbia. See Hypercapnia
Hypercyanotic spells, 413
    prevention and treatment
        measures, 414
Hyperglycemia, 528
    avoidance in perioperative
        management, 153
    effect on post-cardiac arrest neurologic
        function, 8
    effects on perioperative morbidity and
        mortality, 152
Hyperkalemia, 121–122, 232
    as complication of succinylcholine,
        121–122
    ECG manifestations, 232
    treatment, 122, 232
Hyperosmolar nonketotic states, 154
Hyperparathyroidism
    anesthetic considerations for parathyroid
        resection, 164
    causes, 163–164
    postoperative concerns after parathyroid
        resection, 164
Hypertension
    intravenous agents used to treat,
        511, 512
    postoperative, differential diagnosis,
        510–512
Hypertensive heart disease (HHD), 53
Hyperthyroidism
    causes, 157–158
    effects on vital organ function, 155
    intraoperative concerns, 159
    preoperative considerations, 158–159
    primary, 157
    secondary, 157–158
    signs, 156
    symptoms, 156
    tertiary, 158
Hypertrophic cardiomyopathy (HCM),
    39, 52, 53
Hypertrophic obstructive cardiomyopathy
    (HOCM), 39–42, 53
    anatomic abnormalities in, 39–40
    anesthetic management of patient with,
        41, 42
    for labor and delivery, 41–42
    hemodynamic goals in, 40
    monitoring in patients with, 43
    treatment options, 40–41
Hyperventilation, in intracranial
    pressure reduction, 93
Hypocalcemia
    after parathyroid resection, 164
    symptoms, 163
    treatment, 163

Hypocapnia, maternal, effects on fetus, 376
Hypoglycemia
    avoidance in perioperative
        management, 153
    clinical presentation, 152–153
    with ESLD, 183, 186
    treatment, 153, 528
Hyponatremia, during TURP procedure,
        205–206, 207, 209, 227
Hypopnea, 212
Hypotension
    after aortic unclamping, 198
    postoperative, 503–504
        afterload decrease, 504
        contractility decrease, 504
        preload decrease, 504
        rate alterations, 504
        rhythm alterations, 504
    as spinal anesthesia complication, 328
Hypotensive anesthesia, 300, 301
    contraindications, 300
Hypothermia, 513–516
    benefits to mild intraoperative, 514
    definition, 513
    mechanisms leading to, under general
        anesthesia, 513–514
    mild, 513
    modalities to prevent and treat
        perioperative, 514–516
        circulating water-mattresses, 515
        forced-air warming, 515
        gas and fluid heating, 515
        hot-water bottles
            contraindicated, 516
        insulation, 515
        radiation heat loss
            prevention, 514–515
        redistribution prevention, 514
        shivering treatment, 516
    moderate, 513
    physiologic consequences, 514, 515
        deleterious clinical consequences, 514
    physiologic responses, 514
        nonshivering thermogenesis, 514
        shivering, 514
        vasoconstriction, 514
    prevention in patient with central
        neuraxial block, 516
    severe, 513
    temperature monitoring sites, 514
Hypothyroidism
    causes, 158
    effects, 159 on vital organ function, 155
    intraoperative concerns, 159
    preoperative considerations, 158–159
    primary, 158
    secondary, 158
    signs, 156
    symptoms, 156
    tertiary, 158

Hypovolemia, 504
    as cause of postoperative
        hypotension, 504
    severity estimation, 505
Hypoxemia
    causes, 522–523
        diffusion impairment, 522–523
        hypoventilation, 522
        shunt, 522
        ventilation/perfusion (V/Q)
            mismatch, 522
    differential diagnosis, 220
    during one-lung ventilation, treatment,
        80–81, 86–87
Hypoxic pulmonary vasoconstriction
        (HPV), 80
    factors affecting, 80

I

IABP. See Intra-aortic balloon pump
Ibuprofen, in post-laparoscopy pain
        reduction, 223
ICD. See Implanted cardioverter-defibrulator
ICM. See Ischemic cardiomyopathy
ICP. See Intracranial pressure
IDD. See Internal disc disruption
IDDM. See Diabetes mellitus,
        insulin-dependent (IDDM/Type I)
Idiopathic hypertrophic subaortic
        stenosis. See Hypertrophic
        obstructive cardiomyopathy
Idiopathic thrombocytopenic purpura
        (ITP), 380
Implanted cardioverter-defibrulator
        (ICD), 51
IMV. See Intermittent mandatory
        ventilation
Infrared acoustic spectroscopy, in CO_2
        measurement, 74
Infrared light spectroscopy, in CO_2
        measurement, 74
Insulin
    physiologic effects, 150
    preparation properties, 151
Intermittent mandatory ventilation
        (IMV), 524
Internal disc disruption (IDD), 441–442
Intra-abdominal pressure (IAP), 219
Intra-aortic balloon pump (IABP), 54
Intracranial aneurysms, 97–99
    arterial blood pressure control, 98
    management of aneurysm rupture during
        clipping of, 99
    monitoring during craniotomy for
        clipping of, 98
    subarachnoid hemorrhage from ruptured
        aneurysm
        complications following, 97–98
        grading following, 97

Intracranial aneurysms (Continued)
    treatment of cerebral
        vasospasm, 98–99
    treatment options, 98
Intracranial mass
    anesthesia induction and
        maintenance, 95
    contraindications to sitting position,
        94–95
Intracranial pressure (ICP), 89
    effects of anesthetic agents and vasoactive
        drugs, 90–93
    increased
        factors contributing, 90
        signs and symptoms, 93
        treatment, 93, 94
    monitoring, 93
Intra-discal electro-thermocoagulation
        (IDET), 441–442
Intramuscular opioid therapy, advantages
        and disadvantages, 432
Intraocular pressure (IOP), 235
    factors that increase, 236
    factors that lower, 237–238
    mechanism by which maintained,
        235–236
Intraoperative cell salvage, 290–291
    advantages and disadvantages, 295
    controversies and contraindications,
        291–292
    indications, 291
Intraoperative coagulopathies, 279–286
    acquired inhibitors, 282, 283–284
    acquired platelet dysfunction, 283
    blood derivatives used in treatment,
        285–286
        recombinant activated protein C,
            285–286
        recombinant factor VIIa
            (rFVIIa), 285
    blood products to treat, 284–286
        cryoprecipitate, 285
        donor-retested plasma, 284, 285
        fresh frozen plasma (FFP), 285
        liquid thawed plasma, 285
        plasma 24, 285
        platelet concentrate, 284
        plateletpheresis, 284
        solvent/detergent-treated plasma
            (SD-plasma), 284, 285
    dilutional, 281, 282
    disseminated intravascular coagulation
        (DIC), 282, 283, 364–365
    fibrinolysis, 282, 283
    heparin excess, 282
    laboratory tests if PT or APTT
        prolonged, 281
    preoperative evaluation, 279–281
        family history, 279, 280
        laboratory tests, 279, 280

Intraoperative coagulopathies (Continued)
  preoperative evaluation (Continued)
    medications, 279, 280, 281
    patient history, 279, 280
    physical examination, 279, 280
  thrombosis, 282
  vitamin K deficiency, 282
Intraventricular hemorrhage (IVH)
  grades, 422
  in preterm infant, 422
Intubation, difficult. See Difficult airway
IOP. See Intraocular pressure
Ischemic cardiomyopathy (ICM), 52–53
Ischemic optic neuropathy (ION), 112
Isoflurane
  in carotid endarectomy patients, 103
  central nervous system effects, 91, 92
  compared with desflurane, 468
  effect on hepatic blood flow, 189
  hepatic injury following exposure to, 191
Isoproterenol, in allergic reaction
  treatment, 320
ITP. See Idiopathic thrombocytopenic
  purpura
IVH. See Intraventricular hemorrhage

J

Jehovah's Witnesses
  and blood transfusion, 298–299
    in minor, 299
  and cell salvage, 291

K

Ketamine
  in cardiac tamponade treatment, 486
  central nervous system effects, 91, 92
  in cesarean section anesthesia, 352
  in congestive heart failure patients, 23
  in electroconvulsive therapy, 106
  in motor evoked potential
    monitoring, 111
  and nausea and vomiting, 469
  in office setting, 477
  in open-eye injury treatment, 237
  side-effects, 477
Ketorolac, 471
Kidney transplantation. See Renal
  transplantation
Kupffer cells, 186
Kussmaul's sign, 48, 486

L

Labetalol
  central nervous system effects, 91, 93
  in hypertension treatment, 511
  in pheochromocytoma
    treatment, 172

Labor and delivery, 347–354
  analgesia options, 347–348
  general anesthesia for cesarean section,
    351–352
    advantages, 351
    disadvantages, 351
    suggested method, 352
  placental drug transfer, 352–353
  post-cesarean pain relief, 353
  postpartum hemorrhage, 353
  regional anesthetic techniques, 348–349
    combined spinal-epidural (CSE)
      technique, 349
    epidural analgesia, 348–349
    patient-controlled epidural analgesia
      (PCEA), 348–349
    spinal versus epidural anesthesia, 350
  regional anesthetic techniques for
    cesarean section, 350–351
    absolute contraindications, 350
    advantages, 350
    epidural anesthesia, 351
    relative contraindications, 350
    spinal anesthesia, 351
    suggested technique, 351
  retained placenta, 354
    presentation, 354
    treatment, 354
  stages of labour, 348, 349
  treatment for postdural puncture
    headache, 351
  uterine atony, 353–354
    anesthetic management, 353
    hypogastric artery ligation,
      353–354
    hysterectomy, 353–354
    intraoperative cell salvage, 354
    obstetric management, 353
    presentation, 353
    risk factors, 353
  "walking epidural," 349–350
Lactate detoxification, 184, 185
Lansoprazole, 177, 178
Laparoscopy, 217–223
  anesthetic techniques, 222
    general anesthesia, 222
    local, 222
    regional anesthesia, 222
  benefits, 221
  cardiovascular changes associated,
    219–220
    effects of CO_2 absorption, 219
    effects of patient positioning, 219–220
    effects of pneumoperitoneum, 219
  complications, 221–222
    pneumothorax, 221
    subcutaneous emphysema
      (SQE), 221
    venous gas embolism (VGE), 221–222
  during pregnancy, 376

Laparoscopy (Continued)
  etiology and treatment of
    post-laparoscopy pain, 223
    anesthetic factors, 223
    operative factors, 223
    pneumoperitoneum factors, 223
  gas used for insufflation, 218
  initiation, 218
  nausea and vomiting incidence, 468
  nitrous oxide use controversy, 222–223
  regional circulatory changes, 220
    cerebral, 220
    hepatoportal, 220
    lower limb, 220
    pulmonary effects, 220
    renal, 220
  surgical procedures, 217–218
    gynecologic, 218
    intra-abdominal, 217–218
Laplace's law, 195
Laryngeal mask airway (LMA), 255–257,
  258, 464–465
  in asthmatics, 500
  in laparoscopic surgery, 222
  in preterm infants, 423
  ProSeal, 257
Laryngoscopic grades, 252
Laser(s), 265
  argon, 266, 267
  CO_2, 265–266, 267
  KTP, 266
  KTP-Nd-YAG, 267
  Nd-YAG, 265, 266
  parts of laser system, 265
  types used in laryngeal and
    tracheobronchial surgery, 266
  types used in medical practice, 265–266
  YAG, 267
Laser laryngoscopy, 265
  airway fire treatment, 267
  anesthetic techniques, 267
  hazards, 266–267
    to anesthetic equipment, 266–267
    to operating room personnel, 266
    to patients, 266
  indications, 266
Lateral decubitus position,
  complications, 79
Lean body mass, 214
Left ventricular assist device (LVAD), 51,
  54–56
  anesthetic considerations for patients
    supported by, 54–55
  anesthetic drugs used, 55
  aspiration pneumonitis risk, 55
  chest compressions
    contraindicated, 55
  intraoperative considerations, 55
  preoperative considerations,
    54–55, 56

Left ventricular assist device
    (LVAD) *(Continued)*
  description, 54
  intra-anesthetic monitoring for patients
      with, 55–56
    CVP monitoring, 56
    pulmonary artery catheters
        (PACs), 56
    SVR calculation, 56
    transesophageal echocardiography
        (TEE), 56
Left ventricular outflow tract (LVOT),
    obstruction, 39–40
LES. *See* Lower esophageal sphincter
Levobupivacaine
  for brachial plexus anesthesia, 338
  toxic effects, 318
Lidocaine
  for brachial plexus anesthesia, 338
  central nervous system
      effects, 91
  in dental procedures, 319
  for epidural anesthesia, 317
  with epinephrine, 315
  patch, 444
  with sodium bicarbonate, 316
  for spinal anesthesia, 316–317, 326–327,
      333
  for topical anesthesia, 317
  toxic effects, 319
  for tumescent anesthesia, 317
Lithium carbonate, effects, 107
Liver disease, 181–193. *See also* Hepatic
    functions
  anesthetic techniques free of hepatotoxic
      effects, 192
  causes of postoperative hepatic
      dysfunction, 191–192
  coagulation problems anticipated,
      192–193
  end-stage. *See* End-stage liver disease
      (ESLD)
  nonanesthetic drugs affecting hepatic
      blood flow, 192
  preoperative evaluation of patients with,
      188–189
Liver transplantation, 193
  fibrinolysis problems, 283
  intraoperative anesthetic problems, 193
  transfusion requirements, 193
LMA. *See* Laryngeal mask airway
LMWH. *See* Low-molecular-weight heparin
Local anesthetics, 313–320
  allergic reactions to, 319–320
      treatment, 320
  amide, 313, 314
      metabolism, 315
  chemistry, 313–314
  clinical differences between ester and
      amide, 315

Local anesthetics *(Continued)*
  ester, 313, 314
      metabolism, 315
  factors affecting potency, onset, and
      duration of action, 314
  factors influencing blockade, 315–316
  mechanism of action, 314
  mixtures of, 316
  pharmacokinetics, 315
  in pregnancy, 316
  for regional anesthetic procedures,
      316–317
  sequence of anesthesia following neural
      blockade, 314–315
  toxic effects, 317–319
      treatment, 319
Low back pain, 439–442
  clinical presentation of herniated nucleus
      pulposus, 440
  differentiation from spinal stenosis,
      440, 441
  differential diagnosis, 439–440
      intrathoracic/intra-abdominal, 440
      muscular, 439, 440
      neurologic, 439–440
      skeletal, 439, 440
  epidural steroid injections, 441
  facet joint disease, 441
  failed back syndrome (FBS), 442
  incidence, 439
  internal disc disruption (IDD), 441–442
  myofascial syndrome, 440–441
  oral medications for, 442
  sacroiliac disease, 441
Low-molecular-weight heparin (LMWH), 383
  comparison with standard
      heparin, 383
  and neuraxial anesthesia
      anesthetic experience, 384
      recommendations, 311, 384
  use in pregnancy, 383–384
Lower esophageal sphincter, 175–176
  effect on tone of pharmacological agents
      during anesthesia, 178
Lower extremity anesthesia, 341–345
  anesthetic options, 341
      advantages and disadvantages, 341–343
  femoral nerve block, 343
      choice of local anesthetic, 344
      sedation for, 344
  innervation of lower extremity, 342–343
  management of agitated patient, 344
  postoperative pain control, 344–345
  sciatic nerve block, 343–344
      choice of local anesthetic, 344
      necessity for total knee
          arthroplasty, 343
      sedation for, 344
  use of tourniquet in total knee
      arthroplasty, 344

Lumbar plexus, 342–343
Lumbar plexus block, 311–312
Lung resection. *See* Pulmonary resection
LVAD. *See* Left ventricular assist
    device

M

MAC. *See* Minimum alveolar concentration
Macintosh blade, 254
Macroglossia, 249
MADIMS, 394
Magnesium sulfate
  in eclampsia prevention, 358–359
  effects of magnesium at different plasma
      levels, 359
  magnesium toxicity, 359
  properties, 359
  in torsades de pointes treatment, 6, 8
Magnetic resonance imaging (MRI),
    425–427
  devices/objects considered unsafe
      for, 426
  and Down syndrome child, 428
  magnetic field problems associated,
      425–426
  patient-related considerations, 426–427
  problems with physiologic monitors and
      equipment in MRI suite, 426
Maintenance fluid, requirements
    according to weight, 396
Malignant hyperthermia (MH),
    121, 143–147
  characterization of clinical
      episode, 144
  definitive diagnosis, 146–147
  inheritance of susceptibility, 143
  nontriggering agents, 146
  in office setting, 476
  pathophysiology, 143–144
  significance of masseter muscle
      rigidity, 146
  significance of masseter muscle
      spasm, 121
  treatment, 144–145, 146
  treatment of patients with susceptibility
      to, 145–146
  triggering agents, 146
  vs. neurolept malignant syndrome, 147
Mallampati classification of pharyngeal
    structures, 250, 252
Mannitol
  in brain edema treatment, 93
  following renal transplantation, 234
  in IOP reduction, 236
  as irrigating fluid, 208
MAOIs. *See* Monoamine oxidase inhibitors
MAP. *See* Mean arterial pressure
Mask ventilation, difficult. *See* Difficult
    airway

Mass spectrometry, in CO_2 measurement, 74

Masseter muscle rigidity (MMR), 146

Masseter muscle spasm (MMS), 121

Massive transfusion, definition, 281

Mean arterial pressure (MAP), 89
    determination, 503

Mechanomyograph (MMG), 133

Meconium, limitation of neonatal aspiration risk, 390–391

Medullary thyroid carcinoma, 157

MELD. *See* Model for end-stage liver disease

MEN. *See* Multiple endocrine neoplasia (MEN) syndromes

Mendelson's syndrome, 176

Meningitis, following spinal anesthesia, 330

MEP. *See* Motor evoked potential

Meperidine, in shivering treatment, 516

Mepivacaine
    for brachial plexus anesthesia, 338
    in dental procedures, 319
    for epidural anesthesia, 317

Metabolic acidosis, in ESLD, 187, 188

Methemoglobinemia, 319

Methohexital, in electroconvulsive therapy, 106

Methylmethacrylate cement toxicity, 310

Methylparaben, 320

Methylprednisolone
    in allergic reaction treatment, 320
    relative potency, 166

Metoclopramide, 177, 178, 458
    in postoperative nausea and vomiting treatment, 469, 477, 518

Metoprolol, in pheochromocytoma treatment, 172

MG. *See* Myasthenia gravis

MH. *See* Malignant hyperthermia

MI. *See* Myocardial infarction

Micrognathia, 249

Midazolam
    in ambulatory surgery, 462, 463
    as Category D drug, 374
    effects at different dosages, 468
    in moderate sedation, 467
    preoperative administration, 460

Middle ear surgery. *See also* Postoperative nausea and vomiting
    conduction of general and regional anesthesia, 245
    contraindications for long-acting neuromuscular blockers, 244–245
    importance of control of blood loss, 244

Military antishock trousers (MAST), 532

"Mill wheel" murmur, 94

Miller blade, 254

Milrinone
    in congestive heart failure patients, 24
    in right ventricular failure treatment, 34

Mineralocorticoids, 165

Minimum alveolar concentration, in infants, 422

Mitral stenosis, 31–34
    anesthetic strategy in patients with, 33
    etiology and pathophysiology, 31–32
    hemodynamic goals in, 32
    hypotension treatment in patient with, 33
    intraoperative management principles, 32
    intraoperative monitoring, 32–33
    perioperative right ventricular failure treatment, 33–34
    preoperative optimization of patient's condition, 32

Mitral valve prolapse, 37

Mivacurium
    in electroconvulsive therapy, 106
    in open-eye injury treatment, 237
    side-effects, 467
    for tracheal intubation, 467

MMG. *See* Mechanomyograph

MO. *See* Morbid obesity

Model for end-stage liver disease (MELD), 189

Moderate sedation, 466–467

Monitored anesthesia care, 477

Monoamine oxidase inhibitors (MAOIs), effects, 107

Morbid obesity (MO), 211–214
    anesthetic plan for bariatric surgery, 213–214
    definition, 211
    diagnosis of obstructive sleep apnea, 212
    diseases associated, 211–212
    effect on functional residual capacity, 212
    equipment to anesthetize for bariatric surgery, 213
    pathophysiology of obstructive sleep apnea, 212
    as possible indicator for awake intubation, 212–213

Morbilliform rash, 532

Morphine, in subarachnoid space, 327

Motor evoked potential (MEP), 110
    effects of anesthetics on, 110–111

MRI. *See* Magnetic resonance imaging

Multifocal atrial tachycardia, 506
    treatment options, 507–508

Multiple endocrine neoplasia (MEN) syndromes, 163
    type I, 163
    type II, 170, 171
    type IIA, 163
    type III, 170, 171

Multiple sclerosis, and spinal anesthesia, 330

Mustard operation, 414, 416

Myasthenia gravis (MG), 137–142
    anesthetic technique for transcervical thymectomy, 139–140
    confirmatory tests, 138
    diagnosis, 138
    lesion, 137–138
    myasthenic crisis vs. cholinergic crisis, 141
    Osserman Classification System, 138
    postoperative ventilation predictors, 141–142
    premedication for surgery, 139
    resistance to depolarizing muscle relaxants, 139
    sensitivity to nondepolarizing muscle relaxants, 139
    strength assessment following emergence from anesthesia, 140–141
    treatment alternatives, 138–139

Myocardial contractility, 12

Myocardial contusion. *See* Blunt cardiac injury

Myocardial infarction (MI)
    noncardiac surgery following, 15–20
        additional drugs to have available, 19–20
        additional preoperative investigations, 18
        anesthetic technique, 20
        cardiac risk evaluation, 15–18
        implications of prior coronary revascularization for anesthetic management, 18–19
        intraoperative monitoring, 19, 20
        postoperative management, 20

Myocardial ischemia. *See also* Coronary artery disease
    drugs used to treat or prevent, 66
    hemodynamic goals in, 12
    intraoperative detection, 14, 67
    pharmacologic alternatives for treating, 12–13
    risk factors, 195–196

Myocardial steal, 13, 196

Myocarditis, 21

Myofascial syndrome (trigger points), pathogenesis and treatment, 440–441

N

N-acetyl-*p*-benzoquinine imine (NAPQI), 190

Naloxone
    in neonatal resuscitation, 390
    in reversal of opioids, 527–528

NAPQI, 190

Nasogastric tube (NGT), management during induction, 177

Nausea. *See also* Postoperative nausea and vomiting
    cause, 517

Neonatal resuscitation, 387–391
Apgar score in assessment of
need for, 391
equipment for, 391
management in delivery room, 389–391
physiologic changes at birth, 387–389
Neostigmine, 130
risk of bradycardia following
administration, 63
Neuraxial opioids, 434–436
advantages and disadvantages of
subarachnoid and epidural opioids,
435
analgesia-producing mechanism, 434
dosage schedules for commonly used,
435–436
potential side-effects, 434–435
Neuroleptic malignant syndrome, 147
Neuromuscular blockade. See Depolarizing
neuromuscular blockade;
Nondepolarizing neuromuscular
blockade
Neuromuscular junction monitoring,
133–135
accelerography, 134
electromyograph, 133–134
in myasthenia gravis diagnosis, 138
mechanomyograph, 133
need for, 133
patterns of nerve stimulation, 134–135
double-burst, 135
single-twitch, 134
tetanic, 135
train-of-four (TOF), 134–135
phonomyography, 134
Neuromuscular transmission, anatomy and
physiology, 117–118
Nicardipine, in hypertension treatment, 511
NIDDM. See Diabetes mellitus, non-insulin-
dependent (NIDDM/Type II)
Nitric oxide, in right ventricular failure
treatment, 34
Nitroglycerin
central nervous system effects, 91, 93
in hypertension treatment, 359, 511
Nitroprusside, in hypertension
management, 359
Nitrous oxide
central nervous system
effects, 91, 92
hepatic injury following exposure to, 191
and nausea and vomiting, 469
teratogenicity in mammals, 374
Nondepolarizing neuromuscular blockade,
125–128
antagonism of, 128, 129–132
clinical indices of recovery from
blockade, 131–132
clinically relevant acetylcholinesterase
inhibitors, 129–130

Nondepolarizing neuromuscular
blockade (Continued)
antagonism of (Continued)
doses and duration of action of
acetylcholinesterase
inhibitors, 130
mechanism of acetylcholinesterase
inhibition, 130
mechanism of cyclodextrins, 131
metabolic factors affecting, 128
need for antimuscarinics, 130–131
onset of action for acetylcholinesterase
inhibitors, 130, 131
overall strategy, 129
effects of antibiotics on, 126–127
effects of drugs other than antibiotics on,
127–128
factors affecting, 127, 140
interactions of relaxants with other
drugs, 126
mechanism of production, 125
pharmacology of relaxants, 125–126
Nonobstetric surgery during pregnancy,
371–377
anesthetic concerns, 371
anesthetic implications of physiologic
changes, 372–374
cardiovascular system, 372–373
central nervous system, 373–374
gastrointestinal system, 373
hematologic system and blood
constituents, 373
hepatic system, 373
renal system, 373
respiratory system, 372
effects of anesthetic agents in pregnant
patient, 374–375
animal studies, 374
category ratings of anesthetic agents,
374–375
epidemiologic studies, 375
retrospective studies, 375
general recommendations for anesthesia,
376–377
incidence, 371
intraoperative monitors, 376
laparoscopic surgery considerations, 376
precautions to avoid intrauterine fetal
asphyxia, 376
prevention of preterm labor, 376
Nonsteroidal anti-inflammatory drugs
(NSAIDs)
actions, 442
in cancer pain treatment, 452
in low back pain relief, 442
and neuraxial anesthesia, 311
in PHN pain treatment, 445
and renal problems, 308
in rhematoid arthritis treatment, 308
side-effects, 442

Norepinephrine
addition to local anesthetics, 315
metabolism, 170
Norwood I procedure, 417
Novacor LVAS, 54, 55
Novocain, 319
NSAID. See Nonsteroidal anti-inflammatory
drugs
Nucleic acid amplification testing (NAT),
277–278

O

Obstructive sleep apnea
diagnosis, 212
pathophysiology, 212
Octreotide, 228
Oculocardiac reflex, 239–240
treatment, 240
Oculocephalic (doll's eyes) reflex, 529
Oculovestibular reflex, 529
Office-based anesthesia, 475–479
considerations before providing, 476
discharge criteria, 477–479
documentation, 476
equipment, 476
growth in services, 475–476
limitations for types of
patients/procedures, 476–477
malignant hyperthermia
treatment, 476
method/technique, 477
postoperative nausea and vomiting
treatment, 477
Omeprazole, 177, 178
Omphalocele. See Gastroschisis and
omphalocele
Oncologic surgery, cell salvage and, 291–292
Ondansetron
following adenotonsillectomy, 263
in postoperative nausea and vomiting
treatment, 470, 477, 518
One-lung ventilation, 73–83, 86–87
anesthetic evaluation before lung
resection, 73–74
complications of lateral decubitus
position, 79
double-lumen endobronchial tubes for
choice of side, 75–76
clinical problems associated with
placement and use, 79
positioning, 76–78
technique for placing, 76
indications, 75
pleural drainage systems, 81–82
potential post-thoracotomy
complications, 82–83
single-lumen endotracheal tubes for, 75
treatment of hypoxemia during, 80–81,
86–87

One-lung ventilation (Continued)
  ventilation and oxygenation
    monitoring, 74–75
  ventilation and perfusion effects
    during, 79–80
  for video-assisted thoracoscopy, 86
Open-eye injury, 235, 236–238. See also
    Intraocular pressure
  neuromuscular blocking agent choice, 237
  non-anesthetic agents to maximize
    surgical outcome, 237–238
  preoperative evaluation, 236
  relative urgency, 236
  true ocular emergency, 236
Opioids
  in cancer pain treatment, 452
  central nervous system effects, 91, 92
  extended-duration, 452, 453
  prolonged effects, 527–528
  reversal, 527–528
  in subarachnoid space, 327
Oropharyngeal (gag) reflex, 529
Osborn wave, 514
Osmolarity, calculation, 154
Osserman Classification System, 138
Osteoblasts, 161
Osteoclasts, 161
Oxycodone, 471
Oxygen delivery. See DO_2
Oxygen transport, 287–288
Oxygenation, monitoring, 75
Oxyhemoglobin binding factor, 288
Oxyhemoglobin saturation. See SaO_2

P

PABD. See Preoperative autologous blood
    donation
Pacemakers, 43–45
  asynchronous, vs. demand, 43–44
  bipolar, 44
  codes for, 43, 44
  demand, vs. asynchronous, 43–44
  dual-chamber
    in treatment of dilated
      cardiomyopathies, 53
    vs. single-chamber ventricular, 44
  electrocautery interference, 44
    prevention, 44–45
  hysteresis, 45
  indications for, 8
  myopotential inhibition of, 45
  unipolar, 44
  ventricular (single-chamber), vs. dual
    chamber, 44
$PaCO_2$, 89–90, 94, 218, 317
$PaCO_2$–$ETCO_2$ gradient, 218
PACU. See Postanesthesia care unit
PADSS. See Postanesthesia Discharge
    Scoring System

Pancuronium, central nervous system
    effects, 91
PaO_2, 90, 94, 287
Paradoxical pulse, 486
Parathyroid hormone (PTH), in calcium
    regulation, 162
Parathyroid-related protein (PTHrP), 162
Parvovirus B19, 278
Passavant's ridge, 262
Patient-controlled analgesia (PCA),
    432–433, 471
  advantages and disadvantages, 433
  dosage schedules, 433
  following lower extremity surgery, 344
PC. See Pressure control
PCA. See Patient-controlled analgesia
PCE. See Perioperative cardiac events
PCWP. See Pulmonary capillary wedge
    pressure
PDPH. See Postdural puncture headache
PEEP. See Positive end-expiratory pressure
"Pendelluft" effect, 483
Penicillin
  allergy to, 532–533
    and allergic reaction to cephalosporin,
      532–533
    antibiotic to use in patient with,
      532–533
Perfluorocarbons, 301–302
Peribulbar blockade, 240
Pericardial surgery, with VAT, 85
Pericardiocentesis, 48–49
Perioperative bronchospasm, signs and
    causes, 500
Perioperative cardiac events (PCE)
  definition, 16
  predictors of, 16–17
  surgical risk for, 17, 18
Permissive hypercapnia, 401
Pharmacokinetics, 421
Phenoxybenzamine, in pheochromocytoma
    treatment, 171
Phentolamine, in hypertension treatment, 511
Phenylephrine
  addition to local anesthetics, 315, 327
  in cardiac transplantation patient, 63
  in hypotension treatment, 319, 328
Pheochromocytoma, 169–173
  anesthetic choices, 172–173
  clinical presentation, 170
  conditions that may mimic, 170
  description, 169
  diagnostic criteria, 170
  intraoperative management goals, 172
  other syndromes associated, 170, 171
  postoperative problems associated with
    resection of, 173
  preoperative preparation, 170–172
  undiagnosed, management following
    anesthesia induction, 173

PHN. See Postherpetic neuralgia
Phonomyography, 134
Physostigmine
  in myasthenia gravis treatment, 138
  in reversal of sedatives, 467, 527
Placenta previa, 369–370
  anesthesia for emergency cesarean
    section, 370
  clinical presentation, 369
  comparison with abruptio
    placento, 370
  diagnosis, 370
  "double set-up," 370
  obstetric management, 370
Plasma cholinesterase, 119–120
  variants, 120
    incidence, 120
Plasmapheresis, in myasthenia gravis
    treatment, 138
Platelet function tests, 380–381
  bleeding time test, 381
  platelet function analyzer
    (PFA-100), 381, 382
  thromboelastogram (TEG), 381, 382
Pleural drainage systems, 81–82
PMNs. See Polymodal nociceptors
Pneumothorax
  clinical signs and symptoms, 482
  as complication of laparoscopic
    surgery, 221
  diagnosis, 482
  treatment, 482
Poiseuille's law, 420
Polymixin B, effect on neuromuscular
    blockade, 126–127
Polymodal nociceptors (PMNs), 430
PONV. See Postoperative nausea and
    vomiting
Portopulmonary hypertension, 187
Positive end-expiratory pressure (PEEP)
  in ARDS treatment, 523
  in bariatric surgery, 214
  for hypoxemia during one-lung
    ventilation, 86
  in venous air embolism treatment, 94
Positive predictive value, 252
Postanesthesia care unit (PACU). See also
    Postoperative nausea and vomiting
  discharge criteria, 478, 519
    examination, 519
    follow-up, 519
    instructions to patient, 519
  incidence of complications
    in, 518
Postanesthesia Discharge Scoring System
    (PADSS), 478
Post-conceptual age, calculation, 423
Postdural puncture headache (PDPH),
    328–329, 332, 351
  in ambulatory patient, 461

Posterior ischemic optic neuropathy
    (PION), 112
Postherpetic neuralgia (PHN), 444–445. *See
    also* Acute herpes zoster
    incidence, 444
    invasive procedures for treatment, 445
    medications for treatment, 444–445
    patients at risk, 444
    presentation, 444
    prevention, 445
Post-implantation syndrome, 204
Postoperative cell salvage, 294
Postoperative nausea and
    vomiting (PONV)
    cause of nausea and vomiting, 517
    as complication of middle ear
        surgery, 243
    general anesthetic techniques to
        minimize, 243–244
    incidence, 468, 517–518
    risk factors, 468–469, 517
    risk with local anesthesia, 244
    treatment options, 469–470, 518
        dexamethasone, 469, 477, 518
        dolasetron, 243, 477, 518
        droperidol, 469, 477, 518
        ephedrine, 470
        granisetron, 243, 477, 518
        5-HT$_3$ antagonists, 243, 477, 518
        metoclopramide, 469, 477, 518
        multimodal management, 518
        non-pharmacologic therapies, 518
        ondansetron, 470, 477, 518
        prophylaxis, 243, 469–470, 477, 518
        scopolamine, 470, 518
        tropisetron, 477
Postoperative pain, 429–436
    alternative postoperative analgesic
        modalities, 432
    intramuscular opioid therapy, advantages
        and disadvantages, 432
    major afferent pain pathways, 430–431
    neuraxial opioids, 434–436
        advantages and disadvantages of
            subarachnoid and epidural
            opioids, 435
        analgesia-producing mechanism, 434
        dosage schedules for commonly used,
            435–436
        potential side-effects, 434–435
    organ systems affected, 430
    patient history factors impacting
        management, 430
    patient-controlled analgesia (PCA),
        432–433, 471
        advantages and disadvantages, 433
        dosage schedules, 433
        following lower extremity surgery, 344
    physiologic effects, 430, 431
    preemptive analgesia, 436

Postoperative pain (*Continued*)
    primary chemical mediators of
        pain, 431–432
    regional analgesic techniques, 433–434
    undertreatment in past, 429–430
Postoperative vision loss, risk factors, 112
Post-tetanic facilitation, 135
Prazosin, in pheochromocytoma
    treatment, 171
Prednisone
    in poison ivy treatment, 167
    relative potency, 166
Preeclampsia, 355–361
    anesthetic options for cesarean
        section, 361
    as cause of thrombocytopenia, 380
    consequences of epidural anesthesia,
        359–361
    etiology, 356–357
    incidence, 356
    management of hypertension, 359
        comparison of drugs, 360
    mild, 356
    obstetric management, 357–358
    pathophysiologic changes, 357
        cardiovascular, 357, 358
        central nervous system, 357, 358
        hematologic, 357, 358
        hepatic, 357, 358
        pulmonary, 357, 358
        renal, 357, 358
        uteroplacental, 357, 358
    postpartum problems anticipated, 361
    prevention of degeneration into
        eclampsia, 358–359
    risk factors, 356
    severe, 356
    signs and symptoms, 356
Preemptive analgesia, 436
Pregnancy. *See also* Nonobstetric surgery
        during pregnancy
    category ratings of drugs during, 374
    coagulation changes in, 364, 365
    hypertensive disorders of, 355–356
        chronic hypertension, 355
        gestational hypertension, 356
        preeclampsia-eclampsia. *See*
            Preeclampsia
    physiologic changes of, 372–374
        cardiovascular system, 372, 372–373
        central nervous system, 372, 373–374
        gastrointestinal system, 372, 373
        hematologic system and blood
            constituents, 372, 373
        hepatic system, 373
        renal system, 372, 373
        respiratory system, 372
Prematurity
    borderline, 421
    definition, 421

Prematurity (*Continued*)
    moderate, 421
    severe, 421
Preoperative autologous blood donation
    (PABD), 292–294
    contraindications, 293
    disadvantages and risks, 293–294
    indications, 292, 293
    patient criteria, 292, 293
Pressure control (PC), 524
Pressure support (PS), 524
Preterm infant, 419–424
    anatomic and physiologic differences
        between infant and adult, 419–421
        cardiac, 420
        cricoid cartilage, 420
        epiglottis, 420
        hematologic, 420
        larynx, 419–420
        occiput, 419
        pharmacologic, 421
        pulmonary, 420
        renal, 420
        tongue, 419
        vocal cords, 420
    anesthetic options and concerns, 422–423
        continuous caudal anesthesia, 423
        general anesthesia, 422–423
        spinal anesthesia, 423
    definition of prematurity, 421
    discharge home, 423–424
    induction options for general
        anesthesia, 423
    monitoring, 423, 424
    nil per os (NPO) guidelines, 422
    pharmacokinetics and
        pharmacodynamics of anesthetic
        drugs as compared with adults,
        421–422
    postoperative pain control, 423
Prilocaine, toxic effects, 319
Procaine, 319
Propofol, 178
    in ambulatory surgery, 463, 464, 465
    antiemetic properties, 517
    central nervous system effects, 91, 92
    in electroconvulsive therapy, 106
    in moderate sedation, 467
    in nausea and vomiting
        prophylaxis, 470
    in office setting, 477
    as preferred agent in asthmatics, 500
Propranolol
    in hypertension treatment, 511
    in pheochromocytoma treatment, 172
Prostacyclin, in pregnancy, 357
Protamine, 67
Proteinuria, definition, 356
Prothrombin time, 188, 189
Proton pump inhibitors, 177, 178

PS. *See* Pressure support
PT. *See* Prothrombin time
PTH. *See* Parathyroid hormone
Pulmonary artery catheterization (PAC)
    in AAA surgery, 197
    in intraoperative monitoring, 19, 20
Pulmonary aspiration. *See* Aspiration
Pulmonary capillary wedge pressure
        (PCWP), 66, 67, 197
    "v-wave," 67
Pulmonary contusion
    diagnosis, 483, 485
    treatment, 483–485
Pulmonary function tests (PFT)
    in asthma vs. chronic obstructive
        pulmonary disease, 496–497
    before lung resection, 73–74
    in obstructive and restrictive lung
        disease, 496–497
Pulmonary resection. *See also* One-lung
        ventilation
    anesthetic evaluation before, 73–74
    role of thoracostomy tube
        following, 81
Pulmonary vascular resistance
        (PVR), 35–36
Pulse oximeter, 75
Pulseless electrical activity (PEA), 8–9
Pulsus paradoxus, 48
Pupillary response to light, 529
PVR. *See* Pulmonary vascular resistance
Pyloric stenosis, 403–404
    anesthetic considerations, 404
    clinical presentation, 403
    diagnosis, 403
    metabolic derangements, 403–404
    surgical treatment, 404
Pyridostigmine, in myasthenia gravis
        treatment, 138

R

RA. *See* Rheumatoid arthritis
Rabeprazole, 177, 178
Raman spectroscopy, in CO_2 measurement, 74
Ranitidine, 177, 178, 458
Rapid shallow breathing index (RSBI), 525
RCM. *See* Restrictive cardiomyopathy
Re-entry ("paroxysmal supraventricular")
        tachycardia, 507
    treatment options, 507
Reflex sympathetic dystrophy (RSD), 447
Regional anesthesia, 316–317
    central neural blockade, 316–317
    infiltration, 316
    intravenous, 316, 462
    peripheral nerve blocks, 316
    topical, 317
    tumescent, 317
Regional curare test, 138

Regurgitation
    mechanisms for prevention, 175–176
    prevention with cricoid pressure,
        177–178
    risk factors, 176
Remifentanil
    in ambulatory surgery, 462–464
    central nervous system effects, 91, 92
    in electroconvulsive therapy, 106
    in moderate sedation, 467
    in motor evoked potential
        monitoring, 111
    in office setting, 477
Renal transplantation, 231–234
    anesthetic concerns, 232–234
        general anesthesia, 232–234
        regional anesthesia, 234
    effect of diabetes, 231
    implications of long ischemic
        times, 234
    importance of timimg of hemodialysis,
        231–232
    treatment of hyperkalemia and associated
        problems, 232
Renin, 357
Reperfusion injury, treatment, 103
RES. *See* Reticuloendothelial system
Respiratory failure, 521–525. *See also*
        Adult respiratory distress
        syndrome
    definition of postoperative respiratory
        failure, 521
    extubation criteria, 525
    metabolic acidosis, 523
    types, 521–522
        hypercapnic (type II). *See* Hypercapnia
        hypoxemic (type I). *See* Hypoxemia
    ventilatory modes, 524
Respiratory reflex, 529
Restrictive cardiomyopathy (RCM),
        52, 53
Reticuloendothelial system (RES), 186
Retinal detachment, 239–241
    advantages and disadvantages of general
        anesthesia for scleral buckle
        repair, 239
    complications of retrobulbar
        anesthesia, 240
    events during surgery, 240
    intraocular gas
        anesthetic implications,
            240–241
        types, 240
    oculocardiac reflex, 239–240
    treatment, 240
    types amenable to elective
        repair, 240
Retinopathy of prematurity (ROP), 423
Retraction blades, 253–254
Retrobulbar blockade, 240

Rheumatoid arthritis (RA), 307–309
    anesthetic considerations for patient
        with, 308
    anesthetic evaluation of patient with,
        308–309
    diagnostic criteria, 307, 308
    treatment, 307–308
Right ventricular failure,
        treatment, 33–34
Rocuronium
    central nervous system effects, 92
    in open-eye injury treatment, 237
    pharmacology, 125–126
Rofecoxib, in adenotonsillectomy, 263
ROP. *See* Retinopathy of prematurity
Ropivacaine
    for brachial plexus anesthesia, 338
    for epidural anesthesia, 316, 317
    in femoral and sciatic nerve
        blocks, 344
    for spinal anesthesia, 316–317
    toxic effects, 318
RSBI, 525

S

Sacroiliac disease, 441
Samsoon classification of pharyngeal
        structures, 250, 252
SaO_2, 287–288
Sciatic nerve block, 343–344
    choice of local anesthetic, 344
    necessity for total knee
        arthroplasty, 343
    sedation for, 344
Sciatic plexus, 343
Scleral buckle repair. *See* Retinal
        detachment
Scoliosis, 297–301
    classification, 297–298
    curvature assessment, 298
    intraoperative anesthetic considerations
        for posterior spinal fusion surgery,
        299–300
    postoperative anesthetic considerations
        following repair, 301
    preoperative evaluation, 299
    wake-up test, 300
Scopolamine, in postoperative nausea and
        vomiting treatment, 470, 518
Selective serotonin reuptake inhibitors
        (SSRIs), effects, 107
Senning operation, 414, 416
Sensitivity (statistical), 252
Septic shock, 167–168
Sevoflurane, 468
    central nervous system effects, 91, 92
    in electroconvulsive therapy, 106
    in office setting, 477
Shingles. *see* Acute herpes zoster

Shock, 503–508. *See also* Hypotension, postoperative; Supraventricular dysrhythmias
  definition, 504–505
  hemodynamic parameter changes according to etiology, 505, 506
  hypovolemia severity estimation, 505
  transfusion need assessment, 505–506
  types and treatment basics, 505
    cardiogenic, 505
    distributive, 505
    hypovolemic, 505
    obstructive, 505
SHOT study, 271, 276
Shunt equation, 522
Shunted blood, 80
Sickle cell disease, 276
Siker blade, 254
SIMV. *See* Synchronized intermittent mandatory ventilation
Single-twitch stimulation, 134
Sinus tachycardia, 506
  differential diagnosis, 144
  treatment options, 506
Sodium bicarbonate
  addition to local anesthetics, 316
  in cardiopulmonary resuscitation, 4–5, 7
    indications for, 4–5
  in neonatal resuscitation, 390
Sodium citrate, 177, 178
Sodium deficit, calculation, 209
Sodium nitroprusside
  central nervous system effects, 91, 92–93
  in hypertension treatment, 511
Somatosensory evoked potential (SSEP), 110
  as adjunct to wake-up test, 300
  effects of anesthetics on, 110–111
  for neurologic function monitoring, 102
Somatostatin, mechanism of action, 228
Sorbitol, as irrigating fluid, 208
Spinal anesthesia, 323–333
  advantages over general anesthesia, 330–331
  agents commonly used, 326–327
  in ambulatory patient, 461
  approaches to subarachnoid space, 325
  catheter (continuous), advantages and disadvantages, 331–333
  choice of local anesthetic, 316–317
  comparison with epidural anesthesia, 331, 332
  complications, 328–330
  contraindications, 330
  equipment to be available, 323–324
  factors affecting anesthetic spread, 325–326
  lateral decubitus position advantages, 324

Spinal anesthesia *(Continued)*
  in patients on antiplatelet drugs, 329–330
  in patients with liver disease, 192
  sitting position advantages, 324
  spinal tray arrangement, 324
  technique, 324–325
  vasoconstrictor addition advantages, 327–328
Spinal cord ischemia, 491–492
  following spinal anesthesia, 330
Spine surgery, 109–112
  anesthetic considerations for surgery in prone position, 109, 110
  monitors, 109–110
  pain relief modalities after, 112
  postoperative vision loss risk, 111–112
SQE. *See* Subcutaneous emphysema
SSEP. *See* Somatosensory evoked potential
SSRIs. *See* Selective serotonin reuptake inhibitors
Steroids, naturally produced, 165
Stylets, 254
Sub-Tenon blockade, 240
Subacute bacterial endocarditis. *See* Eisenmenger syndrome
Subcutaneous emphysema (SQE), as complication of laparoscopic surgery, 221
Succinylcholine, 118–123
  in carcinoid syndrome treatment, 228
  central nervous system effects, 91, 92
  in cesarean section anesthesia, 352
  contraindications, 122–123
    for renal transplantation, 232
  crossing placenta by, 353
  in electroconvulsive therapy, 106
  factors decreasing normal metabolism of, 119–120
  in laser laryngoscopy, 267
  muscle relaxation action, 118
  myalgias associated, 467
  in open-eye injury treatment, 237
  in patient with full stomach, 178
  pharmacology, 119
  phase II blockade, 120
    treatment, 121
  resistance of myasthenics to, 139
  side-effects, 121–122
  termination of action, 119
Sudeck's atrophy of the bone, 448
Sufentanil
  central nervous system effects, 91, 92
  in subarachnoid space, 327
Sulfonylureas, 151
Supramaximal stimulus, 133
Supraventricular dysrhythmias, 506
  treatment options, 506–508
    in patients with aortic stenosis, 28, 29

Supraventricular tachycardia (SVT)
  following VAT, 87
  risk factors, 87
  treatment, 5–8
SVR. *See* Systemic vascular resistance
SVT. *See* Supraventricular tachycardia
Synchronized cardioversion, 508
Synchronized intermittent mandatory ventilation (SIMV), 524
Syndrome of inappropriate antidiuretic hormone (SIADH), 227
Systemic vascular resistance (SVR), 36
  reduction in as result of ESLD, 187
Systolic anterior motion, cause, 39

T

T_4 ratio, 135
Tacrolimus, 61
TCA. *See* Tricyclic antidepressants
TCD. *See* Transcranial Doppler
TEE. *See* Transesophageal echocardiography
TEF. *See* Tracheoesophageal fistula
Temporomandibular joint (TMJ), 248–249
  translation of, 250–251
Tensilon test. *See* Edrophonium, test for myasthenia gravis
Teratogens, 374
Testosterone, 165
"Tet" spells. *See* Hypercyanotic spells
Tetanic stimulation, 135
Tetracaine
  for spinal anesthesia, 316–317, 325, 326, 461
  for topical anesthesia, 317
  toxic effects, 318
Thalidomide, 374
Thiamylal, in cesarean section anesthesia, 352
Thiazolidinediones, 151
Thiopental
  central nervous system effects, 92
  in electroconvulsive therapy, 106
Third-trimester bleeding, major causes, 363–364
"Thoracic shock," 482.
Thoracic trauma, 481–492. *See also* Cardiac tamponade; Flail chest; Hemothorax; Pneumothorax; Pulmonary contusion; Traumatic thoracic aortic injury
  blunt cardiac trauma, 486. *See also* Blunt cardiac injury
  consequences, 481–482
  transmediastinal gunshot wounds, 492
Thoracoscopy, 85–87. *See also* Video-assisted thoracoscopy
Thoracotomy
  compared with VAT, 85–86
  potential complications following, 82–83

Thrombocytopenia
  causes during pregnancy
    dynamic disorders, 380, 381
    static disorders, 380, 381
  platelet transfusions for, 192–193
  in pregnancy, 379–384. See also Platelet
        function tests
    anesthetic experience with LMWH and
        neuraxial anesthesia, 384
    causes, 380
    concerns when placing epidural
        catheter, 380
    epidural hematoma risk, 380, 382
    evaluation of patient with platelet
        count <100,000 mm^{-3}, 383
    expected platelet count during
        pregnancy, 380
    known cases of epidural hematoma in
        parturient, 382
    lowest "safe" platelet count, 380
    practical recommendations, 383
    recommendations for anesthetizing
        parturient taking
        LMWH, 384
    role of platelets in coagulation, 380
    safety of initiating epidural anesthetic
        when platelet count
        <100,000 mm^{-3}, 382–383
Thromboembolism prophylaxis, and
      neuraxial anesthesia, 311
Thromboplastin, 357
Thromboxane, in pregnancy, 357
Thymectomy
  anesthetic technique for, 139–140
  in myasthenia gravis treatment, 138–139
Thyroid disease, 155–160. See also
      Hyperthyroidism; Hypothyroidism
  conditions associated, 157
  effects of thyroid on vital organ
      function, 155
  evaluation, 156–157
  intraoperative concerns, 159
  postoperative concerns, 159–160
  preoperative considerations in patient
      with, 158–159
  preoperative tests for patient with, 159
  thyroid hormone regulation, 156
  thyroid hormone synthesis and
      release, 156
  thyroid storm, 157
Thyromental distance, 250
Thyroxine (T$_4$), 155
  synthesis and release, 156
TIVA. See Total intravenous anesthesia
TMJ. See Temporomandibular joint
Tolazoline, in preoperative management of
      CDH, 401
Tonsillectomy. See also Adenotonsillectomy
  on ambulatory basis, 458
  without adenoidectomy, 261

Topical anesthesia, 317
Torsades de pointes, 6, 8
Total body water (TBW), 209
  in infants and adults, 421
Total hip replacement. See Hip
      arthroplasty
Total intravenous anesthesia (TIVA),
      111, 465–466
Total knee arthroplasty. See also Lower
      extremity anesthesia
  need for sciatic nerve block, 343
  use of tourniquet in, 344
Total parenteral nutrition (TPN), risk of
      hypoglycemia, 152
Tracheoesophageal fistula
      (TEF), 405–408
  diagnosis, 405
  Gross' classification, 405, 406
  "H" type, 405
  incidence, 405, 406
  incidence of associated anomalies,
      405–406, 407
  intraoperative management,
      406–408
    intubation, 406–407
    occlusion of fistula, 408
    operating room set-up, 407
  postoperative concerns, 408
  preoperative concerns, 405–406
    VACTERL, 405, 407
  presentation, 405
  types, 406
Train-of-four (TOF) stimulation, 134–135
TRALI. See Transfusion-related acute lung
      injury
Transaminase, as indicators of liver
      damage, 188
Transcranial Doppler (TCD), for
      neurologic function monitoring, 102
Transesophageal echocardiography (TEE)
  in endovascular stent placement, 203
  in intraoperative monitoring, 19, 20
  in intravascular volume measurement, 66
  in myocardial ischemia detection, 14, 67
Transfusion reaction, 269–278
  crossmatch types
    antiglobulin, 270
    computer, 270, 270–271
    immediate spin, 270
  delayed reactions, 276–278
    alloimmunization, 276–277
    delayed hemolytic transfusion reaction
        (DHTRs), 276
    graft-versus-host disease, 277
    iron overload, 277
    transfusion-transmitted viral and
        parasitic infection, 277–278
  immediate reactions, 271–276
    acute hemolytic, 271, 272
    allergic and anaphylactic, 271–274

Transfusion reaction (Continued)
  immediate reactions (Continued)
    circulatory overload, 272, 274
    citrate intoxication, 273
    febrile non-hemolytic, 272, 274
    hyperkalemia, 273
    hypotensive, related to
        bradykinin/cytokines, 273, 275
    hypothermia, 273
    sepsis related to bacterial
        contamination, 273, 275–276
    transfusion-related acute lung injury
        (TRALI), 273, 276
  preliminary laboratory
      investigation, 270
  standards for tranfusion practice, 269
  steps to be taken when occurs, 270
Transfusion trigger, 288
Transfusion-associated graft-versus-host
      disease (TA-GVHD), 277
Transfusion-related acute lung injury
      (TRALI), 273, 276
Transient blindness, 208
Transient radicular irritation (TRI), 329
Transmediastinal gunshot wounds, 492
Transsphenoidal hypophysectomy,
      113, 114, 115–116
  advantages, 114
  airway management, 115
  postoperative concerns, 115–116
  structures within transsphenoidal surgical
      field, 115
Transtracheal ventilation, 257–259
Transurethral resection of the prostate
      (TURP), 205–209, 227
  complications, 206–208
    bladder perforation, 206
    bleeding, 207
    coagulopathy, 207
    hypothermia, 207
    toxicity of irrigating fluids, 208
    transient bacteremia and
        septicemia, 207
  general anesthesia, 209
  irrigating fluid types, 208. See also Glycine
  regional anesthesia, 208–209
    benefits, 208–209
    level, 209
  sensory innervation of involved
      structures, 209
  sodium deficit correction, 209
  TURP syndrome, 205–206
    cardiovascular effects, 206
    central nervous system effects, 205–206
    treatment, 206
Traumatic hemopericardium, perioperative
      management options, 485–486
Traumatic thoracic aortic injury
  diagnosis, 489
  mechanism, 489

Traumatic thoracic aortic
    injury (Continued)
    perioperative clinical and anesthetic
        pitfalls, 490–492
    airway management, 491
    central line placement, 491
    diagnostic, 490–491
    related to spinal cord ischemia,
        491–492
    related to use of anesthetic
        drugs, 491
    radiographic findings, 489, 490
    reasons to suspect, 489–490
    surgery prioritization in patient
        with, 490
Trendelenburg position, 219, 222, 319
    reverse, 93, 219
Tricyclic antidepressants (TCAs)
    in cancer pain treatment, 452
    effects, 107, 442
    in PHN pain treatment, 444–445
Trifluoroacetyl (TFA) adducts, 191
Trigger points, 440–441
Tri-iodothyronine (T$_3$), 155
    synthesis and release, 156
Trimethaphan, in hypertension
    management, 359
"Triple H therapy," 99
Trisomy 21. See Down syndrome
Tropisetron, 477
Troponin I, in blunt cardiac injury
    diagnosis, 488
Trousseau's sign, 163
Tumescent anesthesia, 317
Turner syndrome, and coarctation of the
    aorta, 415
TURP. See Transurethral resection of the
    prostate

Tympanomastoidectomy, 243–245. See also
    Middle ear surgery

U

Unfractionated heparin (UH), 383
Uterine tone, monitoring during
    nonobstetric surgery, 376
Uteroplacental ischemia, 356

V

VACTERL, 405, 407
VAE. See Venous air embolism
Vancomycin, 533
Vanillylmandelic acid (VMA), 170
Varicella, 443
Vasomotor paroxysmal syndrome, 226
Vasopressin
    in cardiopulmonary resuscitation, 4, 6
    indication for, 4
    in diabetes insipidus treatment, 115
VAT. See Video-assisted thoracoscopy
Vecuronium, central nervous system
    effects, 91, 92
Venous air embolism (VAE), 94, 95
Venous gas embolism (VGE), as complication
    of laparoscopic surgery, 221–222
Ventilation
    common modes, 524
    monitoring, 74–75
    purpose, 74
Ventricular dysrhythmias, 506
Ventricular fibrillation (VF), 2, 508
    algorithm for, 3
    antidysrhythmic therapy, 5, 6–7
    treatment, 2, 508. See also
        Cardiopulmonary resuscitation

Ventricular tachycardia (VT), 2, 506, 507
    algorithm for, 3
    antidysrhythmic therapy, 5, 6–7
    treatment options, 2, 508. See also
        Cardiopulmonary resuscitation
Ventriculostomy, in intracranial
    pressure measurement, 93
VF. See Ventricular fibrillation
VGE. See Venous gas embolism
Video-assisted thoracoscopy (VAT), 85–87
    advantages compared with thoracotomy,
        85–86
    anesthetic techniques for, 86
    complications, 86, 87
    treatment of hypoxemia during
        one-lung ventilation, 86–87
    types of operations done with, 85
Vitamin D, in calcium regulation, 162
Vomiting. See also Postoperative nausea and
        vomiting
    cause, 517
von Hippel-Lindau syndrome, 170, 171
von Recklinghausen's disease, 170
von Willebrand disease (vWD),
    281, 304–305
    treatment, 305
VT. See Ventricular tachycardia

W

Wake-up test, 111, 300
Warfarin, 311
WHO ladder, 452
Wolff-Parkinson-White syndrome, 8
Wu laryngoscope, 254